TEXTBOOK OF DERMATOLOGY

VOLUME 1

STRUCTURE, FUNCTION, AND COMMON DISEASES OF THE SKIN

Dr. Mariya Kharodawala

ALLIED HEALTH PRESS

Textbook of Dermatology

Volume 1: Structure, Function, and Common Diseases of the Skin

Author: **Dr. Mariya Kharodawala**

Allied Health Press
4164 Lakeshore Road
Burlington ON L7L 1A4
Canada
www.alliedhealthpress.com
Email: orders@arclereducation.com

ISBN: 978-1-77956-825-0

ABOUT THE AUTHOR

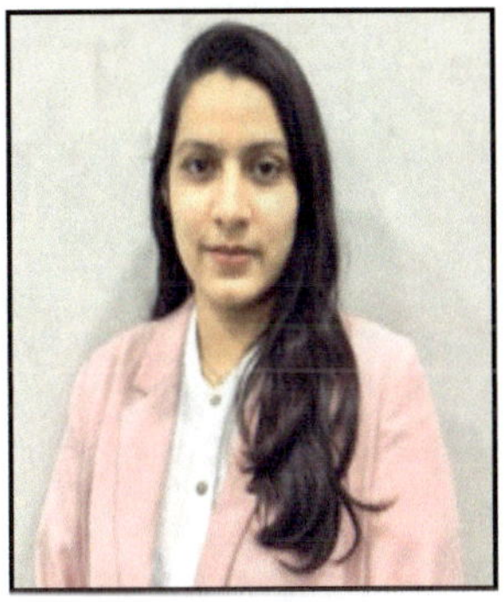

Dr. Mariya Kharodawala holds an MBBS degree with a gold medal from The Maharaja Sayajirao University of Baroda and an MD in Dermatology, Venereology, and Leprosy from B. J. Medical College, Pune, both of which are among the premier medical institutes in India. She is currently working as a Senior Resident in Dermatology. Her areas of interest include clinical dermatology, dermatopathology, and academic writing. Over the years, she has contributed to peer-reviewed journals and actively participated in national and international conferences. Her professional journey is driven by a passion for continuous learning, research, and teaching. Alongside her academic pursuits, she is committed to bridging the gap between medical knowledge and public awareness through digital platforms. Reviewing this comprehensive dermatology textbook has been an intellectually rewarding experience, and she is delighted to contribute to the academic growth of future dermatologists.

Brief Table of Contents

Getting Started with This Book

Chapter Openers

A list of Chapter Outline is presented providing a brief Introduction to what will be covered in the chapter.

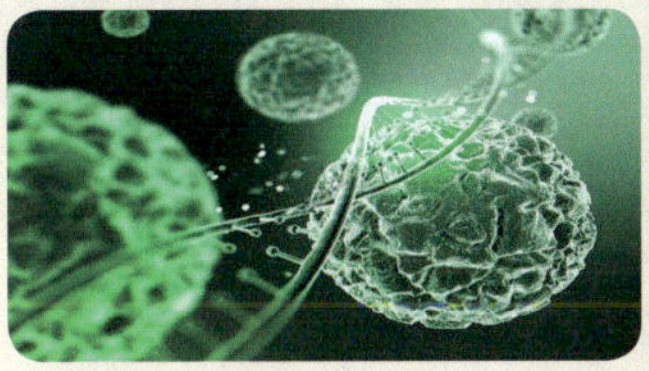

LEARNING OBJECTIVES

After studying this chapter, you will be able to:

1. Discuss the scientific method in biology;
2. Explain the cell theory;
3. Discuss the genetics and heredity;
4. Evolution and natural selection;
5. Focus on ecology and ecosystems;
6. Learn about human biology;
7. Evaluate the plant biology;
8. Explain the microbiology;
9. Focus on current trends in biology.

Introduction

Often referred to as the science of life, biology is a broad field of study aimed at comprehending the several kinds of life on Earth, from tiny creatures to sophisticated multicellular entities. Comprising several subfields, including molecular biology, ecology, and evolutionary biology, each of which advances our knowledge of living systems, this field clarifies the mechanisms controlling life events, including development, reproduction, and interaction with the surroundings, which is the central goal of biology. Moreover, biology fills in the void between the natural sciences and medicine by offering a necessary understanding of health, illness, and the interactions between organisms and their environments. Dealing with urgent global issues such as climate change, biodiversity loss, and new diseases depends on an awareness of these complex biological interactions, therefore highlighting the critical part biology plays in modern civilization. Fundamentally, biology explores and tests ideas about the living world using the scientific method. Through methodical observation and experimentation,

1.1. The Scientific Method in Biology

Learning Outcome

1. Describe the steps of the scientific method;
2. Focus on hypothesis formation;
3. Learn about experimental design.

Learning Outcomes

The beginning of each section of every chapter contains a set of Learning Outcomes that inform students of concepts they should understand. These outcomes help students understand what they should be able to do if they have mastered the material in that section.

Test Your Knowledge

Throughout each chapter, Test Your Knowledge cues you to note which topics have been covered and to self-test your understanding of the material presented.

Test Your Knowledge

1. Explain why correlation does not imply causation in scientific experiments.
2. How does the scientific method help reduce the influence of personal opinions in research?

Chapter Summary

The Summary Section appear at the end of each chapter and summarize main concepts covered throughout the chapter. These points provide key concepts in an engaging and meaningful way.

Summary

The investigation of biological principles highlights the importance of a comprehensive view of life by reflecting the intricate interactions that occur within living systems. The complexity of biology goes beyond individual species or systems, as this essay highlights; it also includes the interactions that mold ecosystems and affect biodiversity. Researchers can conduct in-depth analyses of metabolomic data using sophisticated technologies like MetaboAnalyst, which offer insights into the molecular mechanisms underlying these interactions. As demonstrated by the developments in MetaboAnalyst, for example, the integration of diverse omics data promotes a thorough understanding of metabolic pathways and helps identify important biological markers necessary for research on development and disease (Chong et al., 2018). Additionally, the phenomenon of ecological invasions is a key component of biological research and a vital field of study. The introduction of non-native species into unfamiliar habitats has significant ramifications and calls for multidisciplinary management strategies. Examining the origins and effects of these biological incursions, invasion science has become a crucial field that highlights the need to comprehend ecological dynamics and community interactions. As interest in biological invasions increases, new findings are emerging that put conventional ecological theories and practices to the test. The importance of incorporating various scientific viewpoints is shown by this developing discipline, which also highlights how invasive species shape ecosystems and advances our knowledge of ecological resilience (David et al., 2013). When taken as a whole, these discoveries from invasion science and metabolomics highlight the value of multidisciplinary biology research. Fostering cross-disciplinary collaboration and utilizing technological breakthroughs to improve our comprehension of intricate biological interactions are crucial as we look to the future of biological research. In addition to deepening our understanding of the complexities of life, this method lays the groundwork for tackling urgent environmental issues. Future studies can ensure the continued relevance of biology in a world that is constantly changing by acknowledging the interconnection of biological systems and opening the door to creative solutions that support sustainability and biodiversity conservation. We might imagine a thorough comprehension of life that serves both academia and society at large through ongoing investigation and integration of scientific knowledge.

Knowledge Assessment

The chapter includes material designed to review and reinforce each content. It includes Critical Thinking Questions to help test of your understanding of information presented in the chapter and Short answer Questions to review your understanding of the key concepts presented in the chapter.

Critical Thinking Questions

1. **Who is known as the "Father of Modern Biology"?**
   a. Aristotle
   b. Charles Darwin
   c. Gregor Mendel
   d. Louis Pasteur
2. **What is the basic unit of life?**
   a. Atom
   b. Molecule
   c. Cell
   d. Organism
3. **Which branch of biology studies the interaction of organisms with their environment?**
   a. Genetics
   b. Ecology
   c. Physiology
   d. Botany
4. **Which macromolecule is the main source of energy for living organisms?**
   a. Proteins
   b. Lipids
   c. Carbohydrates
   d. Nucleic acids
5. **DNA is primarily responsible for which function in living organisms?**
   a. Energy production
   b. Protein synthesis
   c. Storing genetic information
   d. Regulating body temperature

Short Answer Questions

1. What is biology, and why is it important to study biology?
2. What are the three main domains of life, and how are they different from one another?
3. Define homeostasis and give an example of how it works in living organisms.
4. What is the cell theory, and why is it fundamental to biology?
5. How do autotrophs and heterotrophs differ in the way they obtain energy?
6. What is the scientific method, and how is it applied in biological research?
7. Discuss how biology helps address global challenges such as climate change, disease, and food security.
8. Explain the levels of biological organization from the smallest unit to the largest. Provide examples at each level.
9. Describe the relationship between structure and function in biology, giving specific examples from cells or organs.
10. How has the discovery of genetics shaped our understanding of inheritance and variation among organisms?

Supplementary Materials

Key Terms: A list of key terms is given for quick reference

KEY TERMS FROM THIS CHAPTER

Annotation enrichment analysis	Biological structure	Cell
Cell theory	Cellular structure	Ecology
Ecosystems	Genetics	Human biology
Microbiology	Natural selection	Organism
Plant biology		

Further Resources: Recommendations for additional readings, websites, and multimedia resources.

References

1. Argelaguet, R., Velten, B., Arnol, D., Dietrich, S., Zenz, T., Marioni, J. C., Buettner, F., et al. (2018). Multi-omics factor analysis—A framework for unsupervised integration of multi-omics data sets. *Molecular Systems Biology, 14*. https://doi.org/10.15252/msb.20178124.
2. Bacher, S., Blackburn, T. M., Essl, F., & Genovesi, P. (2017). *Socio-Economic Impact Classification of Alien Taxa (SEICAT)*. https://core.ac.uk/download/286567949.pdf (accessed on 8th March 2025).
3. Barnett, R., Brace, S., Cucchi, T., & Dobney, K. (2013). *Divergent Evolutionary Processes Associated with Colonization of Offshore Islands*. https://core.ac.uk/download/20664364.pdf (accessed on 8th March 2025).

Detailed Table of Contents

LIST OF FIGURES

PREFACE

The skin is the largest of the body's organs, acting as an external defense system against environmental injuries while at the same time reflecting internal health. Aside from its protective role, the skin is involved in thermoregulation, sensory perception, and immune surveillance. The skin is also an external marker of a person's overall health, often providing early warning signs of systemic disease and serving as an important site for diagnosis. As a result of this double function—as both mirror and shield, skin illnesses have not only physical but also psychological and social consequences. One must learn the anatomy and physiology of this organ to recognize and cure a wide range of dermatological disorders that occur in people of all ages and backgrounds.

The discipline of dermatology encompasses a wide range of conditions, from benign inflammatory rashes to life-threatening infections, hereditary disorders, and neoplastic processes. Each condition has its own patterns, clinical presentations, and treatment modalities, thereby making dermatology both intricate and integral to the practice of clinical medicine. Visual examination and pattern recognition are also heavily reliant on correct diagnosis, facilitated by technological adjuncts and histopathological knowledge. No matter whether one is seeing a patient with chronic eczema, looking for a suspicious lesion, or dealing with skin infections, an informed approach based on sound knowledge of skin biology and diagnostic practice is necessary.

Textbook of Dermatology – Volume 1 is structured as a comprehensive introduction to the fundamental principles and common disorders encountered in dermatological practice. It combines fundamental theoretical knowledge with clinical utility, enabling students, practitioners, and healthcare professionals to develop diagnostic confidence and treatment competence. The book integrates basic science, clinical competence, and disorder-specific management principles within an organized learning pathway across key dermatology topics. Care has been taken to address common conditions and those that require more precise diagnostic accuracy. The purpose of this book is to equip the reader with an understanding that will allow him or her to move forward with dermatologic issues with a sound grasp of the knowledge and clinical skills needed.

Chapter 1 introduces the medical specialty of dermatology, laying the groundwork with an overview of skin anatomy and its key layers. It includes vocabulary, categories, and the scope of dermatological practice in the modern-day clinic setting.

Chapter 2 covers the physiological processes that enable the skin to function in its various ways, such as the maintenance of barrier function, sensation, thermoregulation, and immune protection. The chapter also outlines how their impairment is manifested in the disease.

Chapter 3 offers guidance in taking dermatological histories and conducting physical exams. The chapter points out symptom chronology, lesion morphology, and patient demographics as important factors in arriving at a clinical impression. Techniques like palpation, diascopy, and distribution analysis are also incorporated to aid bedside diagnosis.

Elementary dermatopathology is introduced to readers in Chapter 4, with a focus on the principal cellular and structural changes observed in skin disease. This involves the introduction of histological nomenclature and staining techniques utilized to aid clinical diagnosis.

Chapter 5 provides an overview of diagnostic methods such as dermoscopy, skin biopsy techniques, and non-invasive imaging technologies. Practical guidance as to when and how to use each tool, what they can be expected to produce, and how to make sense of results is given.

Chapter 6 addresses varied forms of eczema and dermatitis, including atopic dermatitis, allergic contact and irritant contact dermatitis, and seborrheic dermatitis. Clinical presentation, precipitants, pathophysiology, and management strategies are explained comparatively to highlight their differences.

Chapter 7 covers psoriasis and other papulosquamous conditions. The chapter includes discussions of chronic plaque psoriasis, guttate psoriasis, and psoriatic arthritis, as well as diseases such as pityriasis rosea. Readers are given information regarding lesion identification, severity assessment, and the implementation of therapeutic interventions.

Chapter 8 addresses urticaria, angioedema, and mastocytosis, all diseases that are most often related to immune or allergic responses. The chapter covers the diagnostic approach in terms of triggers and differential diagnoses, as well as acute and chronic treatment guidelines.

Chapter 9 discusses lichen planus and variants, such as oral and hypertrophic lichen planus. Similar lichenoid disorders are also discussed, allowing readers to differentiate between disorders having similar characteristics.

Chapter 10 discusses facial dermatoses that are prevalent in the population: acne vulgaris and rosacea. Both are discussed with regard to presentation, precipitants, complications, and management, including topical and systemic treatments, lifestyle interventions, and long-term therapy.

Chapter 11 addresses bacterial skin infections, including impetigo, cellulitis, folliculitis, and more severe presentations such as erysipelas and necrotizing fasciitis. Clinical pointers, risk factors, diagnostic investigations, and antimicrobial therapy are outlined to enable early and effective treatment.

Chapter 12 brings the volume to a close with a discussion of viral infections of the skin. Some of the covered topics are herpes simplex virus, varicella-zoster virus, human papillomavirus, and molluscum contagiosum. For each condition, the chapter provides diagnostic features, transmission, clinical course, and treatment.

This Volume 1 is intended for a diverse audience. It will be useful to medical students and dermatology trainees by explaining things clearly and taking them through important issues in an orderly fashion. General practitioners, nurse practitioners, and physician assistants will find it useful for day-to-day consultation and clinical decision-making. Allied health professionals, like nurses and aestheticians working in dermatologic practice, can also use the text to better understand common skin diseases. The book is intended to provide a solid foundation for all those entering or already practicing dermatology, thereby enabling clear diagnosis and assurance of management at the initial stage of clinical training.

INTRODUCTION TO DERMATOLOGY AND STRUCTURE OF THE SKIN

1

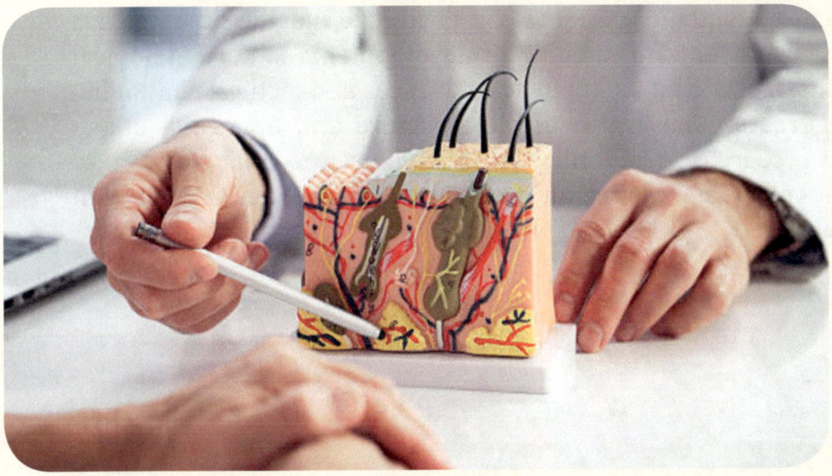

LEARNING OBJECTIVES

After studying this chapter, you will be able to:

1. Know the anatomy of the skin
2. Describe the common skin conditions
3. Understand skin cancer
4. Know the dermatological procedures
5. Describe the advances in dermatology

Introduction

The skin, as the largest organ of the human body, plays an important role in many physiological and structural functions necessary for a person's general well-being. Its complex structure consists of several layers, primarily the epidermis, dermis, and hypodermis, each serving different functions in protection, sensation, and heat regulation. In addition, the skin acts as a critical barrier against external insults, such as pathogens and toxic compounds. Advances in dermatological science point to the multilateral nature of the skin, showing its pivotal role in not just physical barrier functions but also homeostasis and immunity. With an understanding of the skin's intricate structure, physicians are better positioned to assess dermatological diseases and develop effective treatment strategies for superficial as well as systemic skin health-related issues. Dermatology's historical development has been closely linked to advances in our understanding of skin anatomy and pathology. The majority of the information on skin lesions, skin illnesses, and their diagnosis has been derived from research studies, enabling the medical profession to treat various dermatological conditions. In addition, ongoing research has emphasized the necessity of a comprehensive understanding of skin architecture, not just its anatomy, but also the histological attributes that distinguish human skin from that of other animals. This difference is particularly important in veterinary dermatology; there are few studies of non-human primates that reflect a lack of familiarity with the comparative anatomy and pathology, underlining the need for an in-depth investigation into human skin that benefits from the knowledge gained through both human and veterinary dermatology (Ka, 2024). The convergence of dermatology and the structural basis of the skin is crucial to the treatment of not only prevalent dermatological diseases but also to the rising issues surrounding skin health and care. Since the skin is exposed to numerous external environmental stressors, such as ultraviolet light and pollution, the importance of dermatological studies increases. Furthermore, identifying the skin's role in responding to systemic diseases can maximize diagnostic outcomes and therapeutic effectiveness. Scientists must remain watchful for developments in dermatological research, particularly regarding how it intersects with technological advances and medical continuing education. Through the building of a greater knowledge of the structure and operation of the skin from earlier research and current research, dermatology is better placed to offer answers to the complexities of human health and well-being, having an outline for future research into skin science (Couceiro et al., 2024) (Figure 1.1).

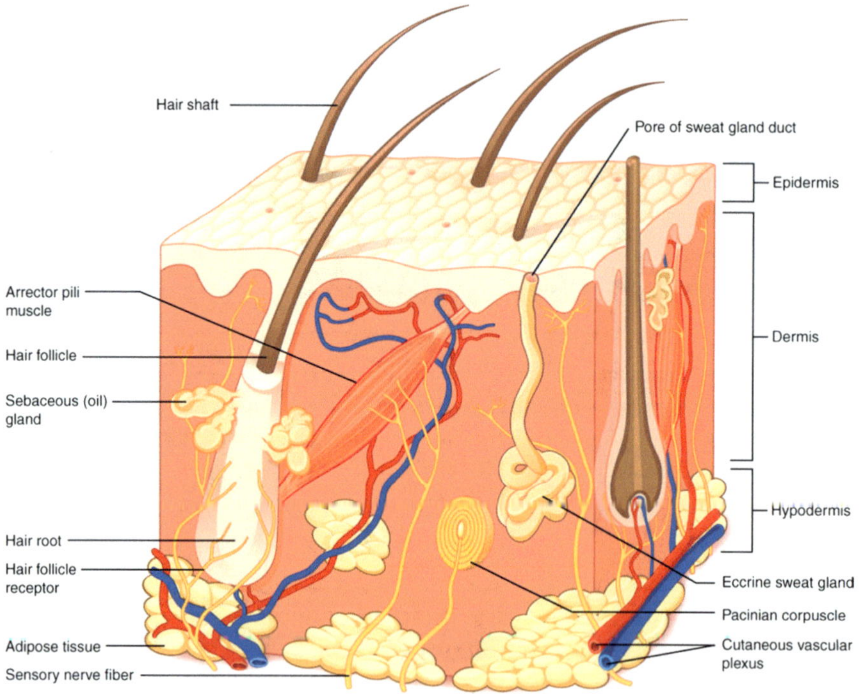

Figure 1.1. The skin is composed of two main layers: the epidermis, made of closely packed epithelial cells, and the dermis, made of dense, irregular connective tissue that houses blood vessels, hair follicles, sweat glands, and other structures. Beneath the dermis lies the hypodermis, which is composed mainly of loose connective and fatty tissues.

Source: https://s3-us-west-2.amazonaws.com/courses-images/wp-content/uploads/sites/1223/2017/02/08004822/501_Structure_of_the_skin-1024x803.jpg.

Definition of Dermatology

Dermatology, a branch of medicine focused on the treatment and research of skin disease, encompasses a very broad range of issues pertaining to skin health and disease. In addition to focusing on matters of beauty, dermatology also addresses potentially life-threatening issues affecting the skin's function. As the primary external protector of the human body, the skin is charged with guarding against noxious external pathogens, and therefore dermatology is instrumental in the prevention and management of diseases. Dermatologists use clinical examination and advanced diagnostic techniques to treat a range of skin disorders, from acne and eczema to more severe diseases such as melanoma. An understanding of the intricate architecture of the skin is essential to dermatologists, as it informs treatment strategies and enhances patient care by sustaining skin homeostasis and health. Part of the practice of dermatology is the full understanding of the skin's architecture. The skin is layered, comprising the epidermis, dermis, and subcutaneous tissue, each with protective and functional roles. The stratification provides the mechanical strength, thermal insulation, and sensory role of the skin. Furthermore, the skin acts as a dynamic organ that interacts with the body's various systems in maintaining homeostasis. The latest studies present the physiologic relevance of the histo-hematic barrier, which regulates metabolic processes among the skin's epithelial and connective tissue. The integrity of this barrier is vital because it prevents invasion by environmental insults and pathogens and permits the required uptake of nutrients and elimination of waste, illustrating the complexity and significance of skin structure in dermatology (Pustovaya et al., 2025). The structure of collagen fibers, a fundamental component of the skin, is significant to dermatological health and disease. Collagen plays a structural, supportive function primarily, and various types control skin elasticity and resilience. Abnormalities in collagen arrangement cause fibrosis or scarring, with a profound effect on the function and appearance of the skin. New imaging methods, such as polarization-resolved second-harmonic generation microscopy, have provided qualitative data on the structure and organization of collagen in normal and scarred skin. Understanding such collagen dynamics is at the core of dermatologists seeking to develop effective treatments for skin diseases. Overall, a refined understanding of the arrangement of the skin and collagen's contribution to that enhances dermatological practice and provides improved outcomes for patients seeking both health and beauty benefits (Zhou et al., 2025) (Figure 1.2).

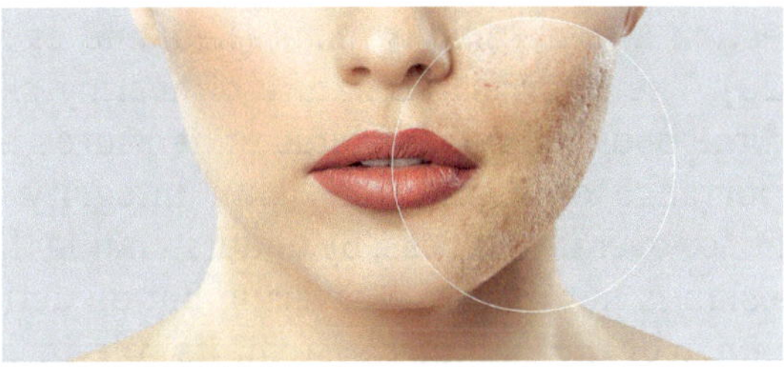

Figure 1.2. Dermatology.

Source: https://media.fmp-data.bliss.build/original_images/Dermatology.jpg.

Significance of Skin in Human Health

Skin plays a very significant role in maintaining human health since it acts as an efficient barrier protecting against environmental hazards. It is primarily responsible for protecting the body from pathogens, chemicals, and physical injury, thereby preventing skin infections and other disorders. Epidermis, the external layer of skin, is made up of tightly packed keratinocytes that secrete keratin, a protein that makes this layer strong. Apart from this, the skin's texture is also maintained by lipids that form a watertight lining, making it even more protective. This barrier function is essential not only for body integrity but also for homeostatic control, i.e., temperature and hydration levels. Changes in the skin, e.g., diabetic foot ulcers, show how its integrity is needed for general health, that damaged skin can lead to severe health problems and loss of quality of life, as shown through various studies (Sawaya et al., 2022). Apart from its protective functions, the skin also plays a critical function in immunological defense. The skin has an advanced system of immune cells, such as Langerhans cells and macrophages, that form the body's first line of defense against pathogenic microbes. When injured or infected, these cells trigger inflammatory responses that allow healing and also stimulate adaptive immunity. For instance, it has been shown that individuals with impaired immune function, usually secondary to impaired skin barrier function, are at increased risk of infection and chronic wounds (Keohane et al., 2020). The interrelated nature of healthy skin and the body's immune status underscores the importance of maintaining skin integrity to enhance overall wellness. By understanding that the skin is not merely a covering but an active member of the immune system, its role in the larger context of human health becomes more notable. Furthermore, the skin is an essential sense organ for human experience with the world. Widely innervated, the skin is the site for the body's sense of touch, temperature, and pain, all of which are essential to protective reflexes and social interaction. The sensory function aids exploration and the response to potential danger in the surroundings, and thus has a health-preventative role. Furthermore, dermatological knowledge contributes to the diagnosis of systemic disorders, as changes in skin sensitivity can be signs of underlying disease. For example, alterations in the sensation or texture of the skin may be indicative of diabetes or vitamin deficiencies, demonstrating how the skin reflects conditions of internal well-being. The intricate balance of the skin's sensory processes and general health reinforces its status as a multi-functional organ required for protecting and sustaining human life.

1.1. Anatomy of the Skin

Learning Outcome

1. Describe the layers of the skin
2. Know the functions of each layer of skin
3. Understand the appendages of skin

The anatomy of the skin is an intricate, interrelated organization of structures that serve crucial physiological functions in the human body. The skin, which consists of three significant layers—epidermis, dermis, and hypodermis—is a protective organ against external aggression and supports thermoregulation and sensation. The epidermis, or the outermost layer, is composed of keratinocytes that produce keratin, a crucial protein that supports the barrier function of the skin. Below it is the dermis, which has collagen and elastin fibers, providing strength and elasticity. The dermal layer contains structures such as hair follicles, sebaceous glands, and sweat glands that are responsible for the skin's homeostasis. The hypodermis, though not actually part of the skin, plays an integral role by anchoring the skin to subjacent tissue, storing fat, and providing major functions in energy storage and heat insulation. Familiarity with the anatomy of the skins is critical when learning dermatologic disease and treatment. Several skin diseases, such as psoriasis, eczema, and acne, result from pathology in these layers and structures. For instance, an abnormal immune response in the skin, leading to scaling and inflammation, is visible in psoriasis. Progress in dermatology procedures generally hinges on an in-depth understanding of the skin layers and their unique roles. Recent findings have underscored the importance of understanding how treatment outcomes vary by age and skin type in dermatology. For the case in point, Brown et al. (2015) inform us that aged skin, particularly in fair skin, responds variably to photodynamic therapy, a therapeutic modality that employs light to activate therapeutic agents. The findings underscore the significance of phototargeting dermatological treatments based on the anatomy and characteristics of particular skin. Besides, advanced studies affirm that technology has the potential to advance our knowledge and treatment of skin ailments. Techniques such as computer modeling and simulation, as presented by Bachynskyy et al. (2018), enable scientists to explore interactions between biological tissues and light therapy. These processes not only enhance knowledge on skin anatomy, but also how low-intensity light initiates beneficial effects, including healing and functional state correction in the skin. With advancing technologies, they open up thrilling avenues for creating targeted treatments that are mindful of the complex anatomy of skin layers and the varied conditions they can suffer from. Towards that end, a thorough understanding of skin anatomy plays a critical role in dermatology, with more effective treatments awaiting design to meet patient-specific needs (Figure 1.3).

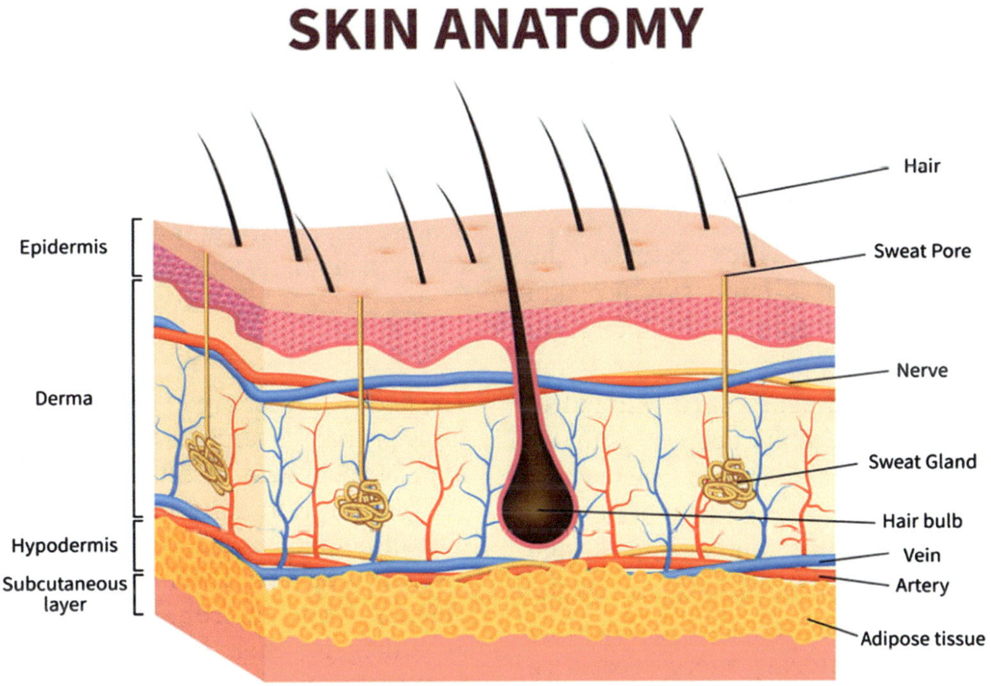

Figure 1.3. Skin anatomy.

Source: https://www.thedermspecs.com/wp-content/uploads/2011/02/skin-anatomy.png.

1.1.1. Layers of the Skin: Epidermis, Dermis, and Hypodermis

Human skin is a multicellular organ consisting of three basic layers: the epidermis, dermis, and hypodermis with characteristic structures and functions. The epidermis, the outer layer, forms the initial defense system against external threats. The epidermis consists primarily of keratinocytes, which manufacture keratin, a protective protein that prevents water loss and serves as a shield against harmful pathogens. This layer also contains melanocytes that synthesize melanin and play a role in skin pigmentation and defense against ultraviolet (UV) radiation. The epidermis is thin but richly organised, being suited for resilience and adaptability, which speaks volumes for its significance in the homeostatic maintenance and defense of inner tissues against harm and infection. Understanding the cellular composition and dynamic nature of the epidermis is of utmost importance in dermatology, especially in treating skin disorders and developing treatment plans. The dermis lies beneath the epidermis, a thicker layer of connective tissue. The dermis is filled with collagen and elastin fibers, which provide structural strength and flexibility, enabling the skin to withstand stretching and pressure. It also contributes to thermoregulation through sweat glands and blood vessels that help the body regulate its temperature. The dermis also contains hair follicles and sebaceous glands, whose functions are skin health and appearance. The vascular supply of the dermis provides nutrients and removes waste, thereby supporting the skin's overall vigor.

The cutaneous interaction between the epidermis and dermis is important for skin health and is a subject of considerable interest in dermatological science, particularly in relation to wound healing and senescence (Ahmad et al., 2017). Below this, at its deepest point, is the hypodermis, or subcutaneous layer, which attaches the skin to deeper structures such as bones and muscles. Comprised largely of adipose tissue and connective tissue, the hypodermis has several functions, including insulating the body, storing energy reserves, and cushioning to protect deeper tissues from damage. The layer also contributes to body temperature regulation by serving as an insulator. Furthermore, the hypodermis contains large blood vessels and nerves that travel into the superficial layers, indicating its function in cellular communication and sensory perception. With advancing dermatology, it is increasingly necessary to understand the complexities of the hypodermis, particularly in the fields of obesity, dermatopathology, and cosmetic procedures (Aliaga et al., 2015) (Figure 1.4).

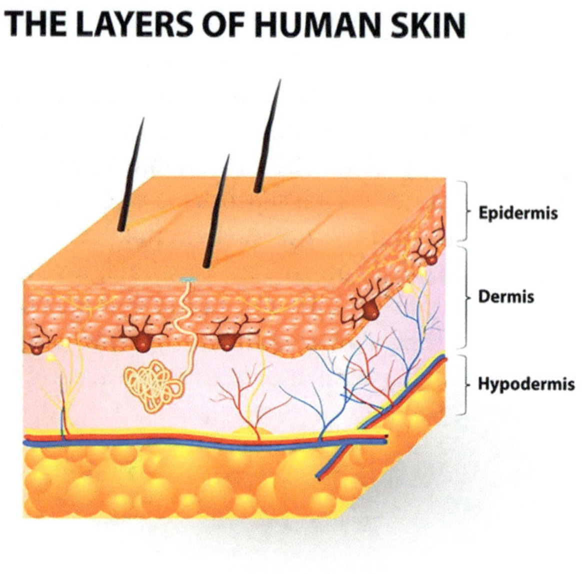

Figure 1.4. Layers of the skin.

Source: https://www.oncobeta.com/fileadmin/user_upload/nmsc-info/skin_structure.jpg.

1.1.2. Functions of Each Skin Layer

The body's largest organ, the skin, is made up of three primary layers: the epidermis, dermis, and hypodermis. Each of these layers has distinct yet similar functions necessary to maintain overall homeostasis and protection. The outer layer, the epidermis, is most associated with defense from environmental elements such as pathogens, chemicals, and physical trauma. Comprising mainly keratinocytes, the epidermis is a process of ongoing renewal, which allows for the shedding of dead cells and the formation of new cells. It is not only necessary for a person's beauty but for the integrity of the skin, thus keeping the barrier intact. Furthermore, elevated epidermal cells such as melanocytes and Langerhans cells are also found to be elevated in pigmentation and immune function, respectively, further indicating the multifunctional role of this dermal layer in maintaining skin health (Lboukili et al., 2023). Subepidermally is the dermis, a thicker layer that consists of shorter connective tissues in a rich matrix, blood vessels, and sensory receptors. The elevated role of the dermis is in thermoregulation and sensation. It is covered with sweat glands and sebaceous glands; the sweat glands regulate moisture and temperature through perspiration, while the sebaceous glands provide essential oils that keep the skin moist and flexible. Additionally, collagen and elastin fibers in the dermis give the skin strength and flexibility, which is very important for its resistance to mechanical stress. Functionally, the dermis also serves as a route for the delivery of nutrients to the epidermis and as a channel for the nervous system to transmit different sensory perceptions. Consequently, the dermis plays a central role in structural stability and in regulating the diversity of physiological responses to environmental changes (Egawa, 2021). The innermost tissue layer, the hypodermis or subcutaneous fat layer, plays an important role in energy storage, insulation, and shock absorption. Composed mainly of adipose and connective tissue, this layer serves as a shock absorber, protecting deeper bones and muscles from injury. The hypodermis also serves as an energy reservoir, mobilizing the body's store of essential fatty acids when needed. Its rich network of blood vessels facilitates the delivery of oxygen and nutrients and the regulation of body temperature, acting as an insulator against heat. Further, this layer supports the superficial skin layers by anchoring them to deeper structures, providing the support and mobility they require. This intricate function illustrates the significance of the hypodermis not only in physical guarding but also in overall metabolic health, thereby making a significant contribution to the whole array of human skin functions (Lboukili et al., 2023).

1.1.3. Skin Appendages: Hair, Nails, and Glands

The rich constitution of human skin extends beyond its external surface to incorporate a variety of appendages that play vital roles in physiological processes. Hair, nails, and glands collectively make up skin appendages for protection, thermoregulation, and sensation. Hair follicles, which are embedded in the dermis, secrete keratinized fibers that serve to shield the scalp and body from the dangers of the environment and serve to insulate. Nails, composed of hardened keratin, protect the distal phalanges and contribute to enhancing tactile sensation, making fine motor functions possible. Their well-being and development are influenced by a variety of factors, including nutrition and overall health, which illustrates the interdependence of skin appendages and overall health. In addition to hair and nails, skin glands play crucial roles in skin homeostasis. Sebaceous glands secrete sebum, with the function of keeping the skin's moisture barrier intact and its antimicrobial defense. Sweat glands, which are of the eccrine and apocrine type, are also in charge of thermoregulation through perspiration as well as excretion. Their activity is regulated by alterations in hormone levels, lifestyle, and external circumstances. The latest evidence identifies the promising potential of using cosmetic treatments with nanoparticles to boost the delivery of active ingredients targeting hair and skin health, underscoring developments in dermatological science. This intersection of skin appendages and cosmetic science underscores the importance of understanding the structure and function of such components. The utility and integrity of skin appendages are closely related to biological and environmental factors. According to the literature, bioactive constituents such as vitamins, minerals, and fatty acids are essential for promoting skin health, influencing conditions such as hydration and elasticity (Michalak et al., 2021). Furthermore, cosmetic formulation development has also offered new ways of utilizing nanotechnology, such as addressing skin absorption and product efficacy issues (Salvioni et al., 2021). This means that tailored skincare regimens, considering individual health profiles and dietary influences, will help maintain these appendages. With advancing dermatological understanding, the focus on skin appendages is sure to further enlighten us about their functions and lead to improved treatments and preventive measures that support their optimal health (Figure 1.5).

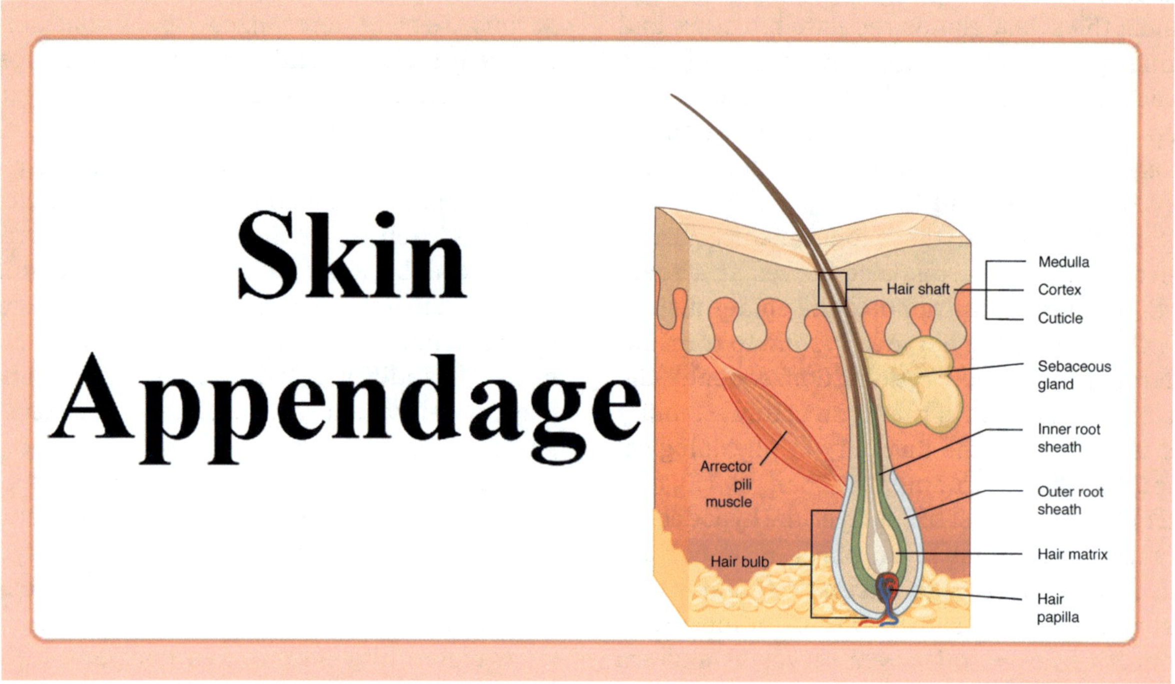

Figure 1.5. Skin appendage.

Source: https://i.ytimg.com/vi/Kw7RhKCTvcY/maxresdefault.jpg.

Test Your Knowledge

1. What are the functions of each layer of skin?
2. What are the appendages of the skin?

1.2. Common Skin Conditions

Learning Outcome

1. Describe the causes and treatments of acne
2. Understand the eczema and its management
3. Know the symptoms of psoriasis

The field of dermatology deals with a large number of common skin disorders that have a major influence on the lives of individuals. Among these diseases, acne is one of the most common ones, occurring mainly in adolescents and young adults. It is caused by the interaction of hormonal shift, excessive sebum secretion, and the availability of *Propionibacterium acnes*, a bacterium that flourishes in plugged follicles. The psychosocial effects of acne can be profound, often producing anxiety and depression in patients with acne. Moreover, the evolution of dermatology has led to the use of various treatment modalities, ranging from topical retinoids to systemic therapy, with greater benefits for patients. With a growing understanding of skin anatomy and acne pathogenesis, treatment is increasingly individualized to address the specific needs of each patient, ensuring appropriate and effective care for this common skin condition (Boffa et al., 2004). Another common skin condition is eczema, and in particular, atopic dermatitis, characterized by inflammation and a disrupted skin barrier. The pathophysiology of atopic dermatitis is multifactorial, encompassing genetic predisposition, environmental triggers, and immune dysregulation. New evidence indicates that cytokines play a crucial role in exacerbating the disease's clinical manifestations, leading to intense itch and rash. Current treatments aim to restore the skin barrier's function and reduce inflammation, while novel treatments are being developed from time to time. There is growing recognition of the role that cornified envelope proteins play in sustaining skin barrier function, and it has been suggested that future treatments will involve upregulating these proteins to effectively inhibit atopic dermatitis (Martyna, 2013). A greater understanding of such underlying mechanisms allows for more directed treatments in dermatology. Another extremely widespread skin condition worthy of consideration is psoriasis, due to its chronic status and its potential to leave patients greatly handicapped. This autoimmune illness presents as red, elevated plaques covered in silvery-white scales, typically on extensor sites such as the elbows and knees. Psoriasis pathophysiology involves an aberrant immune response that accelerates the epidermal cell multiplication cycle, causing them to accumulate rapidly in succession. Recent advances in dermatology have focused attention on the role of inflammatory cytokines in this process, thus offering hints towards potential therapeutic targets. Biologic agents that selectively inhibit such cytokines have revolutionized treatment strategies, allowing patients to achieve significant improvements in quality of life. Additionally, research on the genetic basis of psoriasis can potentially bring more advances in the field of personalized medicine in dermatology, further enhancing the care of patients over the next few years (Boffa et al., 2004) (Figure 1.6).

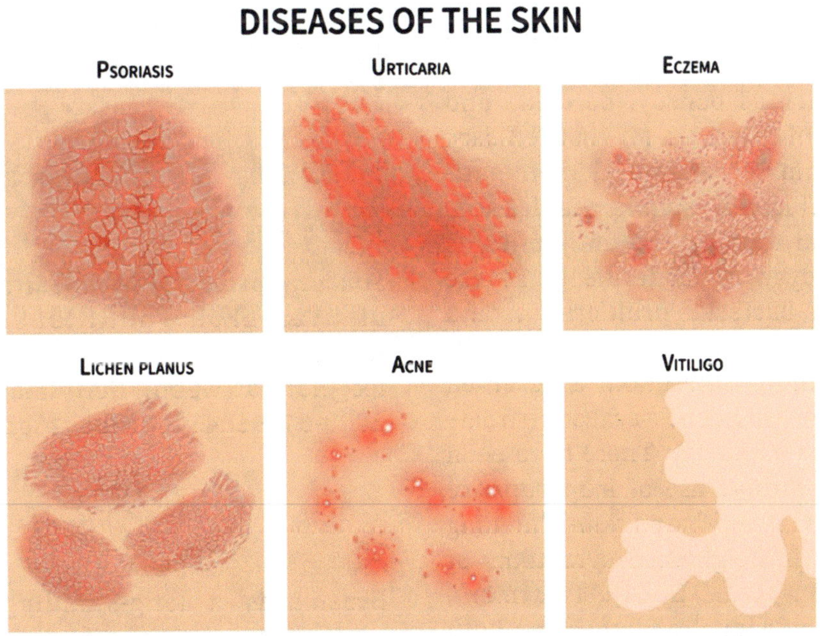

Figure 1.6. Diseases of the skin.

Source: https://www.fionawaring.com/wp-content/uploads/2019/07/shutterstock_1154905705-2-1.jpg.

1.2.1. Acne: Causes and Treatments

Acne, an etiologically multifactorial dermatosis, is most accurately defined as the inflammation of pilosebaceous units of the skin. The pathogenesis of acne is comprehensible to occur as a result of a few interrelated factors, such as hormonal imbalance, genetic susceptibility, and the presence of certain bacteria, i.e., *Propionibacterium acnes*. Endocrine disturbances, typically encountered in puberty, can lead to excessive sebum production, which, when compounded by hyperproliferation of keratinocytes, occludes hair follicles. This blockage creates an ideal niche for bacterial proliferation and attendant inflammation, resulting in the formation of papules, pustules, and cysts. It is recommended that studies indicate that it is important to know these mechanisms for effective treatment, as treatments may need to treat both the inflammatory aspects as well as the cause of these alterations on the skin structure, particularly how to maintain the histo-hematic barrier integrity and its correlation with the immune response (Pustovaya et al., 2025). Acne treatment has a broad spectrum depending on the condition. Topical drugs such as benzoyl peroxide and retinoids are commonly used for their efficacy in reducing sebum secretion and their anti-inflammatory effects. Systemic medication, such as hormonal therapy and antibiotics, is commonly employed in moderate to severe cases to control bacterial proliferation and hormonal effects that cause acne. Importantly, the powerful retinoid isotretinoin is reserved for severe nodulocystic acne because it treats all aspects of acne pathology. There have been instances where chronic use of inappropriate products, such as mercury-based skin-whitening creams, resulted in heightened symptoms of acne (Alsuwaidan et al., 2024). Treatment, thus, should be individual and consider both the physical and psychological impact of acne on patients. Moreover, the compatibility of acne treatment with the structural integrity of the skin should not be overlooked. Because the skin's microbiome stabilizes following treatments, normal flora must be maintained to prevent secondary infections and further inflammatory reactions. Supportive treatments must be introduced into the skin's barriers, like the pilosebaceous complex epithelium, without influencing their functions. Being aware of the adverse impacts of products that disrupt this equilibrium is critical to promoting education on skin health and product use. Globally, management of acne is not only a matter of treating immediate skin lesions but also addressing a systemic program that enhances the skin's protective function and encourages overall dermatological health (Pustovaya et al., 2025) (Figure 1.7).

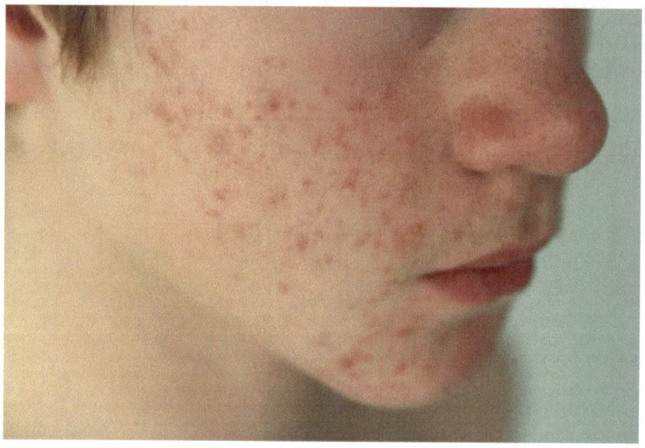

Figure 1.7. Acne.

Source: https://www.health.com/thmb/27qfo5VzSeLF0b9FndNIHbL0HvU=/1500x0/filters:no_upscale():max_bytes(150000):strip_icc():format(webp)/GettyImages-157144963-2000-64093d43108e4bfcaf4b377ac87f5f6a.jpg.

1.2.2. Eczema: Types and Management

Eczema is a long-standing inflammatory skin disease that manifests in various forms, including atopic dermatitis, contact dermatitis, and seborrheic dermatitis. The most typical type is atopic dermatitis, which usually begins in early childhood and is characterized by dry, itchy skin. Contact dermatitis is an allergic reaction to certain irritants or allergens that results in localized inflammation. Seborrheic dermatitis affects predominantly oily areas such as the face and scalp, manifesting as reddish, patchy flakes. It is necessary to understand these differences to effectively manage and treat dermatologically, as each may require a particular management policy based on its unique etiology and presentation. The heterogeneity of eczema demands thorough knowledge of its various types to develop appropriate therapeutic policies. The management of eczema is generally multifaceted, involving pharmacologic treatment, skin care, and lifestyle modifications. Topical corticosteroids and calcineurin inhibitors are typically prescribed to reduce inflammation and mitigate symptoms. Emollients also play an important role in maintaining the skin barrier's hydration and integrity, thereby preventing flare-ups. In extreme situations, systemic treatments in the form of phototherapy or immunosuppressants become imperative. It is making the therapies a part of a patient's daily routine that ensures long-term management. On top of that, patients are urged to identify any culprits, allergens, or irritants that may aggravate their condition. This individualized management plan emphasizes the role of patient compliance and education in achieving optimal results in the management of eczema. Recent developments in dermatological science, best symbolized by the skin barrier and elasticity, have opened up new fronts in the treatment of eczema. Experiments examining the role of exosomes in skin health suggest that these nanoscale vesicles could play an important part in tissue repair and intercellular communication. Examining the biogenic functions of exosomes could open the way to new therapies and interventions specifically designed for eczema. Furthermore, developments in hydrogel technology have led to the creation of multifunctional dressings with wound-healing properties, which could further treat patients with eczema by ensuring optimal moisture retention and enhancing skin barrier protection. This evolving skin care landscape highlights the need for ongoing research and discovery in dermatology, particularly to deepen understanding of the complexities of disorders such as eczema (Dayel et al., 2025; Wu et al., 2025) (Figure 1.8).

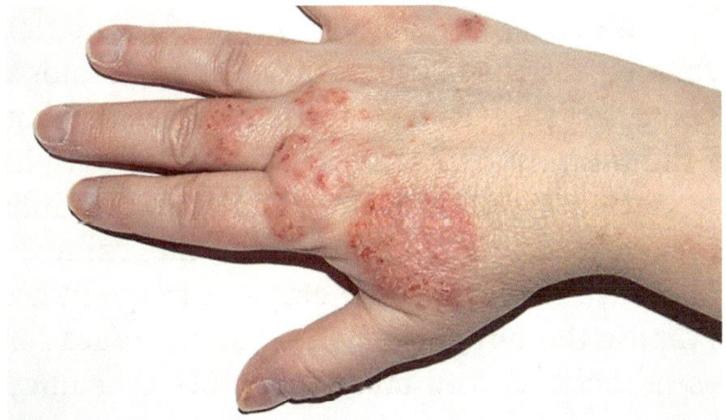

Figure 1.8. Eczema.

Source: https://images.apollo247.in/pd-cms/cms/2024-05/eczema_0.jpg?tr=q-80,f-webp,w-400,dpr-2.5,c-at_max%201000w.

1.2.3. Psoriasis: Symptoms and Therapies

Psoriasis is a chronic inflammatory skin disease characterized by accelerated skin cell growth, resulting in thickened, red, scaly plaques. It causes itching, pain, and elevated plaques that may appear on various body regions, including the elbows, knees, scalp, and lower back. The condition significantly affects the patient's quality of life, causing physical and emotional suffering. The pathogenicity of plaques is a key underlying cause of social stigma and mental illness, and hence can exacerbate the global disease burden. Understanding the pathological mechanisms underlying psoriasis is crucial to designing effective therapeutic regimens. The pathogenic mechanisms involve genetic predisposition, environmental precipitants, and immune dysregulation, illustrating the complexity of disease management. Treatment of psoriasis is diverse and may include topical therapy, phototherapy, and systemic therapy, each tailored to the severity of the disease. Topical treatment, such as corticosteroids and vitamin D analogs, is usually the first-line treatment, intended to cause an anti-inflammatory effect and delay cell turnover. In cases of severe or moderate forms, phototherapy, which uses ultraviolet light to heal the skin, has been effective. Systemic treatments, including oral medications like methotrexate and biologic agents targeted against particular mechanisms of the immune response, are potential options for patients with treatment failure. Notably, most recent studies emphasize the value of adherence to prescribed therapy, as frequent use of topical therapy and effective patient education are associated with more favorable outcomes. Nurse-delivered health education programs can enhance adherence to these regimens and ultimately improve disease management and patient satisfaction (Ali et al., 2025).

Treatment of psoriasis continues to evolve, with new therapies offering hope for patients. Biologic drugs that target specific immune pathways, such as interleukin inhibitors, have demonstrated improved efficacy and safety profiles compared with conventional therapy. New therapeutic modalities, such as small-molecule inhibitors and novel drug-delivery systems using nanoparticle-based carriers, aim to enhance therapeutic performance and patient adherence. Moreover, advances in personalized medicine research have opened the door to biomarkers and multi-omics technologies that can inform treatment decisions and enable health care practitioners to tailor their strategies on a patient-by-patient basis based on individual patient profiles. With ongoing advances in dermatology, coordination among industry stakeholders, practice, and research will be required to bridge the gap between scientific development and clinical translation, ultimately enhancing the quality of life for patients with psoriasis (Masa'deh, 2024) (Figure 1.9).

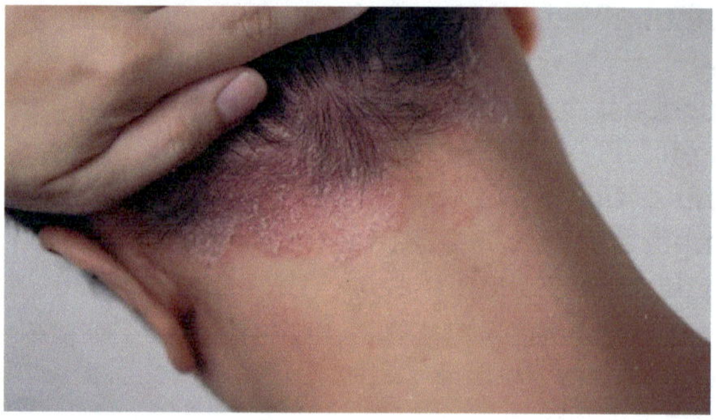

Figure 1.9. Psoriasis.

Source: https://www.health.com/thmb/aEJdBYX_7D88134f1aaKx1yWIB8=/750x0/filters:no_upscale():max_bytes(150000):strip_icc():format(webp)/Health-GettyImages-1604751312-be3c174df1b04084877ff6717123c13f.jpg.

Test Your Knowledge

1. What is acne?
2. What is eczema?

1.3. Skin Cancer

Learning Outcome

1. Describe the types of skin cancer
2. Know the risk factors and prevention strategies of skin cancer
3. Describe the treatment options and prognosis for skin disorders

The increasing prevalence of skin cancer underscores the importance of a good understanding of dermatology and the complex organization of the skin. Skin cancer, which is caused predominantly by uncontrolled cell growth in the epidermis, comprises a number of types, of which melanoma, basal cell carcinoma (BCC), and squamous cell carcinoma (SCC) are the most common. Risk factors include excessive exposure to sunlight's ultraviolet (UV) radiation, genetic influences, and certain lifestyle influences. The epidermis, as the first line of defense against environmental aggressors, is particularly susceptible to UV light and its associated damage, which can cause mutations in skin cells that may be a source of cancer. The interplay between the structure of the skin and the function of defending it against carcinogenic factors is significant in understanding how cancers develop and can be effectively treated. Diagnosis and treatment of skin cancer are based on the ability to recognize its diverse manifestations and to understand the underlying mechanisms. Dermatologists use a range of diagnostic tools, such as dermatoscopy and biopsy, to examine suspicious lesions. Treatment is based on cancer type and stage and involves surgical excision, Mohs micrographic surgery for BCC and SCC, and topical and systemic therapy for advanced lesions. Although the majority of skin cancers are curable with early treatment, education, and awareness remain crucial to the prevention of the disease. For instance, regular skin checks and public campaigns against the dangers of UV exposure help prevent skin malignancies to a great extent. Secondly, understanding the etiology of skin cancers will aid in formulating preventive recommendations, encouraging better skin culture in the populace. New drugs in dermatology have highlighted the importance of understanding the cutaneous effects of antineoplastic treatments, including cyclin-dependent kinase inhibitors. These treatments, while directed against certain types of cancer, induce cutaneous side effects in the form of eczematous papules and pruritus, as studies on the treatments for breast cancer (Sollena et al., 2023) have shown. These developments highlight the necessity of dermatologic monitoring during cancer treatment to avoid disabling side effects while maintaining the efficacy of the cancer treatments themselves. Additionally, research into new modalities, including immunotherapy and targeted therapy, offers greater opportunities for skin cancer treatment but also raises challenges for skin health. With advances in the interface between cancer therapy and dermatology, the identification of skin changes is crucial to enhance treatment and quality of life in patients (Uysal, 2017) (Figure 1.10).

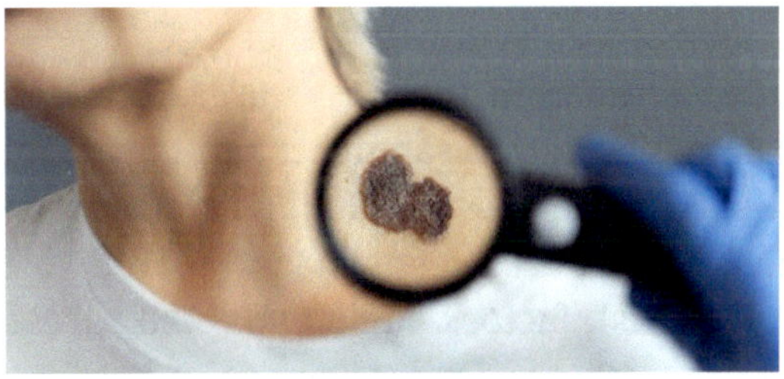

Figure 1.10. Understanding skin cancer.

Source: https://www.kauveryhospital.com/blog/wp-content/uploads/2024/09/How-to-protect-yourself-from-skin-cancer-1200x545_c.jpg.

1.3.1. Types of Skin Cancer: Basal Cell, Squamous Cell, and Melanoma

The spectrum of skin malignancies comprises three major entities: basal cell carcinoma (BCC), squamous cell carcinoma (SCC), and melanoma, each with distinct clinical presentations and prognostic factors. BCC is the most common form of skin cancer, arising from basal cells in the epidermis. It most commonly presents as pearly nodules or pink plaques and is extremely curable by surgical removal. Despite its relatively limited metastatic ability, untreated BCC is capable of invading the tissues around it and producing extensive local devastation. BCC is strongly related to incidental chronic sun exposure, and preventive measures such as sunscreen use and regular skin inspection are most important for identifying potential lesions at an early age. On the other hand, SCC arises from the keratinocytes of the upper layers of the skin and is the second most common form of skin cancer. SCC is likely to manifest as red scaly areas, open sores, or warts that bleed or crust.

Its relationship to ultraviolet (UV) radiation exposure necessitates protective strategies for the skin, such as avoiding tanning beds and wearing protective clothing. While SCC is otherwise more invasive than BCC, its metastatic capacity is generally low relative to melanoma. Certain types of SCC, however, including those in the lip or areas of chronic inflammation, may be at higher risk of spreading and should therefore be followed closely with individualized treatment plans tailored to the patient's risk factors. Melanoma, the rarest of skin cancers, is the most aggressive because of its virulent character and ability to metastasize. Secreted by melanocytes, cells that create skin color, melanoma can present as a new mole or a change in color of an existing mole with features of asymmetry, irregular borders, multiple shades, and a size larger than that of a pencil eraser. Early detection is crucial for effective melanoma management, as prompt treatment significantly improves survival rates. Research has identified various mutations linked to melanoma, particularly in the BRAF and TP53 genes, which further complicate its treatment. Understanding these genetic and environmental risk factors predisposing to skin cancer will assist in developing more effective diagnostic and treatment procedures, as research into the role of cathepsins in skin cancer development has shown (Li et al., 2025; Yost et al., 2025) (Figure 1.11).

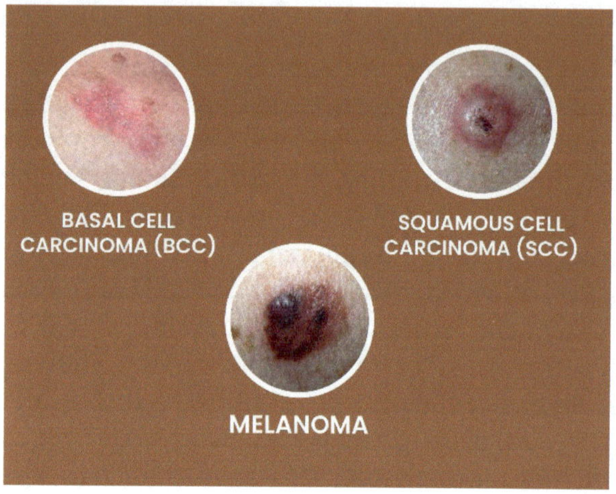

Figure 1.11. Types of skin cancer.

Source: https://drpriyatiwari.s3.amazonaws.com/static/services/skin-types.jpg.

1.3.2. Risk Factors and Prevention Strategies

The health of the skin depends on a range of risk factors that can lead to conditions ranging from minor irritations to severe skin disease. Of these, associated chronic diseases such as cardiovascular disease, diabetes, and obesity may compromise the skin's normal physiology and lead to conditions, including skin failure, in which the protective function is lost. Other determinants, such as age, which compromise skin elasticity and repair processes, also increase skin susceptibility. Environmental determinants such as UV radiation, pollution, and exposure to harmful chemicals also exacerbate skin damage by inducing oxidative stress and inflammation, thereby accelerating skin aging. Identification of risk factors is crucial for both patients and clinicians to establish effective prevention strategies tailored to specific needs (Levine et al., 2022). Effective prevention strategies can mitigate the adverse effects of identified risk factors on skin health. An integrated approach that includes lifestyle modifications, such as a balanced diet fortified with antioxidants, adequate hydration, and physical exercise, is crucial for maintaining skin integrity. Moreover, everyday skin care habits, such as applying broad-spectrum sunscreen, constitute a significant barrier against sun-induced damage. Regular monitoring of skin for the earliest signs of damage or abnormalities allows early physician intervention and averts further complications. Moreover, reducing underlying health complications through medical intervention and lifestyle changes not only improves overall health but also enhances skin resistance. Lastly, routine and highly educated preventive care can significantly reduce the incidence of skin complications across various populations (Renert-Yuval et al., 2021). Education and awareness play key roles in the prevention and management of skin conditions. Risk factors and available preventive interventions must be emphasized to patients through healthcare provider counseling, with a focus on the importance of skin health. Community supports and resources can foster environments where individuals share experiences and approaches, fostering a group approach to preserving skin health. Additional investigation into the pathophysiology of skin disease, e.g., by studying biomarkers for diseases such as atopic dermatitis, can provide greater insight into the potential for individualized prevention. As the understanding of risk factors and skin health increases, it is ever more important that providers and patients alike take active measures not just to address existing skin disease but also to avoid recurrence (Levine et al., 2022) (Figure 1.12).

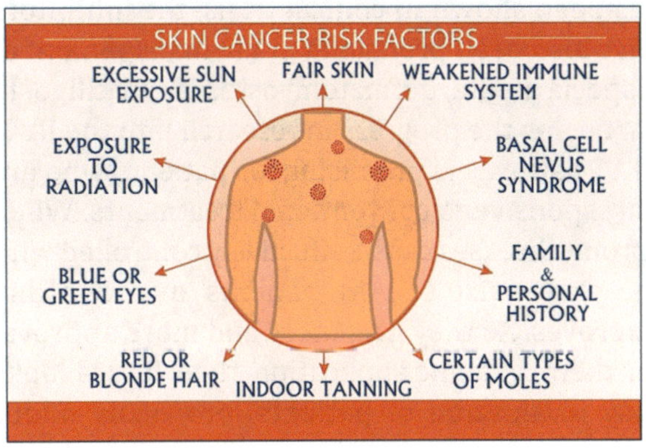

Figure 1.12. Skin cancer risk factors.

Source: https://www.medicoverhospitals.in/images/diseases/skin-cancer-causes-risk-factors.webp.

1.3.3. Treatment Options and Prognosis

The therapeutic approach to the treatment of skin diseases has radically altered with improved understanding of the dermatologic disease at the cellular and molecular levels. Psoriasis and atopic dermatitis are cases in point wherein newer therapeutic methods have been established. Identification of disease-causing elements, particularly cytokines such as IL-17A and IL-23, in psoriasis has transformed clinical practice. These observations underscore the trend toward the use of targeted therapies, especially with Janus kinase inhibitors (JAKi). The potency of JAK inhibitors in blocking multiple cytokine signals simultaneously highlights their value as a general-purpose agent in dermatological treatment. As more research unfolds, such therapy may prove to have both systemic and local applications, improving outcomes in many skin diseases. JAK inhibitors represent a broadly generalizable paradigm for the treatment of skin diseases beyond inflammatory dermatoses. Their mechanism of action is the concomitant modulation of multiple immune pathways, which is most helpful in complex skin disorders with redundant inflammatory signals. Clinically, as has been shown in clinical trials, the inhibitors have also been promising in the management of alopecia areata, dermatomyositis, and vitiligo. In particular, the progress in research into the JAK/STAT pathway is promising for patients who are unresponsive to conventional treatments. When chronic diseases can be effectively controlled with the proper use of JAKi, patients' quality of life improves. As they gain more and more approval for their systemic application, their future looks rosy. Evaluation of patients' prognosis under JAK inhibitor therapy is especially relevant, as the outcome can not only determine treatment efficacy but also its long-term sustainability in terms of its impact on disease management strategy. The preliminary results show that patients report significant alleviation of symptoms and a reduction in disease severity, indicating a positive response rate. However, when assessing prognosis, consideration should be given to treatment duration, potential side effects, and the varying modes of individual ailments. Ongoing research plays a crucial role in simplifying treatment protocols for JAKi to better meet patients' various needs. In light of the need for the development of effective treatments for skin disease, continued research into JAK inhibitors and their long-term consequences will feature centrally in the determination of future dermatological practice and refining prognostic models within clinical settings (Ghoreschi et al., 2019) (Figure 1.13).

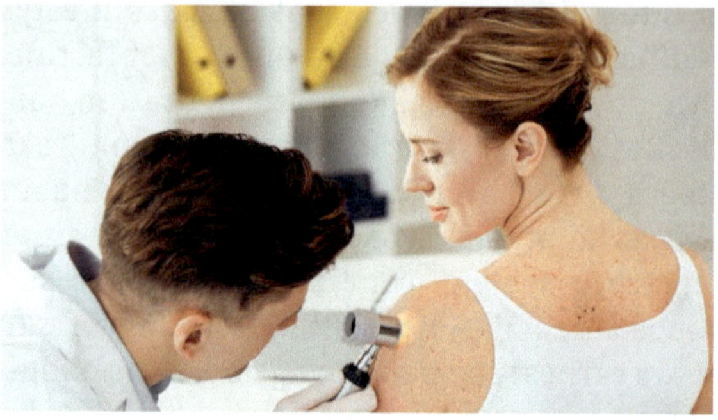

Figure 1.13. The role of dermatologists in skin cancer prevention and treatment.

Source: https://www.pinnacleskin.com/getmedia/880af20d-77f5-4bb6-85dc-43759e82cb8c/Role-Dermatologist-Skin-Cancer_Header-Standard.jpg?width=2000&height=625&ext=.jpg.

Test Your Knowledge

1. List the types of skin cancer.
2. What are the treatment options for skin cancer?

1.4. Dermatological Procedures

Learning Outcome

1. Understand the purpose of skin biopsies
2. Describe the laser treatments for skin conditions
3. Know the procedures of cosmetic dermatology

The branch of dermatological procedures comprises a number of methods that are accountable for the diagnosis and treatment of diseases of the skin, focusing on the development of imaging technologies. Among these developments, photoacoustic dermoscopy (PAD) is a watershed offering noninvasive, high-resolution imaging of skin anatomy. By combining optical excitation principles with acoustic detection, PAD bridges gaps in the resolution of standard imaging methods. PAD is being utilized increasingly in the clinical setting to examine melanoma, psoriasis, and dermatitis and thereby offer clinicians a better tool for anatomical studies. The applications of this approach also extend to the domain of cosmetics, where it is used to evaluate treatment effectiveness, once more emphasizing the skin and its multiple functions in dermatology (Wang et al., 2022). Beyond imaging techniques, dermatological treatments also increasingly use molecular diagnostics to better explain skin pathologies. Traditional diagnostic techniques often rely on subjective tests and invasive biopsies, which may be inadequate for inflammatory conditions (Ibrahim et al., 2022). The development of dermal biomarker patches (DBPs) is a significant advancement, as they have the potential to harvest molecular data using minimally invasive methods. This novel technology can capture the dermal transcriptome and provide data on the molecular "fingerprint" of healthy and psoriatic skin. By reducing the necessity of dolorous biopsy procedures, DBPs both improve patient comfort and create the possibility for sustained surveillance and a deeper understanding of dermatological illnesses. This shift towards molecular diagnostics signals a new era in dermatology, broadening diagnostic and therapeutic options. With the evolution of dermatology, the synergy of advanced imaging modalities with molecular diagnostics holds promising future prospects for the management of skin health. Application of technologies such as PAD and DBPs enables better depth and clarity of skin conditions, which can be tailored to treatment techniques. Physicians now have the potential advantage of applying machine-learning approaches to study difficult phenotypes using these cutting-edge biomarker collection strategies. This brings in technology, not just permits enhanced correctness in diagnosis, but also assists in customization of therapy against individual variation in skin response. As science continues to clarify the complexities of the structure and functioning of the skin, no doubt there will be a possibility of further evolved dermatologic interventions that will revolutionize clinical practice with superior patient outcomes and enhanced quality of care (Ibrahim et al., 2022; Wang et al., 2022) (Figure 1.14).

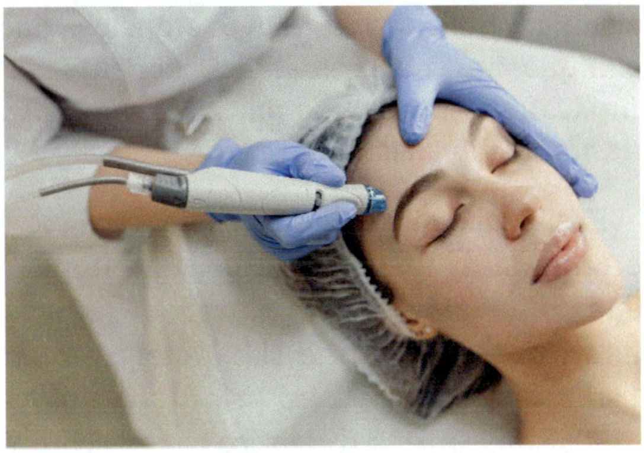

Figure 1.14. Dermatological procedure.

Source: https://thesmarthospital.in/assets/img/services/dermatology.jpg.

1.4.1. Skin Biopsies: Purpose and Process

Skin biopsies are a valuable diagnostic procedure in dermatology that enables dermatologists to obtain skin samples for examination. The initial reason for a skin biopsy is to diagnose a range of dermatological disorders, such as skin cancers, inflammatory disorders, and infections. With the provisional diagnosis, skin biopsies allow clinicians to plan appropriate and effective treatment strategies. Apart from that, histopathologic analysis of biopsy samples helps in understanding the typical structure and morphology of the involved skin in a given ailment. This information is the backbone of dermatology because various diseases have distinct histologic features, which guide therapeutic decisions. For example, detection of atypical cells during a biopsy can confirm malignancy, while detection of inflammatory cells may be associated with autoimmune disorders. This diagnostic utility demonstrates the utility of skin biopsies in clinical medicine and research.

Skin biopsy acquisition is a procedure with careful techniques to avoid causing discomfort to patients and obtain maximal preservation of the tissue. It is commonly performed on an outpatient basis and can be accomplished through various methods such as excisional, incisional, punch, and shave biopsies. Each technique has its indications, benefits, and complications, depending on the size and type of lesion being examined.

Excisional biopsies, for instance, involve the removal of the whole lesion, while punch biopsies involve the removal of a small cylindrical section of the skin. Adequate local anesthesia is administered prior to the biopsy to limit pain. During the process, the acquired tissue is meticulously processed and treated with histological techniques for analysis. Data obtained from the process are valuable for informing skin structure and skin pathology, adding to the knowledge available in overall dermatology practice. In addition to diagnosis, the impacts of skin biopsies also add to research within the skin structure and function domain. As the role of the skin in systemic disease and its intricate immune processes come into sharper focus, biopsies provide a window into the skin's microenvironment.

Examination of skin tissues obtained via biopsies enables researchers to investigate cellular and molecular mechanisms in a number of dermatologic conditions. This is particularly relevant when considering diseases such as urticaria, which is experienced by a large proportion of the population and significantly affects quality of life (Zuberbier et al., 2021). In addition, newer models, including negative-pressure wound-healing studies, help elucidate epithelial regeneration and immune responses within skin lesions, underscoring the multidisciplinary nature of skin biopsies and their role in dermatologic research (Rakita et al., 2020) (Figure 1.15).

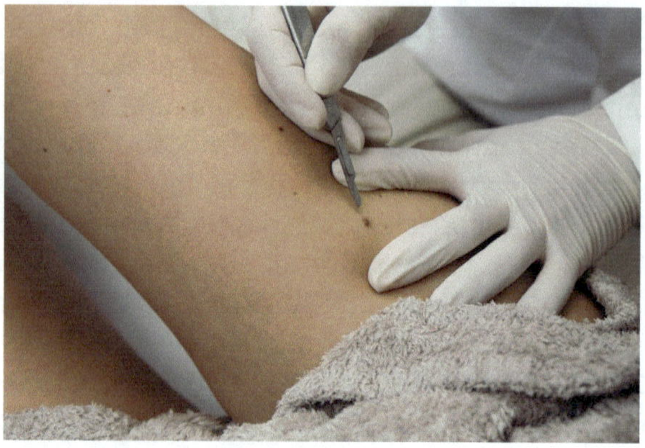

Figure 1.15. Skin biopsy.

Source: https://epidermatology.com.sg/wp-content/uploads/2024/02/skin-biopsy-featured-image-1024x682.jpg.

1.4.2. Laser Treatments for Skin Conditions

Laser development has transformed dermatologic practice, most significantly in the treatment of skin conditions. Laser treatments, which are precise and noninvasive, offer spot solutions for an array of issues from acne marks to blood vessel lesions. Ablative and non-ablative lasers are two of the many types of lasers employed that target specific areas of skin with intense light energy to stimulate changes such as collagen remodeling and the removal of pigmented or vascular lesions. This modality also has the added benefit of minimizing damage to surrounding tissues, allowing rapid healing, and reducing patients' time off work. With dermatologists using these technologies, further study is indicated on their effectiveness and safety profiles to achieve the best possible results and prevent short-term adverse effects in laser therapy for dermatology. Laser therapy for skin conditions is also supported by mounting evidence exploring its numerous uses. For instance, studies have shown promising results for the management of atopic dermatitis (AD), a common inflammatory skin condition, using lasers. Non-UV light therapy, such as low-level laser therapy and intense pulsed light therapy, has emerged as viable alternatives and may be lower risk than traditional UV treatment. Use of laser technology enables a more palpably efficacious intervention, as recent reviews indicate, showing significantly improved outcomes for AD patients, especially since the technology has evolved to meet multiple clinical needs. The discoveries underscore the importance of understanding the various applications of laser therapies in the broader context of skin health and disease treatment (Zablah et al., 2025). Additionally, combining laser treatments with sophisticated model systems enables elucidation of skin diseases at the cellular level.

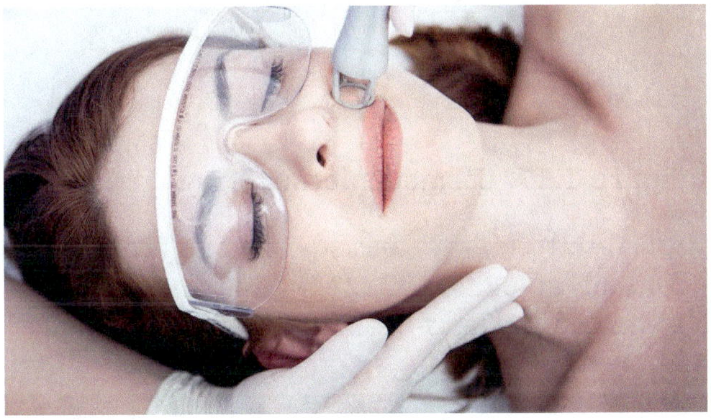

Figure 1.16. Laser treatments for skin conditions.

Source: https://www.manjushasparsh.com/sites/default/files/2023-04/Laser%20Treatments%20for%20Skin%20Conditions.jpg.

The creation of three-dimensional (3D) skin equivalents (FSE) has improved research into the effects of treatments such as laser therapy on skin regeneration and healing. These models mimic the native structure of human skin, enabling researchers to monitor responses to different interventions, such as laser therapies, in real time. Using high-resolution optical devices, scientists can observe metabolic activity in treated tissue, leading to more efficient treatment regimens and individualized strategies for personalized medicine. Using laser engineering and sophisticated skin models in combination, synergy enhances understanding of skin pathology and treatment response, enabling increasingly targeted, individualized dermatologic therapies (Khalid et al., 2024) (Figure 1.16).

1.4.3. Cosmetic Dermatology: Procedures and Ethics

Cosmetic dermatology has experienced astronomical growth over the last few years, with many procedures available to meet clients' aesthetic requirements. From fairly minor interventions like Botox injections to more severe ones like facelifts, cosmetic dermatology procedures are designed to enhance appearance and correct skin blemishes. It is noteworthy that cosmetic dermatology not only targets surface-level enhancement but also requires a profound understanding of the skin's structure, including its dermal and epidermal layers. Practitioners handle these layers but rely on their expertise for generating the maximum output while maintaining healthy skin. But their popularity also creates grave ethical concerns regarding informed consent, potential side effects, and psychological impact of such alterations on self-esteem and identity in patients, especially among younger age groups who may feel compelled to conform to societal beauty standards. The ethics of cosmetic dermatology is a multifaceted problem that warrants earnest consideration. The responsibility of dermatologists extends beyond the procedural aspect; they must ensure that patients are properly informed about the risks and benefits of cosmetic treatments. The rules of good ethics demand an extensive consultation process, in which practitioners should evaluate a patient's motivation for undergoing treatment and provide counseling that sets appropriate expectations. Moreover, professionals need to practice ethical advertising and patient choice, avoiding misleading presentations of the results that can be achieved through such treatments. In the literature, facial attributes identified through various cues significantly influence how individuals respond to cosmetic procedures, demonstrating the intricate connection between skin appearance and social perception. An understanding of these dynamics will guide practitioners in establishing safe, ethical, and effective treatment plans that prioritize the patient's welfare. Furthermore, the convergence of dermatological cosmeticism and evolving societal norms underscores the need for collaboration among dermatologists, patients, and policymakers. Establishing ethical guidelines and standards of practice can help reduce the risks associated with cosmetic treatments and uphold the ideals of beneficence and non-maleficence. Since skin health is related to overall well-being, ensuring that patients make informed decisions in cosmetic dermatology corresponds with the larger objectives of dermatology as a discipline. For instance, maximizing cutaneous health, along with addressing beauty concerns, enhances objective measures of youthfulness, such that parameters like facial contrast influence perceived age, as indicated by studies showing that certain cosmetic interventions can really deliver greater psychological well-being (Mauger et al., 2013). Finally, promoting a culture of ethical responsibility in cosmetic dermatology not only preserves professional integrity but also fosters patient trust, enabling individuals to make choices that speak to their aesthetic and personal objectives (Figure 1.17).

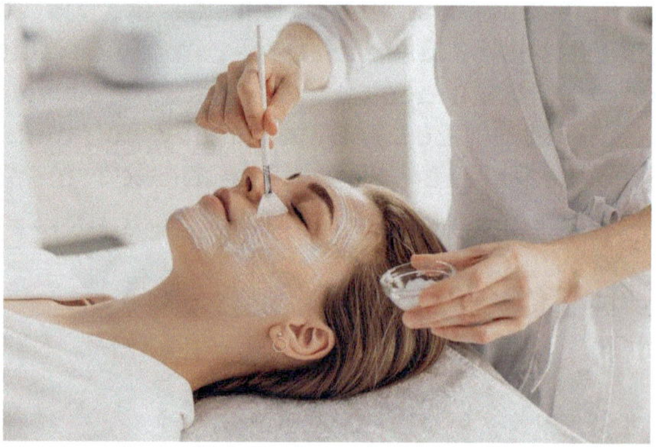

Figure 1.17. Cosmetic dermatology.

Source: https://www.oasisdermatology.com/wp-content/uploads/2022/12/What-is-Cosmetic-Dermatology-Oasis-Dermatology-1000x658.jpg.

Test Your Knowledge

1. What is the purpose of a skin biopsy?
2. How many types of lasers are there?

1.5. Advances in Dermatology

Learning Outcome

1. Understand the role of technology in skin diagnosis
2. Describe the innovations in skin treatment methods
3. Know the future trends in dermatological research

The use of new technologies in dermatology has significantly revolutionized the diagnostic landscape. Among them, the advent of dermal biomarker patches (DBPs) is an excellent example of a new method of understanding skin diseases. Such patches use a minimally painful process to acquire molecular data from the skin, which is superior to conventional biopsy procedures that involve patient discomfort. By leveraging single-stranded DNA modifications to bind to messenger RNA, researchers have employed DBPs to obtain transcriptomic information from healthy and diseased skin (N = 7; 33 unique samples). Not only does this method offer a wealth of information regarding the molecular fingerprint of the skin, but it also offers an ethical alternative to agonizing biopsies, thus improving patient compliance and overall experience. The finding's ability to monitor over time or across varying interventions makes it a core finding in individualized dermatologic treatment (Ibrahim et al., 2022). The second key innovation in dermatology is the growing appreciation of extracellular vesicles (EVs) as mediators of cell-to-cell communication in cutaneous tissues. The nano-scale vesicles secreted from different cell types transport bioactive compounds such as proteins, lipids, and RNA molecules. They also play an important role in modifying the phenotypes of the cells that surround them, and this potentially has therapeutic applications in the treatment of most dermatological diseases. Recent research highlights their potential therapeutic use in wound repair, scar formation, and even cutaneous disease diagnosis, based on analysis of exosome content. The advances in EV bioengineering and therapeutics hold a rosy future in which EVs can be used to develop targeted therapies. These developments mark a revolutionary shift from traditional dermatological treatments to more sophisticated, biologically driven ones, thereby widening the scope of possible treatments for skin disorders (Bobis-Wozowicz et al., 2022). Furthermore, innovation in DBPs and EVs marks an evolutionary revolution in molecular dermatology, enabling more advanced diagnostics and treatment concepts. As these technologies advance, it is essential to reflect on their broader implications for the field, especially regarding scalability and clinical use. The ability to derive rich datasets through non-invasive procedures not only expands our knowledge of various skin diseases but also provides a platform for applying machine learning methodologies in dermatology. With the injection of analytics, dermatology is on the cusp of a new era defined by precision medicine. The intersection of technology, biology, and clinical practice will enable dermatologists to tailor treatment more effectively, paving the way for a future in which skin disease can be cured with unprecedented accuracy and efficiency (Bobis-Wozowicz et al., 2022; Ibrahim et al., 2022).

1.5.1. Role of Technology in Skin Diagnosis

Technological incorporation into skin diagnosis has revolutionized dermatological research, enabling more accurate and timely assessments of dermal conditions. Various non-invasive optical techniques, such as dermoscopy and reflectance confocal microscopy (RCM), have been widely adopted because of their ability to provide high-resolution views of skin lesions. These technologies enhance clinicians' diagnostic ability in the detection of malignant structures at an early stage, with significant effects on patient outcomes. For instance, using high-resolution imaging, clinicians can detect characteristic features that indicate melanoma, something critical with its rising prevalence and resultant fatality. Through the application of these advanced technologies, dermatologists are not only better able to confirm their diagnoses but also to monitor the progression of skin disease over time, promoting more proactive patient care and suggesting possible alleviation of healthcare burdens, as outlined in Al-Ayyad et al. (2024). In addition to traditional diagnostic modalities, artificial intelligence, particularly Convolutional Neural Networks (CNNs), has become a game-changing force in skin diagnosis. With the aid of large-scale databases of skin images, CNNs support the detection of various skin ailments, from benign lesions to melanoma. Such programs are experts at recognizing intricate patterns and specifics that even the best practitioners might overlook, therefore enhancing diagnostic accuracy. Recent studies have demonstrated the capability of CNNs to classify skin disease successfully, enabling swift and accurate diagnosis. Such dermatological technological advancement not only improves clinical practice but also facilitates the need for ongoing learning and adaptation in healthcare fueled by AI interventions, fueling advancements that ultimately translate into improved patient care, as conceptualized in Sayyad et al. (2023). But the integration of such technologies poses a class of issues that must be addressed with prudence. Data quality and diversity issues in training an AI system pose risks of bias that may impact diagnostic outcomes. Additionally, ethical issues of data privacy and algorithmic bias necessitate robust frameworks to ensure patient safety and trust. With dermatology increasingly being merged with new technologies like CNNs and advanced imaging technologies, collaborative efforts between researchers, practitioners, and data scientists are required to address these problems. In so doing, the specialty can reap the full benefits of technological innovation and ensure equal access, while ethical practice ensures patients' continued welfare, further promoting technology's future role in enhancing skin diagnosis and treatment techniques in current dermatology (Figure 1.18).

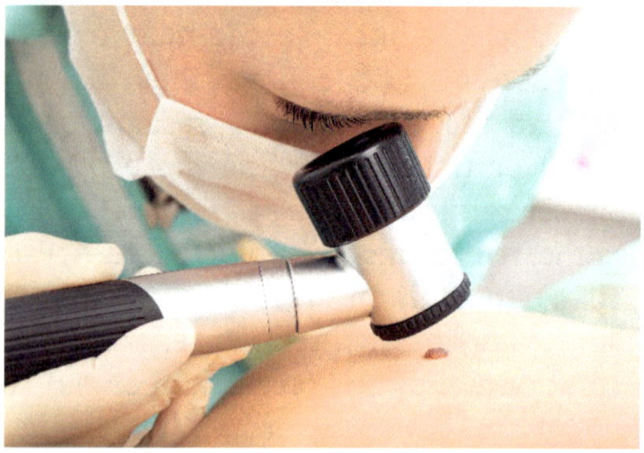

Figure 1.18. Dermoscopy.

Source: https://s3.amazonaws.com/production.scholastica/article/68088/original/depositphotos_26089363_xl.jpg?1674226792.

1.5.2. Innovations in Treatment Methods

The world of dermatology is being revolutionized by the advent of high-technology platforms, i.e., digital twins. It is a technology in which virtual copies are made that represent an individual's skin type with real-time data from various sources, like imaging, genetics, and the environment. Not only do digital twins enhance the diagnostic process, but they also enable personalized treatment approaches, changing how dermatologists diagnose and treat skin disorders. For instance, while treating complicated diseases such as acne or psoriasis, dermatologists can simulate how a patient's skin will respond to different treatments, minimizing trial-and-error that frustrates patients and leads to less-than-ideal care. With the evolution in technology, its ability to provide personalized information and tailored interventions will revolutionize dermatological practice, enhancing patient outcomes and satisfaction within the context of individualized care (Haykal, 2025). Artificial intelligence (AI) further enhances the potential of digital twins in dermatology with greater predictive capability. Computer AI processes vast amounts of information, including imaging and patient history, enabling patterns that most clinicians would miss to be recognized. Specifically, convolutional neural networks (CNNs) can automatically recognize skin-image features important to diagnosis and treatment planning. The ability of AI to learn and refine its categorizations with experience assists dermatologists in making evidence-based decisions, ultimately improving the management of diseases such as melanoma and hyperpigmentation. This shift towards a data-driven, more mechanized approach is a milestone for the field, parallel with what has occurred in other fields of medical imaging, where AI's ability has demonstrated rather large increases over traditional practices. The intersection of AI and dermatology is ushering in a new era of precision and personalization in treatment planning, raising the overall standards of care (Nagendran et al., 2020). Despite the promising advancements, the convergence of the two innovations is fraught with problems. Data privacy issues remain at the heart, with the ongoing collection of confidential patient data raising ethical controversies over security and consent. Moreover, the lack of standardized processes for developing digital twins can hinder widespread adoption in dermatology clinics, particularly among facilities with limited resources and inferior technology. To mitigate such obstacles, collaborative interactions between technology developers, physicians, and regulating bodies must prioritize establishing clear guidelines to facilitate seamless integration as well as ensure patient safety. Emphasizing the necessity to train healthcare professionals on using these technologies properly is also vital. By fostering an environment that enables dermatologists to lead transformations such as digital twins and AI, the industry can set itself up for a future in which patient care is drastically enhanced through data-led, personalized methods (Haykal, 2025) (Figure 1.19).

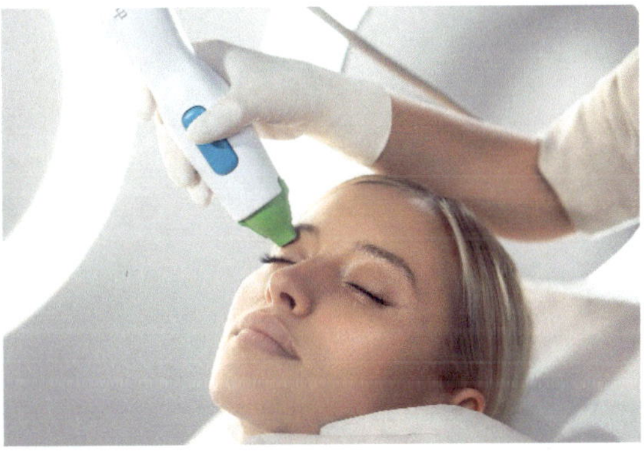

Figure 1.19. The latest innovations in skin treatments.

Source: https://images.squarespace-cdn.com/content/v1/5d52feb1aa6f990001929012/9ae12642-ec45-4639-bb96-5bd01c422e5b/_R5A1556+Kopie.jpg.

1.5.3. Future Trends in Dermatological Research

The future of dermatological research will be greatly influenced by the progress made in the knowledge of melanocyte biology and its implications for several skin diseases. As researchers close the gap in understanding the mechanisms of melanocyte function, novel therapeutic concepts for diseases such as melanoma, vitiligo, and albinism will emerge. The investigation of clinical melanoma research, for instance, is leading to new immunotherapies that activate the body's own immune system to destroy melanoma cells. As research develops with basic melanoma research, it is increasingly becoming possible to develop targeted treatments that address the unique genetic and molecular composition of each tumor. Therefore, the focus on melanocyte biology not only offers new lines of treatment but also highlights significant issues regarding prevention and early management in dermatological disorders, pointing to personalized medicine here (Birlea et al., 2018). In conjunction with these biological discoveries, biomimetic material applications in dermatology are a rapidly developing field that seeks to enhance skin hydration and restore barrier function. Existing literature indicates that biomimetic creams, which replicate the natural lipid structure of skin, moisturize more effectively than traditional moisturizers containing occlusive ingredients such as petrolatum and mineral oil. This indicates a significant shift in dermatological products to address the specific needs of aging skin, particularly among individuals aged over 60 years, where hydration at the appropriate level is critical for skin health. The combination of next-generation formulation methods and knowledge of skin physiology will most probably result in products that not only enhance hydration but also have a proactive role to play in skin barrier repair, highlighting the future of more efficient dermatological treatments and patient-focused treatments (Grant-Ross et al., 2015). Additionally, the convergence of genomics and dermatology research will reshape our comprehension of skin diseases and their treatment. System biology advances facilitate more advanced evaluation of genetic susceptibility to skin diseases and have prompted new developments in risk estimation and therapeutic intervention. Through the application of next-generation sequencing technologies, genomic variations associated with an individual's skin diseases can be identified and used to develop customized therapy. As personalized medicine increasingly becomes an integrated practice, the integration of genetic data into clinical medicine will enable prediction of disease susceptibility and treatment response. This not only indicates a shift towards precision healthcare in general, but also underscores the most urgent requirement for interdisciplinary integration in dermatology, as genetic, biological, and clinical insights converge to formulate new paradigms for the management of skin health (Birlea et al., 2018).

Test Your Knowledge

1. What is the role of technology in skin diagnosis?
2. Discuss the future trends in dermatological research.

SUMMARY

Overall, the intricate structure of the skin not only serves as the body's barrier against injury from the external world but also has a vital role in overall homeostasis. The skin's ability to protect against damage from the external environment, regulate body temperature, and transmit sensations underscores its biological significance. Disruptions of cutaneous homeostasis, whether internal, for instance, change in hormones, or external, for instance, pollution and UV radiation, may lead to numerous skin complications. As described, buffering systems maintaining homeostasis during such imbalances require further research to inform clinical practice as well as formulating skincare products. Thus, a better understanding of these mechanisms will enhance preventive interventions and treatments tailored to individual skin types, thereby ensuring healthier skin. Besides, maintaining skin integrity has consequences beyond physical appearance, affecting psychological well-being and social relationships. Skin illnesses often carry a stigma that has far-reaching implications on an individual's self-esteem and mental health. As evidenced, effective management of skin diseases—through medical and cosmetic modalities—is vital for physical well-being and psychosocial outcomes. Emerging advances in dermatology science indicate mechanisms of skin repair and regeneration, such as inflammatory and immune reactions on wound healing, that can open the door to novel therapies. For instance, the development of new wound care models, as evident in contemporary research, provides insights into cellular behavior during skin healing, highlighting the importance of certain therapeutic methods in dermatology (Rakita et al., 2020). Finally, the future of dermatology holds further advances in understanding the multifaceted functions of the skin. Continued investigation of the microbiome, the neuroendocrine impact on cutaneous diseases, and skin care biotechnologies will be critical to the development of comprehensive treatment regimens. In finding effective treatments for prevalent cutaneous diseases, the combination of dermatological science underlying principles with practical application will be crucial. Beyond better encapsulating the fundamental principles of skin structure and health, this multidisciplinary approach fosters innovation, leading to improved patient outcomes. As we step into the future, compliance with research and innovation in dermatology will be the key to enhancing skin health and quality of life for individuals worldwide (Jiao et al., 2024).

In dermatology, the nature of skin disease necessitates an understanding of human skin anatomy and physiology from multiple perspectives. The key point is the significant relationship between the skin barrier and certain dermatologic diseases. The stratum corneum, the outermost layer of the skin, provides a critical barrier against trans-epidermal water loss and external infection. Disease within this barrier results in skin conditions such as atopic dermatitis, characterized by hyper-inflammatory chronicity and impaired barrier function. This necessitates exploring targeted therapies that restore this barrier—e.g., new therapies to enhance skin hydration and lipid levels can offer new directions for effective management of such disorders, hence the need for dermatology clinics to approach barrier repair as a curative objective. Another key area in dermatology relates to the integration of new therapeutic modalities for treating skin disorders. Phototherapy, for instance, has come up as a non-surgical modality of therapy for conditions like psoriasis and eczema. In reference to limited-resource environments, for instance, Kenya, the introduction of phototherapy services in referral hospitals has been required to effectively control skin diseases. As illustrated by recent programs, training local health personnel in phototherapy application can lead to improved service delivery and greater relief of local health disparities.

The success of such programs depends on collaboration between international dermatological experts and national institutions, demonstrating that with adequate education and the allocation of resources, even areas with underdeveloped healthcare systems can achieve improvements in dermatological therapy, thus bridging treatment gaps. Finally, patient-reported outcomes are at the forefront in guiding dermatological studies and clinical practice, particularly in determining the impact on quality of life from skin disease. Conditions such as atopic dermatitis significantly affect the quality of the patient's daily life, impacting their mental and emotional well-being. Itch and skin pain symptoms have been of particular interest in research, with an emphasis on the role of patient-reported feedback in evaluating therapies. The use of adapted evaluation instruments, such as the Itch NRS and Skin Pain NRS, can provide insight into the intensity of symptoms as perceived by the patient. This patient-centered approach suggests enhancing clinical assessments to better reflect true experiences to guide clinicians in developing effective treatment plans. Patient engagement with dermatology, in addition to maximizing the treatment process, promotes an interactive investigation into how skin wellness has far-reaching implications for quality of life, as evidenced by recent dermatology studies (Abetz-Webb et al., 2019; Beck et al., 2020).

KEY TERMS FROM THIS CHAPTER

- Bacterium
- Dermis
- Genetic predisposition
- Hypodermis
- Langerhans cells
- Propionibacterium acnes
- Skin diseases
- Dermatology
- Epidermis
- Homeostasis
- Immunity
- Macrophages
- Sensory perception
- Skins mechanical resilience

CRITICAL THINKING QUESTIONS

1. **What is the outermost layer of the skin called?**
   a. Dermis
   b. Epidermis
   c. Hypodermis
   d. Subcutaneous layer
2. **Which protein is primarily responsible for the waterproofing of the skin?**
   a. Collagen
   b. Elastin
   c. Keratin
   d. Melanin
3. **What is the primary function of melanocytes in the skin?**
   a. Producing keratin
   b. Generating sweat
   c. Producing melanin
   d. Regulating body temperature
4. **Which layer of the skin contains blood vessels and nerve endings?**
   a. Epidermis
   b. Dermis
   c. Hypodermis
   d. Stratum corneum
5. **What type of sweat gland is involved in thermoregulation?**
   a. Sebaceous gland
   b. Eccrine gland
   c. Apocrine gland
   d. Ceruminous gland

Short Answer Questions

1. Define dermatology.
2. Why is the skin important to the human body?
3. Name the three layers of skin.
4. What are the common skin conditions?
5. What is skin cancer?

Answer to Critical Thinking Questions

1. (b); 2. (c) ; 3. (c); 4. (b); 5. (b)

REFERENCES

1. Newton, L., DeLozier, A. M., Griffiths, P. C., Hill, J. N., Hudgens, S., Symonds, T., Gable, J. C., Paik, J., Wyrwich, K. W., Eichenfield, L. F., Abetz-Webb, L., & Silverberg, J. I. (2019). Exploring content and psychometric validity of newly developed assessment tools for itch and skin pain in atopic dermatitis. *Journal of Patient-Reported Outcomes, 3*(1), 42. https://doi.org/10.1186/s41687-019-0128-zAbuabara, K., Elias, P. M., Lee, C. H., et al. (2019). By protecting against cutaneous inflammation, epidermal pigmentation provided an additional advantage for ancestral humans. https://core.ac.uk/download/323072787.pdf (accessed on 21st July 2025).
2. Adams, B., Belvins, B., Burgess, C., Chotani, R., Chotani, C. M., et al. (2017). Role of cyclooxygenase in the vascular responses to extremity cooling in Caucasian and African males. https://core.ac.uk/download/288395289.pdf (accessed on 21st July 2025).
3. Adeyo, O., Allan, B. B., Barnes, R. H., et al. (2014). Palmoplantar keratoderma along with neuromuscular and metabolic phenotypes in *Slurp1*-deficient mice. https://core.ac.uk/download/323077636.pdf (accessed on 21st July 2025).
4. Affolter, V. K., Bevins, C. L., & Leonard, B. C. (2012). Antimicrobial peptides: Agents of border protection for companion animals. https://core.ac.uk/download/323070658.pdf (accessed on 21st July 2025).
5. Ahmad, S. A., Hadizadeh, M., Marhaban, M. H., et al. (2017). High-frequency ultrasound imaging in wound assessment: Current perspectives. https://core.ac.uk/download/153832795.pdf (accessed on 21st July 2025).
6. Al-Ayyad, M. S., Al-Nabulsi, J., Owida, H. A., et al. (2024). Available medical imaging modalities for melanoma screening. https://core.ac.uk/download/622481089.pdf (accessed on 21st July 2025).
7. Ali, A., Anwar, M., Naeemullah, M., & Hussain, S. (2025). Correlation between nurse-led skin care education and patient adherence to topical treatment regimens in psoriasis. *Physical Education, Health and Social Sciences.* https://www.semanticscholar.org/paper/f3b262acf51bcd92dc68faabe9404c4f8e4fc530 (accessed on 21st July 2025).
8. Aliaga, C., Gutierrez, D., Iglesias-Guitian, J., et al. (2015). A biophysically-based model of the optical properties of skin aging. https://core.ac.uk/download/289983365.pdf (accessed on 21st July 2025).
9. Alsuwaidan, S., Nagshabandi, K. N., & Alajlan, A. M. (2024). Severe nodulocystic acne induced by mercury-containing skin-whitening cream: A case report and call for public awareness. *Case Reports in Dermatology, 16*, 216–220. https://www.semanticscholar.org/paper/6587ab8114c9001b88fd6b3f7777fea597bd1529 (accessed on 21st July 2025).
10. Bachynskyy, M., & Yavorskyy, B. (2018). Informational aspects of the haptic stimulation by the light for correction of the human functional state. https://core.ac.uk/download/286085437.pdf (accessed on 21st July 2025).
11. Beck, K., Bhutani, T., Chang, A. Y., et al. (2020). Implementation of an ultraviolet phototherapy service at a national referral hospital in Western Kenya: Reflections on challenges and lessons learned. https://core.ac.uk/download/323072276.pdf (accessed on 21st July 2025).
12. Bin Dayel, S., & Hussein, R. (2025). Exosomes in dermatology: Emerging roles in skin health and disease. *Pharmaceutics, 17*. https://www.semanticscholar.org/paper/1db86ee43852371b9ae3c314f7f85c58201522e4 (accessed on 21st July 2025).

13. Birlea, S., Bosenberg, M. W., Box, N. F., et al. (2018). Frontiers in pigment cell and melanoma research. http://arxiv.org/abs/1808.01869 (accessed on 21st July 2025).
14. Bobis-Wozowicz, S., & Marbán, E. (2022). Editorial: Extracellular vesicles as next generation therapeutics. *Frontiers in Cell and Developmental Biology, 10*. https://www.semanticscholar.org/paper/732d0232a6adfdf5483d138a9d4ce1fdeef5b999 (accessed on 21st July 2025).
15. Boffa, M. J. (2004). *Dermatology*. https://core.ac.uk/download/46601884.pdf (accessed on 21st July 2025).
16. Brown, C. T. A., Campbell, C. L., Christison, C., et al. (2015). 3D Monte Carlo radiation transfer modelling of photodynamic therapy. https://core.ac.uk/download/30319719.pdf (accessed on 21st July 2025).
17. Bugaevsky, K. A. (2024). Anatomy and histology of the human skin and hair on thematic badges. *Dermatology and Dermatitis*. https://www.semanticscholar.org/paper/d4e5276b89c61b6a4b9e103639b8361e70982ec5 (accessed on 21st July 2025).
18. Cespedes Zablah, A., Griffin, T., & Lio, P. (2025). Beyond ultraviolet: A scoping review of light treatments in atopic dermatitis. *Dermatitis: Contact, Atopic, Occupational, Drug*. https://www.semanticscholar.org/paper/3c2b9aa02efb528f464baa2796d607911f6fb101 (accessed on 21st July 2025).
19. Couceiro, G. A., Benarrós, M. S. C., Rodrigues, A. P. V. C., de Sousa, S. S., da Ribeiro, E. S. C., Bertolo, P. H. L., Muniz, J., et al. (2024). Dermatology in non-human primates: A comprehensive review. *Contribuciones a las Ciencias Sociales*. https://www.semanticscholar.org/paper/8affcfc76626cad335a7ac3490ca5477e8655e64 (accessed on 21st July 2025).
20. Egawa, M. (2021). Raman microscopy for skin evaluation. *The Analyst*. https://www.semanticscholar.org/paper/6f916c1ae0851b766aaf3d1eb742dc207dc92039 (accessed on 21st July 2025).
21. Freer, M., Darling, N., Goncalves, K., Mills, K. J., & Przyborski, S. (2023). Development of a mammalian neurosensory full-thickness skin equivalent and its application to screen sensitizing stimuli. *Bioengineering & Translational Medicine, 8*. https://www.semanticscholar.org/paper/53f9adb686e6cad776fb82c41911dc66e870dbf6 (accessed on 21st July 2025).
22. Gallo, R. L., Irvine, A. D., Kong, H. H., et al. (2019). The microbiome in patients with atopic dermatitis. https://core.ac.uk/download/323064499.pdf (accessed on 21st July 2025).
23. Ghoreschi, K., Meier, K., & Solimani, F. (2019). Emerging topical and systemic JAK inhibitors in dermatology. https://core.ac.uk/download/286097357.pdf (accessed on 21st July 2025).
24. Goriparthi, G. S., Milcovich, G., & Murdan, S. (2011). An assessment of the human nail plate pH. https://core.ac.uk/download/8778791.pdf (accessed on 21st July 2025).
25. Grant-Ross, P., Kurimo, R., Tamburic, S., et al. (2015). An *in vivo* comparison of biomimetic vs. traditional skin moisturization. http://ualresearchonline.arts.ac.uk/8883/1/140625%20IFSCC%202014%20Paper%20Todorova%20et%20al.pdf (accessed on 21st July 2025).
26. Haykal, D. (2025). Digital twins in dermatology: A new era of personalized skin care. *Frontiers in Digital Health, 7*. https://doi.org/10.3389/fdgth.2025.1534859
27. Ibrahim, S., Taft, B. J., Wang, Y., Lee, B. I., Andrade, E., Abaya, C. E., Pramanick, S., et al. (2022). Minimally invasive skin transcriptome extraction using a dermal biomarker patch. *Dermatology and Therapy, 12*, 1313–1323. https://www.semanticscholar.org/paper/15648

7ee4586aae99e6f1ad141a9f61df159612d (accessed on 21st July 2025).

28. Jiao, Q., Zhi, L., You, B., Wang, G., Wu, N., & Jia, Y. (2024). Skin homeostasis: Mechanism and influencing factors. *Journal of Cosmetic Dermatology, 23*, 1518–1526. https://doi.org/10.1111/jocd.16155

29. Keohane, S., Botting, J., Budny, P. G., Dolan, O. M., Fife, K., Harwood, C. A., Mallipeddi, R., et al. (2020). British Association of Dermatologists guidelines for the management of people with cutaneous squamous cell carcinoma 2020. *British Journal of Dermatology, 184*, 401–414. https://doi.org/10.1111/bjd.19621

30. Khalid, A., Dremin, V., El-Tamer, A., Surnina, M., Lancelot, C. L., Rafailov, E., & Sokolovski, S. (2024). Dual-mode OCT/fluorescence system for monitoring the morphology and metabolism of laser-printed 3D full-thickness skin equivalents. *Biomedical Optics Express, 15*, 6299–6312. https://www.semanticscholar.org/paper/c72c08cdfa6014b0b088b50f770ac97c6fd66ceb (accessed on 21st July 2025).

31. Kottner, J., Fastner, A., Lintzeri, D., Griffiths, C., & Blume-Peytavi, U. (2023). Improving skin health of community-dwelling older people: A scoping review protocol. *BMJ Open, 13*. https://www.semanticscholar.org/paper/be6607d2d38e822559c7ed5cde2b83857bf98acb (accessed on 21st July 2025).

32. Lboukili, I., Stamatas, G., & Descombes, X. (2023). Automatic granular and spinous epidermal cell identification and analysis on *in vivo* reflectance confocal microscopy images using cell morphological features. *Journal of Biomedical Optics, 28*. https://www.semanticscholar.org/paper/98cc136ab4f9fc991b3a6f5e9e7ac086aaab7f04 (accessed on 21st July 2025).

33. Levine, J. M., Delmore, B., & Cox, J. (2022). Skin failure: Concept review and proposed model. *Advances in Skin & Wound Care, 35*, 139–148. https://doi.org/10.1097/01.asw.0000818572.31307.7b

34. Li, X., Yang, S., Du, Z., Xie, W., Zhu, M., Han, L., & Zhou, Q. (2025). Cathepsins and skin cancer (*Malignant Melanoma, Basal Cell Carcinoma, and Squamous Cell Carcinoma*): Insight from genetic correlation and Mendelian randomization. *Clinical, Cosmetic and Investigational Dermatology, 18*, 553–566. https://www.semanticscholar.org/paper/6c2287079d24fa1792591062b30dfa8cbae2b3b7 (accessed on 21st July 2025).

35. Masa'deh, Y. K. A. K. (2024). Exploring novel therapies for psoriasis management: A dermatological perspective. *The International Tinnitus Journal*. https://www.semanticscholar.org/paper/5ac7b1e5320c73b371863c0da50a564e8c83eab0 (accessed on 21st July 2025).

36. Mauger, E., Porcheron, A., & Russell, R. (2013). Aspects of facial contrast decrease with age and are cues for age perception. https://core.ac.uk/download/18884264.pdf (accessed on 21st July 2025).

37. Michalak, M., Pierzak, M., Kręcisz, B., & Suliga, E. (2021). Bioactive compounds for skin health: A review. *Nutrients, 13*, 203–203. https://doi.org/10.3390/nu13010203

38. Nagendran, M., Chen, Y., Lovejoy, C. A., Gordon, A., Komorowski, M., Harvey, H., Topol, E. J., et al. (2020). Artificial intelligence versus clinicians: Systematic review of design, reporting standards, and claims of deep learning studies. *BMJ*. https://doi.org/10.1136/bmj.m689

39. Pustovaya, K. N., Piavchenko, G., Kovrigin, V. A., Nozdrin, V. I., & Kuznetsov, S. (2025). Damage of human skin barrier components in exposure of *Demodex* specimens. *Russian Journal of*

Clinical Dermatology and Venereology. https://www.semanticscholar.org/paper/9198ebbbfa404e0aea472adef6b92c38eb562a20 (accessed on 21st July 2025).

40. Rakita, A., Nikolić, N., Mildner, M., Matiasek, J., & Elbe-Bürger, A. (2020). Re-epithelialization and immune cell behaviour in an *ex vivo* human skin model. *Scientific Reports, 10*. https://doi.org/10.1038/s41598-019-56847-4 (accessed on 21st July 2025).
41. Renert-Yuval, Y., Thyssen, J. P., Bissonnette, R., Bieber, T., Kabashima, K., Hijnen, D., & Guttman-Yassky, E. (2021). Biomarkers in atopic dermatitis—A review on behalf of the International Eczema Council. *Journal of Allergy and Clinical Immunology, 147*, 1174–1190.e1. https://doi.org/10.1016/j.jaci.2021.01.013 (accessed on 21st July 2025).
42. Salvioni, L., Morelli, L., Ochoa, E., Labra, M., Fiandra, L., Palugan, L., Prosperi, D., et al. (2021). The emerging role of nanotechnology in skincare. *Advances in Colloid and Interface Science, 293*, 102437–102437. https://doi.org/10.1016/j.cis.2021.102437 (accessed on 21st July 2025).
43. Sawaya, A. P., Stone, R., Mehdizadeh, S., Pastar, I., Worrell, S., Balukoff, N. C., Kaplan, M. J., et al. (2022). *FOXM1* network in association with *TREM1* suppression regulates *NET* formation in diabetic foot ulcers. *EMBO Reports, 23*. https://doi.org/10.15252/embr.202154558 (accessed on 21st July 2025).
44. Sayyad, J., et al. (2023). Exploring the potential of convolutional neural networks in healthcare engineering for skin disease identification. https://core.ac.uk/download/591405140.pdf (accessed on 21st July 2025).
45. Sollena, P., Nikolaou, V., Kotteas, E., Stratigos, A., Fattore, D., Orlandi, A., Mannino, M., et al. (2023). Cyclin-dependent kinase 4/6 inhibitors and dermatologic adverse events: Results from the EADV Task Force "Dermatology for Cancer Patients" International Study. *Cancers, 15*. https://www.semanticscholar.org/paper/9a39643ae0be8ac1f5cd4c14c6d1aa20fefea468 (accessed on 21st July 2025).
46. Uysal, B. (2017). Tumor treating fields for glioblastoma: Review. https://www.semanticscholar.org/paper/bdbdd5e2d635523fd04bf43b8856fb5a349af508 (accessed on 21st July 2025).
47. Wang, Z., Yang, F., Zhang, W., & Yang, S. (2022). Quantitative and anatomical imaging of human skin by noninvasive photoacoustic dermoscopy. *Bio-protocol, 12*(7), e4372. https://www.semanticscholar.org/paper/e55009f3a2273c52406ba2b9161d12c65e0d763b (accessed on 21st July 2025).
48. Wesserling, M. (2013). Role of genetic aspect in pathogenesis of atopic dermatitis. https://core.ac.uk/download/71976799.pdf (accessed on 21st July 2025).
49. Wu, Z., Lu, D., Sun, S., Cai, M., Lin, L., & Zhu, M. (2025). Material design, fabrication strategies, and the development of multifunctional hydrogel composites dressings for skin wound management. *Biomacromolecules*. https://www.semanticscholar.org/paper/9bafc3d4c5e8a2c194844e00db104495605f73b8 (accessed on 21st July 2025).
50. Yost, C., Tripathi, N., Braat, J., Zamora, D., Dinh, H., & González Vélez, M. (2025). Targetable mutations in cutaneous skin cancers: A comparative study across melanoma, squamous cell carcinoma, basal cell carcinoma, and Merkel cell carcinoma. *Journal of Clinical Oncology*. https://www.semanticscholar.org/paper/64631adba5661d3c669cbfc28f8a6c51f9f2aeeb (accessed on 21st July 2025).

51. Zhou, M., Gomes, M. P., Elgersma, A., Korkmaz, H. I., Boekema, B., & Groot, M. L. (2025). Multiscale investigation of collagen structure in human skin and gel matrices using polarization resolved second harmonic generation microscopy. *Scientific Reports, 15*. https://www.semanticscholar.org/paper/60f84d4e2530120c2fa23aa53995efacbe8b9f80 (accessed on 21st July 2025).

52. Zuberbier, T., Abdul Latiff, A. H., Abuzakouk, M., Aquilina, S., Asero, R., Baker, D. R., Ballmer-Weber, B., et al. (2021). The international EAACI/GA^{2}LEN/EuroGuiDerm/APAAACI guideline for the definition, classification, diagnosis, and management of urticaria. *Allergy, 77*, 734–766. https://doi.org/10.1111/all.15090 (accessed on 21st July 2025).

SKIN PHYSIOLOGY AND FUNCTIONS

2

LEARNING OBJECTIVES

After studying this chapter, you will be able to:

1. Understand the skin physiology
2. Know the skin functions
3. Describe the skin health and disorders
4. Know the aging changes in skin

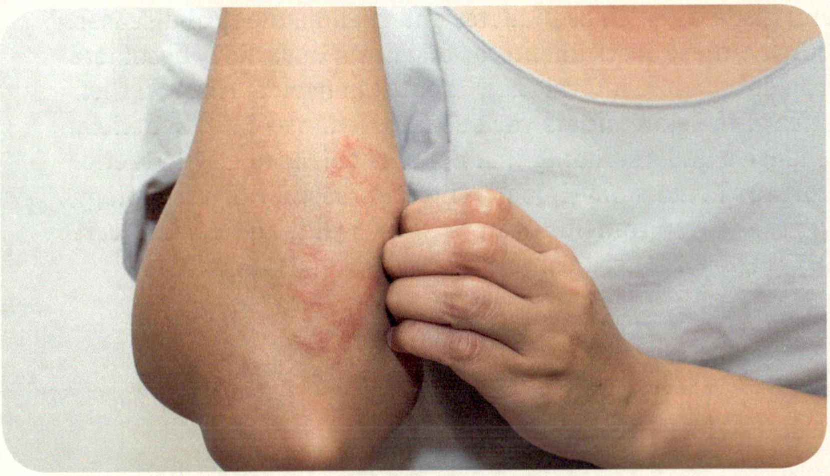

Introduction

Skin, being the largest organ of the human body, performs functions far beyond protection. It functions as a barrier and safeguards internal organs from external threats such as pathogens, toxins, and physical injury. This protective mechanism plays a significant role in maintaining homeostasis and avoiding infections. Also, the skin regulates body temperature through processes such as perspiration and vasodilation, thereby maintaining a stable body temperature. In addition, the skin's complex structure, with layers such as the epidermis, dermis, and subcutaneous tissue, facilitates its multiple functions. The complexities of skin physiology are not only important to skin health but also to broader interpretations of human physiology as a whole, because interaction with the external environment is necessary. One of the novel fields of research in skin physiology is the interpretation of the skin microbiome and its influence on human health. Skin contains millions of microorganisms, including bacteria, fungi, and viruses, which form a unique microbiome required to maintain skin function and integrity.

These microbes help supply the first line of defense against infection, are immunomodulatory, and assist in wound healing. Research emphasizes the complex equilibrium of this microbiome, whereby imbalances lead to skin disorders and systemic disease. As an example, symbiotic relationships between the host human and resident microbes are advantageous for the host's immune function, highlighting the importance of skin health for overall well-being. The role of these microbes in skin physiology underscores the interdependence of microbial life and human health, and, incidentally, has therapeutic implications. In addition, the introduction of new diagnostic techniques has significantly influenced our understanding of skin physiology, particularly in identifying microcirculation and metabolic disorders. Laser Doppler flowmetry and spectroscopy are among the non-invasive diagnostic techniques that have revolutionized how physicians diagnose skin integrity disorders. These technologies provide an opportunity for early diagnosis of microcirculatory disorders, thereby enhancing treatment outcomes in several diseases, such as diabetes and rheumatological diseases. Due to their high sensitivity and specificity, these instruments of diagnosis have now become a part of the clinical practice, and they provide valuable information about skin health. Through their insights into the functional characteristics of the skin and its various interactions—both beneficial and undesirable—we develop a comprehensive understanding that not only guides medical practice but also advances the broader trajectory of human physiology. This intersection of technology, microbiology, and dermatology has the potential to transform our way to health and disease care (Gillen et al., 2017; Dremin et al., 2019) (Figure 2.1) radically.

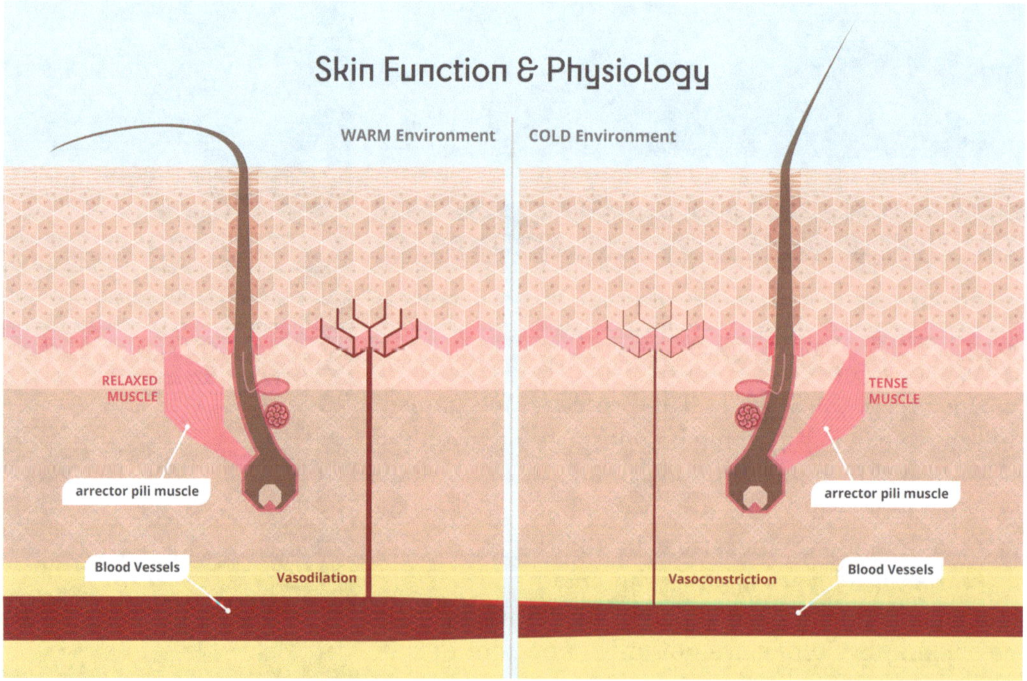

Figure 2.1. Skin: function & physiology.

Source: https://lightskinscience.clinuvel.com/wp-content/uploads/2022/07/lss-skin-function-physiology-01-1536x985.png.

2.1. Skin Physiology

Learning Outcome

1. Understand the role of skin in thermoregulation
2. Describe the skin's barrier function against pathogens
3. Know the sensory functions of the skin

The skin is a critical barrier against the outside world and the inside of the body and is a key part of homeostasis. The three primary layers of the skin—epidermis, dermis, and hypodermis—all contribute significantly to the complicated functions of the skin. The epidermis, the superficial layer, is largely composed of keratinocytes that provide protection against microbial invasion and environmental stress. At the same time, the dermis is filled with connective tissue, blood vessels, and nerves, all of which are crucial for thermoregulation and sensation. The subcutaneous layer, or hypodermis, exists to store fat and act as insulation, and also plays a role in thermal regulation. Awareness of these layers allows for a more complete understanding of how the skin protects against harm while also playing a role in necessary physiological functions, such as wound healing and sensation. Skin microcirculation is crucial for nutrient and oxygen delivery to the dermis and thermoregulation. Cooperation between vascular function and skin physiology is particularly stressed by new diagnostic techniques, e.g., laser Doppler flowmetry, with online registration of blood flow. The non-invasive methods have shown enormous potential in the detection of microcirculatory abnormalities in various diseases, e.g., diabetes mellitus and rheumatic diseases. By evaluating the severity of such disorders with advanced techniques, the clinician can have an improved understanding of the underlying pathophysiologies and, accordingly, can apply effective treatment modalities. Microcirculation evaluation enables us to understand the skin's response to environmental stressors and thus shows that skin physiology is not only structural in nature but also intrinsically linked to the body's overall metabolic status and function (Dremin et al., 2019). Also, in addition to acting as a barrier, the skin is an active component of the endocrine system, participating in hormone synthesis and regulation. Further, through its interaction with ultraviolet light, the skin synthesizes vitamin D, which is crucial for calcium uptake and bone development. The skin also generates a variety of signaling molecules, including cytokines, which are crucial in the orchestration of immune responses. These functions illustrate the complexity of skin physiology as it not only regulates external stimuli but also internal metabolic processes. The coordination between skin function and overall health is evident and highlights the importance of large amounts of research into skin physiology in dermatology and endocrinology. This realization also extends the scope of research to the influence of environmental conditions on skin health, showing that the implications of skin physiology extend well beyond surface considerations (Garshnek et al., 2025) (Figure 2.2).

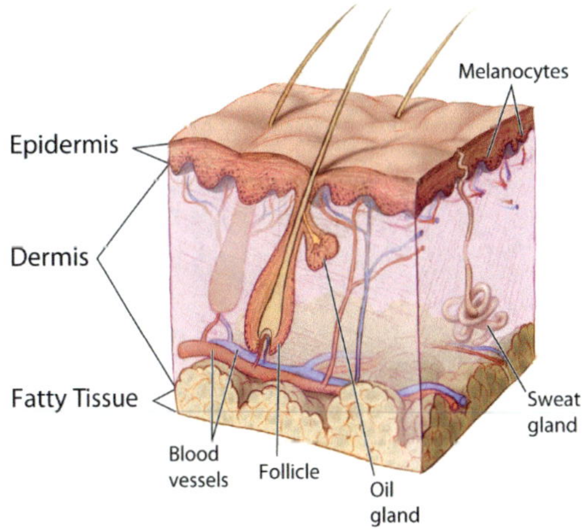

Figure 2.2. Skin physiology.

Source: https://static.wixstatic.com/media/0a9f25_331acab4e5bd4c56be9c3ce27d0cdfab~mv2.jpg.

2.1.1. Role of Skin in Thermoregulation

The skin plays an active role in thermoregulation, not only as a protective layer to the body but also as an actively regulating one, maintaining its temperature. Having multiple layers, the skin uses sweating and vasodilation as cooling mechanisms for excess heat. When body temperature rises due to environmental conditions or metabolic processes, skin sensory receptors detect this, and the hypothalamus is stimulated to initiate cooling. Sweat glands secrete water that evaporates from the skin's surface, cooling the body, while dermal blood vessels dilate to increase blood flow and facilitate heat dissipation. This active process demonstrates the skin's role in maintaining thermal homeostasis, enabling the body to respond effectively to various environmental stresses. In addition to sweating and blood flow regulation, physiological adaptation to environmental stress also influences the skin's thermoregulatory function. For instance, patients with compromised thermoregulatory function, such as those with multiple sclerosis (MS), exhibit considerable difficulty in maintaining appropriate body temperature during physical exertion. Research has shown that MS patients exhibit diminished sweating, which plays a critical role in effective heat dissipation during physical exercise, leading to increased thermal stress. However, the study reported no differences in core body temperature between normal controls and MS patients during exercise, suggesting that, even though the sweat response is impaired, other temperature-regulating mechanisms can maintain homeostasis under some circumstances

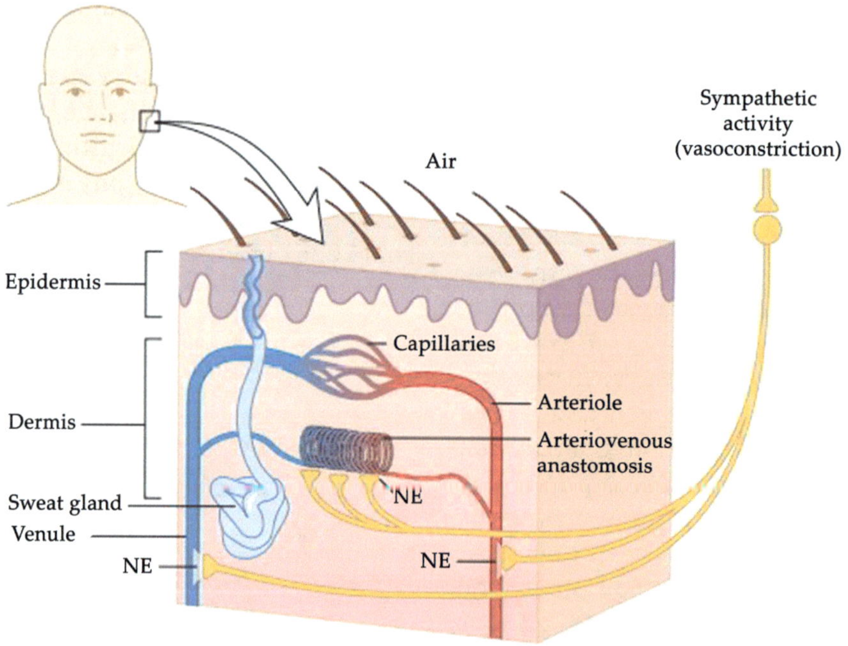

Figure 2.3. Skin thermoregulation.

Source: https://www.earthslab.com/wp-content/uploads/2017/01/011417_1620_Thermoregul1.jpg.

These findings testify to the complexity of the skin's role in thermoregulation and demonstrate how many variables influence its efficiency. Furthermore, the skin's role in thermoregulation is extended to the acclimatization process, where the organism adapts to prolonged exposure to heat. This may involve physiological or behavioral adaptations that enable organisms to survive in extreme heat more easily. It is knowing the functions of the skin in thermoregulation that enables interventions, such as thermal protection systems for space-traveling astronauts, which provide protection through environmental control during space travel. As the literature has highlighted, thermoregulatory responses are not reflexive; they require a good understanding of energy metabolism and the body's capacity to establish equilibrium between heat generation and loss while performing various activities. Therefore, research on the multifunctional role of the skin in thermoregulation provides useful information that extends beyond individual medicine to influence other disciplines, such as occupational safety and environmental physiology (Allen et al., 2018; Greenleaf et al., 2025) (Figure 2.3).

2.1.2. Skin's Barrier Function Against Pathogens

The skin serves as a crucial barrier against pathogens that work to protect the human body from an enormous number of infections. This barrier function is not passive; instead, it is an active, multifunctional system that incorporates physical, chemical, and biological mechanisms to resist potential threats. The epidermis, which is the outermost layer of the skin, consists of compactly arranged keratinocytes, which form a physical barrier against the invasion of pathogens. Beneath this layer, the immune response of the skin enhances the functionality of the barrier by employing immune cells such as Langerhans cells that detect and respond to invaders. Since they are the first line of defense, these cells play a significant role in recognizing pathogens and initiating the immune response, ensuring the invasion of the physical barrier does not result in excessive damage to the organism. In addition to the physical architecture, the biochemical properties of skin also play a significant role in overall barrier function. The skin secretes antimicrobial peptides and lipids, which not only destroy pathogens but also retain an optimal microbiota required for healthy skin. Resident microbiota contributes to the skin's overall immunity by competing against pathogens for substrates and spatial niches.

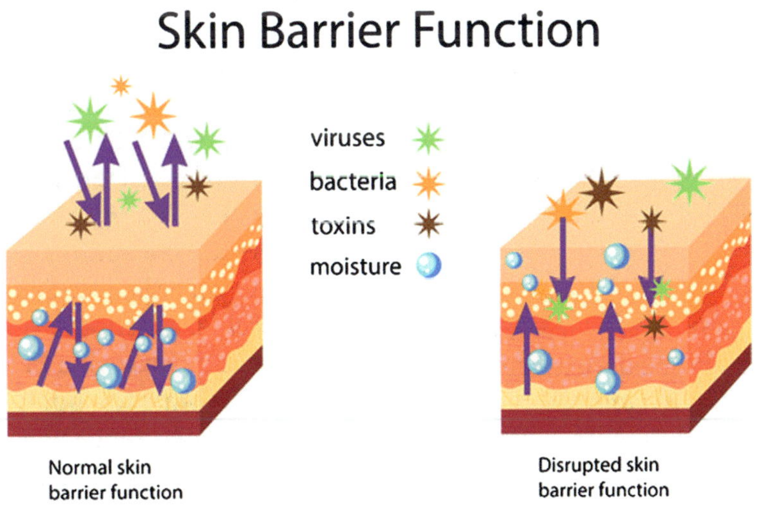

Figure 2.4. Skin's barrier function.

Source: https://cdn.shopify.com/s/files/1/1486/4832/files/Skin_Barrier_Stock_Image_600x600.jpg?v=1682597519.

Along with basic colonization resistance, such host-beneficial microbes have been shown to profoundly influence the pathogenic potential of infections, demonstrating the co-immunity principle whereby the host relies not only on its immune system but also on the resident community of microbes for protection. Both the maintenance of skin integrity and disease prevention depend on cooperative interaction. In addition, skin coloration has been observed to have its evolutionary benefit in terms of barrier function. Evidence indicates that individuals with darker pigmentation have a higher level of resistance to damage and inflammation caused to the skin by external agents, including UV light. This protection is not only apparent but also evidenced by a genetically mediated adaptation to preserve skin integrity. Evidence indicates that pigmented skin exhibits reduced levels of pro-inflammatory cytokines in response to irritants compared to lighter-skinned humans, thereby positively attributing pigmentation to enhanced barrier function. By enhancing a healthier skin microclimate through reduced inflammation, pigmentation would increase resistance to pathogens, highlighting the critical interdependence among skin morphology, immune function, and evolutionary progress (Abuabara et al., 2019). The intersection of these factors highlights the complex function of skin in safeguarding human health (Figure 2.4).

2.1.3. Sensory Functions of the Skin

The skin is an essential sensory interface between the human body and the external world, having a sophisticated system of receptors that allow for the perception of a variety of stimuli. The receptors can be broadly classified as mechanoreceptors, thermoreceptors, and nociceptors, each being specialized to detect a specific kind of sensory stimulus. Mechanoreceptors, for example, respond to touch stimuli like pressure and vibration and enable people to interact with the environment. The somesthetic sense of touch is not just a basic form of interaction; it also plays a key role in social and emotional interaction. The effective transmission of these sensory messages to the brain is enabled by specific nerve fibers that are part of the general somatosensory system that governs human behavior and interaction with the world.

To appreciate the sophistication of human perception, one should be aware of how sensory inputs to the skin are processed. Localization of pain and touch is a complex process that involves numerous neural structures, which attests to the complexity of the somatosensory system. Localization distortions, as recorded by research, show that our perceptual experience depends not merely on the direct stimulation of nerves but also on central processing mechanisms within the brain. Such systematic localization errors may vary widely depending on the skin areas being stimulated, with differing biases in how stimuli affect Aβ and Aδ fibers for touch and pain, respectively. These findings warrant further investigation into the neural maps of sensory information, with a focus on the dynamic interplay between peripheral stimuli and central nervous system processing (Alloway et al., 2011). In addition, the roles of consciousness and perception in sensory functioning cannot be overstated, as they pervade the entire physiological landscape of the human organism. Sensory perceptions are not merely a function of individual inputs but are part and parcel of a broader consciousness that interconnects bodily experience with subjective comprehension. Cellular processes, notably oscillations in membrane potentials, add complexity to our understanding of how sensory function might be a component of conscious awareness. This concept resituates consciousness as an emergent phenomenon rather than a neurocentric one, in which the interconnectedness of skin receptors, nervous pathways, and conscious phenomena takes center stage. Such an integrated perspective affirms that the skin's sensory processes extend well beyond detection, serving as requisite contributors to the emergent character of human consciousness and experience (Barnes et al., 2017).

Test Your Knowledge

1. What is the role of skin in thermoregulation?
2. How is the skin a barrier against pathogens?

2.2. Skin Functions

Learning Outcome

1. Protect skin against environmental hazards
2. Describe the synthesis of vitamin D
3. Understand the role of skin in immune response

Skin is the primary barrier between the body and the environment, playing an important protective function. Comprising a number of layers, predominantly epidermis and dermis, skin guards against pathogens, chemical irritants, and physical injuries. The outermost layer, the stratum corneum, consists of dead, keratinized cells and serves as an extremely effective barrier. The skin is also involved in immune responses because it has resident immune cells that can see and respond to invading foreign elements. Protection does not exist only in the form of physical barriers; it also lies in the skin's ability to retain water, thereby maintaining hydration and homeostasis. Importantly, failure of these defense mechanisms can result in various dermatological conditions, demonstrating the skin's fundamental position in overall health and disease. Thermoregulation is also a simple function of the skin that maintains body temperature within a narrow and steady range. The skin does this by dilating and constricting blood vessels and by exciting sweat glands. When the body is in a heated state, dermal blood vessels expand, and heat is lost; simultaneously, sweat glands produce perspiration that evaporates to cool the skin. In cold temperatures, blood vessels constrict in order to preserve heat. These mechanisms are regulated by a complex interplay of neural and hormonal inputs, hence making the skin an active player in thermoregulation. In addition, changes in hormones and environmental changes can influence these mechanisms, which suggests that the ability of skin to control temperature is adaptive and proportional to the body's general homeostatic needs. Lastly, the skin is also involved in sensory perception as an essential interface between the body and the world. It contains many receptors that can detect touch, warmth, pain, and pressure, enabling human beings to interact meaningfully with the world around them.

These sensory inputs are processed by the central nervous system, allowing for immediate response to potentially threatening stimuli. Current evidence indicates that skin physiology may also affect internal processes, such as stress response based on attachment theory, where emotional and physical states are conveyed through skin-derived information. In addition, the skin plays a role in mediating physiological states through circadian rhythms and hormonal mechanisms, suggesting an interactive communication system between internal health and skin function. In general, the sensory abilities of the skin are essential to survival and well-being and are thus vital to human physiology (Figure 2.5).

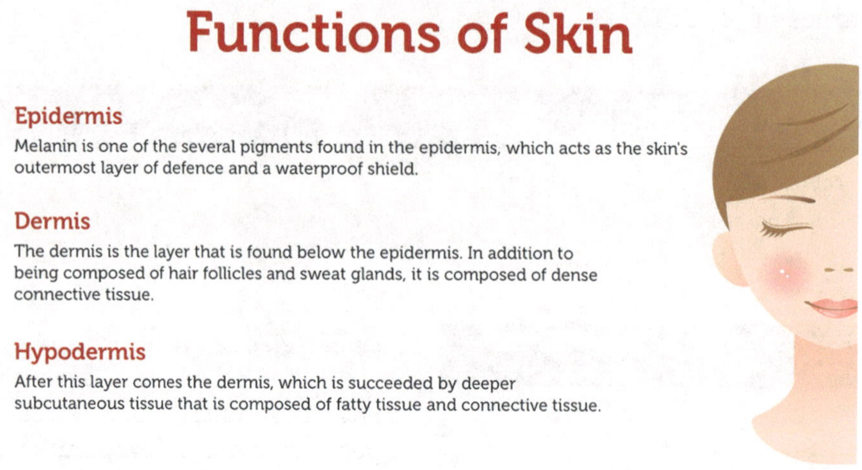

Figure 2.5. Function of skin.

Source: https://assets.lybrate.com/imgs/tic/enadp/function-of-skin.jpg.

2.2.1. Protection Against Environmental Hazards

The skin is the body's first line of defense against a range of environmental hazards, including pathogens, ultraviolet (UV) radiation, and chemical exposure. Its multi-layered structure—comprising the epidermis, dermis, and hypodermis—is essential to its protective role. The outermost epidermis is composed primarily of keratinocytes that produce keratin, a protein that provides structural strength and waterproofing. This barrier is not entirely impermeable; however, it does reduce the penetration of destructive microorganisms and the loss of water. Additionally, melanocytes, which are in the epidermis, release melanin, which absorbs UV radiation, thereby shielding inner tissues from potential damage. These physiological processes illustrate the skin's critical role in shielding the body from physical and environmental assault. In addition to its physical barrier, the skin is also active in immune processes, contributing to protection against environmental pathogens. Immune cells such as Langerhans cells, found in the epidermis, enable the skin to identify and respond to foreign antigens. When the presence of a threat, such as viruses or bacteria, is detected, these cells initiate an immune response, calling other immune cells to the site of exposure. This immunologic aspect of cutaneous physiology plays a vital role in early detection and prevention of infection, highlighting the skin's dual protective role against both direct injury and systemic illness. The interaction of the immune system with the skin is particularly crucial in situations involving a single challenge, such as Extravehicular Activity (EVA) research for lunar missions, where skin protective functions would be key in dangerous environments (Carr et al., 2025). Understanding the complexities in dermal physiology relative to environmental hazard factors extends to the realization of the potential for detrimental effects when such protective mechanisms collapse. Physical contact with pollution, extreme temperatures, and sunlight radiation may lead to skin damage, rendering the person susceptible to skin diseases, including cancer. Ameliorative approaches, such as a proper skincare regimen and the use of sunscreen, can enhance the skin's protective mechanisms against these hazard factors. Also, ongoing research into the human skin's reaction in situations like those of space flights further indicates why this protective layer is so important. Research indexed in scientific databases indicates the depth of the knowledge base across aerospace medicine and cutaneous responses in adverse environments, illustrating the crucial protective role of the skin in varying circumstances (Figure 2.6).

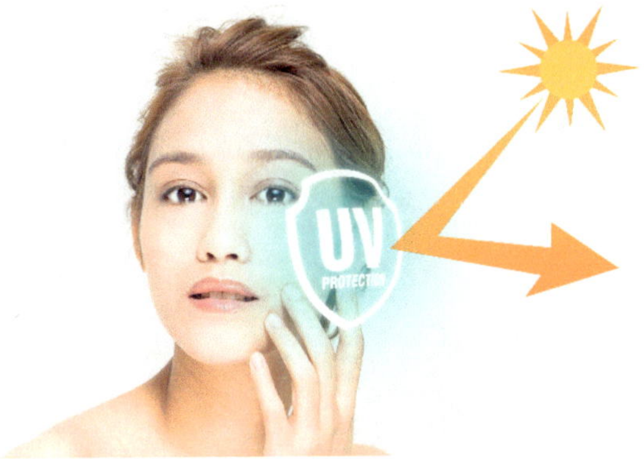

Figure 2.6. The importance of sun protection for safeguarding your skin from harmful UV rays.

Source: https://lirp.cdn-website.com/af397b3f/dms3rep/multi/opt/Untitled+design+-+2024-07-31T101250.920-1920w.png.

2.2.2. Synthesis of Vitamin D

Vitamin D synthesis is a significant process that highlights the fine balance between skin physiology and overall human health. When skin comes in contact with ultraviolet B (UVB) rays from the sun, the substance 7-dehydrocholesterol, which is present in skin, is converted to previtamin D3. This is a critical conversion because it triggers a chain of events that leads to the generation of vitamin D, a fat-soluble vitamin that is a key player in calcium homeostasis and bone metabolism. In populations with limited sunlight exposure, vitamin D production may be reduced, leading to medical conditions such as osteomalacia or osteoporosis. In addition, the skin's ability to produce vitamin D effectively can be influenced by a number of factors, including skin color, age, and geographical location, making it crucial for people to be screened for vitamin D levels and supplemented as needed. Research has increasingly linked vitamin D status with a broad array of health outcomes, irrespective of bone health. Recent research has demonstrated that adequate vitamin D levels are important for muscle function and overall athletic performance, further reinforcing the need to ensure proper levels. A comparison study of serum vitamin D levels in university athletes found that athletes with low vitamin D levels were at high risk of musculoskeletal injury, further underscoring the importance of vitamin D not only for athletic performance but also for injury prevention. The findings revealed striking discrepancies in serum vitamin D content across different populations, with African American athletes possessing far lower content compared to their Caucasian peers. The disparity underscores the importance of targeted health interventions that account for vitamin D synthesis and uptake across various populations, thereby enabling all individuals to benefit from its health-protective effects (McGill et al., 2014). Secondarily, the effects of vitamin D manufacture extend to larger physiological processes that contribute to health and well-being. Vitamin D receptors in numerous body tissues suggest that vitamin D participates in processes ranging from immune responses to mood regulation. As recognition grows that vitamin D's function extends well beyond the mere absorption of calcium, health professionals now actively advocate for more integrated public health policies to address widespread deficiencies. Strategies might include promoting more sun exposure, recommending dietary sources of vitamin D, and supporting supplementation programs, especially in at-risk groups. Such an overall strategy is aimed not only at personal health gains but also at public health resistance to disease caused by vitamin

D deficiency, such as diabetes and cardiovascular disease. With advancing research, vitamin D continues to be highlighted as essential for maintaining normal skin physiology and function in the human body (Garshnek et al., 2025).

2.2.3. Role in Immune Response

Skin is the first line of defense in the immune system, forming a physical barrier that protects the body from harmful pathogens and environmental trauma. This barrier includes layers that contain keratinocytes like the epidermis. In addition to providing mechanical support, keratinocytes also play an active role in immune function by recognizing pathogens via pattern recognition receptors. Once recognized by these receptors, keratinocytes can initiate immune activity by stimulating the production of antimicrobial peptides that eliminate the pathogen.

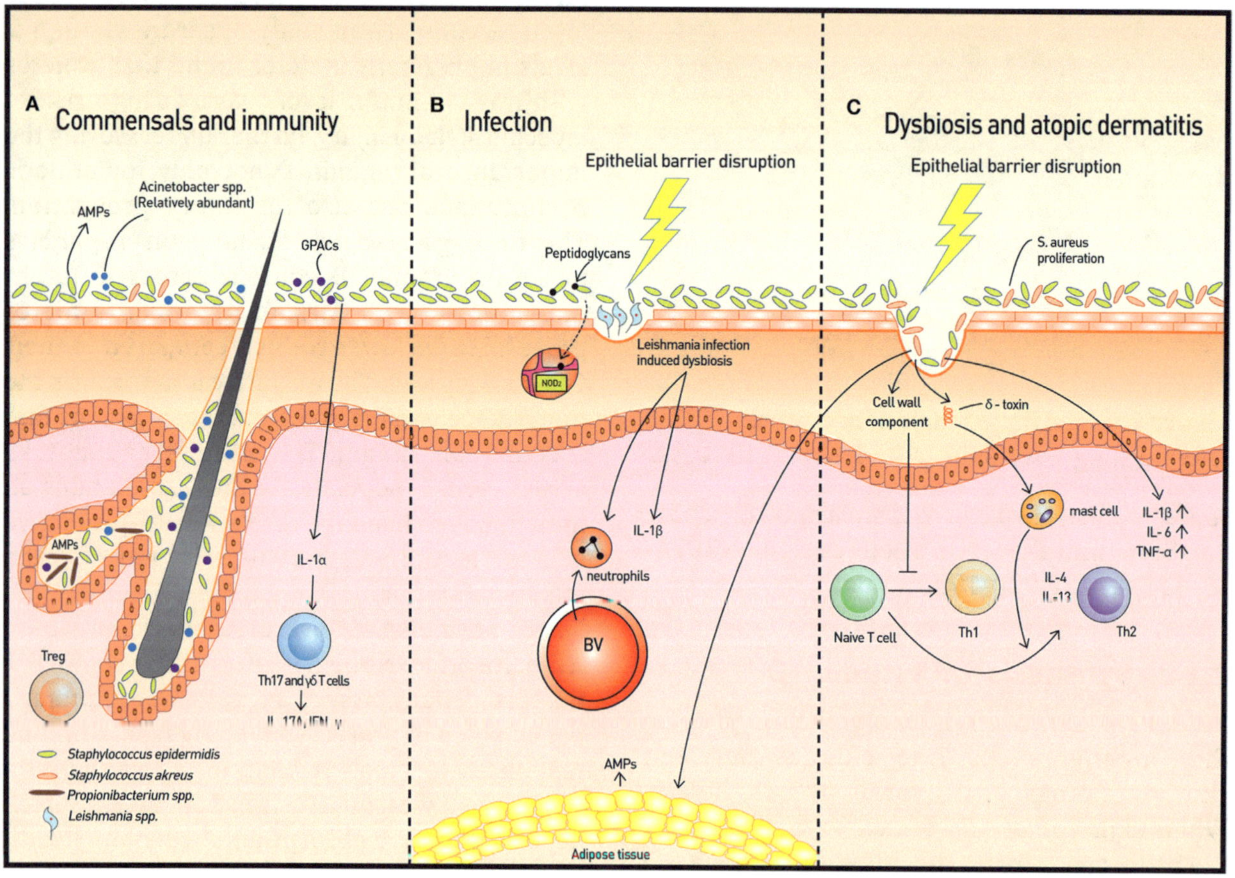

Figure 2.7. Skin microbiota and immunity. (A) The microbiome is more diverse in healthy skin. (B) The dysbiosis induced by Leishmaniasis infection is not only transmissible but also exacerbates skin inflammation via neutrophil recruitment and IL-1β production. (C) In atopic dermatitis, *Staphylococcus aureus* proliferates, and microbial diversity decreases concomitantly.

Source: https://www.frontiersin.org/files/Articles/309715/fimmu-08-01955-HTML/image_m/fimmu-08-01955-g001.jpg.

Secondly, the mechanical and chemical barriers of the skin are complemented by its ability to generate inflammatory signals, thereby mobilizing additional immune cells to the site of infection or injury. Such a multi-faceted approach highlights the fundamental role of the skin in amplifying the innate immune response, underscoring the interaction between physical form and immune function. Beyond its physical impermeability, the skin also contains a rich microbiome that bears significant responsibility in governing the immune response. The commensal presence, for instance, of Staphylococci is a major factor in immunomodulation, particularly in early life, as the body is still acquiring knowledge on how to assemble its immunological pathways. These commensal bacteria communicate with host immune cells to allow a balance that contributes to immune tolerance and minimizes the probability of hypersensitivity responses. The example is the stimulation of antibody production by these microbes, which is essential for preparing the immune system to effectively deal with potential pathogens. This mutual interaction between host immune cells and skin-residing microbes generates an intricate network that not only supports immune health but also underscores the importance of skin microbiome diversity for optimal immune function (Gillen et al., 2017). Moreover, interaction between vitamin D, calcium signaling, and skin physiology further illustrates the immune regulatory functions of the skin. 1,25 dihydroxyvitamin D, the biologically active vitamin D form, regulates numerous features of skin health and the immune system through binding to the vitamin D receptor (VDR). It has been discovered that interference with the VDR pathway can lead to profound epidermal differentiation defects and environmental stress response, hence making the skin vulnerable to infection and inflammatory diseases. Besides, vitamin D's control of calcium homeostasis in the skin is a cornerstone of maintaining an optimal immune response, as calcium signaling is central to keratinocyte function and to the attributes of the skin barrier. Disruption of this pathway has been associated with increased susceptibility to dermatoses and cancer, illustrating convergence of nutrient signaling, skin health, and immune function (Bikle et al., 2016) (Figure 2.7).

Test Your Knowledge

1. How does the skin protect the body from environmental hazards?
2. What is the role of skin in immune response?

2.3. Skin Health and Disorders

Learning Outcome

1. Describe the common skin conditions
2. Know the impact of UV radiation on skin health
3. Understand the importance of skincare and hygiene

The skin's health is inevitably linked to its functions, such as protection, sensation, thermoregulation, and metabolism. As the largest organ in the human body, the skin serves to defend against external pathogens and environmental toxins, and hence it plays a significant role in the immune system. Skin diseases, such as eczema, psoriasis, and dermatitis, undermine these functions and increase the individual's risk of secondary infection. All these conditions often arise from complex interactions between genetic predisposition, environmental precipitants, and immunological problems, illustrating how intricate skin health is. Moreover, skin also reflects an individual's overall health status; therefore, a comprehensive analysis is necessary to identify potential illness and improve function through specific interventions. Non-invasive diagnostic research has significantly enhanced the understanding and management of skin disease. Techniques such as laser Doppler flowmetry and fluorescence spectroscopy have become accessible, providing information on microcirculatory and metabolic derangements of skin diseases. The integration of these optical diagnostic methods has proved to be crucial in the early diagnosis and detection of diseases like diabetic dermopathy and rheumatology-associated diseases, and improving therapeutic responses. The high sensitivity and specificity of these diagnostics ensure early treatment, with the ultimate aim of restoring skin integrity and maintaining its physiological functions. As research in dermatologic diagnosis continues to advance, the implications for skin health practice can redefine clinical approaches to common disorders and, in doing so, improve patients' quality of life. Additionally, the reciprocal relationship between skin health and systemic disease underscores the role of interprofessional approaches in dermatology. For instance, diseases such as diabetes and autoimmune diseases like to present with major dermal features, which would suggest that interventions would have to be holistic in nature to include both systemic and cutaneous management. A better understanding of how systemic health impacts skin physiology can lead medical practitioners to incorporate dermatological assessments into overall health evaluations to deliver more preventive and personalized care. This inter-disciplinary synergy has not only implications for the treatment of existing skin disease but also for future disease prevention. Ongoing research in skin physiology is thus crucial, as it offers a comprehensive perspective that leads to improvements in overall health and well-being, as research advances have demonstrated (Dremin et al., 2019; Garshnek et al., 2025) (Figure 2.8).

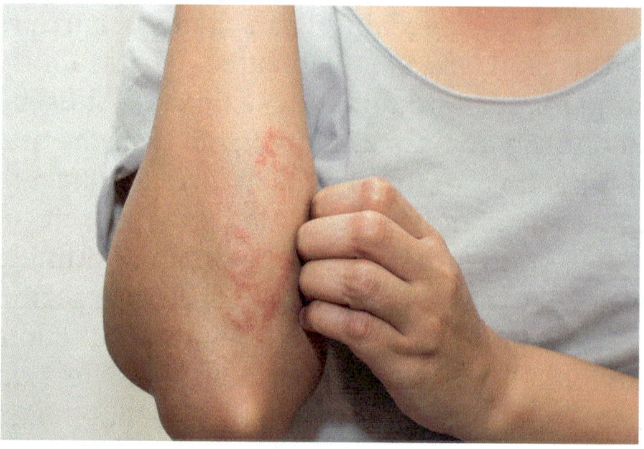

Figure 2.8. Skin disorders.

Source: https://listmyclinic.com/wp-content/uploads/2021/04/SKIN-1.jpg.

2.3.1. Common Skin Conditions: Acne, Eczema, and Psoriasis

The prevalence of common skin disorders such as acne, eczema, and psoriasis underscores the complex interplay between the skin's physiological processes and multiple environmental and genetic factors. Acne vulgaris is primarily caused by the overproduction of sebum, which can result in blockage of the hair follicle and offer a substrate for bacterial growth, such as that of *Propionibacterium acnes*. This condition is most commonly observed in the teen years but can extend into adulthood, greatly influencing one's mental health and self-esteem. The pathogenesis of acne must be identified, as it underpins the need for specific therapeutic measures, including topical retinoids and systemic treatment. Moreover, the psychosocial impact of acne mandates attention to patient education and supportive therapy because patients are typically gravely upset by observable cutaneous lesions, and this suggests an intimate correlation between integumentary integrity and psychological durability. Another powerful dermatologic challenge is eczema, also called atopic dermatitis, which presents with dry, pruritic skin that can be highly annoying. This condition is believed to have an etiology that combines genetic predisposition and environmental provocation by allergens and irritants. Eczema patients' disrupted skin barrier leads to increased water loss and pathogen exposure, driving the issue and a cycle of inflammation and scratching. The role of dermatology nurses becomes increasingly important in the effective management of eczema, as they are tasked with providing valuable patient education on skin care habits, recognizing early symptom exacerbations, and helping develop overall management strategies. Not only does such information alleviate physical discomfort, but it also informs patients with awareness, justifying the nurse-patient relationship that is key to the treatment of chronic skin conditions (Chukwu et al., 2018). Psoriasis is a chronic inflammatory dermatosis with a high sensitivity of skin cell turnover, leading to thick, scaly plaques that severely impact an individual's quality of life.

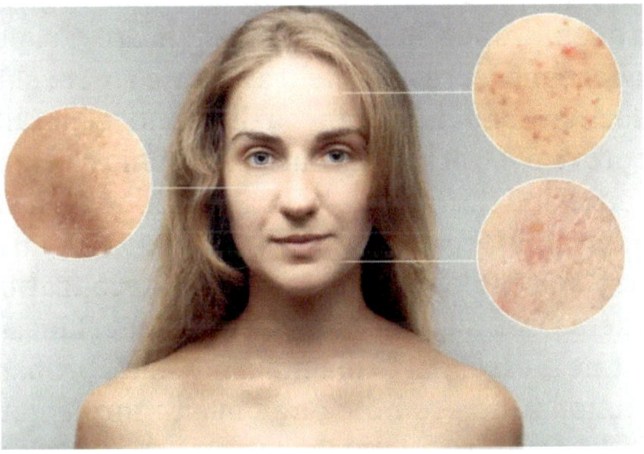

Figure 2.9. The most common skin problems.

Source: https://sa1s3optim.patientpop.com/filters:format(webp)/assets/images/provider/photos/2631986.png.

The underlying immune mechanisms involve hyperactivity of T-cell-mediated responses, which hampers the normal function of keratinocytes. This condition often coexists with comorbidities such as psoriatic arthritis and metabolic syndrome, attesting to the need for holistic treatment addressing both skin and systemic illness. Interestingly, recent evidence suggests an apparent link between the health of the gut microbiome and psoriasis severity, hypothesizing that changes in microbial balance can influence inflammation of the skin (Acharjee et al., 2022). Thus, dermatological professionals are encouraged to consider nutritional factors and to promote measures that favor the preservation of an equilibrium gut-skin axis, thus enhancing patient outcomes in the treatment of skin disease (Figure 2.9).

2.3.2. Impact of Ultraviolet (UV) Radiation on Skin Health

UV radiation, one component of sun exposure, plays an important role in skin health, particularly given its strong impact on skin physiology. Ultraviolet rays, after passing through the epidermis, initiate a wide array of biological processes, including the synthesis of vitamin D, which is used to maintain bone strength and immune function. However, the positive impact of vitamin D production can be negated by the negative effect of overexposure to UV radiation. Continuous exposure to UV radiation leads to damage in the DNA of skin cells, and this causes sunburn and increased susceptibility to the development of skin cancers such as melanoma. This duality refers to the inherent paradox in the interaction between UV radiation and skin health, where the skin's protective mechanisms generally counteract the damaging effects of UV exposure over the long term, underscoring the need for appropriate sun protection. The skin's response to UV radiation includes physiological changes that may affect its appearance or function. Acute effects include redness and inflammation, which are the immediate responses of the skin to injury. Chronic exposure leading to premature aging manifests as photodamage, including wrinkling, loss of skin elasticity, and irregular pigmentation. Such deposition not only impairs the cosmetic appearance of the skin but also alters its barrier function, rendering it more susceptible to environmental irritants and infections. As the skin's natural repair mechanisms are unable to reverse the damage caused by UV radiation, a cycle of injury and repair occurs, and, if left uncontrolled, results in significant long-term sequelae for skin health, highlighting the necessity of protection against UV radiation. In addition to the public health consequences to an individual's skin health, the public health impact of exposure to UV radiation extends beyond individual cutaneous disease, raising concerns about increasing skin cancer rates. Education and public awareness campaigns play an important role in raising the general public's awareness of the hazards of UV exposure and the necessity of sun protection practices, such as the use of broad-spectrum sunscreen and protective equipment.

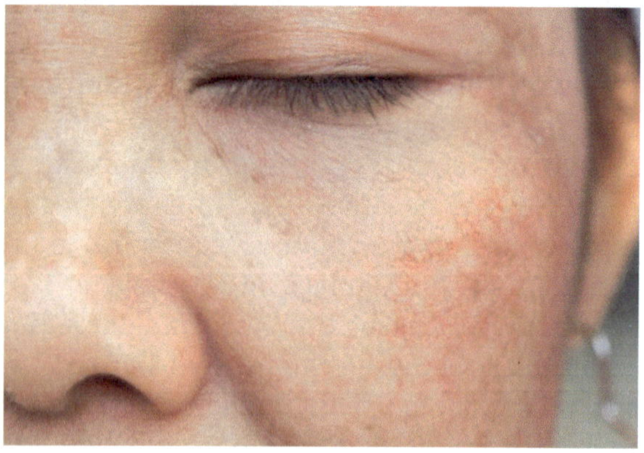

Figure 2.10. Effects of ultraviolet (UV) radiation on skin.

Source: https://www.awnings.com.sg/wp-content/uploads/2022/07/Effects-of-UV-Radiation-on-Skin-2.jpg.

The literature emphasizes the role played by the fact that prevention interventions will lower the incidence of skin cancers, an aspect that makes it important for health care providers to advocate for preventive skin care measures. Furthermore, understanding the genetic vulnerability of certain individuals to skin damage caused by UV radiation can inform individual preventive strategies. As research advances, the significance of knowledge and the dissemination of the contribution of UV radiation to maintaining healthy skin remain central to advocating for a healthier world amid increased UV exposure in contemporary lifestyles (Alving et al., 2012; Barwood et al., 2019) (Figure 2.10).

2.3.3. Importance of Skincare and Hygiene

The importance of skincare and hygiene is strongly rooted in human skin physiology and function, with the focus on the skin as an important barrier and its protective roles. The skin is not only the body's first line of defense against pathogens but also regulates various physiological processes, including thermoregulation and sensation. It becomes necessary, therefore, to maintain skin hygiene through proper cleansing and skincare. Proper hygiene measures can help avert the risk of skin infection, enhance skin quality, and generally improve overall health. Lack of hygiene can lead to acne and dermatitis, which not only seriously undermine the integrity of the skin but also carry psychological impacts. This realization underscores that following a consistent skincare routine is essential to maintain the skin's primary functions and promote one's health throughout life. In addition, systemic determinants such as exercise and environmental exposures play major roles in skin health, and therefore consistent hygiene habits are vital to overall health. Aerobic exercise performed regularly has been shown to enhance blood flow, thereby improving nutrient delivery to the skin and stimulating collagen production, a major contributor to skin firmness and elasticity. Physical exercise may also increase the risk of skin irritation and dryness. Therefore, incorporating proper skincare routines alongside physical exercise is crucial for optimizing skin barrier function. An in-depth understanding of such interactions highlights the delicate balance between physical fitness training and a good skincare regimen to gain full advantage while avoiding potential harms (Fabian et al., 2024).

For older people in particular, skin cleanliness becomes more critical due to increased vulnerability of aging skin towards dryness and impaired barrier function. Experiments have shown that routine hygienic procedures, such as mild cleansing and emollient use, improve skin barrier function, thereby facilitating greater hydration and limiting transepidermal water loss. Studies have shown that inexpensive, simple regimens such as soapy water and glycerin application can successfully reverse xerosis, providing evidence that tailored hygiene procedures can make a considerable leap toward improved skin health. Since the aging population continues to rise, healthcare programs need to focus on promoting proper hygiene and skincare so that the quality of life can be enhanced, as well as skin diseases can be prevented, which is most commonly seen among aged individuals (Ali et al., 2017) (Figure 2.11).

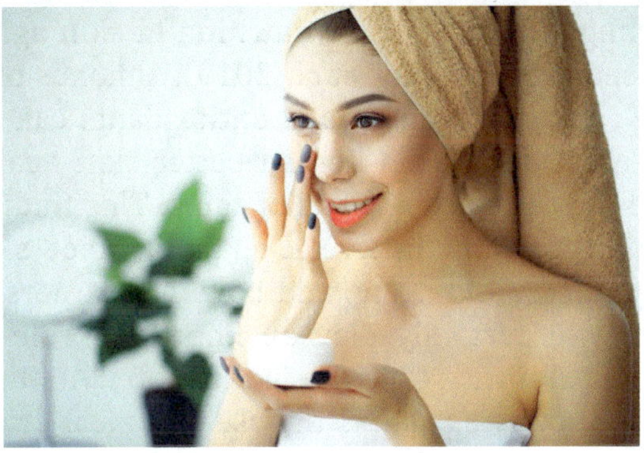

Figure 2.11. Importance of skincare.

Source: https://cdn.shopify.com/s/files/1/0251/2184/9419/files/shutterstock_1051577057_1024x1024.jpg?v=1659125830.

Test Your Knowledge

1. What is the impact of UV radiation on skin health?
2. What is the importance of skincare and hygiene?

2.4. Aging and the Skin

Learning Outcome

1. Describe the changes in skin structure with age
2. Understand the effects of aging on skin function
3. Know the strategies for maintaining skin health in older adults

Aging dramatically affects the skin, leading to a wide range of changes that affect its structure and function. As individuals age, the dermal layer of the skin loses elastin and collagen, which are crucial proteins that keep the skin firm and elastic. This loss results in wrinkles, fine lines, and sagging skin, all features typical of aging. Furthermore, the skin's ability to retain water is impaired through the interference with lipid synthesis and the loss of natural moisturizing factors. This leads to dry and less elastic skin. Knowledge of such changes is essential for formulating effective skincare regimens designed to counteract the effects of aging and improve the overall state of the skin. Identification of the biological basis of skin aging enables targeted measures to maintain skin integrity and help maintain a youthful appearance. Recent research has moved to the effects of nutrients on aging skin, with findings indicating that some nutrients can reverse some components of aging. A prime example is eating almonds, as a randomized controlled trial demonstrated their capacity to reduce the severity of wrinkles in postmenopausal women. Subjects who followed a diet rich in almonds in the current study experienced significant improvement in skin texture after 16 weeks, highlighting the role of nutrition in skin aging mechanisms (Burney et al., 2019). Almonds that are rich in fatty acids and antioxidants can be the possible reason behind better skin health and hence retarded signs of aging. This finding underscores the interrelation among diet, skin physiology, and aging, and how what a person eats will certainly play an important role in skin health and resilience in the future. Another feature of aging skin is the use of topical drugs to enhance skin function and aesthetic appeal.

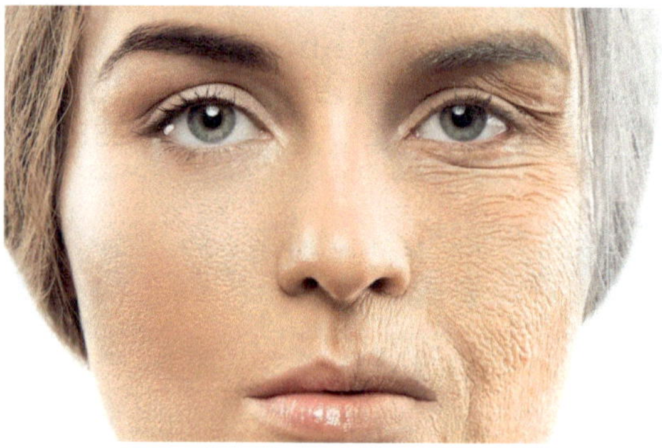

Figure 2.12. Understanding skin ageing: What happens when skin ages.

Source: https://www.kosmoderma.com/wp-content/uploads/2021/07/Blog_Aging-min-1080x675-5.jpg.

One such drug is hyaluronic acid (HA), which is prized for its ability to retain water and moisturize the skin. Low-molecular-weight HA has been found to penetrate the skin more effectively than high-molecular-weight HA, thereby positively affecting skin health without causing inflammation (Malle et al., 2011). Use of LMW HA has also been linked to improved keratinocyte function and cell-cell communication, both of which are important for maintaining the skin's barrier function. Therefore, application of such chemicals in anti-aging cosmeceuticals can induce quantifiable alterations in skin texture, elasticity, and overall cosmetic look of aged skin. Therefore, the application of evidence-based actives in skincare routines can complement lifestyle interventions, contributing to a more harmonized approach to skin well-being during aging (Figure 2.12).

2.4.1. Changes in Skin Structure with Age

With age, the skin's structure and function are severely affected, and several changes become apparent, such as wrinkles, sagging, and loss of elasticity. All these changes result from the continuous breakdown of collagen and elastin fibers, the most important constituents responsible for keeping the skin elastic and firm. The older the person gets, the slower the synthesis rate is, while the breakdown process is more active. Besides, epidermal thickness decreases, weakening the skin's barrier function and its ability to retain water. Not only is this decreased water content responsible for dryness, but it also renders the skin susceptible to environmental stress and irritants. Hence, it is crucial to understand these structural changes to develop potent anti-aging therapies and prophylactic drugs that can maintain skin quality over time. Aside from the loss of elastin and collagen, senescence also affects the skin's microcirculation, which governs nutrient delivery and waste clearance. Decreased density and function of blood vessels within the dermis may lead to inadequate perfusion of the skin, resulting in generalized pallor and diminished healing potential. Studies have also underscored the need to diagnose microcirculatory disorders, particularly in the elderly, as these changes are prone to accelerate skin ailments of aging. For instance, techniques such as laser Doppler flowmetry have gained popularity as a vital method for diagnosing early microcirculatory disorders. By recognizing these changes, researchers and medical practitioners can better treat not only the cosmetic problems but also the intrinsic physiological changes that may happen secondary to aging, ultimately enhancing the health and function of the skin (Dremin et al., 2019). Aging also impairs the skin's immune function and resistance to infection, highlighting yet another crucial aspect of skin physiology. As the skin ages, production of antimicrobial peptides decreases, impairing its resistance to pathogens. This compromised resistance makes it susceptible to infection and slows healing from injuries. The skin's capacity to repair itself also declines as age increases, in part due to reduced cellular turnover and declining metabolic activity of skin tissues. Knowledge of such alterations with age is important for health care professionals, as they develop ways to enhance the skin's protective measures and aid healing in older patients. Overall, a complete awareness of how the architecture of the skin changes with age is important not only for cosmetic purposes but also for the maintenance of the function and health of this vital organ in the elderly individual (Aspden et al., 2015) (Figure 2.13).

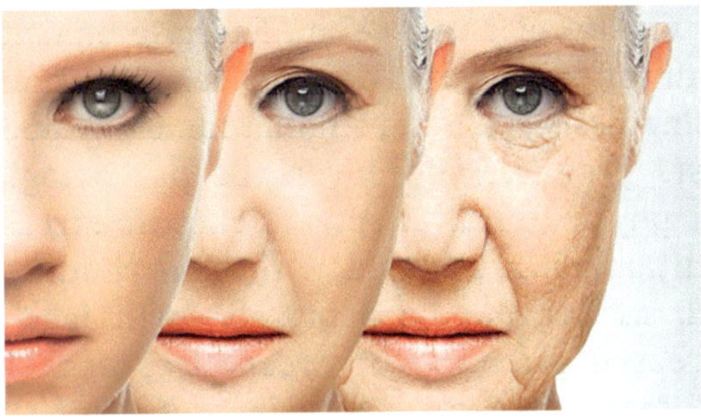

Figure 2.13. Changes in skin structure with age.

Source: https://rewindskinandlaser.com.au/wp-content/uploads/2022/05/Changing-Skin-Care-As-We-Age-768x432-1.jpg.

2.4.2. Effects of Aging on Skin Function

Aging profoundly affects skin function, and these changes are clearly evident in the skin's morphology and physiology. With advancing age, the structural integrity of the skin is lost mainly due to a decrease in collagen and elastin production. The firmness and elasticity of the skin are compromised as a result, and it shows more sagging and wrinkling. Besides, the epidermis also becomes thinner, compromising the integrity of the skin's barrier function and making it more susceptible to environmental stressors such as pathogens and environmental toxins. As a result, older persons may develop heightened sensitivity and more skin ailments. Also, the skin's ability to retain moisture decreases with age, leading to dryness and making aging more visible. These physiological changes underscore the importance of defining the process of skin aging to develop effective dermatological interventions and treatments for improved skin health in aging populations. Microcirculation is essential for maintaining skin health, and its dysregulation is a shared consequence of aging. This capability is significant because impaired microcirculation may reduce nutrient delivery and waste removal in the skin, further accelerating the aging process. Non-invasive optical diagnostic methods have emerged as advanced approaches for evaluating microcirculatory abnormalities in aging skin. Studies have indicated that these diagnostic devices are sufficiently equipped to identify early microvascular alterations, thereby providing information regarding dermatologic conditions associated with aging. For instance, laser Doppler flowmetry has shown reduced perfusion in aging skin, which underlies alterations in skin function such as thermoregulation and inflammation. These advances in diagnostic techniques indicate the potential of targeted therapy to improve microcirculation and, by extension, skin function and health in the elderly (Dremin et al., 2019). Apart from structural changes, the activity of peripheral molecular clocks in skin cells is also affected by aging, influencing hair growth and pigmentation. It has been found that aging alters the expression of central clock genes, such as

BMAL1 and PER1, in hair follicles, leading to disruption of the hair cycle. This disruption can result in protracted phases of alopecia or changes in hair pigmentation, further affecting an individual's appearance and psychological well-being.

Thyroid hormones have been found to be pivotal as peripheral clock regulators; fluctuations in thyroid status can increase the aging effect on the physiology of the skin. Diseases associated with thyroid deficiency or hyperfunction can dysregulate peripheral clock function, further accelerating the overall decline in skin function. Understanding the interaction between endocrine regulation and skin physiology is essential for formulating strategies to mitigate the effects of aging on skin function, thereby enhancing the quality of life among older persons (Farjo et al., 2015).

2.4.3. Strategies for Maintaining Skin Health in Older Adults

The best preservation of skin health among older people involves an interlocking process that takes into consideration both intrinsic and extrinsic effects from the beginning. As individuals age, the skin undergoes significant physiological changes, including decreased elasticity and moisture content due to reduced sebaceous gland activity. Hence, the application of topical moisturizers that have emollients and humectants is essential. Not only do these moisturizers hydrate immediately, but they also create a protective barrier that reduces transepidermal water loss. In addition, sun exposure can exacerbate skin aging through photoaging; therefore, the routine use of broad-spectrum sunscreen can greatly reduce the likelihood of harmful UV effects. The interface of environmental factors, such as irritants and pollutants, further underscores the importance of protective skincare routines tailored to the unique demands of aging skin. By adopting these interventions, elderly people can greatly enhance the cosmetic attractiveness and functional integrity of their skin. In addition to local treatments, nutritional intake is also crucial in order to support the skin health of older individuals. Dietary intake of antioxidants, vitamins, and fatty acids plays a crucial role in enhancing the skin's strength and repair mechanisms. Vitamins C and E are particularly crucial in collagen synthesis and combating oxidative stress, respectively. Besides, omega-3 fatty acids from fish and certain plant oils are involved in maintaining the skin's lipid barrier, ensuring water retention. Hydration is also important, as adequate water consumption maintains cellular function and appearance. Recent research highlights the pivotal role of gut microbiota to the health of the skin, with studies indicating that a disrupted microbiome can increase skin homeostasis. The interaction among diet, microbiota, and cutaneous physiology is consistent with the therapeutic potential of diet modification to produce profound protective effects on skin aging (Hou et al., 2022). Finally, lifestyle choices such as regular physical exercise, smoking cessation, and stress management are necessary for maintaining the vitality of elderly skin. Exercise enhances perfusion and facilitates the delivery of nutrients to skin tissues and the elimination of metabolic waste products. Moreover, the psychological and physiological effects of chronic stress—traditionally associated with skin conditions such as eczema or psoriasis—will lead to increased inflammatory responses and skin disintegration. Stress-reducing activities such as mindfulness, meditation, and yoga can help prevent these adverse effects and improve well-being. Avoiding tobacco usage is also crucial, as these hinder blood circulation and lower oxygen to the skin, inducing premature aging effects. By adopting these holistic lifestyle methods, older individuals can significantly improve the health and appearance of their skin and enhance its physiological functions throughout the aging process (Cryan et al., 2019) (Figure 2.14).

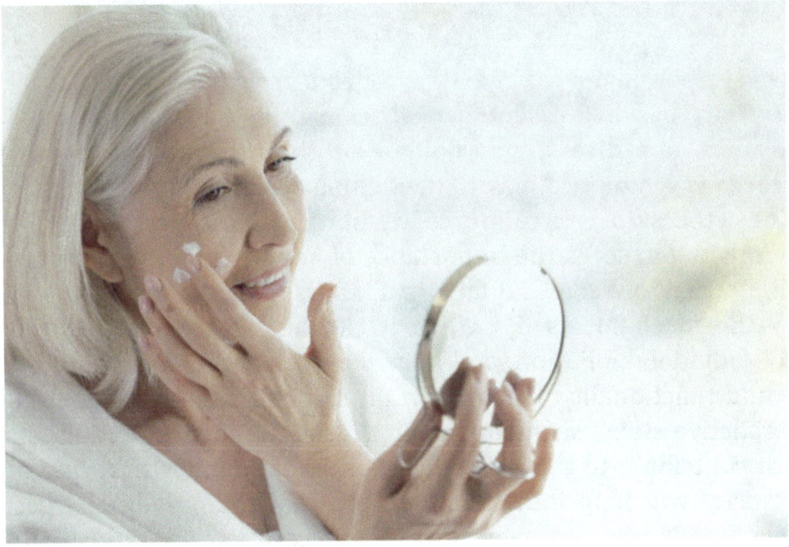

Figure 2.14. The best skin routine for seniors and healthy aging.

Source: https://s11727.pcdn.co/wp-content/uploads/2021/05/skin-care-for-seniors-importance-tips-more.png.

Test Your Knowledge

1. What are the effects of aging on the skin?
2. Describe the strategies for maintaining skin health in older adults.

SUMMARY

In general, the intricate physiology of the skin reflects its many functions in human health. In addition to acting as a barrier, skin is essential for thermoregulation, sensation, and immune response facilitation. The existence of a diverse microbiome on the skin not only helps to maintain these processes but also coexists symbiotically with the human organism, influencing health. By balancing microbial populations, the skin can reinforce its barrier properties and control inflammatory response. Such synergy underscores the importance of adopting a holistic approach to skin health that considers both internal and external factors. Finally, research on skin physiology emphasizes the need to clarify the mechanisms by which it can be affected by environmental stressors. Components like UV radiation, pollution, and lifestyle all have the potential to significantly impair the skin's integrity and functionality. It is important to understand that keeping the skin's health in check involves proactive steps, such as proper hydration, good nutrition, and protection from the sun, all of which contribute to the skin's function as the body's first line of defense. Keeping skin health as a priority will help individuals ensure that their body's largest organ continues functioning optimally. Finally, ongoing scientific research continues to expose the complexity of skin biology, providing ever more advanced understanding of its functions and responses to challenge. For instance, research into the skin microbiome illustrates how these bacterial communities can influence immune function and, indeed, overall well-being. With advancing scientific understanding, new treatments and prevention can be developed to enhance skin health aligned with broader public health priorities. The skin, by the way, remains in the spotlight for more research, with promise that can not only improve dermatological care but also overall human health and well-being, as exemplified in the research of Garshnek et al. (2025) and Gillen et al. (2017).

One important aspect of the physiology of the skin is that it serves as a cover and barrier for the human body. Skin provides the first line of defense against external threats such as pathogens and poisonous substances, thereby maintaining homeostasis. Its structural elements, particularly the epidermis, dermis, and subcutaneous tissue, contribute partly to this protective function. The skin also plays a role in maintaining body temperature through sweating and vasodilation, thereby supporting thermoregulation, which is vital for maintaining internal balance. Given the skin's multifunctional nature, understanding its physiological responses to various stimuli offers insights into overall health, including potential correlations between skin integrity and chronic disease. Scientists continue to study how the skin is involved in communication with internal physiological functions, thereby underscoring its importance beyond merely serving as an outer covering. In addition, skin is closely linked to emotional and psychological well-being, as its impact is influenced by attachment processes and stress. More recent research has shown that attachment styles can affect physiological responses, including skin healing and general health outcomes. For instance, secure attachment can help guard against stress-related skin diseases, whereas insecure attachments can be augmenting, highlighting a key point of convergence between psychology and physiology. This complex interaction is further explored in studies examining how stress influences not just emotional health but also bodily functioning, such as inflammation and wound healing. Such information provides better insight into skin health, with a focus on accounting for both psychological and physical factors in clinics, thus enhancing the outcomes of treatments for skin conditions as part of overall general care. Finally, the environment plays an essential role in regulating skin physiology and function, particularly in relation to temperature fluctuations and their influence on skin health. Environmental stress, such as high temperatures, can significantly affect cardiovascular responses, as illustrated by studies on physiological adaptation to temperature in animals. These studies shed light on probable mechanisms by which environmental factors control skin responses, including alterations in heart rate and skin conductivity, and hence provide clues on how to optimize skin function and wellness across various environments. This connection between environmental factors and skin physiology underscores the need for interdisciplinary research that considers variables from both biological and environmental perspectives. By widening the scope of research to include interactions between the environment and the health of the skin, researchers can devise improved prevention and treatment methods for skin ailments and ultimately enhance quality of life.

KEY TERMS FROM THIS CHAPTER

- Bacteria
- Laser Doppler flowmetry
- Pathogens
- Physical injuries
- Skin health
- Skin physiology
- Subcutaneous tissue
- Fungi
- Microorganisms
- Perspiration
- Skin
- Skin microbiome
- Spectroscopy
- Toxins

CRITICAL THINKING QUESTIONS

1. **Which of the following is NOT a function of the skin?**
   a. Protection against microorganisms
   b. Regulation of body temperature
   c. Production of red blood cells
   d. Sensation
2. **Which layer of the skin plays a major role in thermoregulation by containing sweat glands?**
   a. Epidermis
   b. Dermis
   c. Hypodermis
   d. Stratum corneum
3. **What is the primary function of sebaceous glands in the skin?**
   a. Produce sweat for thermoregulation
   b. Secrete sebum to lubricate and protect the skin
   c. Aid in the synthesis of vitamin D
   d. Facilitate sensory perception
4. **Which of the following mechanisms is used by the skin to maintain body temperature?**
   a. Vasodilation and vasoconstriction
   b. Cellular respiration
   c. Filtration of blood
   d. Active transport of ions
5. **Which vitamin is synthesized in the skin upon exposure to UV radiation?**
   a. Vitamin A
   b. Vitamin B12
   c. Vitamin D
   d. Vitamin E

Short Answer Questions

1. What is skin physiology?
2. What is the sensory function of the skin?
3. Which part of the skin serves as the first line of defense against the external environment?
4. Name the three types of skin disorders.
5. Which skin change occurs with aging?

Answer to Critical Thinking Questions

1. (c); 2. (b) ; 3. (b); 4. (a); 5. (c)

REFERENCES

1. Afonso, N., Kelekar, A., & Alangaden, A. (2020). "I have a cough": an interactive virtual respiratory Case-Based module. *MedEdPORTAL, 16*, 11058. https://doi.org/10.15766/mep_2374-8265.11058Abuabara, K., Elias, P. M., Lee, C. H., Lin, T. K., et al. (2019). By protecting against cutaneous inflammation, epidermal pigmentation provided an additional advantage for ancestral humans. https://core.ac.uk/download/323072787.pdf (accessed on 21st July 2025).
2. Acharjee, M., Akter, S., Akter, S., Banerjee, R., et al. (2022). Impact of gut microbiome on skin health: Gut-skin axis observed through the lenses of therapeutics and skin diseases. https://core.ac.uk/download/558723039.pdf (accessed on 21st July 2025).
3. Ainsworth, M., Avitsur, R., Baumeister, R. F., Beedie, C. J., Biomarker Definitions Working Group, Bolger, N., Bowlby, J., et al. (2014). The attachment system and physiology in adulthood: Normative processes, individual differences, and implications for health. https://core.ac.uk/download/294625964.pdf (accessed on 21st July 2025).
4. Ali, A., Ananthapadmanabhan, K. P., Atrux-Tallau, N., Balaskas, K., Baranda, L., Baranoski, G. V. G., Beauregard, P. B., et al. (2017). Skin cleansing and emolliating for older people: A quasi-experimental pilot study. https://core.ac.uk/download/74236603.pdf (accessed on 21st July 2025).
5. Allen, D., Chaseling, G., Davis, S., Huang, C. J., et al. (2018). Impaired thermoregulatory function during dynamic exercise in multiple sclerosis. https://open.bu.edu/bitstream/2144/32925/3/AllenDR-MSExerciseThermoreg-Manuscript-R2.pdf (accessed on 21st July 2025).
6. Alloway, K. D., Apkarian, A. V., Azanon, E., Batschelet, E., Bentley, D. E., Berens, P., Bookstein, F. L., et al. (2011). A supramodal representation of the body surface. https://core.ac.uk/download/125054.pdf (accessed on 21st July 2025).
7. Alving, K., Asano, K., Basu, S., Fubini, B., Bosquillon, C., Brain, J. D., Brown, J. S., et al. (2012). Toxicity of lunar dust. http://arxiv.org/abs/1206.6328 (accessed on 21st July 2025).
8. Aspden, R. M., Bruel, A., Chen, L., Delville, C., et al. (2015). The effects of graded levels of calorie restriction: I. Impact of short-term calorie and protein restriction on body composition in the C57BL/6 mouse. https://core.ac.uk/download/30435703.pdf (accessed on 21st July 2025).
9. Barnes, V. A., Cearley, S. M., Junca, S., Ravinder, R., et al. (2017). The dynamic role of breathing and cellular membrane potentials in the experience of consciousness. https://core.ac.uk/download/131210584.pdf (accessed on 21st July 2025).
10. Barwood, M., Best, R., Gillis, J., Jeffries, J. A., et al. (2019). Oral application of L-menthol in the heat: From pleasure to performance. https://core.ac.uk/download/287723714.pdf (accessed on 21st July 2025).
11. Bikle, D. D., Jiang, Y., Nguyen, T., Oda, Y., et al. (2016). Disruption of vitamin D and calcium signaling in keratinocytes predisposes to skin cancer. https://core.ac.uk/download/323063349.pdf (accessed on 21st July 2025).
12. Burney, W. A., Chodur, G. M., Foolad, N., Newman, J. W., et al. (2019). Prospective randomized controlled pilot study on the effects of almond consumption on skin lipids and wrinkles. https://core.ac.uk/download/323062627.pdf (accessed on 21st July 2025).

13. Carr, G. P., Neal, V., Pogue, W., Schmitt, H. H., et al. (2025). Advanced extravehicular activity systems requirements definition study. Phase 2: Extravehicular activity at a lunar base. https://core.ac.uk/download/pdf/42829079.pdf (accessed on 21st July 2025).

14. Chukwu, R., & Mankila, J. (2018). Dermatology nurses' job description: Literature review. https://core.ac.uk/download/161432240.pdf (accessed on 21st July 2025).

15. Cryan, J. F., O'Riordan, K. J., Cowan, C. S. M., Sandhu, K. V., Bastiaanssen, T. F. S., Boehme, M., Codagnone, M. G., et al. (2019). The microbiota-gut-brain axis. *Physiological Reviews, 99*, 1877–2013. https://doi.org/10.1152/physrev.00018.2018 (accessed on 21st July 2025).

16. Dremin, V. V., Dunaev, A. V., Goltsov, A., Makovik, L., et al. (2019). Multimodal optical diagnostics of the microhemodynamics in upper and lower limbs. https://core.ac.uk/download/228178569.pdf (accessed on 21st July 2025).

17. Eskin, A., & Riccio, D. C. (2025). The effects of environmental temperature changes on the EKG of the squirrel monkey *Saimiri sciureus*. https://core.ac.uk/download/pdf/85253653.pdf (accessed on 21st July 2025).

18. Fabian, D., Kędziora, F., Siwiec, J., Smyl, P., et al. (2024). The role of physical activity in enhancing and preserving skin health. https://core.ac.uk/download/636386058.pdf (accessed on 21st July 2025).

19. Farjo, B., Farjo, N., Hardman, J. A., Haslam, I. S., et al. (2015). Thyroxine differentially modulates the peripheral clock: Lessons from the human hair follicle. https://core.ac.uk/download/30733998.pdf (accessed on 21st July 2025).

20. Garshnek, V., Hooke, L. R., Radtke, M., Rowe, J., et al. (2025). *USSR Space Life Sciences Digest*, issue 3. https://core.ac.uk/download/pdf/42842161.pdf (accessed on 21st July 2025).

21. Gillen, A. L. (2017). Staph bacteria from first breath: The interweaving of the nasal microbiome with the intricate and complex nose. https://core.ac.uk/download/220159120.pdf (accessed on 21st July 2025).

22. Greenleaf, J. E., & Kaciuba-Uscilko, H. (2025). Acclimatization to heat in humans. https://core.ac.uk/download/pdf/42827514.pdf (accessed on 21st July 2025).

23. Hou, K., Wu, Z. X., Chen, X. Y., Wang, J. Q., Zhang, D., Xiao, C., Zhu, D., et al. (2022). Microbiota in health and diseases. *Signal Transduction and Targeted Therapy, 7*. https://doi.org/10.1038/s41392-022-00974-4 (accessed on 21st July 2025).

24. Malle, B., Baccarani-Contri, M., Bhattacharya, J., Gauglitz, G., Schmitz, G., Korting, H. C., Schwach-Abdellaoui, K., et al. (2011). Fifty-kDa hyaluronic acid upregulates some epidermal genes without changing TNF-α expression in reconstituted epidermis. https://core.ac.uk/download/16432240.pdf (accessed on 21st July 2025).

25. McGill, L. E. (2014). Serum concentration levels of 25(OH)D and injury reports in NCAA Division I football players. https://core.ac.uk/download/211340324.pdf (accessed on 21st July 2025).

DERMATOLOGICAL HISTORY TAKING AND PHYSICAL EXAMINATION

3

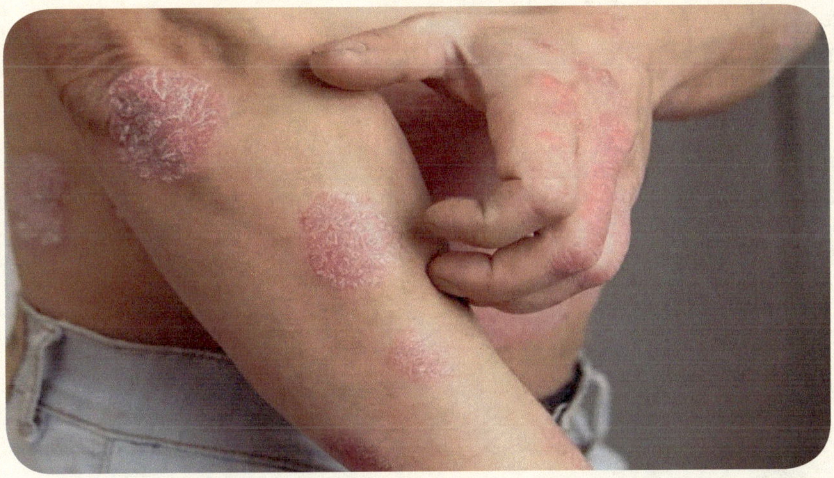

Introduction

In dermatology, methodical history taking and proper physical examination cannot be overemphasized. These are crucial first steps toward a comprehensive picture of a patient's dermatologic disorder. The process of history taking initially allows clinicians to obtain pertinent information such as the history of onset and duration of the signs and symptoms, previous dermatological diseases, family medical history, and how lifestyle factors contribute. Each item of data that is collected serves to distinguish between various skin diseases, treatment methods that then follow, and finally assists in informing clinical decision-making. Secondly, skin disease generally has complex interdependencies with systemic disease, so history is a key element of a good diagnostic approach as clinicians try to elucidate potential correlations and mechanisms relevant to patient care. The physical examination then confirms what has been gathered from the patient's history. A thorough examination involves assessing morphology, distribution, and lesion features such as color, shape, and

LEARNING OBJECTIVES

After studying this chapter, you will be able to:

1. Know the fundamentals of dermatological history taking
2. Describe the patient interview techniques
3. Understand the specifics of dermatological symptoms
4. Understand the patient's past medical and family history
5. Describe the physical examination techniques for accurate diagnosis
6. Understand the role of technology in enhancing documentation and communication

texture. Differential diagnoses are made using this process, a crucial aspect of dermatology in which numerous diseases may present with similar clinical appearances. The integration of history and physical examination enables medical practitioners to identify subtle evidence that can point to complex underlying processes, such as autoimmune diseases or infections. This outcome of the examination is important in crafting a holistic treatment plan that may involve therapeutic interventions ranging from topical therapy to systemic therapy. This integrative approach, marked by collaboration among specialists, enhances patient care and promotes an all-encompassing view of dermatological well-being. Additionally, the significance of adopting a systematic approach to dermatological history-taking and physical examination is underscored by advances in medical practice. For instance, ongoing research and updates to clinical guidelines ensure that practitioners are informed of optimal practices and emerging treatments in the specialty.

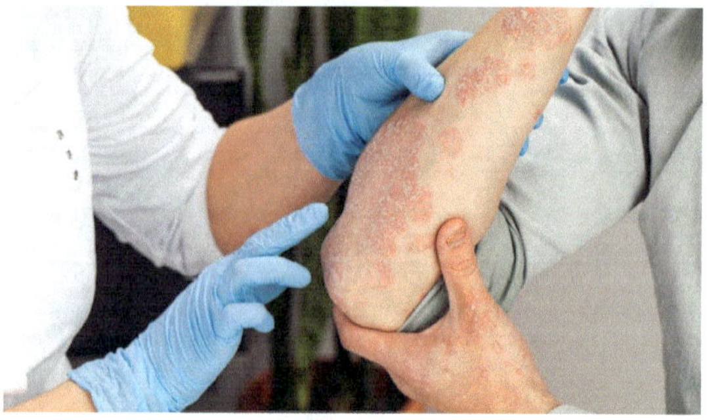

Figure 3.1. Dermatological assessment: examination.

Source: https://www.practicenursing.com/media/mqkn5fnt/adobestock_393573411.jpeg?width=1002&height=564&bgcolor=White&v=1db887b55986fd0.

As noted in recent updates, the management of certain diseases, such as those involving immune checkpoint inhibitors, requires maximum vigilance for dermatological symptoms that may occur during treatment (Schneider et al., 2021). Similarly, vigilance regarding the complexity of conditions such as tuberous sclerosis complex underscores the need for ongoing education in light of evolving diagnostic practices and treatment protocols (Northrup et al., 2021). Thus, the integration of detailed history taking with a competent physical examination essentially improves the clinician's ability to deliver quality dermatological services and thus contribute to patient health outcomes (Figure 3.1).

3.1. Fundamentals of Dermatological History Taking

Learning Outcome

1. Understand the significance of history taking
2. Describe the key components of a dermatological history
3. Describe the common dermatological conditions requiring a detailed history

An appropriate understanding of dermatological history-taking is the core of accurate diagnosis and effective treatment in dermatology. An appropriate dermatological history includes an evaluation of the patient's skin condition, relevant medical, social, and family history. It begins with the clinician obtaining information regarding the nature, duration, and course of the symptoms. This initial step allows the establishment of primary lesions and etiology, which, by extension, may have a bearing on treatment. Furthermore, careful history allows the identification of causal factors like environmental exposure, use of medication, and history of skin disease, thereby enriching the clinical picture with accuracy. By establishing a strong therapeutic relationship through effective communication, clinicians can gain critical information that may otherwise be difficult to obtain, thereby leading to improved outcomes for patients. In addition to the patients' presenting issues, there is a need to gain information on the patients' skin history and previous dermatological diagnoses. These are questions about previous skin disease, treatments undergone, and results. This type of information can help clinicians recognize patterns that are indicative of familial or hereditary factors affecting the patient's current presentation. Secondly, information regarding the patient's psychosocial setting is important, as this can affect follow-through on treatment regimens and overall health.

Stress, for instance, can exacerbate many dermatologic illnesses. In addition, establishing the patient's skin type and sun history is important because recurrent sunburn patients are at higher risk of developing skin cancers such as actinic keratoses, for which careful follow-up is required (Reinehr et al., 2019). By bringing together past data with current clinical evidence, dermatologists can paint the full picture for accurate diagnosis and treatment. Another key component of dermatology history taking is incorporating physical exams in line with information derived from patient history. In physical examination, dermatologists should not only observe obvious skin lesions but also palpate to assess texture, mobility, and tenderness, which can yield valuable diagnostic information. Combining information from both history and examination allows dermatologists to identify subtle, complex conditions that could otherwise go undetected. For instance, faint variations in texture or color can become more apparent when carefully examined, necessitating a methodical approach. Adapting the physical examination to the history obtained can optimize the diagnostic process and enable timely interventions. Ultimately, skill in dermatologic history taking and physical examination provides a solid foundation for honing patient care, connecting treatment to an individual's specific requirements and history (Mulcare et al., 2020) (Figure 3.2).

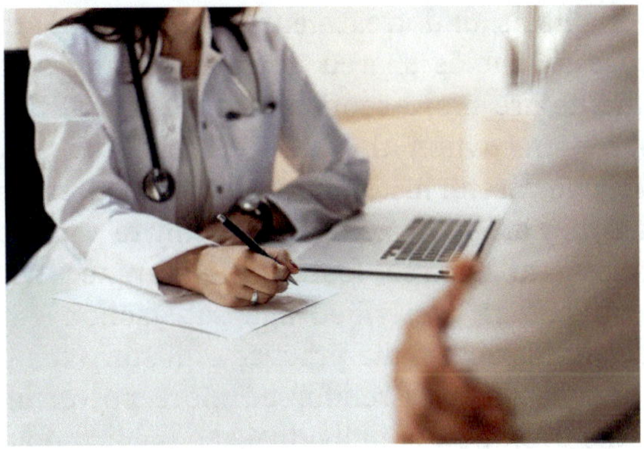

Figure 3.2. History taking of dermatology.

Source: https://idrissderm.com/wp-content/uploads/2025/04/Homepage-4-scaled.jpeg.

3.1.1. Definition and Significance of History Taking

History-taking during dermatological examination is an essential component of patient care, providing useful information about a patient's condition. History taking is the official process of obtaining a patient's history, symptoms, and factors influencing their health, in dermatology, including skin lesion questions, relevant symptoms, and previous treatments administered. This method enables the creation of a holistic view of skin disease and its diagnostic and management options. Clinicians are able to better identify underlying reasons for skin complications through capturing relevant information, including the patient's family history, drug use, and habits. This process also helps clinicians assess the effectiveness of prior measures and tailor treatment options to specific patients, improving overall care. The value of meticulous history-taking extends beyond a diagnostic function; it is essential for establishing patient rapport and trust. Clear communication during this time allows practitioners to demonstrate empathy and compassion, which is particularly significant in dermatology, as patients present with conditions that are sensitive or stigmatizing. An open and respectful environment encourages patients to share issues that could be critical to reaching a diagnosis and treatment plan. Second, the process enables shared decision-making since patients are more confident in managing their care plans when they are directly involved. Through careful histories, dermatologists can be sure they are responding thoroughly to patients' issues and desires, fostering adherence with treatment as prescribed and satisfaction with care. Additionally, the practice of history taking in dermatology is reinforced more powerfully by the evolution of individualized medicine and evidence-based practice. Recommendations for today focus on an organized approach to how body diseases are assessed and managed with a comprehensive patient history. For instance, while generalities are provided for skin diseases, genetics, environmental exposure, and comorbid diseases often dictate individual patient outcomes. New guidelines focus on how history-taking and diagnostic tools can be combined to ensure optimal treatment outcomes. Therefore, the dermatologists are better poised to tailor therapy based on individualized clinical presentations, for example, of complicated cases of diseases such as tuberous sclerosis complex, solidifying the bedrock tenet of total history taking (Northrup et al., 2021). This amalgamation of history and clinical data leads to better outcomes and better patient care (Figure 3.3).

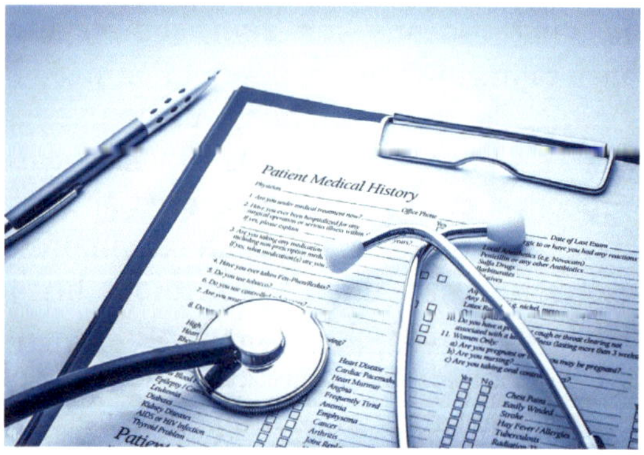

Figure 3.3. Medical history.

Source: https://patientbest.com/wp-content/uploads/2019/07/medical_records.jpg.

3.1.2. Key Components of a Dermatological History

Taking an adequate dermatologic history is a fundamental component of effective clinical dermatology practice. The clinician starts by taking a clean history of the patient's presenting complaint, including the onset and duration of the skin lesions and their character. The history should be specific to features such as lesion size, shape, color, and distribution, as well as any associated symptoms, such as itching or pain. This very first question not only forms the basis for diagnosis but also helps in understanding the probable broader implications on the patient's quality of life. Chronic dermatoses often require a subtle balancing of psychological and emotional considerations, thereby aptly demonstrating the need for thorough history-taking. A skilled clinician appreciates that the subtleties of a patient's presentation can reveal underlying pathology, thereby enhancing the efficiency of follow-up assessments and interventions, as noted by Alsararatee (2025). Besides the history of the presenting condition, there is a need for a complete dermatological history to include a patient's history of present illness and endeavors to consider past medical history, past skin conditions, treatments, and reactions. Special attention should be paid to any family history of dermatological disease, which may predispose individuals to certain dermatoses. The clinician also needs to inquire about sun exposure, occupation exposures, and skincare practices, as these can play a big role in the clinical presentation. A history of drugs is relevant too, since some drugs will induce cutaneous reactions. This hybrid approach not only enhances the diagnostic process but also facilitates the construction of a patient-centered management plan. By situating history within personal, family, and lifestyle factors, clinicians can foster a more comprehensive model of therapeutic dermatology, one consonant with the research outlined in Siviter et al. (2025). Lastly, gathering a detailed social and psychological history is required to create a comprehensive picture of dermatologic disorders. Stress, anxiety, and depression can exacerbate skin ailments, and thus it is important to address these areas during history-taking. In addition, assessment of the impact of skin disease on quality of life can guide treatment and intervention to improve the patients' overall well-being. Therapists need not shy away from discussing sensitive topics such as social stigma surrounding skin diseases, which may have an effect on the patient's mental health and treatment adherence. Overall, integrating psychosocial issues into routine dermatological history-taking highlights the importance of an integrative approach to patient care. This inclusive approach fosters an environment conducive to effective communication and plays an important role in developing a therapeutic relationship between patient and clinician, ultimately leading to improved clinical outcomes and patient satisfaction, as evidenced by Alsararatee (2025) and Siviter et al. (2025).

3.1.3. Common Dermatological Conditions Requiring Detailed History

Detailed history in common dermatological conditions is crucial in the diagnosis and management of such conditions, as it significantly influences the success of treatment. For example, urticaria and wheals, as well as angioedema, require a thorough history to identify potential precipitants, such as drugs, food, or the environment. Acute urticaria, according to new guidelines, has an impressive lifetime prevalence of approximately 20%, underscoring its commonality and the importance of obtaining an adequate history that can elicit information on the nature and duration of the patient's symptoms. Systematic patient assessment of patients' lifestyle, habits, and history of similar skin lesions is essential. Moreover, chronic spontaneous urticarias' impact on quality of life supports the reality that a comprehensive history can directly correlate with successful management, positioning the clinician to mold interventions that promote patient well-being (Zuberbier et al., 2021). Another significant dermatological disorder wherein history-taking must be taken carefully is tuberous sclerosis complex (TSC), a genetically determined disorder that has multiple dermatological manifestations, including angiofibromas and hypomelanotic macules. TSC can be treated well if the variability of presentation, which can be quite wide ranging from one individual to another, is understood clearly. Clinicians need to ask about family history, symptom onset, and any concomitant neurological findings to inform a comprehensive diagnostic examination. Contemporary guidelines emphasize the imperative of immediate screening and continuing surveillance, which parallels the evolution of diagnostic criteria that emphasize the importance of gathering comprehensive patient histories.

Therefore, the difference in how TSC may manifest necessitates a comprehensive history-taking approach to ensure optimal care and a greater understanding of this multifaceted condition (Northrup et al., 2021). Urticaria and TSC are not alone in drawing attention to the need for diligent historical context, as other skin diseases, including eczema and psoriasis, also emphasize this requirement. Eczema patients require inquiry into eczema triggers, family history, and potential allergens, as these can significantly impact treatment plans. Similarly, psoriasis, with numerous different presentations, requires questioning a patient's history about the onset of symptoms, prior treatments, and comorbidities. Such in-depth histories allow clinicians to better assess the probability of severity as well as the disease's overall impact on function. As these conditions necessitate a multifactorial interpretive paradigm, history taking has an unassailable role in not only making diagnoses but also directing therapeutic interventions according to individual patient needs. A complete historical understanding ensures that management plans are appropriately adjusted, maximizing patient engagement and treatment outcomes (Figure 3.4).

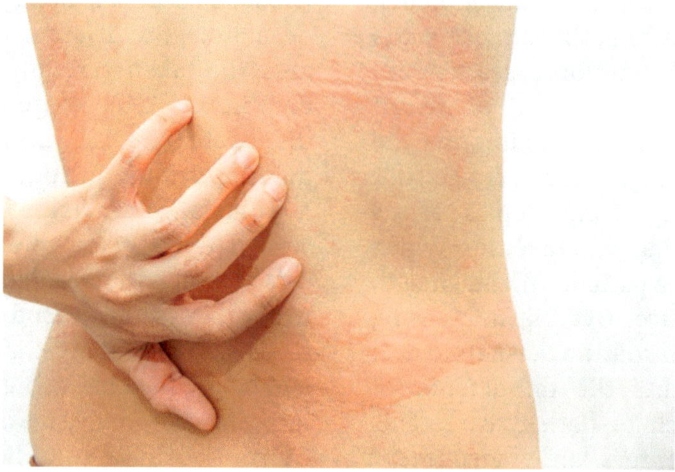

Figure 3.4. Urticaria.

Source: https://media-pierre-fabre.wedia-group.com/api/wedia/dam/transform/u5wa3z31qn5se9mger5maqqna 93rh14d61ik6je/eczema-urticaria- itching-back-patches?t=crop&width= 1.000&height=1.000.

Test Your Knowledge

1. What is the significance of history taking?
2. What are the key components of a dermatological history?

3.2. Patient Interview Techniques

Learning Outcome

1. Establish rapport with the patient
2. Know the effective questioning strategies
3. Understand the importance of active listening

An effective patient interview forms the core of appropriate dermatological history taking and physical examination. Patient-centered communication skills are useful in establishing rapport required to elicit the needed information. Through open-ended questioning, practitioners can persuade patients to describe their symptoms and concerns in their own terms, enabling the clinician to pick up vital details that may otherwise be missed. Open-ended questioning permits a more subtle appreciation of the patient's situation and also empowers patients by validating their experience. For instance, open-ended questions such as " or " Can you tell me what brought you in?" urge patients to share timelines, precipitants, and relevant history, thus providing the dermatologist with important context upon which to make an assessment (Alsararatee, 2025). The wealth of information obtained by this method significantly enhances the clinician's capacity for making an informed decision. Active listening is an important skill for patient interviewing that affects the quality of dermatological assessments. Clinicians need to engage actively with patients, projecting empathy and understanding through non-verbal cues and affirmatory responses. This not only helps grasp the patient's concerns but also fosters a safe environment where patients are comfortable disclosing sensitive details about their skin diseases. Eye contact and avoiding distractions during the interview are also crucial for establishing trust and eliciting honest, holistic responses. This active interaction is especially important in dermatology, where the psychological burden of skin disease can affect a patient's emotional health. Adding these active listening strategies to dermatological history-taking enhances the diagnostic process and ultimately improves patient outcomes (Tasrif et al., 2024). Moreover, the inclusion of guided frameworks in interviewing patients will make history taking more effective. There are a number of models, such as the SOAP (Subjective, Objective, Assessment, and Plan) model, that give a step-by-step way of documenting patient information such that everything important is achieved.

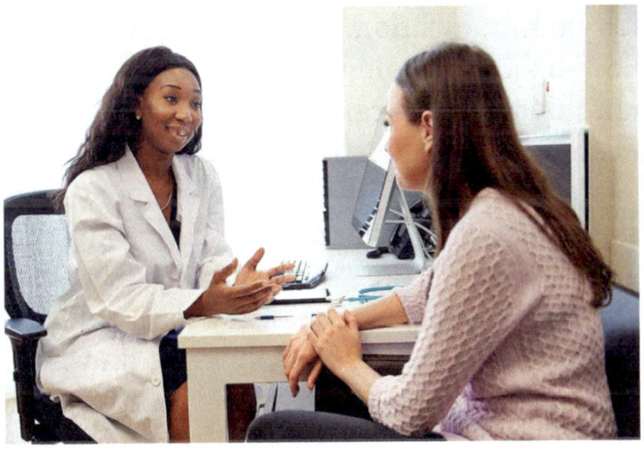

Figure 3.5. Patient interview.

Source: https://cleardermatology.com/wp-content/uploads/Doctor-and-patient-having-consultation.jpg.

For instance, in the subjective component, dermatologists can request information such as skin changes, treatment history, family history, and psychosocial factors, thereby enabling an extensive evaluation. This strategy also enables practitioners to transition seamlessly into the physical examination phase, ensuring that essential information informs clinical assessment. Moreover, the use of diagnostic tools with patient questioning, as highlighted in modern literature, can significantly improve diagnostic efficiency. By incorporating structured interview processes with rigorous physical examinations, dermatologists can potentially improve the quality of their clinical practice, providing holistic and compassionate care to patients (Alsararatee, 2025) (Figure 3.5).

3.2.1. Establishing Rapport with the Patient

Establishing rapport with the patient is a fundamental aspect of dermatologic history and physical examination and significantly affects the validity of the clinical assessment. Patients are more likely to disclose important information about their skin problems when they feel heard and respected by their caregivers. Rapport may be established through empathic communication, active listening, and non-judgment. Especially in dermatology, where patients' conditions may be delicate and affect their self-esteem, establishing an encouraging atmosphere can foster openness and increase the validity of the patient account. Through successful patient engagement, not only do dermatologists demonstrate patient care commitment, but they also ensure adherence to treatment regimens, ultimately resulting in better outcomes. The use of digital health technologies is increasingly being used to enhance patient rapport, especially in healthcare settings today, with the new paradigm established by the COVID-19 pandemic. Telehealth has been the practical solution for maintaining continuity of care while reassuring patients that they are not being abandoned. Experiences under the pandemic demonstrated how effective telehealth on secure platforms is in lowering the anxiety that comes with face-to-face visits, particularly for those afflicted with chronic skin disease. Telehealth facilitates ongoing interaction, and patient satisfaction is often improved because patients can consult from the comfort of their own homes. This level of accessibility confirms the role of maintaining established relationships and providing dermatologists with means to act in a timely manner, thus making patients feel less abandoned, especially during times of limitation and hardship (Ward et al., 2022). Awareness of the limitations of different patient populations still enhances rapport-building in dermatologic practice. Several cultural backgrounds, socioeconomic levels, and age can affect not only patients' perceptions of dermatological conditions but also their treatment expectations. Sensitivity to these allows for individualized communication styles, which can help establish rapport and trust. Informal communication styles, for instance, are more acceptable to younger patients, as outlined in recent telehealth studies (Yeung et al., 2023). By adapting to the preferences of various populations, dermatologists are more likely to identify with their patients, thereby improving health literacy and engagement in self-care and ultimately strengthening the therapeutic alliance, which is crucial to successful clinical outcomes.

3.2.2. Effective Questioning Strategies

Effective questioning strategies are a key component of dermatological history-taking and physical examination because they can significantly enhance diagnostic accuracy and patient rapport. Open-ended questions are particularly beneficial in this context, as they allow the patient to present their symptoms and issues in their own words, providing a richer clinical impression. For example, asking Can you tell me about changes you've noticed on your skin? calls for a more elaborate reply than a yes or no. This approach provides a nonjudgmental setting; hence, the patient feels heard and understood, which can, in turn, stimulate more honest disclosure about his or her symptoms, habits of life, and psychosocial history that may impact the dermatological disease. Overall, the proper use of open-ended questions not only helps extract pertinent information but also improves the clinician-patient relationship, which is the highest priority for quality care. Follow-up questions are equally important in the dermatologic context, clarifying and expanding on initial patient responses. Follow-up questions can potentially add depth to the clinician's understanding of a patient's condition. As a starting point, if a patient complains of itching, the follow-up question would be, When did the itching start, and are you aware of anything that precipitates it? Such targeted questioning may reveal patterns or correlations not apparent on a broad question alone. This is not only helpful for identifying the symptom type but also for excluding potential dermatological conditions, thereby improving the diagnostic process. In addition, the presence of follow-up questions shows the patient that the clinician values their viewpoints, engendering trust and facilitating open communication. Thus, the force of good follow-up questioning is an essential tool for taking dermatological history. Moreover, using a framework in questioning can make the act of history-taking effective and complete without compromising information. By adopting these models, such as the "Zebra" approach, where clinicians have a definite model in which to ask about some symptoms, history, and family history, dermatologists can efficiently gather the necessary information. This sequential approach is especially beneficial given the multifactorial etiology of skin diseases, which are frequently encountered. For instance, in examining a rash, sequential questioning of the history, such as onset, duration, associated symptoms, past treatment, and family history, can guide the examination. Clinicians would also involve questioning about potential psychosocial factors affecting the patient's skin condition, as highlighted by evidence of the significance of such factors in dermatological treatment (Bhatia et al., 2023). To that degree, applying a formalized method to questioning not only provides maximum efficiency in the consultation process but is also aligned with the holistic approach to care necessary in the treatment of dermatological conditions, as evidenced by contemporary case studies (Figure 3.6).

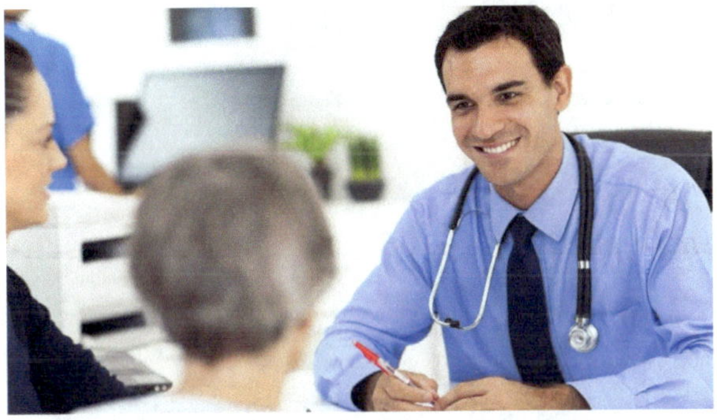

Figure 3.6. consultation one-to-one

Source: https://images.thesouthfirst.com/wp-content/uploads/2023/09/patient-historyfinal_V_jpg--1280x720-4g.webp?sw=1536&dsz=1280x720&iw=750&p=false&r=1.25.

3.2.3. Importance of Active Listening

Active listening is a pivotal skill in dermatological history-taking and physical examination. It not only helps augment the provider-patient interaction but also validates that a genuine and detailed record of information is being gathered during clinical consultations. By interacting closely with patients, dermatologists can obtain significant information about symptoms, history, and contextual factors influencing skin diseases. Active listening fosters a cooperative environment in which the patient is heard and respected, leading to greater care satisfaction and improved treatment adherence. It also allows clinicians to pick up on nuances of patient presentation that might otherwise be missed. Therefore, fostering a trusting dialogue between patient and clinician is key to effective dermatologic examination. The application of strategies such as summarizing, reflection, and clarifying questions can significantly enhance the effectiveness of active listening in clinical practice. By applying them, healthcare professionals, as well as by accepting the patient's viewpoint, are also accepting the patient's concerns. Validating is critical in dermatology, where diseases often have significant psychosocial as well as physical impacts.

For instance, learning a patient's emotional response to conditions like psoriasis or eczema requires both careful questioning and active listening. In this way, providers can provide interventions grounded in a fully textured understanding of the patient's lived experience. Furthermore, by elevating the significance of what they contribute to the treatment conversation, patients will be more apt to engage more deeply in the diagnostic conversation, leading to improved diagnostic quality and outcomes for the patient. The synergy between good history-taking and active listening in dermatology extends beyond the confines of a single consultation; it spills over into broader healthcare dynamics. The importance of effective and clear communication cannot be overstated, particularly in an era of technology where miscommunication or less-than-effective documentation can lead to misunderstandings spreading like wildfire. As evidenced, integrating active listening skills into educational pedagogies such as problem-based and case-based learning enhances medical education by equipping future healthcare providers with essential interpersonal competencies (Wang et al., 2021). In addition, the changing nature of social media as a health communication channel underscores the need for flexibility in listening to and responding to patient needs across varied contexts (Farsi, 2021). With advancing health care, an active-listening practice culture in dermatology will not only lead to better clinical outcomes but also to more comprehensive patient care (Figure 3.7).

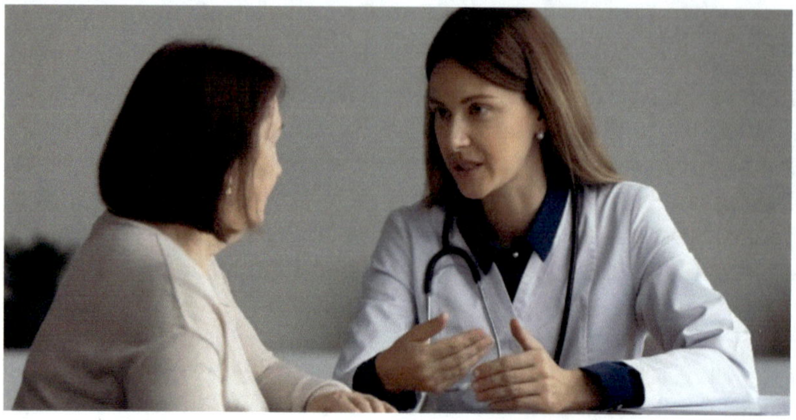

Figure 3.7. Importance of active listening.

Source: https://dermatology-innovation.com/wp-content/uploads/2024/05/doctor-patient-consult-1280x640.jpg.

Test Your Knowledge

1. Describe the effective questioning strategies.
2. What is the importance of active listening?

3.3. Specifics of Dermatological Symptoms

Learning Outcome

1. Describe the types of skin lesions and their characteristics
2. Understand the duration and progression of symptoms for making accurate diagnoses
3. Associate systemic symptoms in establishing a comprehensive diagnosis

A good grounding in dermatological signs is essential for establishing a solid foundation for dermatological history-taking and physical examination. Specific lesion characteristics, such as morphology, distribution, and accompanying symptoms, provide valuable pointers for diagnosis. For instance, papules, plaques, or vesicles are strong indicators of dermatological diseases. The evaluation of molluscum contagiosum, a diffuse viral infection that creates dome-shaped, pearly papules, illustrates the merit of observing attentively. Lesions are typically 2–5 millimeters in size and can begin to itch or become inflamed, particularly in secondary infections. These characteristics are not only required for diagnosis but also for the development of successful treatment regimens, which can include local treatments such as tretinoin to resolve lesions and reduce cosmetic burden (Kumar et al., 2021). Careful attention to the context in which the lesions develop is essential. The patient's age, immune status, and atopic history can significantly affect the course and presentation of skin dermatological manifestations. Molluscum contagiosum is much more prevalent among immunocompromised individuals and pediatric patients, both of whom underscore the importance of age in diagnosis. Furthermore, aggressive patient interrogation of the exposure history—e.g., swimming in public baths or skin-to-skin contact—can help identify potential modes of transmission. This history-taking during the investigation not only helps establish the correct diagnosis but also informs the broader epidemiological context of the disease, which can be used to inform public health interventions aimed at prevention (Kumar et al., 2021). In addition to familiar presentations, dermatological examination must consider atypical and rare conditions such as Papuloerythroderma of Ofuji (PEO). The disorder manifests as extremely pruritic papules that develop into plaques and possibly erythroderma, predominantly in the elderly. The occurrence of such distinctive symptoms, nevertheless, may make a differential diagnosis from other cutaneous diseases feasible, such as cutaneous T-cell lymphoma. Because of the complexity of PEO, the necessity of careful examination—with a corresponding review of lab findings, such as elevated IgE levels and peripheral eosinophilia—is of tantamount importance for determining a precise diagnosis. Successful management of such disorders can involve topical corticosteroids or systemic therapy like methotrexate. An adequate understanding of these facts underscores the critical role of prudent history-taking and systematic examination in the diagnosis and management of diverse dermatoses (Figure 3.8).

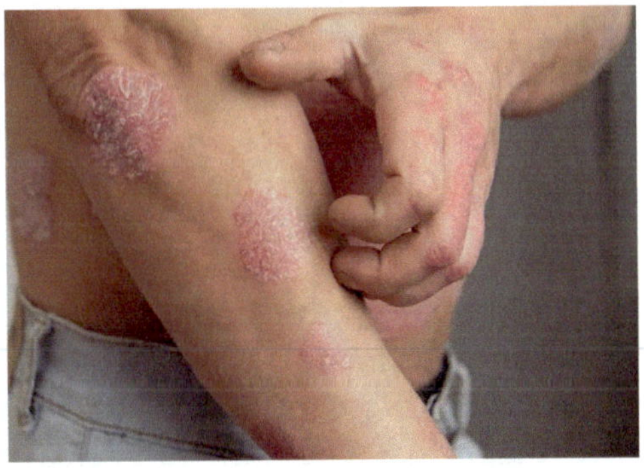

Figure 3.8. Symptoms of psoriasis.

Source: https://kaydermatology.com/storage/2022/12/kaydermatology_Blog_WHAT_IS_PSORIASIS.jpeg.

3.3.1. Types of Skin Lesions and Their Characteristics

Skin lesions present in numerous different ways with distinct characteristics, which could be suggestive of associated dermatologic pathologies. Among the common types are macules, which are flat color changes smaller than 1 cm in diameter and do not consist of an alteration in the skin's texture. They can point to diseases like vitiligo or other pigmentary disorders. Papules, on the other hand, are small lumps on the skin that can be of any size, with a palpable component, typically associated with diseases such as acne or psoriasis. Identification of the fine features of such lesions is required on dermatological history and physical examination, as it leads the clinician to an appropriate diagnosis and effective management. Vesicles and bullae are fluid-filled lesions ranging from a varying diameter, of which vesicles are smaller (less than or equal to 1 cm) and bullae are larger (larger than 1 cm). These lesions are produced by a multitude of etiologies, both infectious and autoimmune, such as herpes simplex and pemphigus vulgaris, respectively. In the presence of blistering disease, note should be taken of flaccid blisters, as these can lead to erosion and affect a patient's quality of life immensely. A thorough physical examination of these characteristics can give significant information about the patient's skin status, allowing for early intervention and treatment modification as prompted by the clinical presentation found during examination (Saffarian et al., 2022). Nodules and tumors are a variety of skin lesions that are characterized by having solid, elevated lesions that may extend further into the dermis. Nodules typically point to lesions greater than 1 cm in size, and they may be indicative of conditions as diverse as benign neoplasms, such as lipomas, to melanoma, which is a malignant growth. Tumors, on the other hand, bring to mind a broader pathological consideration since they typically mandate additional studies such as biopsy or imaging examinations. Moreover, assessment of any associated signs, such as ulceration or color changes, is necessary for the differential diagnosis. Physical examination, combined with comprehensive history taking, significantly aids in distinguishing benign from malignant lesions and facilitates appropriate management for the patient (Schneider et al., 2021) (Figure 3.9).

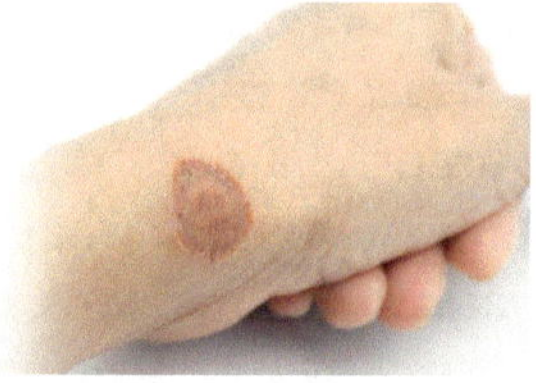

Figure 3.9. Understanding lesion.

Source: https://www.medicoverhospitals.in/images/articles/lesion.webp.

3.3.2. Duration and Progression of Symptoms

The duration and evolution of symptoms are also key aspects to understand in the process of dermatological history taking, as this information is instrumental in making accurate diagnoses. Clinicians have to obtain thorough information about when the symptoms started, the progression rate, and any changes in severity. The temporal aspect facilitates a more comprehensive understanding of the nature of diseases since some dermatologic conditions develop according to certain timelines during their course. As an example, rashes or lesions that develop relatively rapidly can suggest acute inflammatory processes, while those that come on over weeks or months can be indicative of chronic disease. Knowledge of the duration of symptoms and temporal evolution allows dermatologists to distinguish between similar presentations, narrow differential diagnoses, and thus set the stage for a focused physical examination and further investigation. Moreover, symptom evolution can also provide information regarding the underlying etiology and probable precipitants of cutaneous diseases. For example, if the number or size of lesions is increasing, or if secondary symptoms such as pain or pruritus are intensifying, this can suggest an active infectious process or worsening of a chronic inflammatory disease. The clinician's capacity to identify whether symptoms are stable, improving, or worsening over time can guide management and inform patients about the expected course of their disease. It also emphasizes the importance of patient education on symptom monitoring, as such ongoing observation can generate valuable information that will alter treatment or lead to earlier intervention. In addition, temporal dynamics in the course of symptoms can also indicate probable associations with environmental variables to help clinicians better comprehend patients' conditions. Some dermatologic features might be associated with environmental exposures, lifestyle changes, or comorbidities that could influence symptom intensity and duration. This multi-faceted approach is significant in situations where adverse events, as indicated in clinical trial outcomes, reveal findings that symptoms may worsen over time—such as an increase in falls or injuries with specific medications, such as verubecestat (Aisen et al., 2019). A systematic assessment of symptom duration and progression not only guides short-term medical management but also paves the way for future care, enabling an evidence-based response to shifting patient needs (Adaskevich et al., 2014).

3.3.3. Associated Systemic Symptoms

When conducting dermatological skin examinations, determining systemic symptoms associated with is essential in rendering an inclusive diagnosis. The skin is typically an expressive organ, reflecting more generalized systemic conditions that present as dermatologic manifestations. Autoimmune illnesses, infections, and cancers usually present with cutaneous findings and systemic symptoms such as fever, weight loss, or fatigue. For instance, the presence of a new rash and systemic signs might suggest an underlying condition that requires early investigation, such as vasculitis or systemic lupus erythematosus. Identification of such associated signs not only guides the diagnostic process but also determines treatment urgency, which is critical to treatment outcomes. Knowledge of the interconnections between dermatologic diseases and systemic illnesses is also critical to optimizing patient management. Diseases like gastric cancer, for example, are known to have distinct dermatological presentations that are precursors to further disease.

As can be observed in Ajani et al. (2022), gastric cancer is going to be associated with systemic signs at the time of diagnosis of advanced disease, potentially overshadowed by skin findings. The value of a thorough dermatological history becomes apparent, as recognition of these associations can lead to earlier detection of malignancy and improved survival. Clinicians should be careful when assessing these signs of a systemic nature, as early treatment is able to modulate progression and enhance the quality of life of the patients, in addition to treating both cutaneous and overall health status. Patient care for systemically presenting patients also requires a multidisciplinary team, particularly if irAEs develop during immunotherapy. As described by Schneider et al. (2021), immune checkpoint inhibitor-treated patients may experience skin manifestations and a variety of systemic symptoms, for which management strategies must be tailored to each patient. Defining these irAEs and their treatment with multidisciplinary approaches is crucial to complete treatment for both dermatology and systemic health. The treating physicians must be vigilant in observing and responding to symptom severity, and judiciously employ corticosteroids and immunosuppressants. This approach emphasizes the importance of careful dermatological history taking and clinical examination, as it provides the foundation for identifying systemic disease and initiating early therapeutic interventions (Figure 3.10).

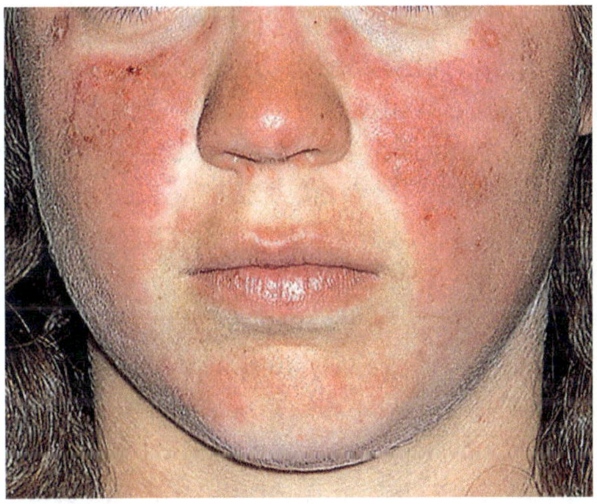

Figure 3.10. Systemic lupus erythematosus.

Source: https://solmed-clinic.com/wp-content/uploads/2023/05/acute_cutaneous_lupus_erythematosus1.jpg.

Test Your Knowledge

1. What are the types of skin lesions?
2. What are the systemic symptoms?

3.4. Medical and Family History

Learning Outcome

1. Understand the relevance of past medical history in dermatology
2. Understand the family history of skin conditions
3. Know the impact of medications and allergies on skin health

Taking medical and family history is a key component of dermatological history-taking because it helps the clinician identify potential predisposing factors for skin disorders. Indeed, taking a thorough medical history includes the patient's history of prior skin conditions, treatments, and allergies, which may provide valuable background for the current dermatological condition. In addition, understanding a patient's prior medical interventions and responses can help clinicians tailor effective treatment regimens. For instance, individuals who have had eczema in the past will respond differently to certain dermatologic medications than individuals with no history of the condition. Establishing these differences makes the treatment individualized and effective, thereby reducing the likelihood of aggravating the conditions or causing side effects. This cautious approach underscores the importance of comprehensive data collection during the initial consultation, as reaffirmed by studies emphasizing history-taking as an important step toward good exams and interventions (Alkhaqani, 2023). Family history has a special bearing on dermatological assessment, as it can detect inherited predisposition to many skin disorders, including psoriasis, melanoma, and acne. Careful history-taking regarding the patient's family relationships might uncover tendencies toward inheritance that are not evident on physical examination. For instance, a patient with a family history of having numerous members who have been diagnosed with skin cancers might need more intensive screening and prevention than those without such a history. Family data are important because they can contribute to the robustness of early detection strategies and warn patients about lifestyle modifications that can reduce their risk factors. Additionally, understanding inherited skin disease can help patients become informed about their susceptibility, enabling them to make appropriate decisions regarding monitoring and preventive treatment (Sonne et al., 2021). This data not only supports the clinician's diagnostic ability but also helps create a collaborative patient-clinician relationship founded upon active health management. Integration of medical and family history enables comprehensive knowledge of dermatologic disease rather than isolated symptomatology.

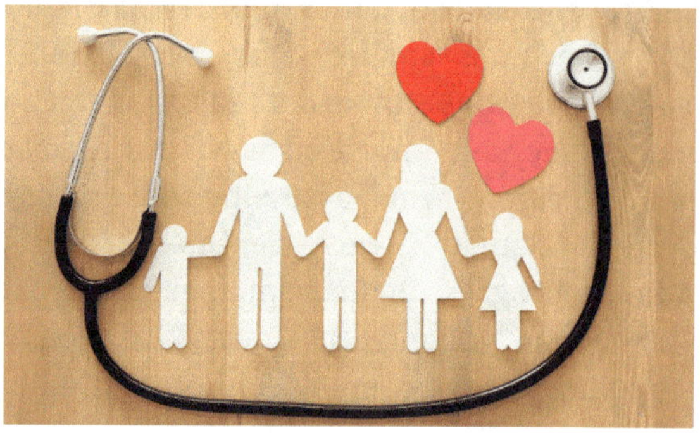

Figure 3.11. Family health history.

Source: https://familytreemagazine.com/wp-content/uploads/2020/09/exploring-family-health-history.png.

By integrating medical data with familial dynamics, clinicians can create a more complete patient profile that supports productive diagnosis and customized treatment planning. These global evaluations can reveal underlying system states that manifest as dermatological manifestations, prompting further investigative efforts. The approach also has the ability to enhance patient education since individuals with skin issues prone to genetics can be guided towards desirable lifestyle alterations and prophylactic practices. Therefore, the significance of the medical and family history cannot be overstated, serving as the bedrock for effective dermatological history-taking and physical exams, ultimately leading to enhanced patient outcomes in dermatology (Alkhaqani, 2023) (Figure 3.11).

3.4.1. Relevance of Past Medical History in Dermatology

In dermatology, history cannot be overemphasized, as it is a cornerstone of accurate diagnosis and appropriate therapy. Proper medical history enables dermatologists to note potential relationships between current skin disease and patients' past illnesses. This is particularly important in relation to chronic or recurrent dermatoses, as most skin diseases are driven by systemic factors. For instance, conditions like eczema and psoriasis often co-occur with comorbidities, such as allergies or autoimmune diseases, which influence treatment regimens. By including background data in the diagnosis, doctors can tailor their interventions to each patient's unique needs, thereby enhancing the overall quality of care and the likelihood of successful outcomes. Further, an understanding of the skin's dermatological history is paramount to determining patterns and predisposing situations related to skin disease. Information regarding family background tends to identify genetic situations and thus indicates why dermatological examination among individuals with a disease history among relatives, like melanoma or atopic dermatitis, is valuable. It is possible to monitor and prevent more aggressively once these patterns are identified, especially in individuals at increased risk. In addition, knowledge of the history of prior treatment and its efficacy helps clinicians to formulate individualized management strategies without duplicating unnecessary procedures that may have failed in the past. This dynamic interaction between past medical history and skin examination provides a more comprehensive approach to dermatological care, ultimately leading to better patient satisfaction and health outcomes. Finally, advances in technology and data management, including the potential use of digital twins, could leverage the value of past medical history in dermatology. Integrating artificial intelligence into assessing complete medical histories can enable a highly individualized paradigm of patient care by correlating many biological and clinical data points. These systems can improve decision-making processes, as evidenced by their use in complex conditions, including multiple sclerosis, where individualized management plans are critical. In dermatology, this technology may improve understanding of the patient's presentation and response to interventions, facilitating the formulation of individualized therapeutic approaches. As the field advances, the careful integration of past medical history with cutting-edge technology will become a revolutionary force in maximizing clinical results in dermatologic practice, marking a significant milestone toward precision medicine.

3.4.2. Family History of Skin Conditions

Dermatologists should always take the family history of skin disease. Knowledge of the family history of skin disorders is a critical component of dermatologic history taking and physical examination. An effective exploration of the patient's family history might reveal trends in inherited skin ailments, such as eczema, psoriasis, or melanoma. Not only does this aid in the making of current dermatological conditions diagnoses, but it can also aid in the prediction of future skin-related health threats for the patient. Because the states of the skin can have genetic origins, the practitioners must thoroughly review the patients' relatives' medical histories and observe any familial tendencies that can be used to direct treatments. Such a thorough examination can make it possible for clinicians to play an active role in the early management of inherited skin diseases, making them more tangible. Last but not least, patient engagement in discussing family history improves collaboration and, consequently, dermatological condition management in a familial setting (Alsararatee, 2025). Moreover, the familial implications extend beyond mere diagnosis; they are used to develop prevention strategies. For instance, individuals with a family history of first-degree relatives with certain skin diseases may be assisted with lifestyle modification or regular skin examinations. Patients must be counseled regarding how their genetic predisposition may influence the development and progression of dermatologic disease. As demonstrated in studies in which incidental findings of dermatologic disease changed management strategies, providers may use family history to perform more targeted examinations and anticipate particular complications. Including anogenital examination in routine assessments can uncover issues not identified through history taking. Adding family history to the diagnostic process thus enhances the quality of care and improves outcomes by managing existing conditions and upcoming threats (Phillips et al., 2025). Finally, the socio-cultural dimension of family history and skin diseases cannot be overlooked. Patients may belong to cultures where family medical history is not the norm to be discussed, and this could result in gaps in data gathered during the consultation. Clinicians, then, need to proceed with such conversations with cultural sensitivity and appreciation of patients' comfort levels. Promoting open discussions about familial skin conditions can help demystify fears and perceptions of skin health that may be prevalent in specific communities. In doing so, healthcare workers can build trust with their patients and therefore obtain a more complete medical history. This not only contributes to more specific interventions but also encourages individuals to take an active interest in their dermatological health, thereby promoting better outcomes in skin condition management (Alsararatee, 2025) (Figure 3.12).

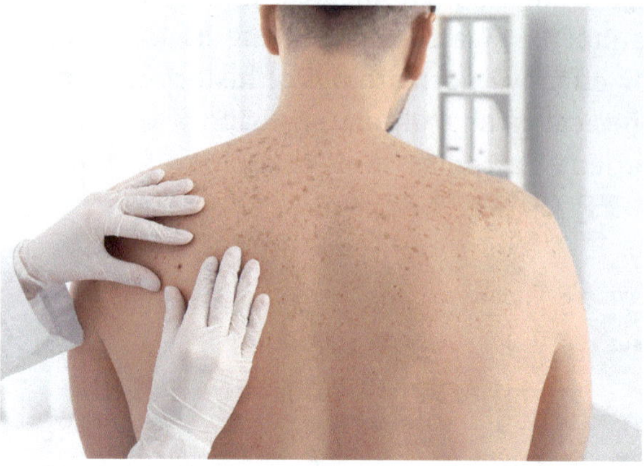

Figure 3.12. Family's history of melanoma.

Source: https://www.thebowmaninstitute.com/wp-content/uploads/2021/02/116150758_s.jpg.

3.4.3. Impact of Medications and Allergies on Skin Health

The influence of drugs on skin health is a significant factor to be addressed while taking the dermatological history and physical examination. Adverse drug reactions (ADRs) significantly influence skin integrity and appearance, typically expressed in various cutaneous drug reactions (CDRs). CDRs can be expressed in numerous ways, including urticaria, maculopapular eruptions, and severe forms such as Stevens Johnson syndrome, which take place with a range of medications. A hospital-based observational study recognized that the causative drugs in cutaneous reactions in children are frequently cotrimoxazole and NSAIDs, which cause a large percentage of cutaneous reactions. Information on offending drugs for skin-related ADRs enables clinicians to better advise patients on potential risks and adjust medications to avoid adverse effects, thereby enhancing patient outcomes and skin health (Alessandro et al., 2020). Besides drugs, allergies play a major role in skin health as they have the potential to trigger allergic reactions that result in various dermatological conditions. Allergic reactions can be initiated by environmental factors such as pollen, animal dander, or food, to produce cutaneous manifestations such as atopic dermatitis, contact dermatitis, or urticaria.

The relationship between skin health and allergies is a good demonstration of how the immune response influences the appearance and barrier function of the skin. In addition, it has been indicated in recent studies that psychological stress caused by an allergy can aggravate skin disorders, including alopecia areata, by weakening the immune system. Individual case reports correlated the onset of alopecia areata with COVID-19 infection, suggesting viral infections could trigger autoimmune responses in genetically predisposed individuals (Alessandro et al., 2020).

Such complex interactions necessitate meticulous dermatological history to explore drug use as well as allergy history in evaluations. It is also important to integrate information on drug effects and allergies into the assessment of skin status in dermatological practice to improve patient care. Clinicians must employ a rigorous system that involves extensive patient interviews, taking into account not only current medications and potential allergens but also patients' past dermatologic issues. This process might lead to improved diagnoses and customized treatment regimens designed to avoid harmful reactions. In pediatric populations, in which the risk of CDPs is typically heightened by the widespread use of antibiotics and other medications, this framework is all the more necessary. Thus, understanding how medications and allergies affect skin health should be an integral component of dermatology education and practice, ultimately improving the quality of patient care (Rahman et al., 2020) (Figure 3.13).

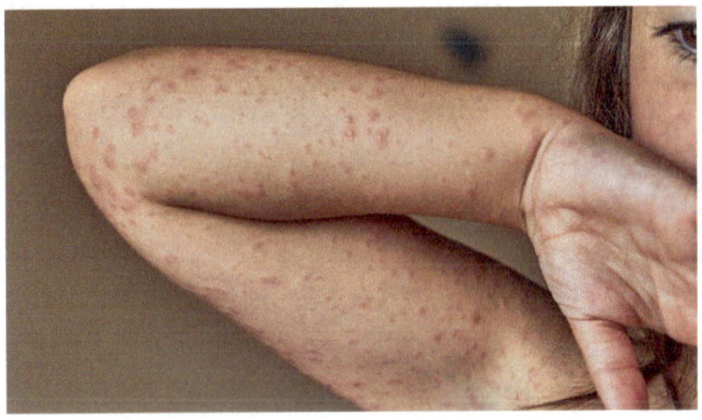

Figure 3.13. Allergic reactions to antibiotics.

Source: https://www.grxstatic.com/4f3rgqwzdznj/2TaXFCCvvdpN2MdWVmTpoE/4e3d68bea6db1eb537556cd181db8a14/cropped_womans_arm_allergic_rash-1337085512.jpg?format=pjpg&auto=webp&width=704.

Test Your Knowledge

1. Describe the family history of skin conditions.
2. What is the impact of medications and allergies on skin health?

3.5. Physical Examination Techniques

Learning Outcome

1. Understand the visual inspection of the skin
2. Understand the palpation and its role in diagnosis
3. Describe the use of dermatoscopy in examination

As components of dermatological history-taking and physical examination, systematic physical examination techniques are most important for providing accurate diagnosis and effective treatment planning. An accurate examination begins with the skin examination, which not only involves naked-eye observation of lesions but also assessment of their characteristics, such as color, shape, size, and pattern. Such observational skills are crucial, as they can provide significant clues to the conditions beneath, thereby enabling practitioners to identify cases of malignancies, infections, and inflammatory skin diseases. Furthermore, palpation can elicit additional information, such as the skin's consistency, temperature, and hydration, which can indicate specific dermatological or systemic conditions. Apart from inspection and palpation, dermatoscopy has also been an invaluable tool in dermatological diagnosis. This is an innocuous procedure that uses a dermatoscope to magnify and light lesions on the skin, allowing clear visual inspection of subsurface structures not visible to the naked eye. Dermatoscopy is useful for differential diagnosis because it improves the visibility of pigment patterns, vascular elements, and other morphological features that may be indicative of specific conditions. It is particularly useful in differentiating benign and malignant lesions, where early detection can be critical to the patient's outcome. The integration of dermatoscopic findings with a patient's clinical history can significantly inform the follow-up management and therapeutic strategy. Furthermore, knowledge of the pathophysiology of skin diseases enriches the physical examination. Knowledge of disease mechanisms allows clinicians to recognize minor signs and symptoms that do not conform to classic presentations. For instance, in immune-mediated adverse reactions to immunotherapy, according to current guidelines (Schneider et al., 2021), the physical examination must be adapted in order to assess known organ system-based toxicities. This comprehensive understanding is reflected in urticaria management recommendations, which emphasize the importance of respecting the multi-dimensional character of the condition (Zuberbier et al., 2021). A holistic approach that combines history-taking and meticulous examination techniques can improve diagnostic yield and provide more effective, patient-targeted treatments for individuals presenting with dermatological symptoms (Figure 3.14).

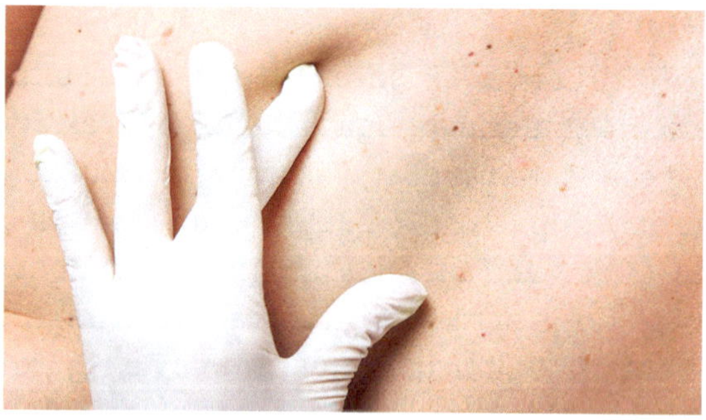

Figure 3.14. Physical examination.

Source: https://www.medline.com/wp-content/uploads/2019/11/STK_SkinAssessment_RGB_840x473.jpg.

3.5.1. Visual Inspection of the Skin

Visual inspection of the skin is a vital component of the physical examination and dermatological history-taking. It involves meticulous scanning of the skin surface for the presence of any abnormality in the form of lesions, pigmentation, and structural changes. It is crucial, as it is often the first port of call for diagnosing many skin diseases, ranging from simple dermatological disorders to more severe pathologies such as skin cancers. Thus, the clinician's ability to detect subtle variations in skin morphology, texture, and coloration can significantly influence patient outcomes. Detailed examinations not only provide essential diagnostic data but also set the stage for further investigation and management planning tailored to the individual patient's disease. Incorporating a structured approach into the visual examination may help the clinician achieve greater diagnostic precision. The ABCDE rule, widely used by dermatologists for mole and pigmented lesion evaluation, focuses on asymmetry, irregular borders, variation in color, diameter, and evolution over time. This approach decreases the risk of missing a diagnosis and brings attention to features representative of malignant changes in those with increased risk for skin cancer. Moreover, visual inspection usually provides an immediate assessment of patients' general health and identifies systemic diseases manifesting as skin changes. On a broader level, employing extensive inspection techniques alongside established guidelines may assist the educational process of health professionals in identifying not just skin disease but also significant underlying conditions requiring interdepartmental management. The arrival of computer-aided diagnosis (CAD) systems once again transforms dermatological practice by introducing technological inputs into visual inspection. Although human experience cannot be replicated, CAD has also gained popularity as an auxiliary tool that helps dermatologists analyze skin lesions more accurately and efficiently. Recent studies highlight the potential of CAD systems to free dermatologists from the vagaries of manual checking, thereby reducing the risk of error, particularly amid a growing patient base with skin problems. The systems have also been instrumental in providing standardized analysis of skin lesions and presenting dermatologists with advanced metrics for evaluation. However, clinical knowledge and visual inspection of the skin remain essential in keeping the optimal level of patient care, as these instruments are ultimately designed to enhance, and not replace, the abilities of observation and decision-making of healthcare professionals (Verkouteren et al., 2021; Hasan et al., 2023) (Figure 3.15).

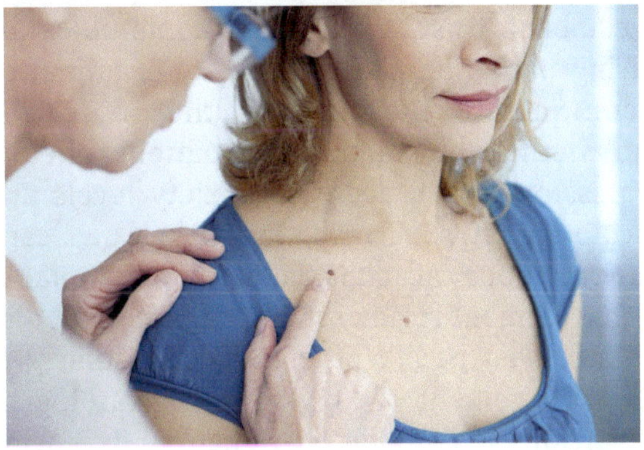

Figure 3.15. Visual inspection of the skin.

Source: https://drhopp.net/wp-content/uploads/2023/10/shutterstock_187808714-1024x683.jpeg.

3.5.2. Palpation and Its Role in Diagnosis

Palpation is a core dermatological tool that functions as a bridge between history and physical findings. By applying various grades of pressure against the skin and underlying tissues, health professionals can assess for texture, warmth, dampness, and tenderness, all significant indicators of dermatological disease. Tactile exploration in this manner allows clinicians to detect normal and abnormal findings and to use them as part of the diagnostic thought process. Moreover, palpation aids in identifying specific dermatological lesions, such as cysts, nodules, or induration, as well as lymphadenopathy, which may signify systemic involvement in skin diseases. Therefore, palpation plays a pivotal role in shortlisting differential diagnoses and deciding further investigation or referral. Apart from enhancing diagnostic efficiency, palpation also promotes a more intimate clinician-patient relationship.

Because dermatology most often involves delicate discussions about the appearance and well-being of the skin, palpation can help reassure patients about the scope of the examination. Dermatologists and nurses, as the literature has emphasized, have an important responsibility to establish trust through clear communication during palpation and other body examination techniques. By explaining the indication and method of palpation to patients, health professionals can decrease anxiety levels and encourage active participation in their own care. Not only does this enhance patient compliance with treatment regimens, but it also contributes to improved health outcomes, particularly in the management of long-term dermatological conditions involving patient participation and partnership. Lastly, the art of palpation is a function of the practitioner's education and experience, highlighting the necessity of formal training in dermatological assessment. Dermatological disorders necessitate delicate palpation techniques best learned through formalized instruction and practice.

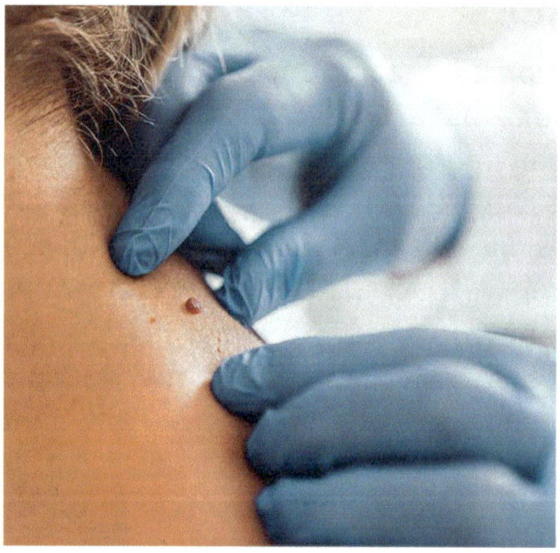

Figure 3.16. Palpation.

Source: https://www.henryford.com/-/media/project/hfhs/henryford/henry-ford-blog/images/mobile-interior-banner-images/2023/05/full-body-skin-exam.jpg?h=600&iar=0&w=640&hash=DA9E46F1643347E109C6F36DF5C6D6DC.

It is evidenced that practitioners and dermatology nurses need professional development to improve such skills. As described by Chukwu et al. (2018), the evolving role of the dermatology nurse is to enhance diagnostic accuracy through extensive patient contact. Moreover, the perceived differences in skin temperature and texture, as with other health examinations, emphasize the value of tactile competence across much of health, including dermatology. The juxtaposition of formal education and field experience positions practitioners to employ palpation as a deciding factor in the diagnostic process, ultimately contributing to better patient care in dermatology (Figure 3.16).

3.5.3. Use of Dermatoscopy in Examination

Dermatoscopy has become a valuable tool in dermatology, greatly enhancing healthcare workers' ability to perform detailed examinations. This photographic technique is innocuous and enables enlarged visualization of the skin lesions, thereby facilitating meticulous assessment of their structure and morphology. As stressed in current studies, dermatoscopy is particularly valuable in differentiating between benign and malignant skin conditions and thus constitutes an essential component of clinical examination. The systematic approach provided by dermatoscopy not just eases diagnosis but also increases diagnostic accuracy, allowing patients to receive timely and accurate treatment. Furthermore, the integration of advanced technology enables healthcare professionals, such as ACPs, to deliver enhanced patient-centered care by improving communication about diagnoses, which may ultimately improve patient outcomes and satisfaction rates (Alsararatee, 2025). The integration of dermatoscopy in the taking of dermatologic history and physical examination represents a paradigm shift in clinical practice. The traditional methods, while helpful, are largely unable to provide comprehensive insight into skin pathology. With dermatoscopy, the clinician can observe features not visible to the naked eye, such as vascular patterns, pigmentary changes, and follicular structures. This extra layer of data is necessary for diseases like malignant melanoma, where early detection is crucial to successful treatment. Aestheticism is only part of dermatoscopy; it is a major player in making the correct diagnosis and therefore in treatment. Such detail is particularly critical when other diagnostic modalities may not work, and the need to include this technique in everyday dermatological practice becomes crucial (Metin et al., 2021). Educational impacts of dermatoscopy should also not be overlooked. As future technologies advance, education of healthcare professionals in dermatoscopic practices is essential to ensure competent, confident practice. With the increasing prevalence of skin diseases, providing formal education to clinicians, especially ACPs, in dermatoscopy can help close the noted performance and knowledge gaps. Training like this provides greater insight into skin diseases and improves accuracy in identifying dermatoscopic characteristics, ultimately resulting in optimal patient care. By integrating dermatoscopy into dermatological practice and education, the specialty has the potential to evolve to meet modern needs and, simultaneously, enhance diagnostic confidence. The role of dermatoscopy is thus not merely pivotal in the context of clinical examination but also pivotal in the professional development of practitioners in the specialty (Alsararatee, 2025) (Figure 3.17).

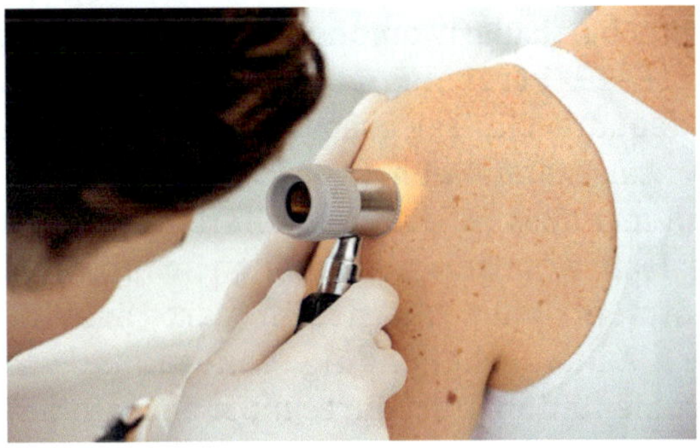

Figure 3.17. Use of dermatoscopy in examination.

Source: https://www.emjreviews.com/wp-content/uploads/2024/11/9am-Derm-5.jpg.

Test Your Knowledge

1. What is palpation?
2. What is the use of dermatoscopy in examination?

3.6. Documentation and Communication

Learning Outcome

1. Understand the importance of accurate documentation
2. Communicate the findings to the patient
3. Know the referral processes for specialized care

Precise documentation and communication are essential aspects of the history-taking and dermatological physical examination. Thorough documentation of patient encounters is not just a legal document but also guarantees continuity of care among healthcare providers. When a doctor carefully documents a patient's history, symptoms, history of past illnesses, and physical findings, it ensures easy, relevant information to use in the future. This is particularly critical in dermatology, where small changes in the patient's skin may presage an underlying systemic issue. Furthermore, the dependability of history-taking and physical examination needs to be complemented by effective physician-to-physician communication, ensuring a concerted approach to managing patients. These elements work together to enhance patient safety and quality of care, emphasizing the importance of systematic communication and documentation in clinical practice. Throughout the COVID-19 pandemic, proper documentation and communication were even more vital. Healthcare workers have had to keep up with evolving clinical guidelines alongside coping with complex diagnostic processes. Studies have shown that diagnostic errors, particularly among patients undergoing COVID-19 screening, often stemmed from inadequate clinical assessment, history, and physical examination (Auerbach et al., 2023). Such mistakes reflect how failure to document can lead to misdiagnosis or an inappropriate treatment plan. As health care providers work under challenging conditions, strict documentation procedures must be maintained not only for the care of unique patients but also for addressing larger public health challenges. It serves to reduce the risk of miscommunication and maintain the health care team's agreement on patient-focused goals. Also, use of technology to enhance documentation and communication cannot be ruled out. Electronic Health Records (EHRs) provide a structured mechanism for capturing patient data, supporting real-time updates and sharing with healthcare teams. In mechanisms such as normalized templates and automated notification tools, EHRs may help mitigate possible inconsistencies in patient data and promote thorough documentation practices. These applications are particularly important in dermatology, where thorough examinations of skin disorders are central to accurate diagnoses and treatment regimens. Moreover, the integration of communication technologies—telemedicine, for example—has transformed the scope of patient interaction, enabling providers to continue care even amid social distancing measures. With advancing healthcare, the harmonious symbiosis of rigorous documentation and sophisticated communication technology remains an essential accompaniment to the provision of effective dermatological care, as the literature emphasizes the importance of effective communication (de Paula et al., 2024) (Figure 3.18).

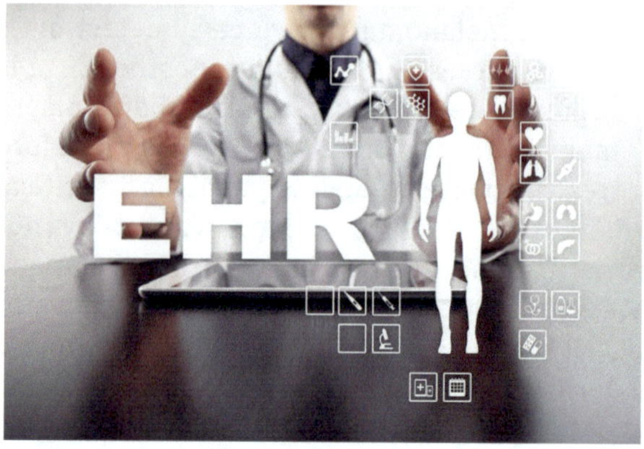

Figure 3.18. Electronic health records (EHRs) for recording patient information.

Source: https://www.medicaltranscriptionservicecompany.com/wp-content/uploads/2022/01/5-ehr-dermatology-practices-use-what-assistance-dermatology-transcription-provide.jpg.

3.6.1. Importance of Accurate Documentation

The importance of proper documentation cannot be overstated in dermatological history taking and physical examination. Documentation is a necessary building block in the clinical practice of dermatology and serves well as a communication tool among health professionals. It ensures continuity of care by providing a record of patient interaction, treatment plans, and clinical findings. Through careful documentation of every meeting, dermatologists and supporting personnel encourage mutual comprehension of a patient's condition, which is paramount in the management of chronic skin illnesses. In addition, good documentation helps monitor the patient's progress through time, enabling appropriate changes to treatment strategies as and when necessary. Through this systematic process, not only is patient care improved but also potential errors are avoided, resulting in improved health outcomes. This is where dermatology nurses are observed rising to prominence, with patient education and treatment regimen adherence front and center, according to a systematic review (Chukwu et al., 2018). Accurate documentation also proves useful in legal and ethical practice in dermatology. Clinical reports are legal documents upon which clinicians may be interrogated in the case of conflict or malpractice. An informative documented case history can justify a clinician's actions and decisions, thereby safeguarding the practitioner and patient. Complete documentation also enables adherence to healthcare law and accreditation requirements. It is possible to establish trends in effectiveness of treatment, which may serve to modify clinical practice for optimal benefit for patients. Given potential complexities in many dermatological diagnoses, accurate record-keeping dispels doubt by providing a firm evidence base for decision-making. In this way, the dermatologist and staff are well-positioned to handle complex cases that often require multi-dimensional management strategies, thereby reinforcing full and accurate record-keeping in practice (Cole et al., 2020). Most critically, accurate documentation goes beyond treating specific patients to inform more extensive public health programs. When dermatologists accurately document cases of skin disease, that information proves highly useful for defining epidemiological trends and incidence of specific conditions in populations. When tallied, researchers can identify risk factors, resulting in preventive measures against diseases such as skin cancer or infectious diseases. Also, accurate data gathering aids in crafting policies to reverse inequalities in dermatologic treatment. Therefore, dermatologists can contribute to developing a larger body of information that influences clinical guidelines and public health policy and improves the dermatology practice as a whole. However, by not following proper documentation procedures consistently, the potential benefits for individual patients as well as public health programs remain unrealized (Chukwu et al., 2018) (Figure 3.19).

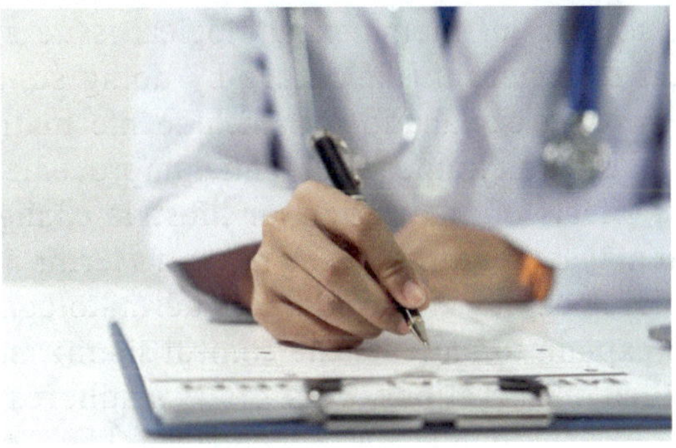

Figure 3.19. The importance of documentation accuracy in patient care.

Source: https://www.proscribemd.com/wp-content/uploads/2024/07/proscribe-313891-documentation-accuracy-patient-blogbanner-1.jpg.

3.6.2. Communicating Findings to the Patient

Good communication of results to the patient is a key part of physical examination and dermatologic history-taking, as it helps enhance the harmonious relationship between the patient and the physician. A proper explanation of the diagnosis ensures that the patient understands and adheres to treatment plans. During consultation, dermatologists must emphasize significant findings pertaining to the patient's condition through aggregation of their observations under physical examination and patient history. For instance, when describing a skin lesion or rash, it is important to note its characteristics, such as size, shape, and color, to give a full picture of the diagnosis. Not only does this candor empower patients, but it also fosters trust, enabling them to actively engage in health care decisions and improving the overall quality of dermatological care. Furthermore, the implications of diagnosed conditions need to be explained in a sensitive yet effective manner. Healthcare professionals should place the results in context, explaining the type of patient condition and potential treatments. Patients will be able to better understand the severity of their dermatological issue and what to expect in the future by doing so. An appropriate explanation can include information about the timeframe for potential improvement, side effects of medication, or lifestyle changes that may be required. Using layman's terms and avoiding excess medical jargon, dermatologists can explain to patients the clinical significance of their observations. This process adheres to best-practice guidelines outlined in authoritative documents and recognizes that successful treatment and patient satisfaction hinge on effective communication (Schneider et al., 2021). Aside from providing clear information, having open conversations with patients about their dermatological outcomes significantly enhances the patient experience. Practitioners must activate patients by asking questions, expressing concerns, and clarifying their condition. Such collaborative discussion not only aids in the eradication of false knowledge but also fosters a sense of patient control over their healthcare. A study found that patients who were proactively involved in discussions about their treatments reported greater levels of care satisfaction (Afonso et al., 2020). Hence, dermatologists need to adopt a sympathetic communication style when answering patients' questions and responding to their emotional responses to their illness. Such an approach not only facilitates a better understanding but also strengthens the provider-patient relationship, ultimately contributing to better adherence to prescribed treatments and improved overall health outcomes.

3.6.3. Referral Processes for Specialized Care

Specialized treatment referral process is an important feature with regard to dermatological history and physical examination, playing an important function to enable patients' access to timely and appropriate intervention. Effective referral systems, when well-organized, can go a long way toward ensuring the transition from general to specialist treatment is highly effective, particularly when skin issues involve complex or systemic ailments. Quality and clarity of the referral are paramount; they can dictate whether the patient's issue is escalated as it should be, or, alternatively, result in inappropriate delays that exacerbate their condition. By incorporating standardized referral protocols, health practitioners can enhance coordination between specialty care and primary care and reduce the vagueness that is traditionally blamed for poor patient outcomes. Further, adaptable clinical care pathways such as those implemented by the Division of Digestive Care and Endoscopy demonstrate good use of referral systems. In a study at Dalhousie University, the use of the SmartPath platform showed a higher rate of accepted referrals than other practices, underscoring the importance of systematic referral pathways for an effective response to patient needs. The ability of such pathways to rank and enable proper investigations equally underscores the importance of including evidence-based tools in the referral process. This reinforces the ability of primary healthcare professionals to make professional judgments about referrals and, consequently, to improve the quality of care provision in dermatology. In addition, remedial improvement of referral process failures extends beyond protecting access to care; it also involves a serious consideration of the quality of the initial assessment by primary healthcare providers. Studies have proven that errors in history taking and physical examinations can lead to inappropriate referrals for patients with complex dermatological presentations. For example, the evaluation of lower gastrointestinal symptoms revealed that most traditional referrals did not include thorough investigative techniques, which may have comparable consequences for dermatological practice (Park et al., 2025). It is thus significant to enhance training and resource allocation for primary care providers, alongside implementing better referral systems. This promise ensures not only that patients in need of advanced dermatology treatment are referred on time but also that they are prepared for proper examination upon arrival at specialized settings (Arsenault et al., 2024) (Figure 3.20).

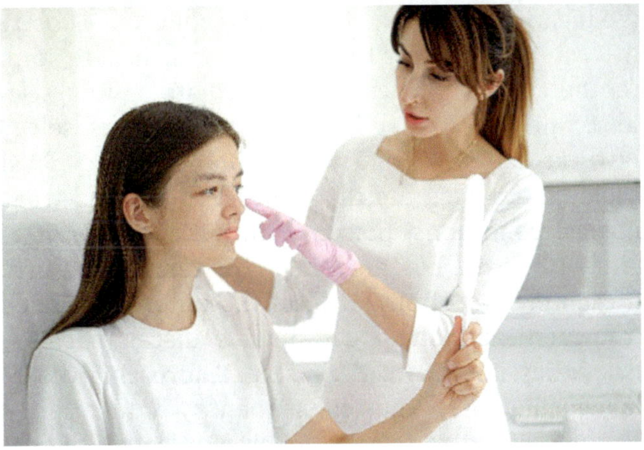

Figure 3.20. examination of the patient

Source: https://facetdermatology.com/cdn/shop/articles/derm-referral_2400x.jpg?v=1736542236.

Test Your Knowledge

1. What is the importance of accurate documentation?
2. Describe the referral processes for specialized care.

SUMMARY

Generally, good dermatological history taking and physical examination are paramount in the diagnosis and management of skin disorders. By gaining a full understanding of patients' histories, health workers are able to obtain vital information that informs clinical decisions and interventions. Patient-dermatology nurse interaction is particularly important because nurses play a crucial role in patient education, thereby supporting adherence to treatment regimens. This enables increased patient-provider relationships, which translate to improved health outcomes. As noted in the literature, the changing roles of the dermatology nurse reflect their significance not only in curing medical conditions but also in facilitating patients' self-management and healing from skin diseases (Chukwu et al., 2018). Further, combining rigid physical exams with myriad history-taking methods yields more accurate diagnoses and tailored treatment plans. Meticulous examination of dermatological conditions, paired with patient interviews, can uncover nuances crucial to understanding individualized health needs. This complementarity is critical, particularly in dermatology, as visual examination often parallels the differential tales patients bring to their illnesses. For instance, the identification of compliance discrepancies usually originates from patients' ignorance of issues they have with their skin. Addressing these voids through effective communication can enhance adherence and, consequently, reduce long-term complications. As such, health professionals must prioritize the art of communication over technical skills to ensure the patient feels heard and directed (Gauci et al., 1997). In addition, ongoing advancements in dermatologic practice encompass technological and research developments, underscoring the necessity for ongoing professional education for healthcare providers. With increasing treatment modalities and knowledge of skin disease, a strong foundation in history taking and physical exam is even more critical. The ongoing development gives a working environment that allows patient-centered care to thrive. It allows dermatology clinicians to remain adaptable and responsive to patient needs, resulting in proactive, rather than reactive, actions to prevent skin disease. Lastly, the commitment to improving dermatologic practice—through careful history-taking, perceptive physical examination, and fostering healthy patient relationships—provides the foundation for exceptional patient care and improved quality of life (Gauci et al., 1997; Chukwu et al., 2018).

In dermatological evaluation, careful history-taking plays a pivotal role in accurate diagnosis and effective treatment. Key factors to consider when moving forward with history-taking include the patient's medical history, family history, and social history that may contribute to skin diseases. For example, careful observation can reveal correlations between systemic infections and cutaneous features. A good example is Mycoplasma pneumoniae, where extrapulmonary manifestations such as skin eruptions may present alongside a primary lung infection, and an accurate history must be taken to identify such complex interrelations (Chan et al., 2024). Besides that, understanding the significance of family history can also give hints regarding hereditary dermatoses and, therefore, allow proper differential diagnoses. Physical examination helps to supplement history-taking by allowing physicians to see and inspect skin lesions more effectively. Dermatologists typically emphasize the need for a systematic approach to inspection, palpation, and dermoscopy in order to properly assess skin abnormalities. For instance, inspecting characteristics such as location, size, color, and texture can facilitate differentiation between various conditions, both infectious and non-infectious ones. An illustrative example is eruptive pseudoangiomatosis, which presents with characteristic lesions that are concerning but self-limiting. Through these educational points of investigation, clinical professionals can avoid ineffective investigations and provide the reassurance patients seek (Mancy et al., 2023). Thus, a systematic physical examination complements history-taking and supports effective clinical decision-making. The integration of physical examination and history-taking provides a well-rounded picture of patients' dermatologic health and emphasizes prevention and management. Conditions like *Mycoplasma pneumoniae*-induced rhabdomyolysis emphasize the need for early detection and intervention to prevent complications in the form of acute renal injury. Similarly, appreciation of benign yet confusing conditions such as eruptive pseudoangiomatosis can help healthcare providers instill confidence and reassurance in the affected. It is significant that clinicians retain these salient points in mind to enhance diagnostic accuracy and maximize the effectiveness of patient care. Lastly, the incorporation of historical findings and formal physical examination enhances depth of insight into dermatologic issues, allowing for precise treatments and improved patient outcomes.

KEY TERMS FROM THIS CHAPTER

Autoimmune diseases
Distribution
Family history
Medical practices
Patient care
Physical examination
Skin disorders
Dermatological health
Environmental exposures
Infections
Morphology
Patients history
Skin cancers
Stress

CRITICAL THINKING QUESTIONS

1. **What is the first step in taking a dermatological history?**
   a. Conducting a physical examination
   b. Asking about the patient's medical history
   c. Identifying the chief complaint
   d. Reviewing the patient's family history
2. **Which of the following questions is most relevant when assessing a patient's skin condition?**
   a. Do you have a history of diabetes?
   b. Have you noticed any changes in your skin lesions?
   c. What medications are you currently taking?
   d. All of the above
3. **When evaluating a skin lesion, the acronym "ABCDE" is used to assess which condition?**
   a. Psoriasis
   b. Melanoma
   c. Eczema
   d. Fungal infections
4. **What does the "D" in the ABCDE rule for melanoma stand for?**
   a. Depth
   b. Diameter
   c. Distribution
   d. Duration
5. **In dermatological history taking, which aspect of the lesion is crucial to document?**
   a. Onset and duration
   b. Progression and associated symptoms
   c. Exacerbating and relieving factors
   d. All of the above

Short Answer Questions

1. What is the dermatologic history taking?
2. Why is history taking important in dermatology?
3. What are patient interview techniques?
4. What are dermatological symptoms?
5. What are the physical examination techniques?

Answer to Critical Thinking Questions

1. (c); 2. (d) ; 3. (b); 4. (b); 5. (d)

REFERENCES

1. Adaskevich, V. P., Katsina, M. A., & Tsikhanouskaya, I. V. (2014). *Basic Dermatology*. https://core.ac.uk/download/80151520.pdf (accessed on 21st July 2025).
2. Afonso, N., Kelekar, A., & Alangaden, A. (2020). "I have a cough": an interactive virtual respiratory Case-Based module. *MedEdPORTAL, 16*, 11058. https://doi.org/10.15766/mep_2374-8265.11058Aisen, P. S., Cummings, J. L., Egan, M. F., Furtek, C., et al. (2019). Further analyses of the safety of verubecestat in the phase 3 EPOCH trial of mild-to-moderate Alzheimer's disease. https://core.ac.uk/download/228082265.pdf (accessed on 21st July 2025).
3. Ajani, J. A., D'Amico, T. A., Bentrem, D. J., Chao, J., Cooke, D. T., Corvera, C. U., Das, P., et al. (2022). Gastric cancer, version 2.2022, NCCN clinical practice guidelines in oncology. *Journal of the National Comprehensive Cancer Network, 20*, 167–192. https://doi.org/10.6004/jnccn.2022.0008 (accessed on 21st July 2025).
4. Alkhaqani, A. L. (2023). Nursing assessment of cardiovascular system: Importance of history taking and physical examination. *Cardiology Research and Reports*. https://www.semanticscholar.org/paper/e1bf2090af75cbb7c36465f780c0a1b6ae41f49b (accessed on 21st July 2025).
5. Alsararatee, H. H. (2025). Dermatological assessment: History-taking and examination. *Practice Nursing*. https://www.semanticscholar.org/paper/a9b6629e181830c76a91101c82a411845ed909d3 (accessed on 21st July 2025).
6. Alsararatee, H. H. (2025). Diagnostic tools and methods for dermatological assessment. *British Journal of Nursing, 34*(10), 502–512. https://www.semanticscholar.org/paper/ae08b26fe2d5e778641269080861808c9894fd6b (accessed on 21st July 2025).
7. Arsenault, C., Mfeka-Nkabinde, N. G., Chaudhry, M., Jarhyan, P., Taddele, T., Mugenya, I., Sabwa, S., et al. (2024). Antenatal care quality and detection of risk among pregnant women: An observational study in Ethiopia, India, Kenya, and South Africa. *PLOS Medicine, 21*. https://www.semanticscholar.org/paper/be9e099294c2269a3c8a18ccac335feed05fab53 (accessed on 21st July 2025).
8. Auerbach, A. M. M. D., Astik, G. J. M. D., O'Leary, K. J. M. D., Barish, P. N. M. D., Kantor, M. A. M. D., Raffel, K. R. M. D., Ranji, S. R., et al. (2023). Prevalence and causes of diagnostic errors in hospitalized patients under investigation for COVID-19. *Journal of General Internal Medicine, 38*, 1902 1910. https://www.semanticscholar.org/paper/ab1390ec4e235cfeecd91f0bdd1c39cd2c7d8480 (accessed on 21st July 2025).
9. Bhatia, S., Pappo, A. S., Acquazzino, M., Allen-Rhoades, W., Barnett, M., Borinstein, S. C., Casey, R., et al. (2023). Adolescent and young adult (AYA) oncology, version 2.2024, NCCN clinical practice guidelines in oncology. *Journal of the National Comprehensive Cancer Network, 21*, 851–880. https://doi.org/10.6004/jnccn.2023.0040 (accessed on 21st July 2025).
10. Capalbo, A., Giordano, D., Gagliostro, N., Balampanos, C. G., Flavia, P., Orrù, F., & Severino, P. (2020). Alopecia areata in a COVID-19 patient: A case report. *Dermatologic Therapy, 34*. https://www.semanticscholar.org/paper/8c803521b8f0accb2090e831c125feda1e16f13d (accessed on 21st July 2025).

11. Chan, J., Biddle, K., Gray, A., & Fernando, M. (2024). P24: A case of mycoplasma-induced rhabdomyolysis. *Rheumatology Advances in Practice, 8*. https://www.semanticscholar.org/paper/4f0f155824a6c5bad4beeeed1f7c2fd2005f1840 (accessed on 21st July 2025).
12. Chukwu, R., & Mankila, J. (2018). Dermatology nurses' job description: Literature review. https://core.ac.uk/download/161432240.pdf (accessed on 21st July 2025).
13. Coelho de Paula, B. A., Haberland, D. F., Guilherme, F. J. A., Barbosa, B. L., Oliveira, A. B., & Monteiro da Silva, T. A. S. (2024). Aerospace nurses' competencies in disaster situations: A scoping review. *Revita Latino-Americana de Enfermagem, 32*. https://www.semanticscholar.org/paper/a9c90b39a92633f610d705ddb86839dd6abfced8 (accessed on 21st July 2025).
14. Cole, S. A. (2020). Individual and collective identification in contemporary forensics. https://core.ac.uk/download/323082704.pdf (accessed on 21st July 2025).
15. Farsi, D. (2021). Social media and health care, part I: Literature review of social media use by health care providers. *Journal of Medical Internet Research, 23*, e23205–e23205. https://doi.org/10.2196/23205 (accessed on 21st July 2025).
16. Gauci, M., & Vella, N. (1997). Occupational screening. https://core.ac.uk/download/46601749.pdf (accessed on 21st July 2025).
17. Hasan, M. K., Ahamad, M. A., Yap, C. H., & Yang, G. (2023). A survey, review, and future trends of skin lesion segmentation and classification. *Computers in Biology and Medicine, 155*, 106624–106624. https://doi.org/10.1016/j.compbiomed.2023.106624 (accessed on 21st July 2025).
18. Kumar, R. G. S., Parvathi, N. C., Suresh, R., Vinay, N., & Vivekananda, I. (2021). Efficacy and safety of povidone iodine with dimethyl sulfoxide vs 0.05% tretinoin in treatment of molluscum contagiosum: A randomized case control study. *Our Dermatology Online*. https://www.semanticscholar.org/paper/70b95dd14f636323281a6f5bf4895906ae8442eb (accessed on 21st July 2025).
19. Mancy, A., Awad, M., & Hafedh, Z. (2023). Eruptive pseudo angiomatosis: An epidemiological and clinical study. *Our Dermatology Online*. https://www.semanticscholar.org/paper/893a3260d9e825975705245aaee2570bd149a020 (accessed on 21st July 2025).
20. Metin, Z., & Metin, M. (2021). Role of food allergy in the etiology of infantile eosinophilic pustular folliculitis. *Pediatric Allergy and Immunology, 33*. https://www.semanticscholar.org/paper/fdba6042affd3df624a7479b68f75f80f640cdb0 (accessed on 21st July 2025)
21. Mulcare, M. R., Naik, N., Greenwald, P., Schullstrom, K., Gogia, K., Clark, S., Kang, Y. H., et al. (2020). Advanced communication and examination skills in telemedicine: A structured simulation-based course for medical students. *MedEdPORTAL*. https://doi.org/10.15766/mep_2374-8265.11047 (accessed on 21st July 2025).
22. Northrup, H., Aronow, M. E., Bebin, E. M., Bissler, J. J., Darling, T. N., de Vries, P. J., Frost, M., et al. (2021). Updated international tuberous sclerosis complex diagnostic criteria and surveillance and management recommendations. *Pediatric Neurology, 123*, 50–66. https://doi.org/10.1016/j.pediatrneurol.2021.07.011 (accessed on 21st July 2025).
23. Park, G., Stewart, M., Jones, J., & Willett, N. (2025). A103 GUTLINK SMARTPATH: An online tool to improve patient care. *Journal of the Canadian Association of Gastroenterology, 8*, i40–i41. https://www.semanticscholar.org/paper/91b14733282efe0aa2c0ff4d07ce5506e26543e3 (accessed on 21st July 2025).

24. Phillips, R., & Crock, C. (2025). Value of whole skin examination in older children presenting with skin conditions. *Pediatric Dermatology*. https://www.semanticscholar.org/paper/29edbd9730b3ad7c57dbf40a1635e3320560e0fe (accessed on 21st July 2025).

25. Qureshi, F., Hughes, A., & Natkunarajah, J. (2020). Methotrexate for papuloerythroderma of Ofuji. *Clinical and Experimental Dermatology, 45*. https://www.semanticscholar.org/paper/d4eb59f0f606d39dd4a5b7905a6ac6c430e173ea (accessed on 21st July 2025).

26. Rahman, M., Khan, A., Chandra, P., Sharmin, L., Rahman, F., & Jamil, A. (2020). Cutaneous drug reactions in children attending a tertiary care hospital. *Taj: Journal of Teachers Association, 33*, 56–62. https://www.semanticscholar.org/paper/f0a6d5f722627c76e6e3037cfd11b090209caf58 (accessed on 21st July 2025).

27. Reeve, J. (2018). The diagnostic approach to coughing in dogs and cats. https://core.ac.uk/download/616484685.pdf (accessed on 21st July 2025).

28. Reinehr, C. P. H., & Bakos, R. M. (2019). Actinic keratoses: Review of clinical, dermoscopic, and therapeutic aspects. *Anais Brasileiros de Dermatologia, 94*, 637–657. https://doi.org/10.1016/j.abd.2019.10.004 (accessed on 21st July 2025).

29. Saffarian, Z., Samii, R., Ghanadan, A., & Vahidnezhad, H. (2022). *De novo* severe pemphigus vulgaris following *SARS-CoV-2* vaccination with *BBIBP-CorV*. *Dermatologic Therapy, 35*. https://doi.org/10.1111/dth.15448 (accessed on 21st July 2025).

30. Schneider, B. J., Naidoo, J., Santomasso, B., Lacchetti, C., Adkins, S., Anadkat, M. J., Atkins, M. B., et al. (2021). Management of immune-related adverse events in patients treated with immune checkpoint inhibitor therapy: ASCO guideline update. *Journal of Clinical Oncology, 39*, 4073–4126. https://doi.org/10.1200/jco.21.01440 (accessed on 21st July 2025).

31. Siviter, P., & Scott, C. (2025). An approach to the incidental sick pig: A toolkit and case discussion. *Livestock*. https://www.semanticscholar.org/paper/2b28a730e2561d89c6488909754b356c370504cf (accessed on 21st July 2025).

32. Sonne, C., Persch, H., Rosner, S., Ott, I., Nagy, E., & Nikendei, C. (2021). Significant differences in written assessments as a result of a blended learning approach used in a clinical examination course in internal medicine: A randomized controlled pilot study. *GMS Journal for Medical Education, 38*. https://www.semanticscholar.org/paper/29bce1a0dd0030519059728ebe918b07f8192d74 (accessed on 21st July 2025).

33. Tasrif, S. M., Imtiaz, D. S. N., Rahman, M. M., Hasan, T., Harun, M., Ur Rashid, H., Sakender, S., et al. (2024). Outcome of myringoplasty with temporal fascia and with sliced tragal cartilage graft—A comparative study. *Medicine Today*. https://www.semanticscholar.org/paper/c49da2c9d525bce8b73362669b36175d2dea1a39 (accessed on 21st July 2025).

34. Verkouteren, B. J. A., Cosgun, B., Reinders, M. G. H. C., Keßler, P., Vermeulen, R. J., Klaassens, M., Lambrechts, S., et al. (2021). A guideline for the clinical management of basal cell naevus syndrome (Gorlin–Goltz syndrome). *British Journal of Dermatology, 186*, 215–226. https://doi.org/10.1111/bjd.20700 (accessed on 21st July 2025).

35. Voigt, I., Inojosa, H., Dillenseger, A., Haase, R., Akgün, K., & Ziemssen, T. (2021). Digital twins for multiple sclerosis. *Frontiers in Immunology, 12*. https://doi.org/10.3389/fimmu.2021.669811 (accessed on 21st July 2025).

36. Wang, H., Jing, X., Liu, L., Shen, X., & Xiong, Y. (2021). Problem-based learning and case-based

learning in dental education. *Annals of Translational Medicine, 9*, 1137–1137. https://doi.org/10.21037/atm-21-165 (accessed on 21st July 2025).

37. Ward, K., Vagholkar, S., Sakur, F., Khatri, N. N., & Lau, A. (2022). Visit types in primary care with telehealth use during the COVID-19 pandemic: Systematic review. *JMIR Medical Informatics, 10*, e40469–e40469. https://doi.org/10.2196/40469 (accessed on 21st July 2025).

38. Yeung, A. W. K., Torkamani, A., Butte, A. J., Glicksberg, B. S., Schuller, B. W., Rodríguez, B., Ting, D. S. W., et al. (2023). The promise of digital healthcare technologies. *Frontiers in Public Health, 11*. https://doi.org/10.3389/fpubh.2023.1196596 (accessed on 21st July 2025).

39. Zuberbier, T., Abdul Latiff, A. H., Abuzakouk, M., Aquilina, S., Asero, R., Baker, D. R., Ballmer-Weber, B., et al. (2021). The international EAACI/GA^{2}LEN/EuroGuiDerm/APAAACI guideline for the definition, classification, diagnosis, and management of urticaria. *Allergy, 77*, 734–766. https://doi.org/10.1111/all.15090 (accessed on 21st July 2025).

BASIC DERMATOPATHOLOGY

4

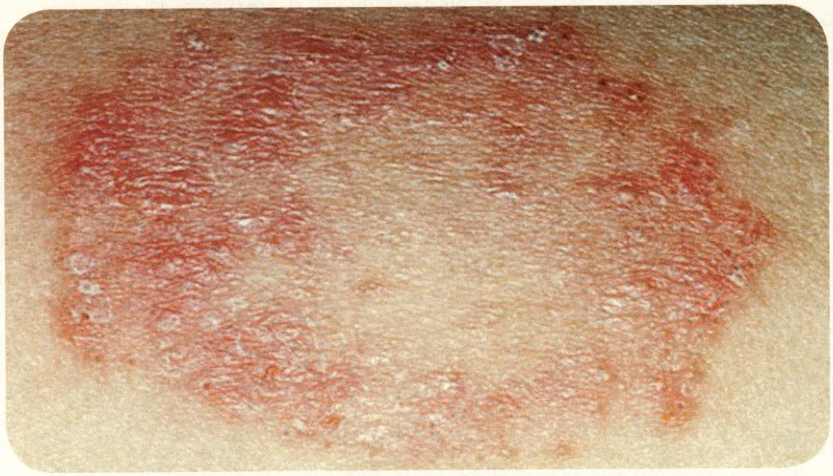

LEARNING OBJECTIVES

After studying this chapter, you will be able to:

1. Know the common skin diseases
2. Understand the diagnostic techniques in dermatopathology
3. Know the inflammatory skin conditions
4. Describe the infectious skin diseases
5. Understand the neoplastic skin conditions

Introduction

The field of dermatopathology stands at the intersection of pathology and dermatology, where the diagnosis of a broad diversity of skin diseases is based on the microscopic analysis of skin lesions. The field emphasizes integrating clinical findings with histopathological data. Dermatopathologists analyze skin biopsies using their expertise to differentiate benign from malignant and inflammatory processes. The method requires a very good command of skin histology, along with an appreciation of complex immunohistochemistry staining procedures. This skill enables such professionals to identify specific markers associated with skin conditions and, consequently, ensure accurate diagnosis and guide effective treatment. Without this blend of learning, accurate dermatological diagnoses would be significantly reduced, underscoring the discipline's significance in clinical practice. In recent years, technological development and imaging techniques have further refined the field of dermatopathology. The employment of high-precision microscopes, digital pathology, and telepathology has transformed pathologists' practices for examining and sharing histology reports. Through these advanced techniques, dermatopathologists can now collaborate regardless of geographic location, providing consultation on problematic cases from a global perspective. These technologies also facilitate the development of artificial intelligence tools to assist in diagnostic processes. Digital pathology not only enhances diagnostic accuracy but also the education component of dermatopathology, enabling better training for future specialists in the specialty. With more dermatopathology becoming a part of this shift, it remains a core element within the broader healthcare system, illustrating the indispensible role that technology plays in patient care. Education and research in dermatopathology play a key role in managing looming challenges in the specialty. Since some dermatological conditions have become commonplace, particularly due to changing environmental factors and heredity, the demand for specialists with current knowledge and competencies has become more urgent day by day.

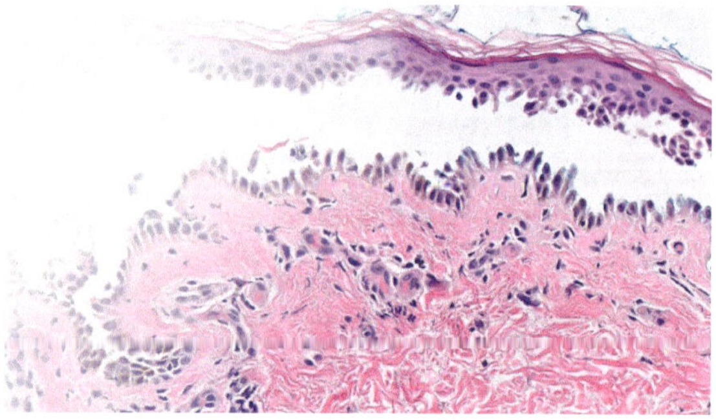

Figure 4.1. Dermatopathology.

Source: https://stanfordlab.com/content/dam/stanfordlabs/marquee-service-pages/banner-dermatopathology.jpg.

Training institutions are responding by expanding their dermatopathology training courses and incorporating the latest research into educational programs, ensuring newly qualified dermatopathologists are well prepared for the demands of current practice. Research programs typically utilize new modeling techniques to forecast workforce supply and demand, emphasizing the impact of emerging technologies and demographics on the specialty. With comprehensive education, the specialty is poised to capitalize on the evolving healthcare landscape. This direct correlation between greater training and improved patient outcomes speaks to the need for ongoing investment in education and research in dermatopathology (+8 other authors et al., 2015; +13 other authors et al., 2015) (Figure 4.1).

4.1. Common Skin Diseases

Learning Outcome

1. Describe the inflammatory skin disorders
2. Learn about infectious skin diseases
3. Describe the neoplastic skin conditions

The multifocal dermatopathology of common skin disorders necessitates a profound understanding of the underlying dermatopathologic mechanisms. Among them, inflammatory dermatoses such as eczema and psoriasis are particularly prevalent and important. Eczema, characterized by red, pruritic lesions, usually arises from genetic factors and may be exacerbated by environmental factors. In contrast, psoriasis is caused by hyperproliferation of the skin cells and the formation of scaling plaques that cause significant distress. Both conditions are expressions of complex interactions between immune response and cutaneous physiology that need to be addressed with targeted therapy directed at these processes in order to treat the symptoms and promote the patient's quality of life. Infectious cutaneous diseases also constitute a significant field of dermatopathology and encompass a range of bacterial, fungal, and viral infections. Infections caused by bacteria, such as impetigo, are most commonly found in children and manifest as crusted lesions caused by *Staphylococcus aureus* or *Streptococcus pyogenes*. Fungal infections, such as those caused by dermatophytes, produce illnesses like tinea corporis (ringworm) that develop in warm, humid climates. Significantly, reflectance confocal microscopy (RCM) has become a useful diagnostic tool that enables real-time visualization of skin lesions caused by these pathogens. Through RCM, clinicians can identify changes in the epidermis and upper dermis, providing insights similar to those of conventional histopathology, thereby improving the overall treatment plan and management strategies for these infections (Arzberger et al., 2020). Further, the study of melanocytic and pigmentation abnormalities underscores the need for ongoing research in dermatopathology.

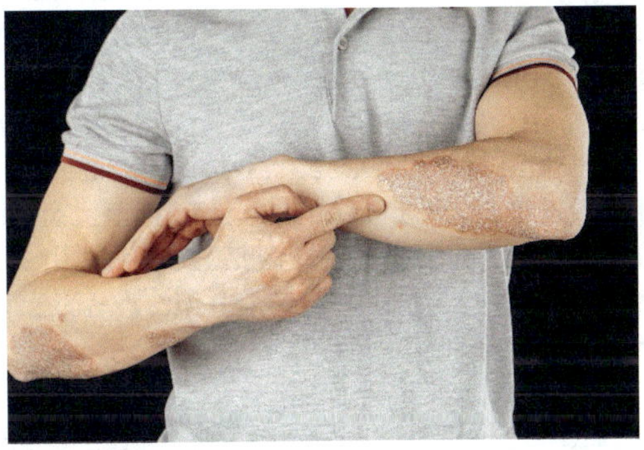

Figure 4.2. Common skin diseases.

Source: https://medanta.s3.ap-south-1.amazonaws.com/blogs/December2024/b3oDWt01ULD2UJxQUDhq35TadOqMkW-metaU2tpbiBEaXNlYXNlcy5qcGc=-.jpg.

Melanoma, an aggressive melanocytic alteration, is a serious danger due to its ability to cause invasive metastasis and mortality. Identification of early melanoma signs through clinical assessment and newer techniques, such as dermoscopy, enables early treatment. In addition, basic research in this area has generated new opportunities to investigate the knowledge of pigmentary disorders such as vitiligo and albinism, which significantly affect physical health and psychosocial quality of life. As scientists aim to learn more about the biology of melanocytes, the results achieved can potentially make treatment processes easier and improve outcomes for patients suffering from these diseases (Birlea et al., 2018) (Figure 4.2).

4.1.1. Inflammatory Skin Disorders

Inflammatory skin diseases are a heterogeneous group characterized by erythema, edema, and often pruritus. These features result from complex inflammatory processes triggered by various etiologic agents, including genetic predisposition, environmental insults, and immune system dysregulation. Some of the most prevalent inflammatory skin diseases include psoriasis, eczema, and dermatitis, which share and possess specific histopathological features. Familiarity with these features is crucial for accurate diagnosis and effective treatment interventions. For instance, psoriasis involves hyperproliferation and dysdifferentiation of keratinocytes, resulting in thickened plaques, while eczema is usually described as involving spongiosis and a lymphocytic infiltrate in the dermis. Distinguishing between the two conditions is crucial, as they require different therapeutic interventions to manage inflammation and re-establish skin barrier function. Reflectance confocal microscopy is now a valuable diagnostic tool in the practice of inflammatory cutaneous conditions. RCM is a completely noninvasive imaging technique that captures high-resolution images of skin lesions in real time, without the need for traditional biopsies. RCM has also been useful in enhancing the diagnosis and treatment of various cutaneous infestations and infections, as it can reveal specific epidermal alterations, such as spongiosis in eczema or the inflammatory infiltrate observed in psoriasis. RCM also allows clinicians to monitor the response to therapy in real-time, reducing unnecessary interventions that can be unhelpful. As such, the integration of RCM into daily dermatologic practice can significantly improve patient outcomes in inflammatory skin diseases (Arzberger et al., 2020). The multifaceted nature of the inflammatory process in the skin is further illuminated by the genetic underpinnings of such diseases as basal cell carcinoma (BCC). Studies have identified genetic differences, particularly in the melanocortin 1 receptor gene (MC1R), that are significantly associated with both BCC susceptibility and inflammatory features of the lesions in involved individuals. Such an association suggests that patients predisposed to inflammatory hyperreactivity, as characterized by their phenotype and genes, may form exaggerated inflammatory responses to environmental incitants and thereby expose themselves to additional risk for malignancies. It is acknowledged that the relationship between carcinogenesis and inflammation reveals shared pathways of dermatopathology that require individualized prevention and monitoring based on unique risk factors, particularly for early-onset BCC cohorts (Bale et al., 2012) (Figure 4.3).

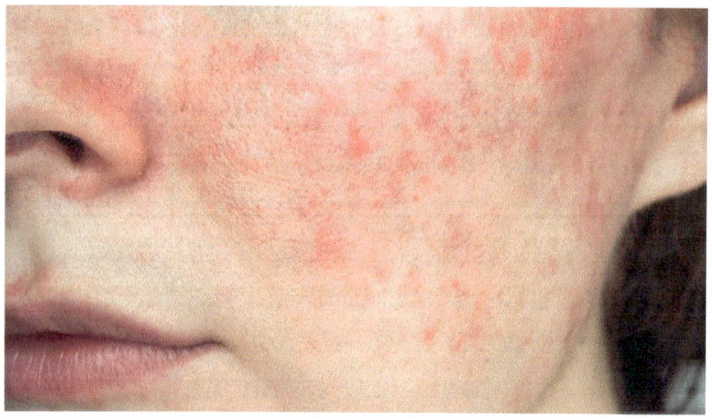

Figure 4.3. Inflammatory skin diseases.

Source: https://cdn.accentuate.cloud/images/59165638808/2-(1)-v1713829848408.webp.

4.1.2. Infectious Skin Diseases

Infectious skin diseases are a significant part of dermatopathology because they encompass a wide variety of diseases caused by a wide array of pathogens, including bacteria, fungi, viruses, and parasites. Bacterial infections such as impetigo and cellulitis tend to be seen as erythematous, tender lesions and can become complicated by systemic spread if not treated. Fungal infections, such as tinea corporis (ringworm), are characterized by annular plaques and can rapidly spread in group settings. The diversity of infectious agents and their related clinical presentations highlights the importance of a solid background in dermatopathology principles for sound diagnosis and treatment planning. Since antimicrobial resistance is on the rise, it becomes essential for doctors to recognize emerging pathogenic strains and to ensure proper management procedures in outpatient and inpatient departments. Reflectance confocal microscopy (RCM) is one such new technology that is changing the face of diagnosis and management of infectious cutaneous diseases. This noninvasive imaging technique enables live imaging of skin structures at the cellular level, which can profoundly enhance diagnostic accuracy. RCM has been most beneficial in evaluating inflammatory and infectious skin diseases because it delineates epidermal and upper dermal alterations. For instance, even though it is impossible to detect viruses directly due to their size, RCM can reveal viral cytopathic effects on keratinocytes, thereby aiding in the diagnosis of viral illnesses like herpes simplex virus. Besides, RCM serves as a strong tool for monitoring treatment outcomes, potentially minimizing unnecessary therapy and improving patient outcomes in the management of infectious skin disease (Arzberger et al., 2020). The dynamic situation of infectious skin diseases also emphasizes the interplay among various microbial agents and host reactions, which demonstrates the complexity of dermatopathology. Scabies, caused by infestation with the mite *Sarcoptes scabiei*, demonstrates how parasitic infestations can trigger severe immune reaction with significant pruritus and secondary infections. In chronic forms, such infections can weaken skin barriers and induce heightened inflammatory responses, culminating in complications like secondary bacterial infections or dermatitis. It is thus crucial to understand the pathophysiology of such interactions to ensure successful treatment regimens. The integration of advanced diagnostic modalities, as reported in available research, offers a perspective into improved management of these conditions and customized interventions based on individual patient needs (Ruiz et al., 2014). Overall, advances in dermatopathology provide fundamental knowledge for preventing and managing infectious cutaneous diseases (Figure 4.4).

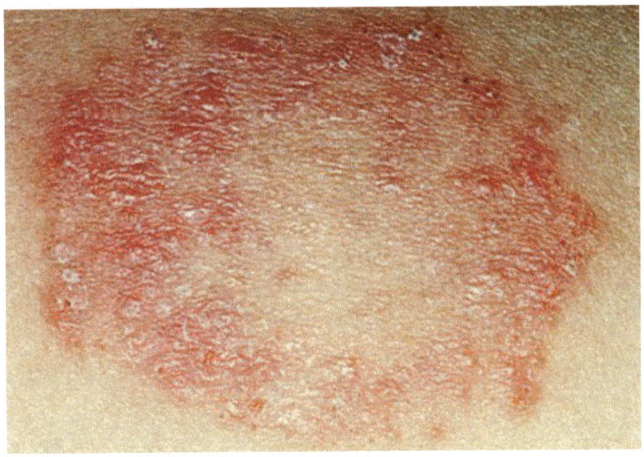

Figure 4.4. Skin Fungal Infection.

Source: https://www.cozmoderm.com/wp-content/uploads/2022/06/skin-infection.jpg.

4.1.3. Neoplastic Skin Conditions

Neoplastic skin disease encompasses a heterogeneous group of diseases involving the pathological development of cells within the skin. The disease may be benign or malignant, with some risk of invasion and metastasis. Among the most common neoplasms are basal cell carcinoma, squamous cell carcinoma, and melanoma, and they differ markedly in cellular origin, appearance, and biological behavior. It is important to respect those differences in making a correct diagnosis and treatment. For instance, while basal cell carcinoma usually presents as an unhealing lesion with a rolled edge, squamous cell carcinoma may present as more painful and aggressive ulceration. The importance of early diagnosis cannot be overstressed, as the diseases are extremely amenable to early intervention procedures, which significantly improve patient outcomes. Sophisticated diagnostic procedures are most useful in the accurate diagnosis of neoplastic skin disease. Dermatopathologists play a pivotal role here, employing a series of laboratory procedures to reach a final conclusion. One such method gaining popularity is cyanoacrylate skin surface stripping (CSSS), in which the stratum corneum and related structures may be harvested minimally invasively. A major benefit of this procedure is that it may be performed painlessly in addition to being minimally hazardous, thus being feasible to administer to patients across any age group. Beyond its potential utility in diagnostics, CSSS can also have applications in experimental dermatology and cosmetology, yielding data on processes such as xerosis and skin barrier function. Such technology has a progressive impact on dermatopathology, ultimately informing patient care and management plans. Treatment for neoplastic skin diseases depends on the specific type and grade of the tumor. The most common treatments are surgical removal, cryosurgery, and topical chemotherapy, each designed to destroy the cancer cells with minimal loss of healthy tissue. Melanoma, as the more dangerous tumor, generally requires more integrated treatment modalities, such as immunotherapy or molecularly targeted therapy, in addition to surgery. The research today is committed to identifying the molecular and genetic bases of the tumors to inform more tailored treatment modalities that hold the promise to transform patient prognosis profoundly. Furthermore, an emphasis on lifestyle determinants such as exposure to UV radiation and genetic predisposition underscores the need for preventive interventions in high-risk groups. As therapeutic modalities evolve, the integration of new modalities has the potential for better control of neoplastic skin diseases (Figure 4.5).

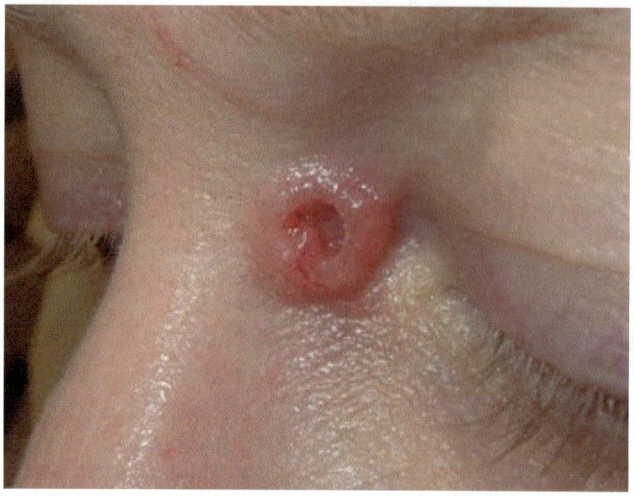

Figure 4.5. Neoplastic skin lesions in the elderly patient.

Source: https://media.springernature.com/lw685/springer-static/image/chp%3A10.1007%2F978-3-540-89656-2_55/MediaObjects/978-3-540-89656-2_55_Fig1_HTML.jpg.

Test Your Knowledge

1. What is the most common inflammatory disorder of the skin?
2. What is a neoplastic skin condition?

4.2. Diagnostic Techniques in Dermatopathology

Learning Outcome

1. Describe the histopathological examination
2. Understand the immunohistochemistry
3. Know the molecular techniques in dermatopathology

The complexity of skin illnesses calls for a diverse array of diagnostic techniques under dermatopathology. Histopathological examination remains the best approach, as microscopic analysis of skin biopsies diagnoses a variety of dermatological conditions. Specialized dermatopathologists interpret tissue architecture, cell morphology, and immunohistochemical profiles to distinguish benign from malignant lesions. Digital pathology developments, more recently, have enhanced the traditional practice of using high-resolution digital images from skin specimens in innovative ways to examine them. With digital imaging, remote consultation and collaborative diagnosis are possible through high-resolution images generated by pathologists. This shift to digital platforms not only increases access to expert opinion but also the pedagogical value of dermatopathology, thereby increasing understanding of dermatological disease among new doctors. The inclusion of these sophisticated methods is critical in increasing diagnostic accuracy and maximizing patient outcomes for dermatology. In addition to histopathology, molecular diagnostic techniques have also emerged as salient in dermatopathology, providing insights at the genetic level.

Techniques such as polymerase chain reaction (PCR) and next-generation sequencing (NGS) may detect specific genetic mutations typically associated with cutaneous cancers. Molecular diagnosis is of great value, particularly where histopathological appearances may be ambiguous or tumors are present uncommonly. Detection of biomarkers may be pivotal in guiding treatment, thereby enabling personalized medicine in dermatology. Furthermore, improvements in in situ hybridization techniques enable localization of specific RNA or DNA sequences in tissue specimens, thereby creating a more specific image of disease processes. As dermatopathologists increasingly incorporate molecular diagnostics into their repertoire, the possibilities for improved prognostic and therapeutic interventions become clearer.

Furthermore, the integration of artificial intelligence (AI) into diagnostic techniques is transforming the field of dermatopathology. Artificial intelligence computer programs have shown promise in evaluating dermatopathological images, aiding pathologists in identifying patterns in various skin diseases. For instance, machine learning algorithms can aid robust analysis of big data, resulting in more consistent and precise diagnostic findings. In a study on examining digital pathology practice, researchers highlighted that scanning and zooming methods play a crucial part in improving detection precision for pathologists viewing breast biopsy images. The distinction between scanning and zooming underscores the need for pathologists to adapt their visual search approach when investigating diverse skin lesions, emphasizing the dynamic nature of diagnosis in this area (Ruiz et al., 2014; Brunyé et al., 2021). As these technologies continue to evolve, their integration into routine practice is poised not only to accelerate the diagnostic process but also to enhance the accuracy of dermatopathological evaluation (Figure 4.6).

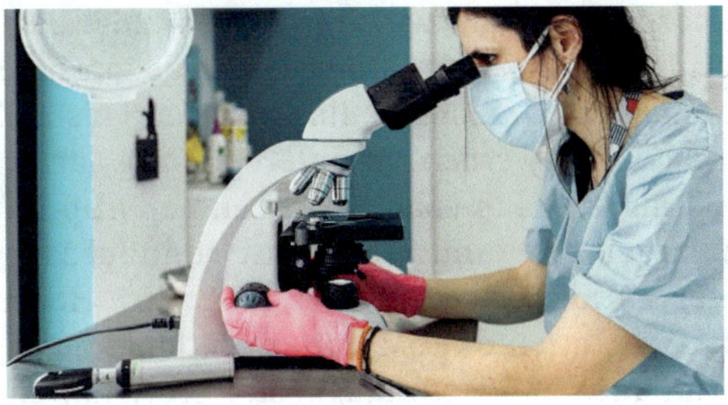

Figure 4.6. Diagnostic techniques in dermatopathology.

Source: https://media.post.rvohealth.io/wp-content/uploads/2022/06/female-scientist-looking-through-microscope-1200-628-facebook-1-1200x628.jpg.

4.2.1. Histopathological Examination

Histopathological examination is a cornerstone of dermatopathology and enables clinicians to make informed diagnoses based on microscopic examination of skin biopsies. It involves studying tissue samples stained by a variety of techniques, including hematoxylin and eosin (H&E), which reveal cellular architecture and pathology. After studying these samples, dermatopathologists can identify malignancies, inflammatory diseases, and infectious diseases. Specifically, the understanding of histopathological findings is based on thorough familiarity with normal skin anatomy and the changes that define many dermatologic conditions. Furthermore, novel imaging tools have been developed to complement traditional histopathology in an effort to increase diagnostic accuracy and predictability in dermatological practice. Recent years have seen advances such as reflectance confocal microscopy (RCM) serving as valuable adjuncts to histopathological examination. RCM enables non-invasive, real-time imaging of the skin and provides detailed information on its architecture and pathologies without exposing the patient to excisional biopsies. RCM's high resolution has been demonstrated by research to reveal minute alterations in the epidermis and superficial dermis, which is comparable to the accuracy of histopathology in the diagnosis of cutaneous infections or infestations. This skill is particularly crucial in differentiating various skin disorders to enable early and appropriate management and rule out unnecessary interventions (Arzberger et al., 2020). Hence, the integration of RCM with traditional biopsy techniques enhances diagnostic precision and marks the future of dermatopathology in the developing world. Also, the use of nonlinear optical microscopy, such as second-harmonic generation (SHG), has revealed new avenues for investigating the cellular and structural composition of skin lesions. The technique effectively maps the collage network and enables investigation of changes associated with granulomatous diseases, such as sarcoidosis and tuberculoid leprosy. Research has highlighted the limitations of standard histopathological techniques for differentiating between such conditions, indicating the need for additional methods (Cesar et al., 2020). By combining SHG with histopathology, dermatopathologists can enrich their diagnostic arsenal, enabling a more comprehensive understanding of disease pathology and improved patient outcomes. This multidisciplinary approach underscores the central role of histopathologic evaluation in the rapidly evolving field of dermatopathology.

4.2.2. Immunohistochemistry (IHC)

IHC is a cornerstone technique in dermatopathology that accurately localizes proteins in tissue sections. By using target antigen-specific antibodies, IHC enables pathologists to visualize where the molecules of interest are located and expressed. This technique is particularly helpful in differentiating neoplastic from non-neoplastic lesions, thereby correctly identifying malignant and benign skin tumors. Identification of specific cellular markers allows one to distinguish very similar-looking lesions, thus informing appropriate treatment procedures. Consequently, IHC not only improves diagnostic quality but also has applications in prognostic evaluation and therapeutic management, further underscoring its significance in dermatopathology. The value of immunohistochemistry extends beyond diagnostic utility; it also helps elucidate the molecular mechanisms underlying skin conditions. Based on the expression levels of various biomarkers, such as cytokines and growth factors, pathologists can infer the underlying pathophysiological processes in inflammatory skin diseases. This information can enable better management of patients by enabling personalized therapy to be initiated based on the molecular signature determined by IHC analysis. Furthermore, advanced IHC techniques, such as multiplex assays, have improved the ability to analyze multiple markers simultaneously.

This is one area of IHC that further enriches the understanding of data achieved through tissue samples, speeding up the shift towards individualized dermatology. Apart from diagnostic and research applications, immunohistochemistry also significantly impacts the evaluation of treatment response in many dermatologic conditions. The ability to quantify changes in protein expression after treatment can guide clinicians in assessing efficacy and adjusting treatment protocols as needed. For instance, in assessing skin cancers, IHC can help determine the extent to which a tumor is responding to targeted therapy and thus guide subsequent interventions. Additionally, as highlighted in recent studies, the use of imaging techniques such as reflectance confocal microscopy (RCM) in combination with immunohistochemistry is likely to enhance diagnostic and treatment monitoring, enabling non-invasive lesion analysis (Arzberger et al., 2020). Such multiple applications underscore immunohistochemistry's pivotal role in advancing dermatopathology and optimizing patient care across a range of skin disorders (Figure 4.7).

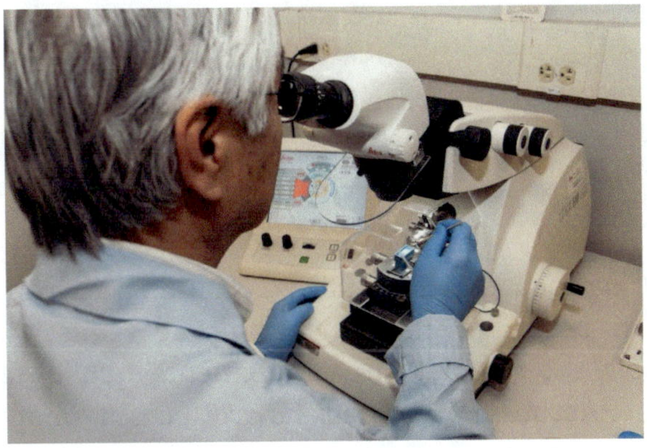

Figure 4.7. Immunohistochemistry (IHC).

Source: https://www.metropolisindia.com/upgrade/blog/upload/2023/07/Demystifying-Immunohistochemistry.jpg.

4.2.3. Molecular Techniques in Dermatopathology

Molecular techniques in dermatopathology represent a crucial milestone in the precision of diagnosis and in the understanding of skin diseases at the cellular level. Such techniques, including polymerase chain reaction (PCR), in situ hybridization, and next-generation sequencing, enable the detection of genetic mutations, microbial DNA, and viral genomes in skin lesions. By analyzing these molecular markers, dermatopathologists can differentiate among dermatological conditions that may histologically appear similar, thereby improving diagnostic accuracy.

This shift towards molecular diagnosis not only optimizes treatment strategies but also enhances disease outcome prediction based on genotypic features. Lastly, the integration of molecular techniques into routine dermatopathology practice will transform the diagnosis and treatment of skin disease, as part of a larger trend toward personalized medicine in dermatology. In the past, the integration of molecular techniques into dermatopathology has been concurrent with advancing technology and expanding knowledge of the genetic etiology of most skin diseases. For instance, melanoma has been positively impacted by molecular diagnostics, with the identification of individual genetic mutations such as BRAF and NRAS having a direct bearing on targeted therapy. Moreover, the techniques not only assist in establishing clinical suspicion but also in identifying emerging pathogens causing chronic skin infections. Such instancesas mycetoma indicate the significance of molecular and histological evaluations in differentiating actinomycetoma and eumycetoma infections, where correct diagnosis is a critical factor in both therapeutic management and prognosis for the patient (Colagrande et al., 2021). This indicates the significant role molecular techniques play in refining dermatopathology's diagnostic model. The dynamic field of molecular techniques has potential in shedding light on dermatopathology areas that were previously unknown or not well understood.

More recent research emphasizes the significance of applying genomic and epigenomic profiling to define diseases such as psoriasis and atopic dermatitis, thereby revealing the immunopathogenic processes involved. Gene expression profile alterations, for example, can be used to detect inflammation and barrier dysfunction pathways and thus present opportunities for more precise therapeutic intervention. Moreover, the fusion of classical histopathological analysis with molecular data improves understanding of skin disease, enhancing diagnostics and research. When these methodologies are combined, they will help increase understanding of disease heterogeneity and open doors to new therapeutic strategies (Ruiz et al., 2014). Lastly, the embracement of molecular techniques in dermatopathology is a significant step towards improved clinical outcomes and patient management in dermatology.

Test Your Knowledge

1. What is an immunohistochemistry test for?
2. What are the molecular techniques used in dermatopathology?

4.3. Inflammatory Skin Conditions

Learning Outcome

1. Understand the histological features of psoriasis
2. Describe the types and diagnostic criteria of eczema
3. Know the causes of dermatitis

Inflammatory skin diseases are a wide range of diseases that are dominated by the dysregulation of the immune system, which primarily brings significant discomfort as well as various degrees of skin damage. These conditions encompass a range of disorders, from atopic dermatitis and psoriasis to more severe variants like cutaneous lupus erythematosus. Pathogenesis is multifactorial, with both genetic predispositions and environmental factors, and complex interactions between the immune cells and skin components. Moreover, recent findings suggest that specific genetic determinants, such as variants in the melanocortin 1 receptor (MC1R) gene, may contribute to susceptibility to inflammatory dermatoses, particularly among people with light skin phenotypes. Unraveling these mechanisms is crucial for the development of targeted treatments that aim to modulate the immune response and suppress inflammation efficiently.

Epidemiologic studies reveal the need for early diagnosis and treatment of inflammatory skin diseases in order to minimize physical as well as psychological impact on patients. Skin diseases like psoriasis and eczema not only affect the external appearance of the skin but also bring about social stigma and emotional distress. The recurrent phases of flare and remission pose the greatest threat to patients' quality of life. Accordingly, physicians are focusing more on patient education to empower patients with self-management techniques, especially during exacerbation, to ensure that they receive maximum emotional support. Further, research into new therapeutic strategies, such as biologics, has shown positive outcomes in severe cases. By targeting the very complex nature of these conditions with an integrated approach, treatment efficacy and overall patient well-being can be maximized. Technological advancements in diagnostic techniques have also contributed to improved outcomes in inflammatory skin disorders. Some of these are reflectance confocal microscopy (RCM), a new tool for the dermatopathology armory, which provides real-time, non-destructive imaging of the skin.

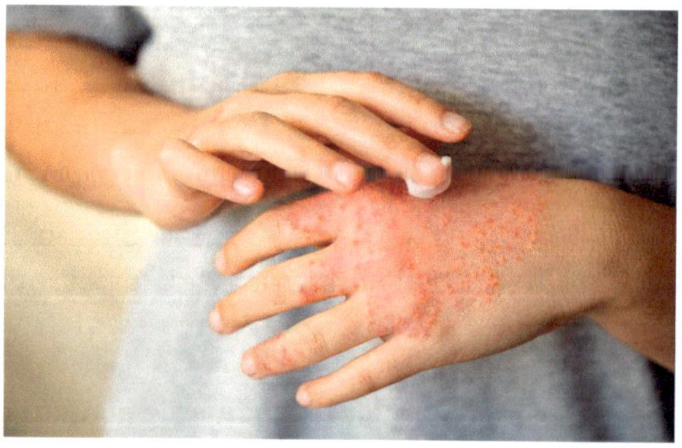

Figure 4.8. Inflammatory skin conditions.

Source: https://cached.imagescaler.hbpl.co.uk/resize/scaleWidth/743/cached.offlinehbpl.hbpl.co.uk/news/2MM/GettyImages-1864570924.jpg.

By enabling visualization of epidermal and superficial dermal alterations typical of most inflammatory diseases, RCM is reported to rival the diagnostic capabilities of standard histopathology protocols. Such an advancement facilitates early and precise disease diagnosis with minimal invasive intervention. RCM also plays a significant role in monitoring treatment response, thus preventing unnecessary and possibly exacerbating treatments. With the advancement of dermatopathology, the incorporation of such new technologies will enhance the understanding and management of inflammatory skin conditions, highlighting the need for research and development in the field (Bale et al., 2012) ; Arzberger et al., 2020(Figure 4.8).

4.3.1. Psoriasis: Pathophysiology and Histological Features

The pathophysiology of psoriasis is complex, with an immunodysregulation and a defective reaction to environmental stimuli. Psoriasis is characterized by a dysregulated inflammatory reaction driven through the T-helper 1 (Th1) and Th17 cell pathways. These inflammatory cells secrete pro-inflammatory cytokines such as tumor necrosis factor-alpha (TNF-α) and interleukin-17 (IL-17), which play key roles in initiating accelerated keratinocyte proliferation.

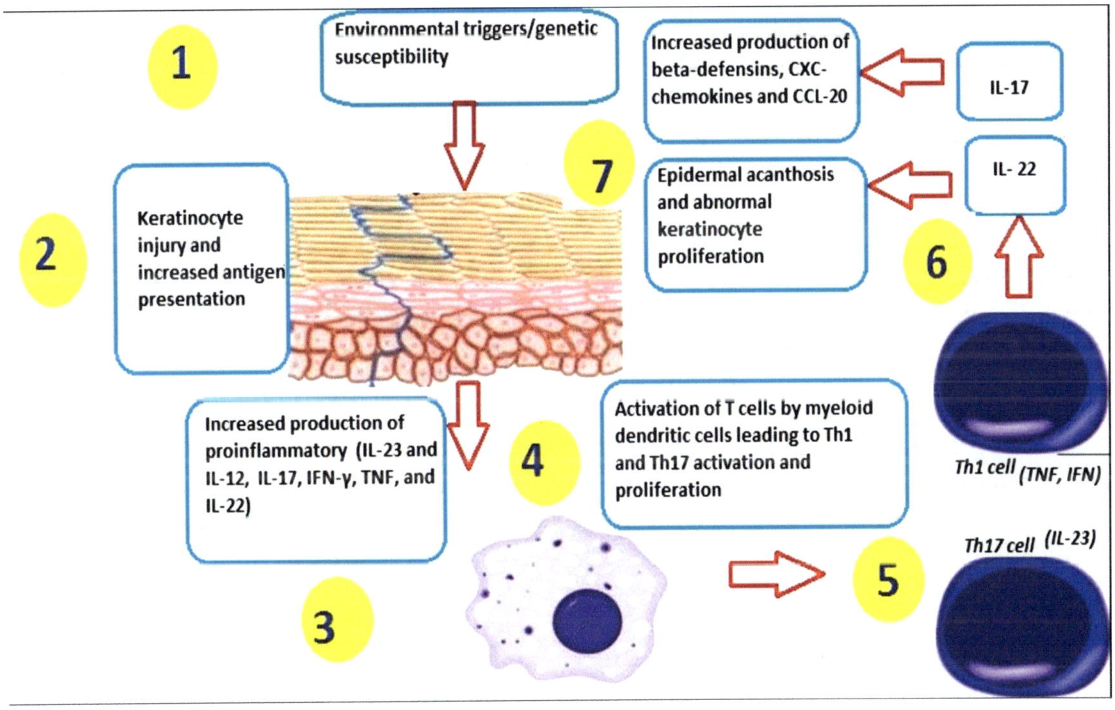

Figure 4.9. Pathogenesis of psoriasis.

Source: https://s3.amazonaws.com/static.wd7.us/4/45/Psorpatho.gif.

This hyperproliferation explains the characteristic thick, scaly plaques observed in psoriasis lesions. More recent evidence has also highlighted genetic and epigenetic factors that may contribute to the pathogenesis and maintenance of the disease. Consequently, understanding these mechanisms enables the establishment of targeted treatments using biologics that inhibit key inflammatory mediators, thus representing a major leap in psoriasis treatment. Histologically, psoriasis has distinct features that are significant for the diagnosis and differentiation from other dermatoses. The epidermis demonstrates marked hyperplasia of the stratum corneum, a parakeratotic scaling pattern, and nuclei in corneocytes. This pathologic keratinization results in the formation of the psoriatic plaques. The dermis is characteristically infiltrated by inflammatory cells, including T lymphocytes, neutrophils, and dendritic cells, which contribute to the disease's inflammatory environment. Increased angiogenesis with elongated dermal capillaries also contributes to the complexity of inflammation. These histological features not only assist in the diagnosis of psoriasis but also provide critical information regarding the underlying pathophysiologic mechanisms that underpin the interaction between immune mechanisms and keratinocyte function (Ring, 2019). The interaction among genetic, environmental, and immunologic determinants provides a multifaceted platform for understanding psoriasis. The role of environmental precipitants, such as infection, stress, and cutaneous trauma, serves to exemplify the complexity of this disorder. Genetic predisposition is evidenced by the elevated heritability measures in familial cases, underscoring the importance of individual gene loci linked to immune response pathways. The greater prevalence of comorbidities such as cardiovascular disease and metabolic syndrome in psoriatic patients also underscores the significant impact of this disease beyond cutaneous expression. These connections call for an integrated approach to management that not only addresses the skin lesions but also addresses the systemic implications of psoriasis, underlining the need for integrated care for the patient (Figure 4.9).

4.3.2. Eczema: Types and Diagnostic Criteria

Eczema, a blanket term for numerous inflammatory dermatoses, primarily includes atopic dermatitis, contact dermatitis, dyshidrotic eczema, and nummular eczema. The most common of these is atopic dermatitis, especially in children, which presents with dry, itchy plaques that may become inflamed. Contact dermatitis, on the other hand, results from skin exposure to allergens or irritants, leading to local inflammation and irritation. Dyshidrotic eczema presents as small, itchy blisters on the hands and feet that are typically set off by environmental factors, while nummular eczema is defined by coin-shaped patches of inflamed skin. Recognition of these distinctive forms not only helps with accurate diagnosis but also guides treatment planning. Due to the diversity of eczema forms in dermatopathology, physicians are required to use a multi-faceted approach to successfully manage patients and design appropriate interventions, underscoring the necessity of reflective diagnostic criteria. Diagnostic criteria for eczema help differentiate among its various forms and inform appropriate management strategies. A thorough patient history, including onset timing, symptoms, and potential precipitants, directs diagnosis. Practitioners also use published criteria, including the Hanifin and Rajka criteria, to classify atopic dermatitis, which address specific symptoms and their duration. Patch testing can also be utilized to identify contact allergens in contact dermatitis. Observational testing and histopathological examination are also imperative in rendering definitive diagnoses because they provide information regarding the inflammatory processes and skin architecture that characterize different eczemas. Due to the complications of dermatitis, application of broad diagnostic criteria is very helpful in differential diagnosis, guiding healthcare workers in the demarcation of treatment protocols for optimal patient outcomes (Chukwu et al., 2018). In addition to the clinical assessment and criteria, an understanding of the pathophysiological underpinnings of eczema is necessary in order to enhance diagnostic accuracy and treatment efficacy. Eczema is believed to result from a combination of genetic, immunologic, and environmental factors. For instance, mutations in genes that affect the skin's barrier function result in water loss and exposure to irritants and allergens. Inflammation is typically mediated by dysregulated immune responses, resulting in increased cytokine levels in the involved tissues. This simultaneous interaction between genetic predisposition and immune response clinically manifests as the varied symptoms of eczema. The insight gained in such a study of the mechanisms is essential not just to improve the diagnostic criteria but also for the development of targeted therapies according to the etiology of eczema, hence improving the overall management plan for eczema patients. (Figure 4.10).

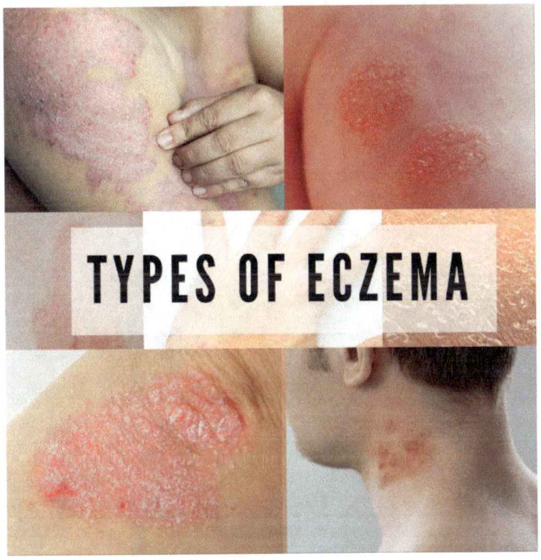

Figure 4.10. Types of eczema.

Source: https://banish.com/cdn/shop/articles/cover_photo_7_types_of_eczema.png?v=1575586990&width=2048.

4.3.3. Dermatitis: Causes and Treatment Options

Dermatitis, a catchall term for a variety of inflammatory cutaneous diseases, may result from numerous causes, including inherited predisposition, environmental factors, and immunocompromised states. An example is atopic dermatitis, often associated with allergic and asthmatic histories, in which the skin's barrier function is disrupted, leading to heightened transepidermal water loss and increased permeability to irritants. Also, direct contact with allergens such as nickel or certain skincare products or irritants such as soaps and detergents may cause contact dermatitis. Such a form of dermatitis demonstrates how environmental changes can trigger an inflammatory response, thereby complicating skin healing. Besides, the role of gut microbiota in the development of dermatitis, as observed in children, particularly is a fascinating correlation; microbiota imbalance may precipitate aggravation of conditions like atopic dermatitis, highlighting the importance of a holistic approach towards understanding the external and internal factors influencing skin health (Liu et al., 2022). Therapeutically, various strategies are employed depending on the type and severity of dermatitis. Initial treatment usually includes topical corticosteroids, which help damp inflammation and relieve symptoms such as itching and redness. For chronic situations, non-steroid options such as calcineurin inhibitors may be recommended to prevent the side effects of steroids. In recent years, the use of biologics has increased, particularly for severe-to-moderate atopic dermatitis, with good results in immunomodulation. In addition, probiotic supplementation in treatment is on the rise; evidence suggests that restoring gut microbiota balance may be an important contributor to the management of dermatitis, through enhanced skin barrier function and immune system modulation. However, despite growing interest, additional high-quality research is needed to document the efficacy and safety of probiotic use for this purpose (Liu et al., 2022). Furthermore, patient education and lifestyle modification are integral components of successful dermatitis care. Patients with dermatitis are typically advised to avoid known precipitating factors, e.g., certain allergens or irritants, and to adhere to a rigorous skincare routine with regular moisturizing to reinforce the skin's barrier function. Mild cleansing products that do not strip the skin of useful oils are also critical. Moreover, lifestyle modifications like stress management can also have a tremendous effect on the disease, as it is a well-documented exacerbating factor in most dermatological conditions. The use of community resources and educational materials increases patient comprehension and adherence to their treatment regimen, encouraging an active role in skin health. As our understanding of dermatitis continues to advance, the emphasis is on developing more effective therapies that incorporate these diverse methodologies while respecting the importance of each patient's unique circumstances (Figure 4.11).

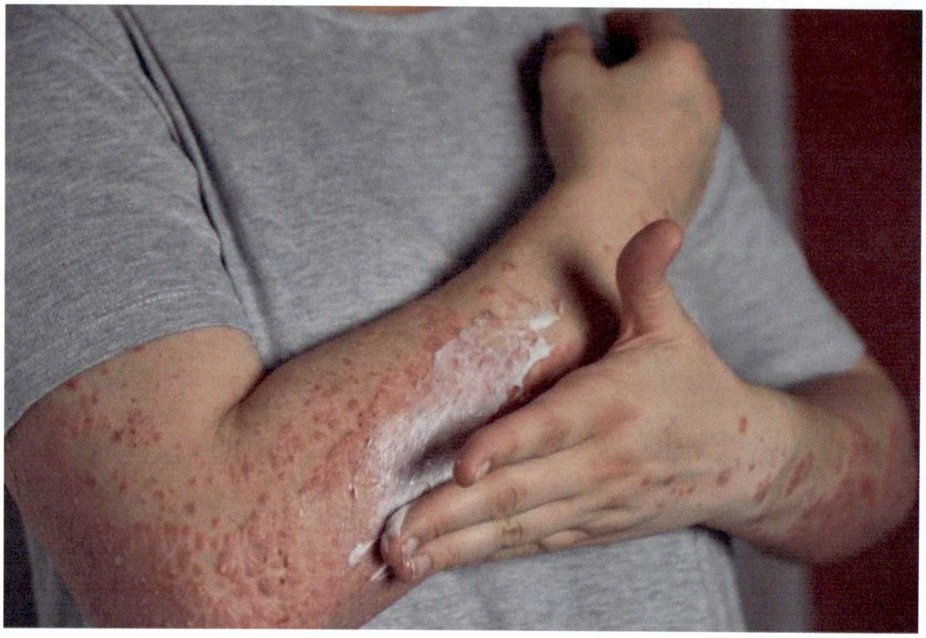

Figure 4.11. Allergic dermatitis

Source: https://www.oasisdermatology.com/wp-content/uploads/2023/03/Best-Contact-Allergic-Dermatitis-Treatment-Oasis-Dermatology-1000x658.jpg.

Test Your Knowledge

1. What are the histologic features of psoriasis?
2. What are the diagnostic criteria for eczema?

4.4. Infectious Skin Diseases

Learning Outcome

1. Describe the common types and treatments of bacterial infections
2. Understand the characteristics and management of viral infections
3. Describe the diagnosis and therapeutic approaches for fungal infections

Infectious dermatological diseases are a significant growing challenge in dermatopathology, involving clinical practices with sophisticated histopathological evaluation. They are mainly due to a range of pathogens, including bacteria, fungi, viruses, and parasites, leading to a varied pattern of presentation from focal eruptions to systemic infection. Accurate identification of such conditions is extremely important, as misdiagnosis can lead to inappropriate therapy and further compromise the patient's condition. For instance, bacterial infections like impetigo may mimic other cutaneous lesions and require individualized antimicrobial treatment. Therefore, complete knowledge of the histopathological features of infectious diseases by the dermatopathologist is necessary to provide an accurate diagnosis and to guide treatment planning. In addition, advances in diagnostic technology, such as reflectance confocal microscopy (RCM), have significantly enhanced the evaluation of infectious cutaneous conditions. RCM is a non-invasive imaging technique that can assess cutaneous infections directly in real time, allowing a glimpse into the epidermis and superficial dermis where infectious processes typically become apparent. RCM has been shown to be equivalent to standard histopathology in detecting changes associated with infectious disease. With its resolution capabilities, RCM enables visualization of numerous skin parasites and fungi and therefore enhances diagnostic accuracy. Although it cannot visualize viruses, which are microscopic, it can reveal viral cytopathic effects in keratinocytes. The utility of RCM not only enables diagnosis but also tracks treatment response, thereby optimizing patient care and minimizing unnecessary interventions (Arzberger et al., 2020). Moreover, the ecological environment of infectious skin infections is constantly changing due to fluctuating environmental conditions, antibiotic resistance, and the emergence of new pathogens. The recurrent recrudescence of new causative infectious pathogens, such as antibiotic-resistant bacteria, complicates the control of diseases such as cellulitis and folliculitis. Furthermore, the increasing prevalence of fungal infections, particularly among immunocompromised patients, necessitates greater caution and more advanced diagnostic methods for dermatologists. Integration of evidence from different sources, including clinical experience and contemporary research, with dermatopathological practice is crucial in addressing these challenges. As knowledge accumulates, the importance of an interdisciplinary approach that integrates clinical dermatology, histopathology, and advanced imaging modalities will be critical for maximizing diagnostic and treatment effectiveness in patients with infectious skin disease (Ruiz et al., 2014).

4.4.1. Bacterial Infections: Common Types and Treatments

Bacterial infections, including dermatopathology, are diverse and encompass a range of skin diseases that significantly impact skin health. Cellulitis, impetigo, and folliculitis are common bacterial infections, each with distinct presentations. Cellulitis occurs as reddening, swelling, and warmth of the affected area following a penetration of bacteria through the skin's opening. Folliculitis, an inflammatory reaction of hair follicles, can be caused by numerous bacterial etiologies and can present as painful pustules. Impetigo, which is most commonly seen in children, is a contagious infection that causes yellow, crusted lesions. Identification of such infections is critical in dermatopathology, as the correct diagnosis dictates the treatment course to avoid complications and ensure skin integrity. For bacterial infections, a combination of antibiotic therapy and adequate wound care is required to achieve favorable results. Topical antibiotics such as mupirocin may be used for localized infections, whereas systemic antibiotics may be utilized for severe infections such as cellulitis. For diseases involving abscess formation, drainage procedures can be performed to remove the source of infection. The choice of antibiotic is based on the bacterial pathogen, highlighting the importance of microbial culture and sensitivity testing. Furthermore, treatment of primary conditions such as diabetes or immunocompromised states is a part of bacterial infection control, as these conditions will increase susceptibility to skin infection. New technologies have opened doors for new diagnosis and treatment approaches for bacterial skin infections.

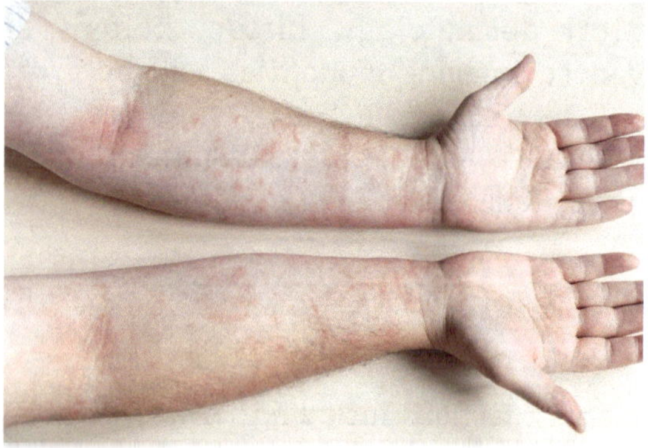

Figure 4.12. Bacterial skin infections.

Source: https://thelifesciencesmagazine.com/wp-content/uploads/2024/10/1.1-What-are-Bacterial-Skin-Infections.jpg.

The application of deep learning models to dermatopathology has yielded promising results in enhancing the accuracy of the diagnosis of numerous skin ailments. A recent study reports an extensive framework with a high validation accuracy rate of 99.44%, underpinning the ability of computational intelligence to assist dermatologists in decision-making. Not only are these technologies facilitating easy diagnosis of bacterial infections, but they are also enabling targeted therapy, which is important in anti-microbial resistance. With further advancement, the integration of technology with dermatopathology will definitely lead to improved patient outcomes and a deeper understanding of bacterial skin infections, and will also become a platform for future research and clinical practice (Adegoke et al., 2022; Lyle et al., 2022) (Figure 4.12).

4.4.2. Viral Infections: Characteristics and Management

Viral infections exhibit a broad range of characteristics that significantly affect dermatopathology. The infections can be presented with various cutaneous appearances, often making them challenging to diagnose, particularly because they can mimic other skin conditions. For instance, viral infections such as herpes simplex and human papillomavirus present vesicular rashes clinically indistinguishable from other inflammatory dermatoses. The histopathological diagnosis, therefore, plays a crucial role in accurately diagnosing causative viral pathogens. By employing immunohistochemistry and polymerase chain reaction techniques, clinicians can differentiate the virus from other dermatoses, thereby improving diagnostic accuracy and informing subsequent management protocols. Such information facilitates achieving better patient outcomes and underscores the crucial need for dermatopathologists to remain well apprised of the evolving dynamics of viral pathologies. Treatment of viral diseases in dermatopathology is a multidisciplinary approach, as treatment regimens often depend on the etiologic agent and the severity of infection. Antiviral therapy, e.g., acyclovir for herpes simplex virus, has been proven effective in lowering the severity of symptoms and shortening the duration of lesions. Vaccination against human papillomavirus has also been proven to be beneficial in preventing the onset of related diseases, such as cervical carcinoma and anogenital warts. In cases of viral exanthem, supportive therapy, such as analgesia and hydration, may be sufficient for convalescence, but treatment should be tailored to individual patient needs and comorbidities. Best management also involves educating patients about the risk of recurrent infection and the need for active prevention of transmission and overall skin health.

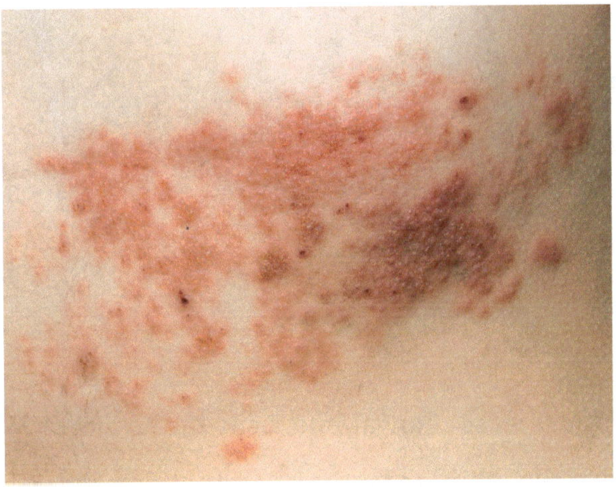

Figure 4.13. herpes zoster infection

Source: https://wchh.onlinelibrary.wiley.com/cms/asset/1f8091ee-234c-4225-9bbf-fd2470274bec/psb1907-fig-0002-m.jpg.

Further, the incorporation of community-based interventions enhances control over viral diseases, as contemporary studies have estimated. By involving patients at the community level, public health schemes can enhance awareness regarding viral dermatological diseases and early warning signs. Public health programs foster a sense of empowerment among people and enhance compliance with vaccination programs and follow-ups. For instance, the role of educational campaigns in endemic regions has been shown to positively impact the epidemiology of non-communicable skin diseases (NTDs) and common skin diseases (Emeritus et al., 2019). Successful community outreach programs not only aid disease control but also contribute to more integrated health solutions, ultimately building resilience against viral infections that otherwise tend to linger in the population. Dermatopathology, in this context, remains at the forefront of the management of viral skin infection, with a twofold priority placed on clinical and community health perspectives (Figure 4.13).

4.4.3. Fungal Infections: Diagnosis and Therapeutic Approaches

Fungal infections are a frequent dilemma in dermatopathology, with variable presentations and a risk of severe complications, especially in immunocompromised patients. Accurate diagnosis is paramount, often requiring synergy between clinical evaluation, histopathological examination, and microbiologic culture techniques. Clinicians must be vigilant for atypical presentations, particularly in those receiving immunosuppressive regimens. Such patients are susceptible to more virulent infections and exhibit heterogeneous cutaneous expression due to impaired immune status. Multidisciplinary treatment involving dermatologists and infectious disease specialists is recommended to ensure appropriate, individualized therapy and improved patient outcomes, particularly for individuals with special vulnerabilities, i.e., recipients of solid organ transplants (Züleyha Özgen et al., 2020). The delay in initiating appropriate treatment can lead to widespread morbidity, underscoring the need for education and awareness among healthcare workers regarding fungal infections. Treatment of fungal infections varies with the organism's class and host immunity. While local infections like tinea can be treated with topical antifungals, more extensive or systemic infections may need treatment through oral or intravenous methods. Choosing the antifungal agent must consider the organism's species, the site of infection, and potential drug interactions in immunosuppressed patients. More modern antifungals and combination regimens are continually under investigation, further emphasizing the evolving treatment landscape. Clinicians should also be adept at identifying patterns of resistance that can complicate the picture. Overall, understanding the pharmacodynamics and pharmacokinetics of antifungal therapy is crucial to achieve optimal treatment outcomes and reduce the risk of adverse effects in affected patients, especially those with special medical histories, such as transplant patients (Züleyha Özgen et al., 2020). On a broader scale, fungal infections cannot be overemphasized as areas that require care by community health programs, particularly in endemic regions. Active involvement of the local healthcare community and patients is the foundation of effective disease control programs, according to new research in skin NTDs. Improved awareness, timely detection, and access to treatments play a key role in stemming the incidence of these diseases. Advanced diagnostic technologies have the potential to enable timely interventions, thereby improving therapeutic outcomes. Additionally, understanding the epidemiology of dermatophyte fungal infections provides useful information for public health programs aimed at reducing the burden of disease among vulnerable populations. The incorporation of strategies grounded in community and clinicians' expertise is thus very important to facilitate a holistic approach to the challenges posed by fungal infections and to improve overall health status (Figure 4.14).

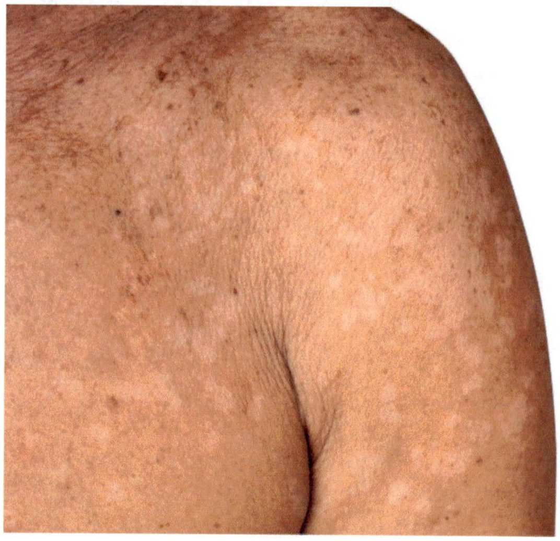

Figure 4.14. Fungal infections of the skin.

Source: https://coastdermatology.com/wp-content/uploads/sites/13/2023/06/fungal-skin-infection.jpg.

Test Your Knowledge

1. What is the most common treatment for a bacterial infection?
2. What is a characteristic of a viral infection?

4.5. Neoplastic Skin Conditions

Learning Outcome

1. Describe the types and clinical significance of benign tumors
2. Describe the malignant tumors
3. Understand the role of early detection and treatment strategies in dermatopathology

Neoplastic skin diseases are a group of tumors arising from skin cells, particularly those related to epidermal growth and differentiation. Of the non-melanoma skin cancers (NMSCs), basal cell carcinoma (BCC) and squamous cell carcinoma (SCC) are the most frequent. Both are usually associated with prolonged sun exposure, which induces DNA damage to skin cells. The new study suggests that human polyomavirus 6 (HPyV6) contributes to the tumor's etiology and pathogenesis. For instance, one study examining an extensive series of NMSC samples found an extremely high prevalence of HPyV6 DNA in BCCs and KAs, with a striking correlation between this polyomavirus and the neoplastic proliferation of keratinocytes (Haugg et al., 2016). These results could be alarming to our understanding of viral contributions to skin cancer carcinogenesis and underscore the need for further insight into viral oncogenesis. Melanoma, unlike NMSCs, is a more aggressive form of skin cancer that develops from melanocytes, the pigment-producing skin cells. The complex interplay between environmental exposures, such as ultraviolet radiation, and genetic predisposition plays a central role in melanoma pathogenesis. Current studies have shown that extrafollicular dermal melanocyte stem cells (MSCs) are involved in this process and that their UV-induced damage can lead to malignant transformation. This is particularly concerning since repeated UV exposure can weaken the integrity of DNA repair functions in such cells, rendering them melanoma stem cells (Bradley et al., 2012). Clarifying the mechanisms of MSC damage and their subsequent conversion into melanoma cells is pivotal to the design of targeted therapies aimed at curing recurrence and enhancing treatment outcomes. Apart from the well-studied roles of HPV and environmental factors, the genetic landscape of the neoplastic skin diseases is increasingly crucial in guiding treatment approaches. Molecular tumor analysis has begun to reveal specific mutations responsible for cancer growth, paving the way for targeted therapies. For instance, treatments that target specific genetic alterations in melanoma, such as BRAF mutations, have shown efficacy in improving patient outcomes. Such advances in the precise identification of neoplastic skin conditions provide for more effective surveillance and therapy. In all, ongoing research in dermatopathology is needed not only to illuminate the mechanisms underlying skin cancers but also to translate such findings into new clinical practices for treating neoplastic skin diseases in patients.

4.5.1. Benign Tumors: Types and Clinical Significance

Dermatopathology encompasses a broad range of benign tumors with varying histopathological features and clinical implications. Among the most common benign tumors is melanocytic nevi, characterized by proliferations of melanocytes—melanin-producing cells. Melanocytic nevi can be further categorized into several subtypes, including congenital melanocytic nevi, acquired melanocytic nevi, blue nevi, and Spitz nevi. Each of these subtypes has distinct genetic and clinical characteristics. For instance, while acquired melanocytic nevi are likely to harbor oncogenic BRAF mutations, congenital and blue nevi have been known to harbor NRAS and GNAQ mutations, respectively. These differences are relevant to note, as they highlight that the tumors are benign and may follow particular pathways toward malignant transformation, underscoring the importance of monitoring their development in clinical practice (Finnerty et al., 2001). In addition to discrete categories, clinical usefulness of benign tumors extends beyond histological classification. Melanocytic nevi, although benign, need meticulous monitoring and management due to their potential to develop melanoma. Clinicians opt to apply criteria such as the ABCDE mnemonic (Asymmetry, Border irregularity, Color variation, Diameter over 6 mm, and Elevation) to raise suspicion for early lesion detection. Moreover, benign tumors can be evidenced by apparent signs, such as changes in pigmentation or growth patterns, which are crucial for further study. The nevi maturation process, as characterized by the expression of protein markers such as S100A6, is crucial for differentiating between benign neoplasms and potential malignancies. Thus, an integrated understanding of the clinical features of benign tumors is important for effectively managing patients and outcomes (Finnerty et al., 2001).

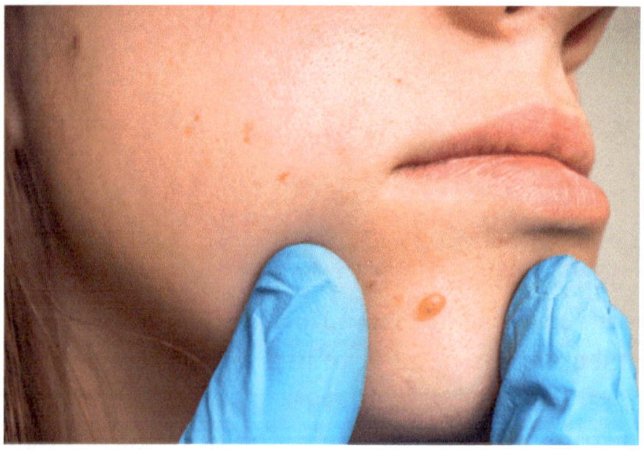

Figure 4.15. Benign tumors.

Source: https://factdr.com/wp-content/uploads/2018/06/Benign-tumours-skin.png.

Both intervention and surveillance are components of the management of benign tumors in dermatopathology. Routine excisions, particularly in cosmetically sensitive locations, are common interventions, whereas close surveillance for evidence of malignant transformation is expected. As the literature explains, development from benign neoplasia to malignancy involves additional tumorigenic changes that can enable escape from senescence in the presence of oncogenes. Such transitions are essential for clinicians and dermatopathologists to understand because they influence overall cancer prevention strategies and patient education. This aspect necessitates further studies to gain deeper insight into the molecular and genetic etiology of benign tumors, thereby enhancing diagnosis, therapy, and predictive models for patient management in dermatopathology (Figure 4.15).

4.5.2. Malignant Tumors: Melanoma and Non-Melanoma Skin Cancers

Malignant tumors, and particularly melanoma and non-melanoma skin cancers, are significant challenges to contemporary dermatopathology. Melanoma, or melanocytic tumor, has attracted particular attention due to its malignity and increasing prevalence. It is the result of exposure to UV radiation, genetic predisposition, and immunological status. Non-melanoma types, such as basal cell carcinoma and squamous cell carcinoma, are more frequent and most often exhibit an indolent course. Even with their relatively lesser malignancy, these cancers emphasize the utmost importance of early detection and treatment. The rising incidence of skin cancers globally demands further research into their pathophysiology as a measure to improve screening, diagnosis, and management strategies, as highlighted by current research aiming at delineating the biological underpinnings of these cancers (Birlea et al., 2018). Diagnosis of malignant skin tumors is primarily based on histopathology, which is central to accurate classification and treatment planning. In the case of cutaneous malignant melanoma (CMM), histopathological features are supplemented by immunohistochemical techniques to provide more detail regarding tumor proliferation and the cell cycle. This measures CMM cell replicative ability and helps to distinguish between high- and low-risk types based on their growth rate and associated histological characteristics. Moreover, the correlation between cancer stem cell growth and transient amplifier cells indicates a complex interplay of cellular mechanisms underlying melanoma development (Piérard et al., 2012). Identification of correlations contributes not only to better prognostic assessment but also to therapeutic intervention in patient-specific oncological portraits. Recent advances in melanomas and non-melanomas of the skin have the promise to revolutionize the field of dermatopathology by combining genetic, molecular, and immunological data. An excellent example is the identification of aberrant pathways, such as the mitogen-activated protein kinase (MAPK) pathway, which provides insight into tumor biology and therapeutic response. This also allows targeted molecular endpoints to be identified, leading to better treatment outcomes.

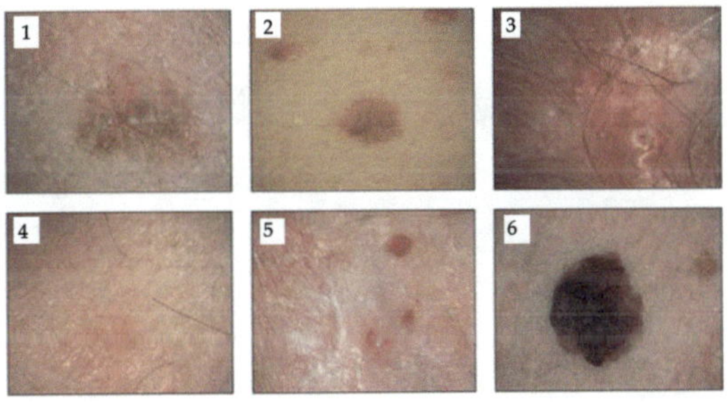

Figure 4.16. Examples of melanoma and non-melanoma skin cancer taken in a clinical setting from six different patients.

Source: https://www.researchgate.net/profile/Thomas-Johansen-2/publication/332580134/figure/fig1/AS:910538787811328@1594100772715/Examples-of-melanoma-and-non-melanoma-skin-cancer-taken-in-a-clinical-setting-from-six.png.

Continued research into skin cancer's intricate biology, including recent developments in melanoma immunotherapy and systems biology, validates the collaborative initiatives aimed at overcoming existing clinical challenges (Birlea et al., 2018). Ultimately, these initiatives ensure improved outcomes in patients and advance knowledge of the pathogenesis that leads to malignant skin tumors, which enhances diagnostic and therapeutic routines in dermatopathology (Figure 4.16).

4.5.3. Role of Early Detection and Treatment Strategies

Early detection in dermatopathology is essential, particularly for cutaneous malignancies such as melanoma. Early identification of suspicious lesions can significantly enhance treatment, and therefore the utilization of screening protocols becomes essential. Various imaging technologies, such as dermatoscopy, have proven to improve diagnostic accuracy, allowing practitioners to more accurately distinguish benign from malignant skin lesions. Public health interventions encouraging regular screening can also facilitate detection by reminding clients to return for examination of changes in their skin. Such anticipation can lead to interventions that not only cut down the disease course but also optimize survival in patients with skin cancer. Early detection thus becomes a pivotal element in successful dermatological disorder management, underscoring the role of ongoing education and awareness. Alongside early detection is the implementation of appropriate treatment measures to guarantee optimal patient results in dermatopathology. Emerging studies recognize novel therapeutic strategies, including targeted therapies and immunotherapies, that have revolutionized treatment for high-risk patients. These advancements not only enhance the efficacy of therapies but also minimize side effects due to traditional modalities. For instance, the use of combinatorial treatment regimens has been very promising in the treatment of drug-resistant melanoma, with a more individualized treatment option based on patient profile. Furthermore, integration of research results at the basic level with clinical practice has the potential for developing new therapeutic pathways, thereby accelerating the translation of scientific advances to clinical application. Closing the gap between early detection and specific treatment modalities is therefore essential for advancing dermatopathology as a field and improving patient care. Foremost in the development of an integrative approach to early detection and treatment is interdisciplinary cooperation among dermatologists, pathologists, and oncologists. By creating synergistic interactions between these fields, practitioners can share knowledge about new findings in melanocyte biology and how these influence patient management. By collaborating, clinical guidelines can be generated, including best practices for detection as well as treatment, and the outcome is improved standards of care. Moreover, collaborative research within such collaborations can add value to research activities aimed at exploring the mechanisms of skin diseases, more effectively informing the design of therapeutic strategies. The current literature emphasizes challenges and prospects within this multidisciplinary research, singling out areas such as melanoma immunotherapy and the study of pigment cells, which hold much promise for the future growth of dermatopathology (Birlea et al., 2018; Ruiz et al., 2014). Thus, a cooperative atmosphere promotes innovation and enhances the general efficacy of early detection and treatment techniques in dermatological practice.

Test Your Knowledge

1. What is the clinical significance of a benign tumor?
2. What is the role of early detection in dermatopathology?

SUMMARY

As an overview of the investigation of basic dermatopathology, it is evident that the field has witnessed significant progress, particularly with the integration of technology in diagnostic processes. This improvement is best exemplified by the transition from traditional microscopy to computerized methods, which enable more accurate analysis and more efficient diagnosis. The application of technology such as virtual reality (VR) microscopes is a milestone, enabling pathologists to improve observational skills and broaden their understanding of complex dermatopathological features. The data indicate that the right technology can streamline the diagnostic process, paving the way for better patient care through faster, more accurate results. As dermatopathology becomes more and more accepting of these technologies, paradigm-shifting models for diagnosis become increasingly possible, encouraging investigation into the applied topics of these emerging technologies, which are also deserving of examination. Moreover, the interaction of traditional knowledge and modern practice is designed to enrich the learning process of clinicians and researchers. By demystifying the interplay between past knowledge and current advances, one may fully appreciate the variability of dermatopathology. The transition from digital pathology platforms, as noted in the contrast between conventional and VR systems, is not only technological but pedagogical. Such a transition results in a rethinking of learning methodologies within the field. Continued research on the optimal use of VR microscopes and magnification methods will further enhance diagnostic accuracy, ultimately improving patient outcomes. Overall, the application of technology here augurs well for a prosperous future in which innovation is aligned with core knowledge to drive growth and development in dermatopathology. Lastly, the implications of the developments extend beyond absolute diagnostic efficiency; they have educational models and interdisciplinary practice implications in dermatopathology. As highlighted, the most important findings regarding the VR microscope underscore a pressing need for ongoing research into user experience and real-world applications in clinical settings (Gilbertson et al., 2013). Further, the importance of understanding the effects of digital slide production on diagnostic features should not be overstated, which supports the necessity for inter-disciplinary collaboration in the purposeful optimization of these technologies. It then becomes the responsibility of professionals in the specialty to be receptive to change and to accept new practice, ensuring they use these tools effectively to maximize their expertise. Through the combination of new technology and age-old dermatopathological principles, future possibilities are promising, offering increased diagnostic ability that will mutually benefit practitioners and patients. As we reflect on these developments, the pursuit of excellence in dermatopathology is a continuous collaborative venture that will shape its future for many years to come (Ruiz et al., 2014).

Dermatopathology, the microscopic examination of skin lesions, unites clinical dermatology with histopathology. At the heart of field lies the examination of skin tumors, which may be benign or malignant. Melanoma, of particular interest, is aggressive and on the rise. Histopathologic diagnostic criteria include measuring melanoma thickness, mitotic rate, and extent of local invasion. Apart from melanoma, basal cell carcinoma and squamous cell carcinoma are also of interest due to their frequency and varied histologic appearances. By describing such characteristics, dermatopathology enables accurate diagnoses that guide clinicians to appropriate treatment for patients based on the type and stage of cancer. Furthermore, a critical component of dermatopathology is the examination of inflammatory cutaneous illnesses, which involve a spectrum of conditions such as psoriasis, eczema, and dermatitis. Such illnesses present with a variety of histopathological alterations, such as epidermal architectural abnormalities and dermal changes. For instance, psoriasis is not only hyperkeratotic but also characterized by a marked infiltrate of immune cells, with evidence of an inappropriate immune response. Inflammatory reactions can also lead to complications such as infection and scarring, validating the need for adequate management regimens. Recognizing these histological characteristics enables dermatopathologists to make important contributions to the identification of the underlying causes of skin inflammation, thereby enabling the development of site-directed therapies and improving patient outcomes in the management of chronic cutaneous disorders. Finally, dermatology nurses play an important role in the overall scope of dermatopathology. As exemplified through current literature, these specialty nurses contribute to patient advocacy and education, enhance treatment compliance, and patient outcomes for various dermatological conditions. Dermatology nurses assist with clinical assessment and also cultivate patient relationships that are critical to effective dermatological management. Their role encompasses assessing skin lesions, administering topical therapy, and providing key education on skin care regimens. By facilitating communication between patients and dermatopathologists, nurses become care facilitators, navigating patients through the complexity of their illnesses, ultimately leading to improved treatment adherence and health outcomes (Chukwu et al., 2018). Their function is even more vital with dermatopathology's ever-evolving nature that resembles the sensitive balance between clinical practice and the education of patients.

KEY TERMS FROM THIS CHAPTER

- Albinism
- Dermatopathology
- Digital pathology
- Healthcare system
- Infectious skin diseases
- Reflectance confocal microscopy
- Streptococcus pyogenes
- Artificial intelligence
- Dermoscopy
- Fungal infections
- High-resolution microscopy
- Melanocytic disorders
- Staphylococcus aureus
- Elepathology

CRITICAL THINKING QUESTIONS

1. **What is the term for the thickened outermost layer of the epidermis observed in hyperkeratosis?**
   a. Stratum basale
   b. Stratum corneum
   c. Stratum granulosum
   d. Stratum spinosum
2. **Acanthosis refers to:**
   a. Thickening of the epidermis, particularly the stratum spinosum
   b. Thinning of the epidermis
   c. Accumulation of fluid in the dermis
   d. Loss of intercellular connections between keratinocytes
3. **Which histological feature is characteristic of psoriasis?**
   a. Basal cell vacuolization
   b. Parakeratosis and elongated rete ridges
   c. Subepidermal blister formation
   d. Lichenoid infiltrate
4. **The presence of multinucleated giant cells in a Tzanck smear is indicative of:**
   a. Fungal infection
   b. Herpes simplex virus (HSV) infection
   c. Psoriasis
   d. Melanoma
5. **What is the hallmark histological feature of lichen planus?**
   a. Basal cell degeneration and a band-like lymphocytic infiltrate
   b. Subepidermal blisters
   c. Neutrophilic abscesses in the stratum corneum
   d. Presence of multinucleated giant cells

Short Answer Questions

1. What is dermatopathology?
2. What are the diagnostic techniques in dermatopathology?
3. What is the most common inflammatory skin condition?
4. What are the infectious diseases of the skin?
5. Name the different types of neoplastic tumors.

Answer to Critical Thinking Questions

1. (b); 2. (a) ; 3. (b); 4. (b); 5. (a)

REFERENCES

1. Omotosho, L., Sotonwa, K., Adegoke, B., Oyeniran, O., & Oyeniyi, J. (2022). AN AUTOMATED SKIN DISEASE DIAGNOSTIC SYSTEM BASED ON DEEP LEARNING MODEL. *Journal of Engineering Studies and Research*, *27*(3), 43–50. https://doi.org/10.29081/jesr.v27i3.287Akaishi, S., Huang, C., Murphy, G. F., Ogawa, R., et al. (2014). Keloids and hypertrophic scars: Update and future directions. https://core.ac.uk/download/28951986.pdf (accessed on 21st July 2025).
2. Arzberger, E., Bastos, P. M., Ferreira, J., Leal-Filipe, T., et al. (2020). Reflectance confocal microscopy for the diagnosis of skin infections and infestations. https://core.ac.uk/download/322493878.pdf (accessed on 21st July 2025).
3. Bale, A. E., American Cancer Society, Molinaro, A. M., Arits, A. H. M. M., Bakos, R. M., Bastiaens, M. T., Bath-Hextall, F. J., et al. (2012). Host phenotype characteristics and *MC1R* in relation to early-onset basal cell carcinoma. https://core.ac.uk/download/323074698.pdf (accessed on 21st July 2025).
4. Birlea, S., Bosenberg, M. W., Box, N. F., Brash, D. E., et al. (2018). Frontiers in pigment cell and melanoma research. http://arxiv.org/abs/1808.01869 (accessed on 21st July 2025).
5. Bradley, P., Casillas, A., Chambers, D., Denholm, R., et al. (2012). Extrafollicular dermal melanocyte stem cells and melanoma. https://core.ac.uk/download/pdf/8731590.pdf (accessed on 21st July 2025).
6. Brunyé, T., Drew, T., Trafton, J. G., Elmore, J. G., Kerr, K., et al. (2021). More scanning, but not zooming, is associated with diagnostic accuracy in evaluating digital breast pathology slides. https://core.ac.uk/download/613720906.pdf (accessed on 21st July 2025).
7. Cesar, C. L., Cintra, M. L., Damiani, G. V., França, K., et al. (2020). Second-harmonic generation imaging analysis can help distinguish sarcoidosis from tuberculoid leprosy. https://core.ac.uk/download/296938886.pdf (accessed on 21st July 2025).
8. Chukwu, R., & Mankila, J. (2018). Dermatology nurses' job description: Literature review. https://core.ac.uk/download/161432240.pdf (accessed on 21st July 2025).
9. Colagrande, A., Cimmino, A., Demarco, A., Foti, C., Arezzo, F., Cazzato, G., Ingravallo, G., et al. (2021). Skin mycetoma in an 11-year-old African boy: Case presentation with emphasis on histopathological features and differential diagnosis. https://core.ac.uk/download/541257906.pdf (accessed on 21st July 2025).
10. Finnerty, B., Fullen, D. R., McNutt, N. S., Reed, J. A., et al. (2001). S100A6 preferentially labels type C nevus cells and nevic corpuscles: Additional support for Schwannian differentiation of intradermal nevi. http://deepblue.lib.umich.edu/bitstream/2027.42/75660/1/j.1600-0560.2001.028008393.x.pdf (accessed on 21st July 2025).
11. Gameiro, A., Gouveia, M., Moreno, A., Tellechea, Ó., et al. (2014). Childhood hypopigmented mycosis fungoides: A commonly delayed diagnosis. https://core.ac.uk/download/75985973.pdf (accessed on 21st July 2025).
12. Giacomel, J., Marghoob, A. A., & Zalaudek, I. (2015). Metaphoric and descriptive terminology in dermoscopy: Lessons from the cognitive sciences. https://core.ac.uk/download/155237859.pdf (accessed on 21st July 2025).

13. Gilbertson, L., Miles, R., Rojo, S., Treanor, D., et al. (2013). Virtual reality microscope versus conventional microscope regarding time to diagnosis: An experimental study. https://core.ac.uk/download/13504976.pdf (accessed on 21st July 2025).

14. Haugg, A. M., Kurz, A. K., zur Hausen, A., Diaz, C., Rennspiess, D., Speel, E. J. M., Beckervordersandforth, J., et al. (2016). Frequent detection of human polyomavirus 6 in keratoacanthomas. https://core.ac.uk/download/pdf/81069513.pdf (accessed on 21st July 2025).

15. Hay, R., Asiedu, K., Hay, R. J., Singh, A., John, W., McBride, H., Govan, B., et al. (2019). Skin-related neglected tropical diseases (Skin-NTDs)—A new challenge. *MDPI eBooks*. https://doi.org/10.3390/books978-3-03921-254-5 (accessed on 21st July 2025).

16. Jargin, S. V. (2024). Fascism in medicine and everyday life. *Authorea (Authorea)*. https://doi.org/10.22541/au.170869975.50200047/v1 (accessed on 21st July 2025).

17. Liu, Y., Du, X., Zhai, S., Tang, X., Liu, C., & Li, W. (2022). Gut microbiota and atopic dermatitis in children: A scoping review. *BMC Pediatrics, 22*. https://doi.org/10.1186/s12887-022-03390-3 (accessed on 21st July 2025).

18. Lyle, L. (2022). Medical school watercooler newsletter–August 12, 2022. https://core.ac.uk/download/588434171.pdf (accessed on 21st July 2025).

19. Molina Ruiz, A. M. (2014). Immunohistochemistry in the diagnosis of cutaneous viral and bacterial infections. https://repositorio.uam.es/bitstream/10486/662932/1/molina_ruiz_ana_maria.pdf (accessed on 21st July 2025).

20. Özgen, Z., & Özer, E. C. (2020). Skin and mucosa in patients with solid organ transplant: Risks and precautions. *Mucosa, 3*, 83–92. https://doi.org/10.33204/mucosa.762566 (accessed on 21st July 2025).

21. Piérard-Franchimont, C., Piérard, G. E., Radermacher, J., Delvenne, P., Paquet, P., & Hermanns-Lê, T. (2014). Cyanoacrylate skin surface stripping and the 3S-biokit advent in tropical dermatology: A look from Liège. https://core.ac.uk/download/192729479.pdf (accessed on 21st July 2025).

22. Piérard, G. E. (2012). Cell proliferation in cutaneous malignant melanoma: Relationship with neoplastic progression. https://core.ac.uk/download/pdf/8674378.pdf (accessed on 21st July 2025).

23. Ring, J. (2019). Progress in dermatology and venereology–Editor's pick of the year 2018. *Journal of the European Academy of Dermatology and Venereology, 33*, 7–10. https://doi.org/10.1111/jdv.15394 (accessed on 21st July 2025).

24. Roth, C. J., Clunie, D., Vining, D., Berkowitz, S. J., Berlín, A., Bissonnette, J. P., Clark, S. D., et al. (2021). Multispecialty enterprise imaging workgroup consensus on interactive multimedia reporting current state and road to the future: HIMSS–SIIM collaborative white paper. *Journal of Digital Imaging, 34*, 495–522. https://doi.org/10.1007/s10278-021-00450-5 (accessed on 21st July 2025).

DIAGNOSTIC TOOLS IN DERMATOLOGY: DERMOSCOPY, BIOPSY, AND IMAGING

5

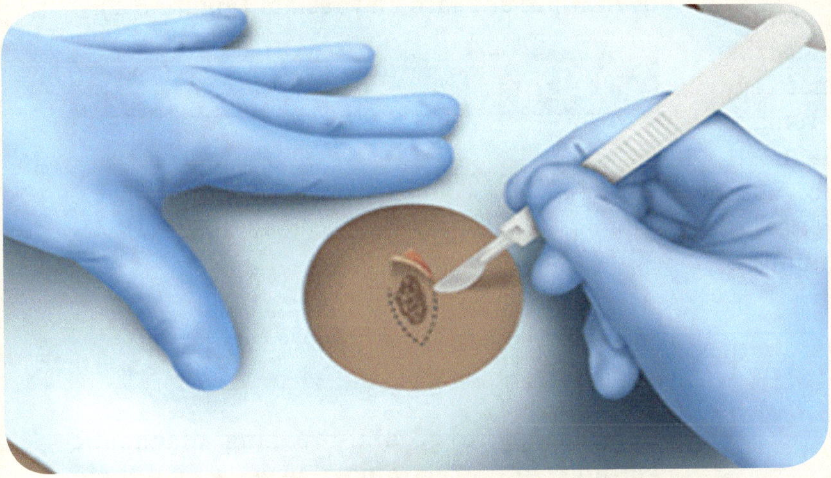

LEARNING OBJECTIVES

After studying this chapter, you will be able to:

1. Learn about dermoscopy and biopsy
2. Understand the importance of advanced imaging techniques in dermatology
3. Compare the diagnostic tools in dermatology
4. Describe the clinical applications of diagnostic tools in dermatology

Introduction

The art of dermatology has experienced a vast transformation in diagnostic tools, effectively enhancing the accuracy of skin lesion assessments. Traditional skin examination methods have been augmented by modern technologies that allow the clinician to visualize and inspect skin pathology more effectively. Among these, dermoscopy, biopsy, and imaging techniques such as line-field confocal optical coherence tomography (LC-OCT) have emerged as essential tools in the diagnosis of skin disorders ranging from benign to malignant. The use of these technologies not only helps distinguish between skin cancers and benign lesions but also reduces the need for invasive tests. As such, an understanding of the strengths and limitations of each tool is imperative for dermatologists to ensure accurate and timely diagnoses. Dermoscopy has become a cornerstone of dermatologic diagnosis due to its ability to visualize structures below the skin surface that are not visible to the naked eye. The technique enhances the clinician's ability to diagnose various skin tumors and benign lesions by examining characteristic patterns and pigmentation. Current studies have likewise indicated that high-magnification and routine dermoscopy provide complementary information to support accurate diagnoses. For instance, salient dermoscopic patterns such as blue–white veils and irregular dots can significantly enhance diagnosis accuracy for conditions such as lentigo maligna melanoma and lentigo maligna, as observed in research studies (D'Onghia et al., 2025). This twin modality of employing both basic and advanced modalities illustrates differentiated cellular features necessary for precision, emphasizing the need for a dynamic practice of dermatology. As a secondary to dermoscopy, biopsy remains the gold standard for definitive diagnosis, particularly if clinical findings are ambiguous. The biopsy provides histological evidence for the diagnosis, enabling effective planning of therapy.

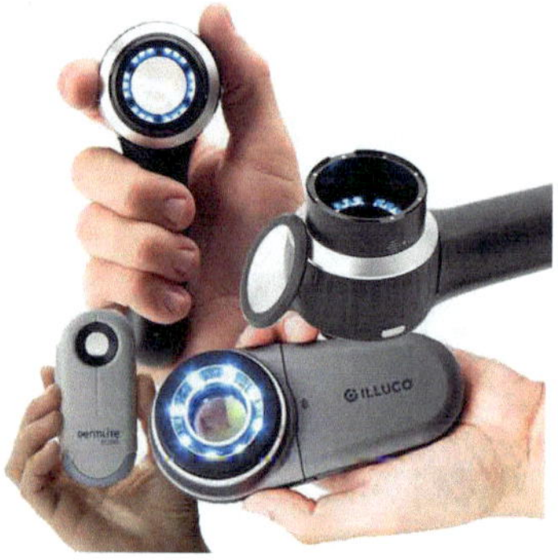

Figure 5.1. Diagnostic equipment in dermatology.

Source: https://zonemedical.com.au/cdn/shop/collections/Diagnostic-Equipment-_-Dermatoscopes-Dermlite.jpg?v=1702899114&width=1296.

However, the invasive nature of biopsies intimidates both the patients and complicates clinical procedures. That's where imaging modalities like LC-OCT are useful, acting as a virtual non-invasive biopsy that can record cellular structure in real time. With growing evidence supporting the use of LC-OCT in various dermatological diseases, such as malignant skin cancer and inflammatory diseases, it serves as a bridge between dermoscopy and classical histopathology (Cappilli et al., 2024). By using such innovative approaches, dermatologists can strategically reduce the need for invasive treatments with improved diagnostic effectiveness, thereby improving overall patient care and results (Figure 5.1).

5.1. Dermoscopy

Learning Outcome

1. Understand the purpose of dermoscopy
2. Describe the techniques and types of dermatoscopes
3. Know the advantages of dermoscopy in skin diagnosis

Dermoscopy, a ground-breaking diagnostic method in dermatology, uses a handheld instrument equipped with a magnification lens and light to maximize visualization of skin lesions. With this method, clinicians can visualize structures and patterns that are imperceptible to the naked eye, greatly improving diagnostic accuracy for most skin diseases, particularly skin cancer. With the growing incidence of melanoma and non-melanoma skin cancer in the world, the adoption of dermoscopy has become more and more necessary. Dermoscopy significantly enhances discrimination between benign and malignant lesions and is therefore a non-invasive diagnostic tool for examining skin changes. Although beneficial, the method has its downsides; dermoscopic image interpretation training remains a constraint, particularly for medical staff who are not specifically trained in dermatological use. Advances in technology have subsequently further optimized the efficiency of dermoscopy, integrating artificial intelligence (AI) to aid in diagnostics. AI algorithms, particularly machine learning and convolutional neural network (CNN)-based models, have been shown to be highly effective at interpreting dermoscopic images. These algorithms can classify skin lesions accurately at or beyond the level of skilled clinicians, overcoming some of the constraints of intrinsic human interpretation of dermoscopy (Liopyris et al., 2022). Thanks to the availability of large datasets, such as those supplied by the International Skin Imaging Collaboration (ISIC), researchers have been able to develop and validate AI systems that have substantial effects in the detection of early skin cancer.

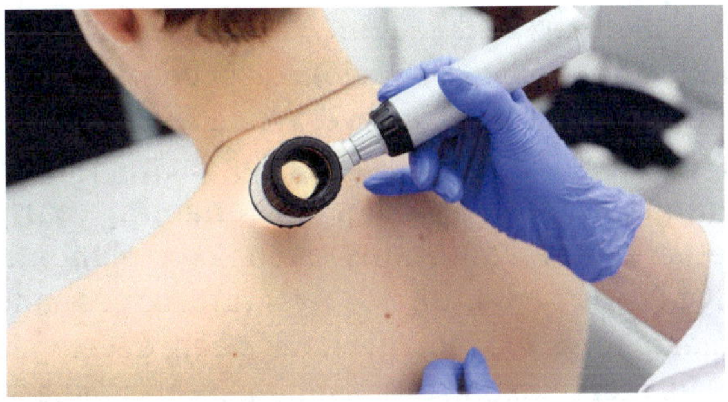

Figure 5.2. Dermoscopy.

Source: https://eledia.sumy.ua/wp-content/uploads/2019/12/dermatolog-01.jpg.

Through the use of AI, the future potential of dermoscopy also includes not just easing clinical workload but also improving patient outcomes through accelerated, more accurate diagnoses. Cooperative work and research in dermoscience continue to be necessary to help developments improve its application in clinical practice further. These programs, such as the ISIC, provide a baseline for developing machine learning models that can guide clinicians' decision-making based on dermoscopic analysis (Cassidy et al., 2021). However, with most technologies, there are challenges, and in this case, they involve data quality and the need for curated datasets free of redundancy. The veracity and validity of the AI models depend largely upon the training data provided, and any discrepancies can lead to spurious conclusions in clinical practice. As researchers address these challenges, integrating dermoscopy with AI and high-quality datasets is an encouraging direction for dermatology to usher in a future in which diagnostic procedures are less laborious, more accurate, and more readily available to healthcare personnel and patients (Figure 5.2).

5.1.1. Definition and Purpose of Dermoscopy

Dermoscopy is a highly advanced non-surgical diagnostic tool that enhances the visualization of skin lesions. Using a special handheld instrument referred to as a dermatoscope, skin specialists can magnify skin details and inspect numerous types of pigmentation patterns, blood vessel structures, and surface textures. This method significantly increases the accuracy of skin condition diagnosis compared with standard visual examinations. Its principal objective is to facilitate the early diagnosis of skin cancers, particularly melanoma, which may appear in very early stages in subtle ways. With the global rise in melanoma, the role of dermoscopy in dermatology has become increasingly significant, enabling clinicians to differentiate malignant from benign presentations and thereby improve patient outcomes (Al-Ayyad et al., 2024). As a result, dermoscopy has revolutionized dermatology, becoming indispensable for on-site examinations and management decisions. The use of dermoscopy is not just for identifying potential malignancies; it also serves as a crucial educational tool for dermatologists. By allowing physicians to view the fine details of skin lesions, dermoscopy enhances practitioners' understanding of dermatopathology and improves their diagnostic skills. Besides melanoma, this method helps assess a wide range of skin conditions, including benign nevi, basal cell carcinoma, and psoriasis. The fact that dermoscopy is non-invasive allows for serial inspections, making it possible to track changes within the lesions over time, which is crucial in early intervention. Besides, the integration of dermoscopy with advanced imaging equipment, such as optical coherence tomography, fosters interdisciplinarity in dermatological diagnosis through comprehensive patient assessments and patient-tailored treatment protocols (Xu et al., 2021). Consequently, the practical and educational advantages of dermoscopy underscore its utility in contemporary dermatology clinics. In addition, dermoscopy enhances the rate and reliability of dermatologic evaluations and serves as a valuable tool both for clinicians and patients. The method allows better stratification of the requirement for biopsy versus those who do not require it, thus maximizing management. As an illustration, by targeting lesions with features more likely to contain malignancy, clinicians can concentrate on at-risk patients for further investigations, e.g., biopsies.

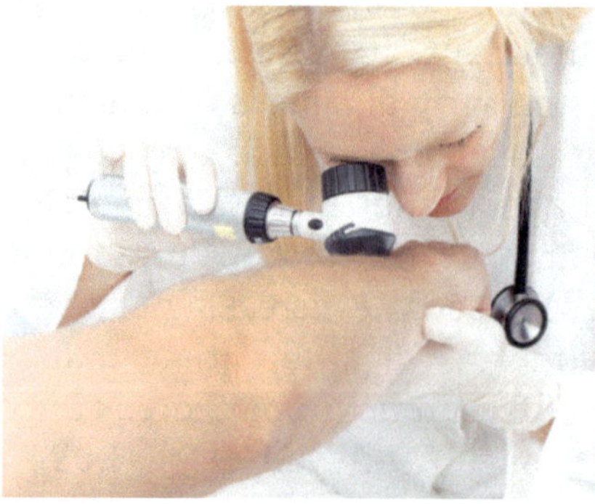

Figure 5.3. Dermoscopy diagnosis: To treat your skin with best medication.

Source: https://www.mayraskinclinic.com/wp-content/uploads/2021/10/Dermoscopy_Mayra.png.

The ability to provide immediate visual feedback also enables patient communication, builds patient confidence, and increases knowledge about their conditions. By incorporating dermoscopic findings into clinical decision-making, doctors can minimize unnecessary invasive diagnostic procedures, reduce patients' anxiety, and optimize resource utilization in the healthcare environment. Thus, dermoscopy is not only a diagnostic tool but also a vital component of the overall process of treating patients in dermatology, indicating its significant contribution to dermatological diagnosis and management (Al-Ayyad et al., 2024) (Figure 5.3).

5.1.2. Techniques and Types of Dermatoscopes

The evolution of dermatoscopes has enhanced the precision of dermatology diagnosis, most notably in the evaluation of skin lesions. Traditional dermoscopy uses handheld devices that light up and magnify the skin, enabling clinicians to identify various aspects of lesions not visible to the naked eye. Visual enhancement is essential for differentiating benign from malignant lesions, thereby enabling early detection of conditions such as melanoma. In addition, handheld dermatoscopes and smartphone technology have been developed to further maximize convenience, particularly in rural areas where dermatologists may not be readily available. Such technology is key not only to maximizing early detection but also to maximizing patient involvement in prevention programs, as noted in recent reviews of health apps for aiding skin cancer screening (Cook et al., 2015). Later innovations have been marked by the creation of digital dermatoscopes, which offer capabilities beyond conventional imaging. Digital dermatoscopes use high-resolution cameras to capture images of skin lesions and enable extensive documentation and digital storage of results. Artificial intelligence algorithms in digital dermatoscopes are intended to improve diagnostic accuracy. For instance, AI-based image classification technologies scan dermoscopic images, aiding clinicians in distinguishing various types of skin cancers with remarkable accuracy (Betz-Stablein et al., 2024). Embedding such technologies also facilitates the easy implementation of teledermatology, enabling dermatologists to review images forwarded by patients or primary care professionals. Such is particularly beneficial in reducing health access inequalities, facilitating timely intervention regardless of geographical limitations. But this transition to sophisticated dermatoscopic techniques is not without its challenges. The dependence on technology, while being favorable, raises concerns about overdiagnosis and what to do with false positives. Further, the accuracy of algorithms largely depends on the quality, diversity, and quantity of training data, which are typically limited by bias and heterogeneity (Betz-Stablein et al., 2024). Therefore, as dermatoscopes evolve, it is crucial for practitioners to maintain a solid understanding of clinical dermatology concepts together with technological advancements. This in turn ensures that clinical judgment is prioritized, thereby overall enhancing the effectiveness of dermoscopic techniques in dermatology as an essential diagnostic tool in the management of skin diseases (Figure 5.14).

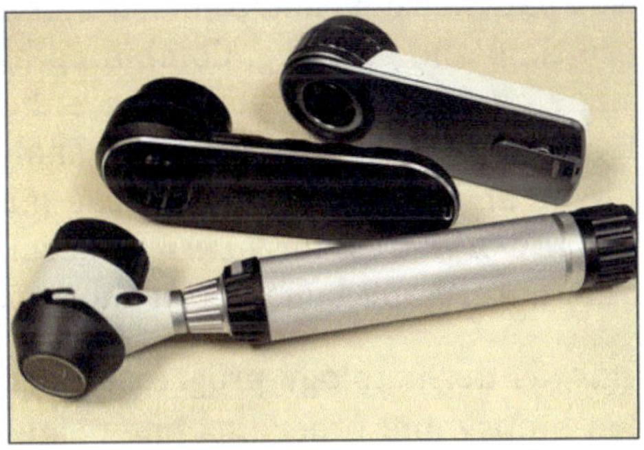

Figure 5.4. Dermatoscopes are hand-held tools used to evaluate skin lesions.

Source: https://www.cmaj.ca/content/cmaj/186/15/1167/F1.medium.gif.

5.1.3. Advantages of Dermoscopy in Skin Diagnosis

The advantages of dermoscopy to the diagnosis of skin are vast, particularly in the early detection of skin cancers such as melanoma. This non-invasive imaging modality allows physicians to examine skin lesions at higher magnification, providing deeper insights into pigmentation and lesion structure not possible with the naked eye. Increased visualization of dermal structures by dermoscopy improves diagnostic accuracy to a large degree, thus facilitating timely interventions that can significantly reduce morbidity associated with skin cancers. Research indicates that dermoscopy increases sensitivity and specificity for detecting malignant lesions compared with traditional examination methods. Such an enhancement not only enables timely diagnosis but also maximizes management outcomes, thereby improving the quality of patients' prognoses, as evidenced by research linking early detection to higher survival rates and lower healthcare costs (Mahumud et al., 2022). Besides, dermoscopy is crucial for differentiating among several skin lesions, particularly when the certainty of visual diagnosis is in doubt. This is particularly valuable in differentiating malignant tumors from benign moles, as the latter can lead to overdiagnosis and unnecessary surgery if misdiagnosed. The details exposed by dermoscopy, such as pigmentation patterns and vascular structures, are central to this differentiation. Studies have shown that dermoscopy significantly enhances the ability to recognize histopathologic subtypes of skin cancers, such as basal cell carcinoma (BCC) and melanoma, thereby supporting tailored treatment strategies that consider the individual nature of the cancer (Li-wen Zhang et al., 2022). Thus, in addition to its role in three-dimensional visualization of skin lesions, dermoscopy enhances diagnosis and optimizes patient care by enabling informed clinical decision-making. In addition, dermoscopy technology is improving with the integration of new developments, such as teledermoscopy, which enhances the availability of specialized dermatologic services, particularly for people in far-flung or underserved areas. Through teledermoscopy, healthcare workers can remotely examine skin lesions captured by patients on handheld devices, thereby enhancing access to quality care without physical visits. Such a shift is especially beneficial for the timely identification of melanoma in populations with limited access to dermatologic care. Furthermore, the use of artificial intelligence in dermoscopy marks an era of precision medicine, with algorithms capable of assisting physicians in real-time clinical decision-making by comparing lesion morphology against enormous databases. Lastly, these developments ensure that dermoscopy not only contributes to dermatology's diagnostic armamentarium but also has a significant impact on healthcare equity and efficiency in patient care management (Mahumud et al., 2022).

Test Your Knowledge

1. What is the purpose of a dermoscopy?
2. What are the different types of dermatoscopes?

5.2. Biopsy

Learning Outcome

1. Define the skin biopsies
2. Know the indications for performing a biopsy
3. Interpret biopsy results

Biopsy is a valuable diagnostic tool in dermatology, as it provides immediate information about skin lesions that are not adequately assessed by clinical inspection. Biopsy is an invasive technique in which a minute amount of tissue is removed from the skin and may be examined histopathologically. The strength of a biopsy in identifying various types of skin diseases, both benign and malignant tumors, cannot be overestimated. While dermatologists are trained to identify morphological patterns, subjectivity cannot be eliminated in diagnosis. By using biopsy, clinicians can make a definitive diagnosis, reducing the risk of misdiagnosis that can lead to inappropriate or delayed treatment. The role of biopsy in ensuring that patients and dermatologists alike cannot be overstated, as it offers a confirmed technique for establishing clinical suspicion and guiding subsequent therapeutic interventions in the right direction. In addition to its diagnostic use, the biopsy procedure could at times be therapeutic. For instance, excisional biopsies allow for both histological study and the removal of the lesion in full, and this can provide both therapeutic benefit and diagnostic insight. Secondarily, the development of biopsy techniques such as punch and shave biopsies has improved patient safety and comfort, shortening recovery time and scarring. Combining biopsy with imaging modalities yet again enhances its effectiveness, particularly while analyzing complex or ambiguous lesions. These merged approaches can give comprehensive information about the nature and behavior of the lesions.

Thus, as dermatology progresses, synergy between biopsy and other imaging techniques forms an essential component in accurate diagnosis and management of skin diseases. All in all, while pattern recognition remains the foundation for dermatological diagnoses, it is biopsy that provides objective quantification to such conclusions. Such objective quantification as histological evaluation gained through biopsy enables doctors to confirm diagnoses made through subjective visual evaluation. Furthermore, as diagnostic technology advances, it serves to further streamline dermatologic practice, and the role of biopsy also evolves. Techniques such as autofluorescence imaging and optical coherence tomography provide complementary information that may validate biopsy findings and further enhance diagnostic accuracy. Yet, a strong understanding of these heterogeneous yet interconnected diagnostic tools is necessary for practicing dermatologists, as the addition of biopsies alongside emerging technologies can potentially improve patient outcomes and enable more targeted treatment protocols in dermatology (Adabi et al., 2017; Aigner et al., 2020) (Figure 5.5).

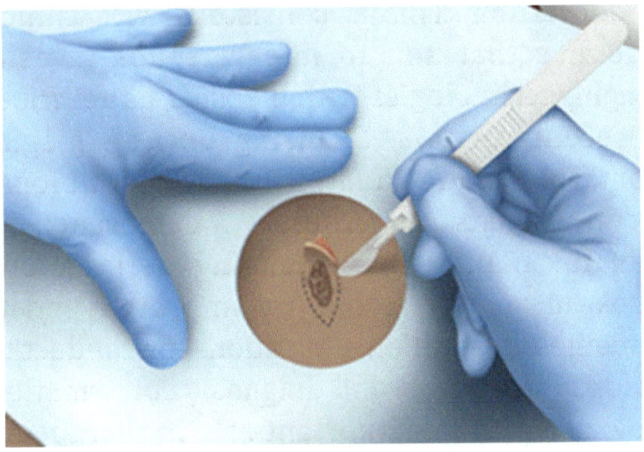

Figure 5.5. Excisional (or incisional) biopsy.

Source: https://images.ctfassets.net/1ny4yoiyrqia/355tQovuuReL7I3wJEfw6x/074791e41ceaa6ba8658598e2f8c8a3b/skin-biopsy-excisional.png?w=450&h=450.

5.2.1. Definition and Types of Skin Biopsies

Skin biopsies are a valuable diagnostic tool in dermatology, allowing for direct examination of the tissue in order to accurately diagnose a number of skin diseases. Skin biopsy is the removal of a skin sample for histopathological analysis, allowing dermatologists to differentiate between benign and malignant lesions with greater precision. Such an approach is especially crucial in diagnosing most skin cancers, such as basal cell carcinoma (BCC), which can often be confused with benign skin lesions, posing a challenge for clinical assessment. Skin biopsies enhance the likelihood of making clinical diagnoses through histopathological analysis, thereby centralizing their role in planning effective treatment protocols tailored to individual patients. Different skin biopsies are available, each suited for different diagnostic needs. The most frequent forms are punch biopsies, oval excisional biopsies, and shave biopsies. Punch biopsies use a round blade to excise a small core of skin, thereby removing an entire specimen thickness without too much trauma to the overlying tissue. On the contrary, elliptical excisional biopsies involve excising large areas of skin in the form of an oval, which may provide extensive information about deeper structures of skin. Shave biopsies, however, involve scooping away superficial layers of skin by scraping, which is most often used for raised lesions.

Each biopsy technique has specific indications and advantages, so selecting the appropriate technique based on the lesion's clinical presentation is crucial for dermatologists. Biopsy techniques not only provide a diagnosis of skin diseases but also provide valuable information that will guide treatment regimens and the patient's management. For example, histopathological examination following biopsies can provide critical information regarding a lesion's inflammatory potential and risk of malignancy. Line-field confocal optical coherence tomography (LC-OCT) is another imaging technique that enhances the diagnostic capability of biopsy by offering real-life virtual skin examinations that can improve diagnostic accuracy and training for dermatology professionals. By combining traditional histological examination with new imaging modalities, dermatologists can increase diagnostic precision and enable early intervention, thereby improving patient outcomes in dermatology practice (Navas et al., 2024; Cinotti et al., 2025) (Figure 5.6).

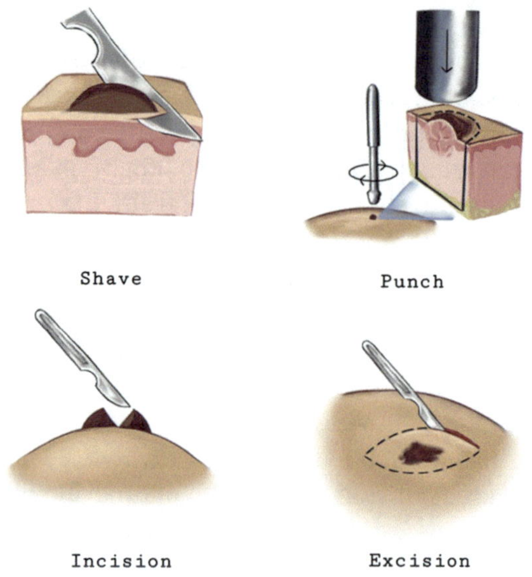

Figure 5.6. Illustration of different types of skin biopsies.

Source: https://www.frontiersin.org/files/Articles/1476685/fmed-12-1476685-HTML/image_m/fmed-12-1476685-g001.jpg.

5.2.2. Indications for Performing a Biopsy

The only indication for performing a biopsy in dermatology is primarily based on the need for a certain diagnosis when non-invasive methods are inadequate. Biopsy techniques are important diagnostic tools for various skin lesions, particularly when distinguishing benign from malignant conditions. For instance, in melanoma suspected cases, a biopsy is then essential for diagnosis, as the condition also possesses a high incidence of metastasis if left untreated. According to recommendations, any lesion that presents atypically clinically is worthy of further investigation via biopsy to classify it, so that proper management can be decided (Bastiaannet et al., 2018). The rising incidence of skin cancer, particularly in European fair-skinned individuals, acts to validate these interventions in early detection and timely treatment (Bastiaannet et al., 2018). The requirement for biopsy is thus paramount when lesions present with suspicious characteristics, thereby further validating the need for organized dermatological treatment. Moreover, biopsy is highly useful as it pertains to surveillance and monitoring results to treatment for already existing dermatological illnesses. For patients with skin diseases such as psoriasis, cutaneous lymphoma, or autoimmune conditions, a biopsy can provide data on both disease evolution and treatment outcome. The histopathological analysis of biopsies allows doctors to diagnose cellular changes indicative of disease worsening or alleviation. This is consistent with clinical pipelines that aim to integrate non-invasive imaging technologies with biopsies, as described in recent reviews. By using optical imaging biomarkers and validating results with biopsy, dermatologists can generate a comprehensive plan for managing challenging dermatologic cases, ultimately leading to improved patient outcomes. In addition, indications for conducting a biopsy extend beyond diagnosis confirmation; they also play an important role in therapeutic decision-making.

Histopathological results play a crucial role in generating personalized treatment plans by informing clinicians about tumor type, stage, and molecular characteristics. This is particularly evident in the management of advanced melanoma, where treatment regimens vary considerably based on histological results (Bastiaannet et al., 2018). Access to specialist facilities that provide multidisciplinary treatment and use high-tech diagnostic equipment is required to optimize patient management. By adhering to established guidelines and ensuring timely performance of biopsies when indicated, health care clinicians are better able to navigate the subtleties of cutaneous pathology and thereby enhance the quality of dermatologic care overall. Ultimately, biopsy taking is based within a system of patient-centered diagnostic and therapeutic approaches for optimizing survival and quality of life for patients.

5.2.3. Interpretation of Biopsy Results

Interpretation of biopsy results is a crucial step in the diagnostic evaluation of dermatoses, particularly in distinguishing benign from malignant lesions. Histopathological analysis of biopsy material provides useful information on cellular morphology and tissue architecture, enabling the clinician to make informed treatment decisions. In cases of suspected skin malignancies such as lentigo maligna melanoma (LM/LMM) and cutaneous squamous cell carcinoma (cSCC), the biopsy not only serves a diagnostic purpose but is also a key determinant of tumor behavior and staging. While dermoscopy offers helpful initial assessment techniques, integrating biopsy results into the final diagnosis improves accuracy and reduces the risk of misinterpretation, ultimately improving patient outcomes in dermatology care (D'Onghia et al., 2025). In addition, new imaging technologies are enhancing the interpretation of biopsy results. Imaging techniques such as confocal microscopy, multiphoton tomography, and optical coherence tomography provide real-time, high-resolution images of skin lesions, allowing a better appreciation of the histological features involved. These imaging modalities complement routine histopathology by providing "optical biopsies," which can be extremely useful in patients with multifocal cSCC, where multiple lesions must be assessed. By employing advanced imaging techniques in combination with histological analysis, dermatologists can optimize diagnostic precision in such challenging cases. By reducing unnecessary surgical and biopsy procedures, the combination is a promising evolution in dermatological diagnostics (Gaikwad, 2025). The importance of accurate interpretation of biopsy results cannot be overemphasized, particularly in matters of deciding on follow-up treatment modalities. This information from biopsy tissue guides not only the nature of the lesion but also the risk of recurrence and metastasis. In aggressive skin cancers, such as cSCC, knowledge of the tumor's biological behavior, as obtained through advanced histopathological analysis, is essential for developing an individualized treatment plan. Furthermore, multidisciplinary teamwork involving pathologists, imaging specialists, and dermatologists augments diagnostic accuracy by merging conflicting perceptions of lesion features. With greater advancements in dermatology, integration of traditional biopsy interpretation and new imaging technologies will certainly enhance clinical practice, ultimately leading to improved patient care in skin disease management and diagnosis (D'Onghia et al., 2025) (Figure 5.7).

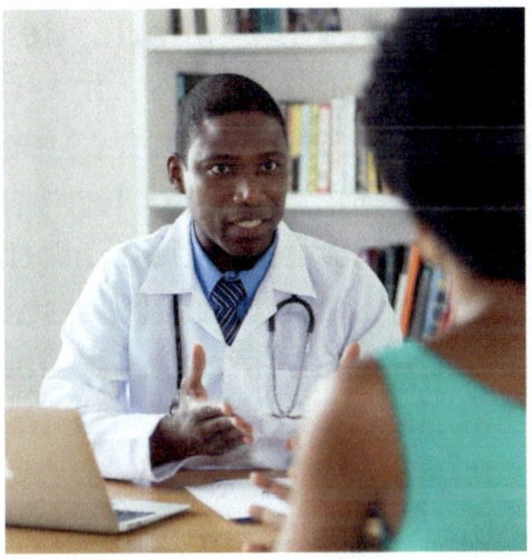

Figure 5.7. Understanding your biopsy results and pathology report.

Source: https://news.cancerconnect.com/.image/ar_1:1%2Cc_fill%2Ccs_srgb%2Cfl_progressive%2Cq_auto:good%2Cw_1200/MTg3Mjc2MDU4ODA0ODg5NDg2/shutterstock_1450907009.jpg.

Test Your Knowledge

1. List the types of skin biopsies.
2. What are the indications for a biopsy

5.3. Imaging Techniques

Learning Outcome

1. Give an overview of imaging modalities in dermatology
2. Understand the role of high-frequency ultrasound in skin assessment
3. Describe the emerging technologies in dermatological imaging

The importance of advanced imaging modalities in dermatology cannot be overstated, especially for accurate diagnosis of complex skin lesions. Routine dermoscopy, while excellent, is limited by its inability to provide cellular-level information. This drawback has been overcome in recent literature with the development of high-magnification dermoscopy and fluorescence-advanced videodermatoscopy (FAV), which significantly improves diagnostic sensitivity by revealing subtle dermoscopic features not apparent at lower magnifications. For instance, in the examination of facial lesions such as lentigo maligna and lentigo maligna melanoma, high-magnification methods have been shown to reveal characteristic features more frequently than standard dermoscopy, thereby enabling clinicians to make more effective decisions. Integration of all these varied imaging devices into clinical practice is required to optimize patient care and avoid unnecessary biopsies, ultimately optimizing the treatment of dermatological disease (D'Onghia et al., 2025). Confocal reflectance microscopy (RCM) and optical coherence tomography (OCT) also play significant roles in dermatology imaging. Both imaging modalities provide high-resolution images of the skin without invasion, enabling high-resolution visualization of cellular structures. RCM enables real-time imaging for differential diagnosis of malignant versus benign lesions, which is particularly helpful in populations with diverse skin types. This skill is critical since skin cancer detection is oftentimes marred by color variation, particularly in Black women, who may present in diverse ways compared to lighter races. The incorporation of RCM and OCT into dermatologic treatment protocols has the potential to revolutionize early detection and intervention, illustrating the imperative for dermatologists to be competent in applying these new tools (Lima et al., 2024). Moreover, the subspecialty training role simply cannot be overstressed as dermatologists remain willing to adopt the latest imaging technologies.

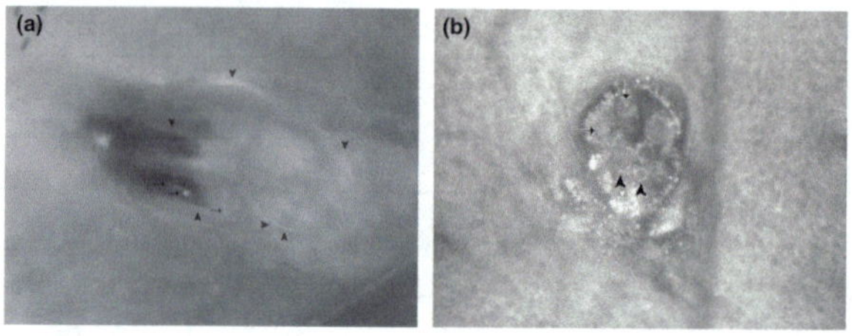

Figure 5.8. (a) Fluorescence-advanced videodermatoscopy (FAV) from a patient with pityriasis folliculorum. Five tubular structures, correlating to demodex mites, are present, occupying a hair follicle. A whitish halo (arrowheads) surrounds every demodex and corresponds to the external layer, the exoskeleton. Bright structures (black arrows) can be observed inside the opisthosoma of some demodex, corresponding to gut cells. (500× magnification). (b) The same external layer (arrow heads) and internal structures (black arrows) can be observed in reflectance confocal microscopy (RCM).

Source: https://www.researchgate.net/publication/345490667/figure/fig1/AS:11431281472881102@1748535078932/a-Fluorescence-advanced-videodermatoscopy-FAV-from-a-patient-with-pityriasis.png.\

Accurate interpretation of images obtained with techniques such as multispectral imaging and electrical impedance spectroscopy requires not only technical expertise but also an understanding of the complex presentations of skin lesions across various populations. With a focus on enhancing health disparities, particularly in the context of detecting skin cancer among the marginalized, tailored training programs will further augment the authority of these diagnostic tools. By empowering practitioners to read results carefully and in context, medical systems can seek equity in care that is appropriate to dermatological diagnoses. Thus, imaging modalities in dermatology coupled with focused educational efforts are a bright future for improved patient outcomes (Lima et al., 2024; D'Onghia et al., 2025) (Figure 5.8).

5.3.1. Overview of Imaging Modalities in Dermatology

The field of dermatology has advanced significantly with the introduction of various imaging modalities that enhance diagnostic accuracy and facilitate treatment. Traditional methods rely heavily on visual examination, which, while helpful, is subjective and can lead to variations in diagnosis due to perception. The introduction of non-invasive imaging modalities revolutionized dermatological examination by providing objective information to assist clinical judgment. Optical coherence tomography (OCT), on the other hand, is currently a principal imaging technique that provides high-resolution cross-sectional imaging of the skin without tissue removal. It is this type of function that enables real-time assessment of the microstructure of skin lesions and is, therefore, a basic tool in today's dermatology for the diagnosis and monitoring of skin disorders (Adabi et al., 2017). Its high penetration depth and spatial resolution are further strengths of OCT in dermatology compared with current imaging methods. OCT operates on interferometric principles, enabling rapid imaging of complex skin architecture and pathology. One important advantage of OCT is that it can provide instant feedback during treatment, for example, by guiding biopsies, which can improve the precision of lesion excision and patient outcomes. There is evidence available that demonstrates its utility for diagnosis of various cutaneous pathologies, ranging from skin neoplasms such as melanoma to inflammatory conditions such as psoriasis. The ability to visualize skin morphology and monitor treatment outcomes has rendered OCT a valuable addition to the dermatologist's diagnostic arsenal (Xu et al., 2021). Beyond OCT, there are various other imaging modalities, such as dermoscopy and reflectance confocal microscopy, that also provide valuable contributions to dermatologic diagnosis. Dermoscopy improves , making the distinction between benign and malignant lesions simpler by observing surface topography and color patterns under magnification that are not visible to the naked eye. Reflectance confocal microscopy is applied for non invasive skin imaging at cellular resolution, providing information on epidermal and papillary dermal alterations. These modalities, which are usually used in conjunction with OCT, enhance dermatologists' diagnostic role and support informed decision-making in patient treatment. Increased utilization of sophisticated imaging equipment necessitates the integration of such equipment into dermatological practices and thereby increasingly renders accurate diagnoses and individualized treatment regimens (Adabi et al., 2017) (Figure 5.9).

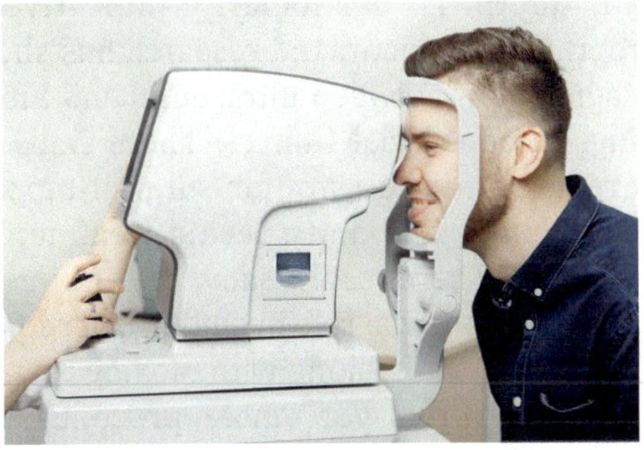

Figure 5.9. Optical coherence tomography.

Source: https://davidhmyers.com/wp-content/uploads/2021/08/OCT-min.jpg.

5.3.2. Role of High-Frequency Ultrasound in Skin Assessment

High-frequency ultrasound is increasingly being used in dermatology because it is noninvasive and can provide high-resolution imaging of skin structures. Clinicians can visualize the epidermis, dermis, and subcutaneous structures in greater detail than with traditional imaging equipment. By employing high-frequency ultrasound, dermatologists can investigate various skin diseases, including tumors and inflammatory disorders, thereby enabling a more precise diagnosis without the need for biopsies. The method's sensitivity in differentiating between superficial and deep lesions improves clinicians' decision-making process and, consequently, patient outcomes and treatment. In the context of lesions that may simulate serious conditions, the precision offered by high-frequency ultrasound is a welcome addition to the diagnostic team, supplementing the current dermatological arsenal of dermoscopy and histopathological examination. High-frequency ultrasound is particularly useful for evaluating certain skin cancers, such as superficial basal cell carcinoma (sBCC). Research has also indicated that this imaging technique is 0.87 sensitive and 0.80 specific for sBCC diagnosis, reflecting its utility in differential diagnosis. Accuracy in measuring tumor depth is particularly indicative of appropriate treatment, and research has shown high agreement between ultrasound and biopsy findings in superficial tumors. These skills not only reduce the necessity for surgical biopsies but also allow safe and specific treatment of sBCC lesions. These results show high-frequency ultrasounds' potential role in guiding subsequent treatment protocols, along with moving towards more conservative yet viable procedures in dermatology, furthering a trend consonant with current advancements in non-invasive diagnostics as suggested (Cheng et al., 2015). Even though the role of high-frequency ultrasound is evolving, it is also necessary to be aware of its integration with other diagnostic modalities, such as dermoscopy and total body photography. Use of these modalities in combination provides us with a general impression regarding the patient's skin condition and informs us regarding the risk factors involved in malignant lesions. For patients who have several dysplastic nevi or are at high risk for developing melanoma, using high-frequency ultrasound in combination with conventional methods might further improve the diagnostic accuracy for melanoma. Such a combination is consonant with guidelines that support a thorough skin examination enabled by newer imaging modalities in addition to clinical assessment. With the constantly evolving nature of dermatology, high-frequency ultrasound will play a significant role in simplifying diagnostic pathways, thereby enhancing early detection and, ultimately, patient prognosis (Soyer et al., 2010) (Figure 5.10).

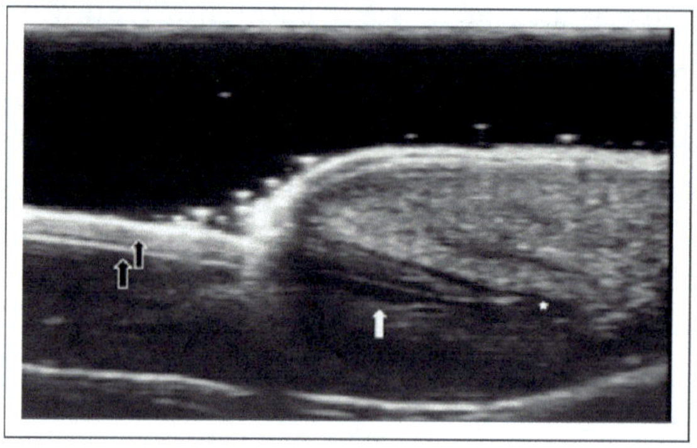

Figure 5.10. Ultra-high frequency ultrasonography (UHFUS) application in dermatology. Ultrasonographic aspect of the proximal part of the index finger nail under there 70 MHz probe. The nail matrix (*) and the nail bed (white arrow) are clearly recognizable as hypoechoic structures. The nail plate is characterized by 2 parallel hyperechoic bands (black arrows).

Source: https://www.researchgate.net/profile/Teresa-Oranges/publication/343270586/figure/fig2/AS:1152310239592455@1651743578634/Ultra-high-frequency-ultrasonography-UHFUS-application-in-dermatology-Ultrasonographic.png.

5.3.3. Emerging Technologies in Dermatological Imaging

New dermatologic imaging technologies enhance dermatologists' diagnostic capabilities, providing noninvasive approaches to improved detection and disease management of cutaneous disorders. Among the new technologies, reflectance confocal microscopy (RCM) is among the most significant, providing high-resolution imaging of skin lesions at the cellular level. RCM enables clinicians to visualize the microstructure of skin in real time, allowing them to differentiate benign from malignant lesions without invasive biopsy. This feature is especially important in skin cancers, where early intervention is paramount in patient care. As noted in current research, these imaging methods are much more sophisticated and are playing a more central role in overall skin cancer management, thereby potentially reducing the incidence of unnecessary surgical procedures (Conforti et al., 2020). Another new imaging device that is increasingly being employed is line-field confocal optical coherence tomography (LC-OCT), which is a "virtual biopsy" of the skin. This technique provides real-time images of skin tissue that are highly akin to traditional histopathology, presenting clinicians with a picture of numerous skin diseases, including inflammatory and neoplastic conditions. Recent research has demonstrated the efficacy of LC-OCT in diagnosing numerous skin tumors, reaffirming its value as an adjunct diagnostic modality. Whereas LC-OCT bridges the gap between dermoscopy and histopathology, it enables dermatologists to quantify lesion features without immediately resorting to invasive procedures. Thus, LC-OCT's use in clinical practice marks a shift towards greater diagnostic accuracy, tailored treatment techniques, and improved patient satisfaction (Cappilli et al., 2024). Furthermore, the advent of multispectral imaging technology and artificial intelligence (AI) in dermatologic imaging is another milestone in the evolution of diagnostic capabilities. Multispectral imaging enables images to be acquired across multiple wavelengths, providing high-resolution information about the composition and characteristics of skin lesions. This additional layer of information enables more accurate diagnoses and skin condition evaluations through fine variation detection not available to the naked eye. AI systems complement these imaging modalities by performing pattern and anomaly detection on large datasets quickly and effectively, assisting dermatologists in discovery. These new technologies all contribute to a more sophisticated and subtle understanding of dermatological conditions, maintaining their revolutionary potential for use in clinical practice and enabling the onset of an era of precise and efficient dermatological treatment (Conforti et al., 2020) (Figure 5.11).

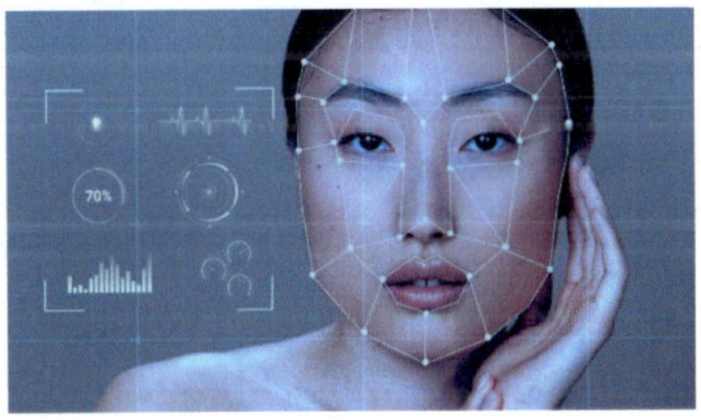

Figure 5.11. Artificial intelligence (AI) in dermatology: Revolutionizing skin care and treatment.

Source: https://itmunch.com/wp-content/uploads/2024/07/facial-recognition-collage-concept-1200x675.jpg.

Test Your Knowledge

1. What are the imaging modalities in dermatology?
2. What is the role of high-frequency ultrasound in skin assessment?

5.4. Comparison of Diagnostic Tools

Learning Outcome

1. Describe the strengths and weaknesses of dermoscopy
2. Know the strengths and weaknesses of biopsy
3. Understand the strengths and weaknesses of imaging techniques

A thorough comparison of dermatological diagnostic tools should account for the continuously evolving nature of non-invasive techniques, particularly in the context of diseases such as melanoma and basal cell carcinoma. Dermoscopy is a separate advancement, enhancing the visibility of skin lesions for the dermatologist. It provides high-resolution images that allow for the identification of patterns indicative of malignancy. Further, dermoscopy, supported by clinical observation, is increasingly being adopted as a useful standard reference for lesion detection that requires further histopathological investigation. By contextualizing these findings within the patient's history and risk factors, dermatologists can better prioritize which lesions require biopsy, optimizing both patient care and resource allocation in clinical settings (Soyer et al., 2010). The collaborative use of dermoscopy and patient history illustrates the diagnostic synergy necessary for effective melanoma screening. In contrast to the non-invasive approach of dermoscopy, traditional biopsy remains a cornerstone of definitive diagnosis in dermatology. While biopsies provide histological evidence and detailed information about the cellular composition of lesions, they are invasive and need not be performed for every suspicious lesion. Evolution of imaging modalities such as optical coherence tomography (OCT) provides an intriguing alternative that combines the advantages of non-invasive diagnosis with the accuracy hitherto the prerogative of invasive methods. Current research indicates that OCT has very good sensitivity and specificity for diagnosing superficial basal cell carcinoma, enabling a more focused patient assessment. More specifically, OCT correlates strongly with histopathological findings, particularly at thicknesses below 0.4 mm, making it a helpful diagnostic modality that may reduce the need for biopsies (Cheng et al., 2015). The integration of novel diagnostic modalities continues to revolutionize the image of dermatologic examination, highlighting the utility of an integrated approach. Non-invasive imaging techniques, including reflectance confocal microscopy and digital dermoscopy, complement the dermatologists' diagnostic arsenal by providing real-time, high-resolution data on lesion characteristics. Each tool has its own strength; e.g., total body photography allows systematic follow-up in high-risk patients for skin cancers, while computer-based diagnostic systems have the potential to enhance diagnostic performance through computational intelligence. This dual approach, which uses both technological advancements and traditional methods, ultimately aims to further improve diagnostic accuracy in dermatology. With advances in technology, it will be critical to examine the efficacy and utility of these tools across various clinical settings to optimize patient outcomes and address the increasing incidence of skin cancer (Soyer et al., 2010).

5.4.1. Strengths and Weaknesses of Dermoscopy

Dermoscopy has emerged as a significant diagnostic tool in dermatology with multiple advantages that enhance clinical practice. One such important advantage is its ability to visualize subsurface skin structures, which cannot be done by traditional visual inspection. Increased visualization aids clinicians in detecting subtle changes in skin lesions, thus earlier detection of malignant conditions like melanoma. For instance, systematic reviews have shown that the ABCD dermoscopy rule is highly sensitive and specific and can be used to rule out melanoma across various patient populations. Besides, dermoscopy is more minimally invasive and sometimes can preclude the need for more invasive procedures, such as biopsy, thereby allowing quicker examination and treatment of skin lesions. The advantages point towards dermoscopy's role in maximizing decision-making processes in dermatological investigations, ultimately towards better patient outcomes (Armstrong et al., 2017). Despite its strengths, dermoscopy also has its weaknesses that can preclude its application in given situations. One limitation is that a great deal of training and experience is needed to correctly interpret the varied dermoscopic patterns. Misinterpretation can occur, leading to inaccurate diagnoses that adversely affect patient care. In addition, the quality of acquired images affects the accuracy of dermoscopy; poor-quality images can obscure critical details, thereby compromising diagnostic accuracy. Compared with computerized image analysis techniques, increasingly applied in dermatology, dermoscopy can also be hampered by artifacts that make lesion assessment more challenging. Management of such disadvantages involves ongoing education for the clinician and possibly developing more robust training modules to ensure appropriate application of this diagnostic tool (Dato et al., 2023). Finally, while dermoscopy is a valuable addition to the dermatological diagnostic arsenal, it is only right that both its strengths and limitations are recognized. The ability to obtain an intimate insight into the lesion will facilitate more accurate diagnosis, particularly in conditions such as melanoma, where early diagnosis is key to a successful outcome. Conversely, operator skill dependence and potential for misinterpretation highlight the need for continuing professional education in dermoscopy. With advances in technology and increased interconnectivity with automated networks, it is important to balance dermoscopy's strengths with an understanding of its limitations. That balance will ultimately translate into the establishment of dermatological diagnostics, enabling practitioners to use the tools available to them in the most effective manner in patient care (Armstrong et al., 2017) (Figure 5.12).

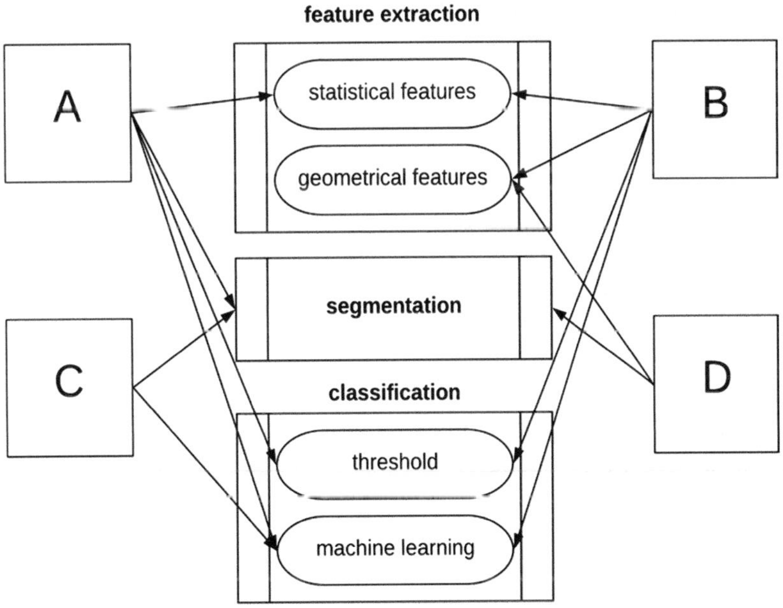

Figure 5.12. Dermoscopic image analysis stages involved in the ABCD rule traits.

Source: https://www.researchgate.net/publication/340993515/figure/fig4/AS:885480405098496@1588126388276/Dermoscopic-image-analysis-stages-involved-in-the-ABCD-rule-traits.ppm.

5.4.2. Strengths and Weaknesses of Biopsy

Biopsy is a cornerstone diagnostic procedure in the field of dermatology, well known for its accuracy in establishing diagnoses for skin conditions. One of the major strengths of biopsy is that it provides histopathological confirmation of an inferred diagnosis, which is critical before initiating a specific treatment program. By removing tissue samples for microscopic study, dermatologists can accurately differentiate between benign and malignant lesions, thereby appropriately treating the patient. With advances in methods—e.g., punch or excisional biopsies—there is greater potential to remove sufficient tissue without excessive scarring. This is particularly so when there is diagnostic doubt, as with the investigation of numerous skin malignancies. In general, the ability to verify diagnoses at the cellular level solidifies biopsy as a necessary instrument, despite the procedure's risks, i.e., scarring or infection at the biopsy site. All the same, biopsy also has its flaws, which discount its value as a diagnostic instrument. Its biggest drawback is sampling error, in that the biopsy cannot accurately represent the entire lesion. This is particularly relevant in cases where lesions have heterogeneous features, which may result in misdiagnosis. Also, the invasive procedure deters patients, particularly those who are apprehensive about surgery. Further, the need for experienced practitioners to read histopathology creates yet another level of complexity, with misreading being a risk factor that complicates diagnostic procedures. In addition, there usually is a wait for results, which can extend patient anxiety or postpone necessary treatment. Such problems underscore the necessity of a multimodal diagnostic approach that combines biopsy with other diagnostic methods. Advances in imaging technology have highlighted both the virtues and the limitations of biopsy in dermatology. For instance, optical coherence tomography (OCT) has emerged as a powerful adjunct to biopsy, enabling non-invasive assessment of skin lesions. In a study examining the efficacy of OCT for the delineation of basal cell carcinoma (BCC) mapping, OCT was shown to accurately define tumor margins, leading to better Mohs micrographic surgery with reduced numbers of surgeries required. These advancements reflect the need to integrate technological progress with conventional methods to compensate for biopsy limitations and increase diagnostic accuracy. Furthermore, incorporating dermoscopy with biopsy will help advance lesion characterization, reducing dependence on surgical procedures in isolation. The interaction between these imaging modalities and biopsy describes an extensive method to dermatological diagnosis, with the goal of optimizing patient outcomes while compensating for the intrinsic limitations of a single diagnostic approach.

5.4.3. Strengths and Weaknesses of Imaging Techniques

Imaging techniques have revolutionized the practice of dermatology, with both strengths and limitations in diagnosis. One of their biggest strengths lies in the fact that they are non-invasive, allowing real-time visualization of skin lesions without removal by way of excisional biopsies. This capability enhances clinicians' ability to diagnose melanomas and other skin conditions more accurately and effectively, ultimately improving patient outcomes. Furthermore, advanced imaging techniques are increasingly being integrated with machine learning algorithms to improve diagnostic accuracy. For instance, models like SegAN and MultiResUNet have achieved improved performance in dermoscopic segmentation, achieving up to 92% accuracy in skin lesion detection, thereby potentially reducing diagnostic errors due to human interpretation. The techniques mentioned above, however, are prone to being image quality dependent and are limited by sensitivity and specificity constraints, which result in false positives or negatives.

Despite the clear advantages, imaging modalities do possess inherent limitations that must be taken into account. Methods like dermoscopy can frequently be operator-dependent and dependent on the quality of the dermatoscope. There is also the issue of differentiation between lesions that can look alike, when border visual signals can get lost or misplaced. Besides, while imaging has improved early detection rates, it has not adequately replaced biopsies, especially when histopathological evaluation is necessary for diagnosis. Imaging reliance at times may lead to overdiagnosis and unwarranted anxiety and treatment for patients (Gao et al., 2025). Moreover, variations in technology and imaging protocols may lead to discrepancies in diagnostic results among different clinical settings, further compounding these issues. Integration of new imaging techniques into dermatology practice also holds the potential to overcome some of their existing limitations. For instance, advances in machine learning and artificial intelligence can enhance the reliability of imaging analysis, further upgrading accuracy. MultiResUNet and SegAN models aim to extract contextual information from dermoscopic images, thereby addressing the limitations of traditional approaches in detecting subtle features of skin lesions (Gao et al., 2025). Moreover, novel transdermal drug delivery systems might be used to supplement imaging techniques by ensuring more effective treatment upon proper diagnosis, particularly for chronic diseases like psoriasis, where patient compliance to treatment is an issue (Gao et al., 2025). Yet dermatologists ought to know how to balance the advantages and disadvantages of these imaging modalities to optimize patient care, so that imaging is employed as an adjunctive tool rather than a replacement for appropriate clinical assessment and histopathological examination (Figure 5.13).

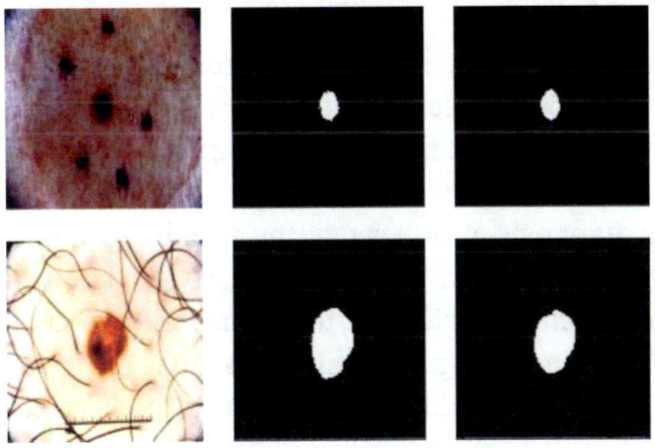

Figure 5.13. Example results of our SegAN (right) with corresponding input (left) and ground truth (middle) on the ISIC 2017 test set.

Source: https://www.researchgate.net/profile/Yuan-Xue-5/publication/325522635/figure/fig1/AS:1169457498079232@1655831803299/Example-results-of-our-SegAN-right-with-corresponding-input-left-and-ground-truth.ppm.

Test Your Knowledge

1. What are the limitations of dermoscopy?
2. What are the strengths of a biopsy?

5.5. Clinical Applications

Learning Outcome

1. Describe the use of dermoscopy in melanoma detection
2. Understand the role of biopsy in diagnosing skin cancers
3. Learn about the imaging in monitoring chronic skin conditions

Clinical applications of diagnostic devices in dermatology, such as dermoscopy, biopsy, and imaging methods, are important for enhancing patient outcomes. Dermoscopy has transformed the diagnosis of skin cancer by enabling clinicians to visualize skin lesions with greater accuracy. The machine facilitates discrimination between benign and malignant lesions because it provides magnification and polarized light imaging, highlighting structural features not discernible by the naked eye. Further, dermoscopy is used in the diagnosis of dermatological diseases other than skin cancers, including inflammatory dermatoses and vascular lesions. Coupled with other modalities of diagnosis, dermoscopy enhances conventional visual inspection and enables earlier and more accurate diagnosis, ultimately reducing the impact of late-stage skin cancers on patient populations. Biopsy remains a mainstay in dermatology diagnostics and renders an absolute histopathological diagnosis of skin disease. Although dermoscopy provides a helpful non-invasive technique, biopsy renders definitive diagnoses feasible by examination of skin specimens under the microscope. Techniques such as shave, punch, and excisional biopsies are used for various dermatologic conditions, providing specific diagnoses and therapeutic modalities for patients. Although effective, a biopsy is invasive by nature and has risks such as scarring and infection. The application of virtual biopsy techniques, such as line-field confocal optical coherence tomography (LC-OCT), is increasingly prominent in clinical settings. LC-OCT acts as a "bridge" between dermoscopy and histopathology by enabling real-time visualization of skin anatomy, allowing pathological features to be inspected without invasive intervention (Cappilli et al., 2024). The innovation is a significant step forward to the provision of holistic care in dermatology. Besides, emerging imaging and data analysis technologies are expanding the clinical scope in dermatology. Deep learning algorithms introduce a fresh approach to skin disease classification, particularly in efficient and effective skin cancer detection. By making use of big data that combines clinical information and smartphone-acquired images, these algorithms enable non-invasive, scalable screening. Combining intermediate fusion techniques across different modalities enhances diagnostic accuracy by using advanced algorithms to classify conditions with greater precision. Results indicate a marked improvement in classification accuracy, surpassing traditional standards (Effendie et al., 2024). The use of imaging technology and AI holds the key to broader access to dermatological services, particularly for low-income communities, thereby addressing disparities in healthcare access. As a result, not only are the clinical applications of these methods enhancing the care of individual patients, but also the broader dermatological landscape (Figure 5.14).

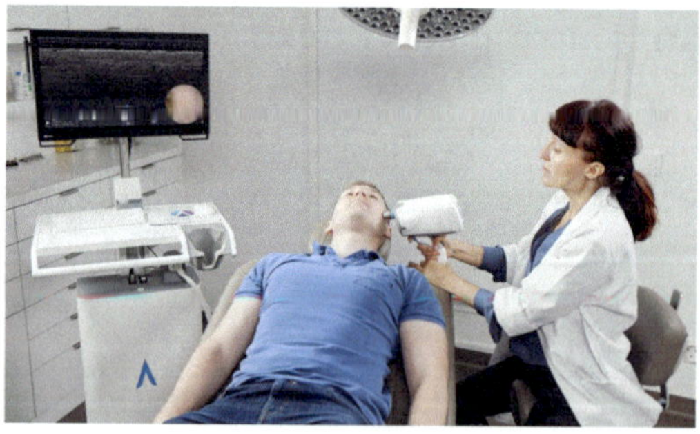

Figure 5.14. Line-field confocal optical coherence tomography (LC-OCT) device.

Source: https://www.mdpi.com/life/life-13-02268/article_deploy/html/images/life-13-02268-g001.png.

5.5.1. Use of Dermoscopy in Melanoma Detection

Dermoscopy is now an invaluable tool for melanoma detection, significantly enhancing dermatologists' diagnostic accuracy. This imaging technique does not require skin incision and enables accurate visualization of skin lesions, revealing minute morphological features that would otherwise be beyond the naked eye. Using a dermatoscope, clinicians can more effectively examine pigmented lesions and distinguish benign nevi from malignant melanomas. Early diagnosis is also of prime concern in the management of melanoma; it has been shown that if diagnosed early, the prognosis is greatly enhanced. Clinical inspection, along with dermoscopy, is therefore considered a criterion point of reference for identifying skin lesions warranting further histopathological examination (Soyer et al., 2010). Beyond primary melanoma detection, dermoscopy also plays a crucial role in monitoring patients with known risk factors. High-risk patients, especially those with large numbers of dysplastic nevi or a family history of melanoma, can be helped by a routine dermoscopically-assisted skin examination. Using total body photography in conjunction with digital dermoscopy can improve follow-up regimens for such patients, allowing dermatologists to monitor lesion changes over time in an anticipatory manner. This approach ensures that any new or changing lesions are detected early, enabling timely intervention. The integration of higher-order imaging modalities further solidifies the position of dermoscopy as a cornerstone in dermatological diagnosis (Soyer et al., 2010). Aside from its real-time use, continued development of dermoscopy and other non-invasive imaging technologies has the potential to alter the playing field of melanoma detection. Techniques such as optical coherence tomography and reflectance confocal microscopy add to dermoscopy additional layers of diagnostic information without the need for invasive biopsy. Although histopathological examination is the standard for diagnosis, the quality of imaging provided by dermoscopic techniques enables faster, economically viable screening. This shift towards non-surgical methods not only enhances diagnostic accuracy but also improves patient satisfaction, making early-stage treatment more feasible. As the art keeps unfolding, it is important for practitioners to remain knowledgeable in these technologies to identify and treat melanomas effectively for their patients (Figure 5.15).

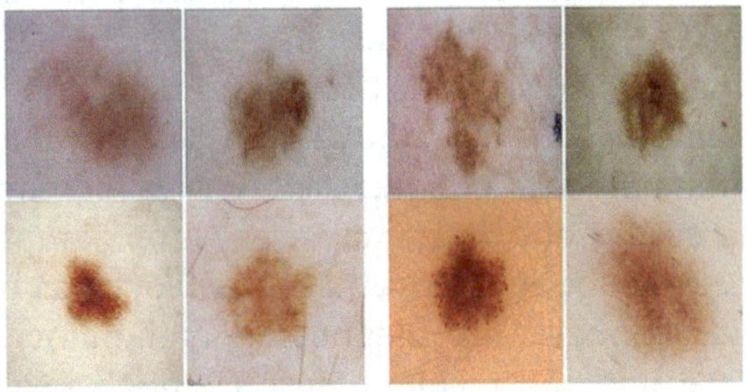

Figure 5.15. Dermoscopy, the microscopic examination of the skin surface, has been used to evaluate skin lesions and the detection of melanoma. Its value, however, has been questioned for melanoma-*in-situ* (MIS). Examples of a lesion classification task. Left example dermoscopic images of melanoma. A right example of dermoscopic images of benign nevi.

Source: https://www.researchgate.net/profile/Athanasios-Valavanidis/publication/340477926/figure/fig2/AS:877597458198528@1586246947420/Dermoscopy-the-microscopic-examination-of-the-skin-surface-has-been-used-to-evaluate.jpg.

5.5.2. Role of Biopsy in Diagnosing Skin Cancers

The application of biopsy in the identification of skin cancers remains paramount despite advances in non-invasive imaging techniques. When clinical evaluations and dermoscopic examination yield inconclusive findings, a biopsy is the definitive diagnostic procedure to determine the presence of malignancy. This entails removing an infinitesimal tissue sample from the lesion for histological examination. In this instance, the pathologist identifies cell alterations characteristic of malignancies such as melanoma, squamous cell carcinoma, and basal cell carcinoma. Though biopsies are invasive and can lead to discomfort or complications, they provide the most precise diagnosis and thus dictate treatment options. As highlighted by advances in imaging modalities, the complementarity of biopsy results with non-invasive approaches has become critical for augmenting diagnostic accuracy and treatment planning (Gust et al., 2024). Despite advances in imaging devices like reflectance confocal microscopy and optical coherence tomography, these cannot entirely replace the biopsy as the gold standard for diagnosing malignancies. These imaging technologies, although useful for differentiating between benign and malignant lesions, at times yield inconclusive or ambiguous results, particularly in intricate cases. To illustrate, in the differential diagnosis between basal cell carcinoma (BCC) and other skin lesions, standard histology remains the gold standard for accurate diagnosis. Studies reveal that integrating biopsy information with that of non-invasive devices can improve overall diagnostic confidence and reduce unnecessary surgical interventions (Bakos et al., 2018). Therefore, the biopsy remains at the core of the diagnostic cascade of skin cancers, particularly when clinical suspicion is strong and imaging results are inconclusive. Secondly, a biopsy not only yields a confirmatory diagnosis but also helps choose the appropriate treatment modality. The histopathological analysis gives crucial information regarding tumor type, grade, and invasion depth, which are critical for both staging and treatment planning. For instance, in melanomas, Breslow thickness, as measured from biopsy specimens, is helpful for risk stratification and planning the subsequent steps of therapy. Follow-up phases can be very helpful with biopsies to assess response to therapy in recurrent or residual lesions. Even with new imaging techniques that potentially enhance skin cancer treatment, biopsy remains the gold standard for accuracy and therapeutic guidance in dermatology (Gust et al., 2024) (Figure 5.16).

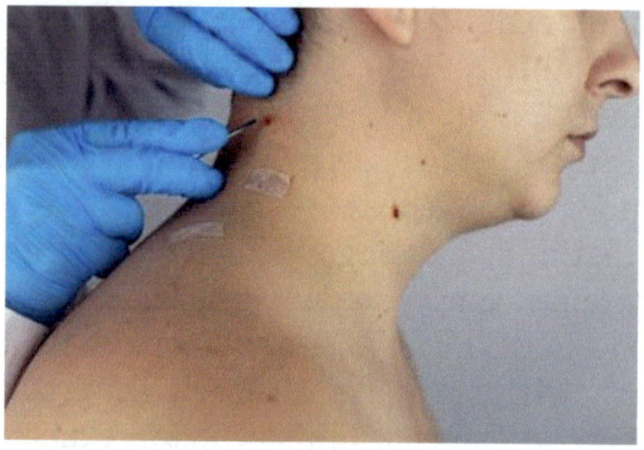

Figure 5.16. The role of a skin biopsy in diagnosing skin cancer.

Source: https://smb.ibsrv.net/imageresizer/image/article_manager/1200x1200/202277/1252194/heroimage0.1851190017334 28273.jpg.

5.5.3. Imaging in Monitoring Chronic Skin Conditions

The advent of advanced imaging modalities has revolutionized the assessment of chronic skin disease so that dermatologists are now able to better appreciate skin pathology. Among the techniques used, autofluorescence imaging (AFI) is especially beneficial because it can identify endogenous fluorophores within tissue without adding exogenous dyes. AFI is a non-invasive procedure that can be applied in real-time to assess skin health and provide vital information on cellular function and tissue integrity. Recent studies have demonstrated that AFI can be employed as an effective surrogate to assess other metabolic conditions and thereby provide a superior understanding of diabetic skin complications. Implementing AFI in daily dermatological practice will enable healthcare practitioners to enhance their early diagnosis and intervention capabilities, leading to superior patient outcomes in chronic skin diseases. Moreover, imaging utility extends beyond initial assessment; it is critical for ongoing follow-up and evaluation of the effectiveness of treatment for chronic cutaneous disorders. For instance, longitudinal studies using imaging modalities, such as dermoscopy and high-frequency ultrasound, have demonstrated their potential to capture fine changes in the disease course over time.

Such advanced imaging techniques empower dermatologists to track disease flare-ups, monitor treatment responses, and adjust therapeutic regimens in real time. Specifically, imaging modalities can define the histological features of diseases such as psoriasis and eczema, enabling more specific therapeutic strategies that account for individual patient requirements. The dynamism of dermatology requires that such advanced monitoring techniques be available, as they yield key information to guide clinical decisions and improve patient management. The application of imaging devices in clinical dermatology reflects the universal tendency toward personalized medicine, in which treatment protocols are increasingly tailored to the unique characteristics of the individual patient's condition. Finally, the application of imaging in dermatology facilitates a greater understanding of chronic skin diseases, as it not only clarifies morphologic alterations but also helps establish impairment of skin function. As seen in the existing literature, ongoing research on the application of AFI methods holds promise for chronic skin disease management, as evidence supports its efficacy in monitoring several dermatological conditions and comorbidities (Aigner et al., 2020). While the future of imaging in dermatology is promising, there is still a critical need for established protocols and research to maximize these technologies in practice (Edwards et al., 2020) (Figure 5.17).

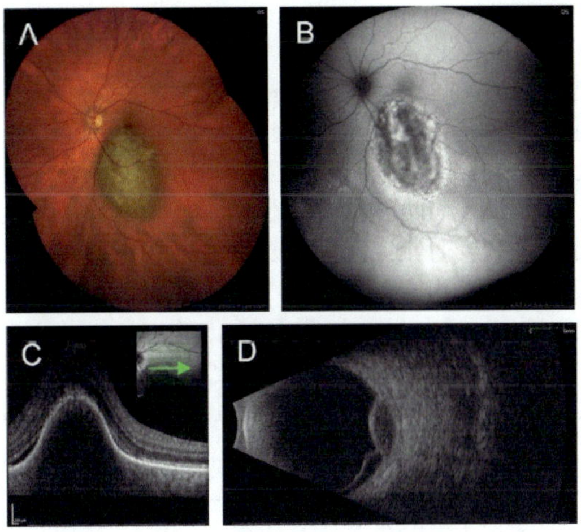

Figure 5.17. Multimodal imaging of a choroidal melanoma in a 51-year-old male patient presenting with metamorphopsia. (A) The fundus photograph shows a pigmented lesion (diameter > 5 mm) with overlying orange pigment, and (B) With marked changes of the signal seen on fundus autofluorescence (illumination with 500–585 nm, FAF-Green). (C) An OCT scan at the tumour's margin shows a subretinal cleft due to malignant exudation. (D) Exudation is also seen on ultrasonography as exudative retinal detachment.

Source: https://www.mdpi.com/cancers/cancers-14-01809/article_deploy/html/images/cancers-14-01809-g001.png.

Test Your Knowledge

1. What is the use of dermoscopy in melanoma detection?
2. What is the role of biopsy in diagnosing skin cancers?

SUMMARY

In dermatological diagnosis, the integration of advanced diagnostic tools such as dermoscopy, biopsy, and imaging has significantly changed the dynamics of skin cancer identification and management. Each of these methods has its own advantages, targeting varying aspects of diagnosis. Dermoscopy, for example, allows clinicians to visualize skin lesions at a higher level of detail, revealing important morphological information that enhances diagnostic accuracy. Biopsy remains, however, the gold standard for the definitive identification of malignancies, based on histopathological evidence, and cannot be substituted. Imaging modalities, particularly those based on deep learning algorithms, are also emerging as powerful adjuncts, making processes more economical and enabling the rapid identification of skin cancers (Naeem et al., 2024). The merging of these technologies not only increases diagnostic accuracy but also improves patient outcomes by enabling earlier intervention. Additionally, the integration of AI with traditional diagnostics, as in recent studies, underscores the potential for significant breakthroughs in early detection of skin cancer. Models such as SNC_Net and DVFNet achieve high precision in discriminating among various skin cancers, with metrics of 97.81% and 98.32%, respectively. These advancements portend a brighter future not only where AI is utilized in aiding diagnosis but also in improving the ability of dermatologists, particularly for ambiguous lesions. By training on extensive datasets such as ISIC 2019, these technologies can learn and develop over time, eventually becoming capable of handling the intricacies of real clinical settings (Naeem et al., 2024). Continuous development provides a strong case for sustained investment in dermatological diagnostic research and development. Overall, the dermatological diagnostic landscape is one of exponentially speeding up multidisciplinary approaches in which old and new technologies find a place. As much as time-tested old favorites such as dermoscopy and biopsy remain valuable, stable image-guided and AI-based tools in our hands mean that a golden era of diagnostic accuracy and curative efficacy is now here. The additive potential of human intelligence and machine-learning technology represents a good case of how dermatology can enhance its operations, provide interventions in a timely manner, and improve patient care. As skin cancer incidence rises worldwide, it becomes ever more essential to have efficient and effective diagnostic methods. Therefore, research and development of diagnostic apparatus must not cease to enable health professionals to be able to counteract skin cancer effectively.

In dermatology, diagnostic aids such as dermoscopy, biopsy, and imaging are crucial for the adequate evaluation of skin lesions. Dermoscopy has the additional benefit of complementing visual inspection by , enabling them to visualize subsurface skin structures more sensitively and specifically. Clinical prediction rules (CPRs) are ancillary tools, triaging patients by assessing symptoms that refer to malignant melanoma. Notably, the ABCD dermoscopy rule has also demonstrated high sensitivity (0.85) and specificity (0.72) in melanoma detection, indicating its potential for application in the clinic. Systematic review of CPRs emphasizes the need to include these tools to improve early diagnosis and, in turn, patients' outcomes. Therefore, evidence-based diagnosis criteria are the linchpin in achieving optimum melanoma detection and management, a necessity in an industry plagued by the risk of death from late detection (Armstrong et al., 2017). A biopsy remains an essential element in the final diagnosis of cutaneous lesions, after an initial clinical assessment, where histopathological confirmation is sought. Despite advances in non-invasive imaging techniques and dermoscopy, biopsy remains the gold standard for distinguishing benign from malignant disease. Punch, shave, and excision biopsies are among the modalities dermatologists use to tailor treatment to lesion categories while accounting for patient comfort and diagnostic accuracy. However, clinicians should remain aware of the risks of biopsy procedures such as scarring and infection. This subtle identification is paramount to making sound decisions on patient treatment. Lastly, integrating biopsies with diagnostic imaging and dermoscopy ensures a complete approach to dermatologic evaluation, paving the way for appropriate treatment modalities (Armstrong et al., 2017). Advances in imaging technology over the past several years have provided novel means of enhancing the diagnosis of skin disease, particularly melanoma. One such emerging technique involves the tensor decomposition-based feature extraction from clinical color images, which preserves both spectral and spatial information of skin lesions. The method shows encouraging results, with an overall sensitivity of 82.1% and specificity of 86.9% for melanoma classification. Such advancements are not only increasing diagnostic precision but also providing a non-surgical method over traditional biopsy methods. Further, they enable the integration of machine learning methods to automate procedure analysis, which could accelerate diagnosis and treatment planning. With dermatology becoming more sophisticated with the use of technology, synergy among dermoscopy, biopsy, and new imaging modalities is bound to enhance the methodology for skin cancer diagnosis and usher in better patient outcomes.

KEY TERMS FROM THIS CHAPTER

- Artificial intelligence
- Biopsy
- Communication
- Dermoscopy
- Irregular dots
- Lentigo maligna melanoma
- Skin examination
- Benign lesions
- Blue-white veils
- Convolutional neural networks
- Inflammatory diseases
- Lentigo maligna
- Machine learning
- Skin tumors

CRITICAL THINKING QUESTIONS

1. **Which diagnostic tool is primarily used for magnified examination of skin lesions?**
   a. Biopsy
   b. Dermoscopy
   c. Imaging
   d. Microscopy
2. **What is the main purpose of a skin biopsy in dermatology?**
   a. To magnify skin lesions.
   b. To assess the internal organs for skin-related conditions.
   c. To extract and examine tissue samples for histopathological analysis.
   d. To provide real-time imaging of skin layers.
3. **Which imaging technique is commonly used for detailed visualization of deeper skin structures?**
   a. X-ray
   b. Ultrasound imaging
   c. Dermoscopy
   d. Fluorescence microscopy
4. **Dermoscopy is most useful for diagnosing which of the following?**
   a. Internal organ damage.
   b. Skin infections.
   c. Pigmented skin lesions, such as melanoma.
   d. Systemic autoimmune diseases.
5. **Which of the following is a limitation of dermoscopy?**
   a. It cannot detect pigmented lesions.
   b. It requires tissue extraction for analysis.
   c. It only provides surface-level skin examination.
   d. It cannot magnify lesions effectively.

Short Answer Questions

1. Define the dermoscopy.
2. What are the advantages of dermoscopy in skin diagnosis?
3. What is a biopsy?
4. What is an imaging technique?
5. Describe the strengths and weaknesses of imaging techniques.

Answer to Critical Thinking Questions

1. (b); 2. (c) ; 3. (b); 4. (c); 5. (c)

REFERENCES

1. Adabi, S., Hosseinzadeh, M., Noei, S., Conforto, S., Daveluy, S., Clayton, A., Mehregan, D., & Nasiriavanaki, M. (2017). Universal in vivo Textural Model for Human Skin based on Optical Coherence Tomograms. *Scientific Reports*, *7*(1), 17912. https://doi.org/10.1038/s41598-017-17398-8Aigner, F., Pratschke, J., Schumann, T., Stockmann, M., et al. (2020). Recent advances and the potential for clinical use of autofluorescence detection of extra-ophthalmic tissues. https://core.ac.uk/download/323257980.pdf (accessed on 21st July 2025).
2. Akella, S. S., Lee, J., May, J., Puyana, C., Kravets, S., Dimitropolous, V., Tsoukas, M. M., et al. (2024). Using optical coherence tomography to optimize Mohs micrographic surgery. *Scientific Reports, 14*. https://doi.org/10.1038/s41598-024-53457-7 (accessed on 21st July 2025).
3. Al-Ayyad, M. S., Al-Nabulsi, J., Owida, H. A., Turab, S., et al. (2024). Available medical imaging modalities for melanoma screening. https://core.ac.uk/download/622481089.pdf (accessed on 21st July 2025).
4. Armstrong, L., Bennett, H., Clyne, B., Fahey, T., et al. (2017). Diagnosing malignant melanoma in ambulatory care: A systematic review of clinical prediction rules. https://core.ac.uk/download/83917582.pdf (accessed on 21st July 2025).
5. Bakos, R. M., Blumetti, T. C. M. P., Roldán-Marín, R., Salerni, G., et al. (2018). Noninvasive imaging tools in the diagnosis and treatment of skin cancers. https://core.ac.uk/download/293632338.pdf (accessed on 21st July 2025).
6. Bastiaannet, E., Beishon, M., Catalano, O., Costad, P., et al. (2018). ECCO essential requirements for quality cancer care: Melanoma. https://core.ac.uk/download/157587653.pdf (accessed on 21st July 2025).
7. Betz-Stablein, B., Cerminara, S. E., D'Alessandro, B. M., et al. (2024). The SLICE-3D dataset: 400,000 skin lesion image crops extracted from 3D TBP for skin cancer detection. https://www.zora.uzh.ch/id/eprint/270318/1/41597_2024_Article_3743.pdf (accessed on 21st July 2025).
8. Bohndiek, S., Fitzpatrick, C. R. M., O'Connor, J. P. B., Pogue, B., et al. (2019). A roadmap for the clinical implementation of optical-imaging biomarkers.
9. Cappilli, S., Paradisi, A., Di Stefani, A., Palmisano, G., Pellegrino, L., D'Onghia, M., Ricci, C., et al. (2024). Line-field confocal optical coherence tomography: A new skin imaging technique reproducing a "virtual biopsy" with evolving clinical applications in dermatology. *Diagnostics, 14*. https://www.semanticscholar.org/paper/b0d3f8a8de1cc20bee2483bbea926570af821c34 (accessed on 21st July 2025).
10. Cassidy, B., Kendrick, C., Brodzicki, A., Jaworek-Korjakowska, J., & Yap, M. H. (2021). Analysis of the ISIC image datasets: Usage, benchmarks and recommendations. *Medical Image Analysis, 75*, 102305–102305. https://doi.org/10.1016/j.media.2021.102305 (accessed on 21st July 2025).
11. Cheng, H. M. (2015). Diagnostic accuracy of optical coherence tomography in superficial basal cell carcinoma. https://core.ac.uk/download/41241524.pdf (accessed on 21st July 2025).
12. Cichocki, A., Jukić, A., & Kopriva, I. (2013). Noninvasive diagnosis of melanoma with tensor decomposition-based feature extraction from clinical color image. https://core.ac.uk/download/33995247.pdf (accessed on 21st July 2025).

13. Cinotti, E., D'Onghia, M., Cartocci, A., Lo Conte, S., Barbarossa, L., Tavernier, C., Rubegni, G., et al. (2025). Line-field confocal optical coherence tomography: Is one hour of training sufficient for diagnosing basal cell carcinoma? *Cancers, 17.* https://www.semanticscholar.org/paper/b690fe470b11706a3770c04e20f292a472262ea2 (accessed on 21st July 2025).

14. Conforti, C., Deinlein, T., Di Meo, N., Giuffrida, R., Guida, S., & Zalaudek, I. (2020). Use of noninvasive imaging in the management of skin cancer. https://core.ac.uk/download/286077367.pdf (accessed on 21st July 2025).

15. Cook, S. E., Palmer, L. C., Shuler, F. D., et al. (2015). Smartphone mobile application to enhance diagnosis of skin cancer: A guide for the rural practitioner. https://core.ac.uk/download/232725616.pdf (accessed on 21st July 2025).

16. D'Onghia, M., Falcinelli, F., Barbarossa, L., Pinto, A., Cartocci, A., Tognetti, L., Rubegni, G., et al. (2025). Zoom-in dermoscopy for facial tumors. *Diagnostics, 15.* https://www.semanticscholar.org/paper/9aeacead561e57109fb1d3815c6a708c08696200 (accessed on 21st July 2025).

17. Edwards, G., Freeman, K., Harward, G., Llewelyn, M., et al. (2020). What diagnostic strategies can help differentiate cellulitis from other causes of red legs in primary care. https://core.ac.uk/download/237942601.pdf (accessed on 21st July 2025).

18. Effendie, M., & Aguiar-Pulido, V. (2024). Multi-modal AI approach for multi-class skin disease classification. *2024 International Conference on Machine Learning and Applications (ICMLA).* https://www.semanticscholar.org/paper/66db0ccb659dee4aad6f22d39e266257efdd28a5 (accessed on 21st July 2025).

19. Ergin, F., Parlak, İ. B., Adel, M., Gül, Ö. M., & Karpouzis, K. (2024). Noise resilience in dermoscopic image segmentation: Comparing deep learning architectures for enhanced accuracy. *Electronics, 13,* 3414–3414. https://doi.org/10.3390/electronics13173414 (accessed on 21st July 2025).

20. Gaikwad, P. (2025). Skin cancer cutaneous squamous cell. *International Journal for Research in Applied Science and Engineering Technology.* https://www.semanticscholar.org/paper/0c7f95f4a3d01f2d7deaeab68068d466b543581c (accessed on 21st July 2025).

21. Gao, Y., Xu, T., Wang, Y., Hu, Y., Yin, S., Qin, Z., & Yu, H. (2025). Pathophysiology and treatment of psoriasis: From clinical practice to basic research. *Pharmaceutics, 17,* 56–56. https://doi.org/10.3390/pharmaceutics17010056 (accessed on 21st July 2025).

22. Gust, C. (2024). *In-vivo* evaluation von Hauttumoren und inflammatorischen Dermatosen mittels nicht invasiver Bildgebung. https://core.ac.uk/download/636729922.pdf (accessed on 21st July 2025).

23. John-Otumu, A., Ekemonye, R., Ewunonu, T., Aniugo, V., & Okonkwo, O. (2024). Optimizing CNN kernel sizes for enhanced melanoma lesion classification in dermoscopy images. *Machine Learning Research.* https://www.semanticscholar.org/paper/7e524a022c37367130890371d28b6650e97a5fac (accessed on 21st July 2025).

24. Krišto, M., Čeović, R., & Šitum, M. (2020). Noninvasive imaging techniques for the diagnosis of nonmelanoma skin cancers. https://core.ac.uk/download/541035537.pdf (accessed on 21st July 2025).

25. Lima, B. M., Machado, G. C., Destefani, A. C., & Destefani, V. C. (2024). Advances in non-invasive diagnostic methods for early detection of skin cancer in Black women: A comprehensive

review of dermoscopy, reflectance confocal microscopy, optical coherence tomography, electrical impedance spectroscopy, multispectral imaging, and adhesive patch biopsy. *Revita Ibero-Americana de Humanidades, Ciências e Educação*. https://www.semanticscholar.org/paper/1505f4b0882f9a35c06c0f912160b81b9c31e5f6 (accessed on 21st July 2025).

26. Liopyris, K., Gregoriou, S., Dias, J., & Stratigos, A. (2022). Artificial intelligence in dermatology: Challenges and perspectives. *Dermatology and Therapy, 12*, 2637–2651. https://doi.org/10.1007/s13555-022-00833-8 (accessed on 21st July 2025).

27. Mahumud, R. A., Janda, M., Soyer, H. P., Fernández-Peñas, P., Mar, V., & Morton, R. L. (2022). Assessing the value of precision medicine health technologies to detect and manage melanoma. *The Medical Journal of Australia, 217*, 275–278. https://doi.org/10.5694/mja2.51696 (accessed on 21st July 2025).

28. Naeem, A., & Anees, T. (2024). DVFNet: A deep feature fusion-based model for the multiclassification of skin cancer utilizing dermoscopy images. *PLoS ONE, 19*, e0297667–e0297667. https://doi.org/10.1371/journal.pone.0297667 (accessed on 21st July 2025).

29. Naeem, A., Anees, T., Khalil, M., Zahra, K., Naqvi, R. A., & Lee, S. W. (2024). SNC_Net: Skin cancer detection by integrating handcrafted and deep learning-based features using dermoscopy images. *Mathematics, 12*, 1030–1030. https://doi.org/10.3390/math12071030 (accessed on 21st July 2025).

30. Navas, M., Farisa, P. M., Rishad, C. M. A., & Gopinath, V. P. K. (2024). Inflammatory foot dermatoses: The correlation among morphological patterns, histopathological findings, and patch test positivity. *Cureus, 16*. https://www.semanticscholar.org/paper/a91cb3be1424d29b56cac199f5d3947cadc4d029 (accessed on 21st July 2025).

31. Nurhayati, R., Oentari, W., Sari, A. K., Siregar, R., et al. (2021). Noninvasive diagnostic modality for skin cancer. https://core.ac.uk/download/639382379.pdf (accessed on 21st July 2025).

32. Plana Dato, M. (2023). Evaluation of different segmentation-based approaches for skin disorders from dermoscopic images. https://diposit.ub.edu/dspace/bitstream/2445/199302/1/TFG_Maria_Plana_Dato.pdf (accessed on 21st July 2025).

33. Salmivuori, M. (2020). New options for non-invasive imaging and non-invasive treatment of skin cancers. https://core.ac.uk/download/322611574.pdf (accessed on 21st July 2025).

34. Soyer, H. P., & Wurm, E. M. (2010). Scanning for melanoma. https://core.ac.uk/download/15101188.pdf (accessed on 21st July 2025).

35. Xu, Q. (2021). The advanced applications for optical coherence tomography in skin imaging. https://core.ac.uk/download/548674568.pdf (accessed on 21st July 2025).

36. Zhang, L., Shen, X., Fu, L., Meng, H., Lu, Y., Chen, T., & Xu, R. (2022). Dermoscopy, reflectance confocal microscopy, and high-frequency ultrasound for the noninvasive diagnosis of morpheaform basal cell carcinoma. *Skin Research and Technology, 28*, 766–768. https://doi.org/10.1111/srt.13197 (accessed on 21st July 2025).\

ECZEMA AND DERMATITIS (ATOPIC, CONTACT, SEBORRHEIC)

6

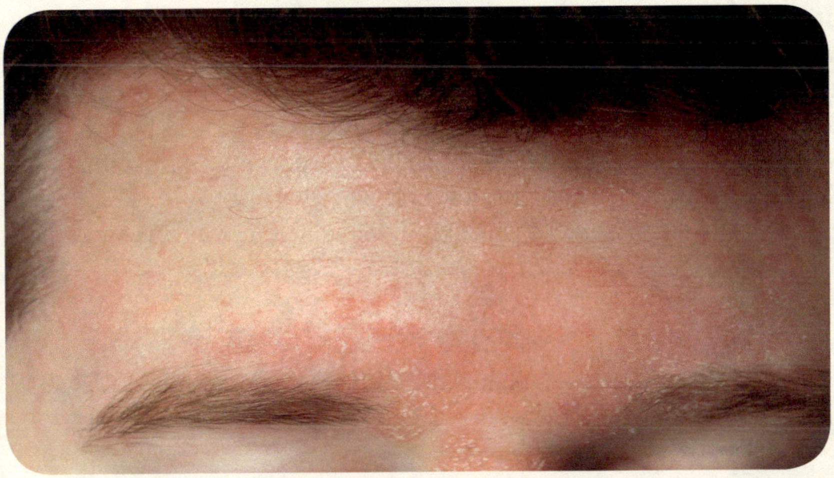

LEARNING OBJECTIVES

After studying this chapter, you will be able to:

1. Understand the eczema
2. Describe the atopic dermatitis, contact dermatitis, and seborrheic dermatitis
3. Know the psychological and social impact of eczema and dermatitis

Introduction

Eczema and dermatitis constitute a group of inflammatory skin conditions, the most significant subtypes of which are atopic dermatitis, contact dermatitis, and seborrheic dermatitis. Their dissemination is delineated by increasing global prevalence, significantly impairing people's quality of life. Eczema may be differentiated by its inflamed and pruritic skin, typically coupled with considerable psychological distress as well as somatic symptoms. An understanding of the pathophysiology of these diseases is relevant because most of them result from an interplay among genetic, environmental, and immunological factors. With advancing dermatological research comes greater recognition of the role of external stimuli, e.g., allergens and irritants, in initiating these dermatoses. Thus, there is a need for a thorough investigation of all types of dermatitis to explain their unique presentations and treatment regimens, and to demonstrate the need for tailor-made therapeutic interventions. Atopic dermatitis, the most common form, is of particular interest because it can be associated with other atopic diseases such as asthma and allergic rhinitis. The immune system dysfunction in patients with atopic dermatitis leads to dysregulation of skin barrier function and an overresponse to environmental stimuli. The disease is chronic, and usually develops during childhood, but often continues into adulthood, which requires lifelong care that not only controls the acute flare but also the systemic disease. Conversely, contact dermatitis results from exposure of the skin to allergens or irritants and is a localized reaction, whereas seborrheic dermatitis is an inflammatory reaction associated with the activity of oil glands. By identifying these types, health professionals can implement more effective interventions tailored to each type of dermatitis, based on its distinct features, thereby maximizing patient outcomes and quality of life. New studies have highlighted the intricate relationship of the skin's microbiome with other skin conditions, including atopic dermatitis and other types of dermatitis.

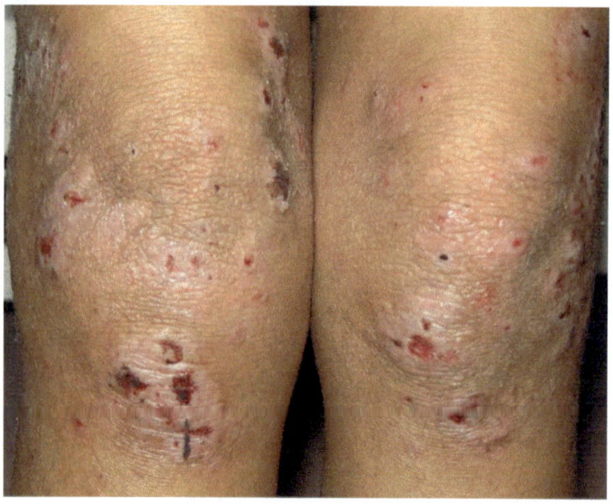

Figure 6.1. Eczema and atopic dermatitis.

Source: https://www.health.com/thmb/wZjgaUmC9fbZADi-VTVOgu5IeQM=/750x0/filters:no_upscale():max_bytes(150000):strip_icc():format(webp)/Health-156.atopic-dermatitis-0004-8adfbb743d474a6784b514b25af5c6fb.jpg.

The gut-skin axis describes the two-way interaction between the gut and skin and how malfunction in one can be caused by disruption in the other, typically evident through skin manifestations. Dysbiosis, or microbial imbalance, is increasingly recognized as an etiological factor in skin disease that significantly affects immune system function and skin integrity. With growing scientific knowledge of this complex interaction, it is important that future research explore the impact of microbial well-being on the etiology and treatment of eczema and dermatitis. This perspective foretells a shift toward integrating dermatological care within a systemic framework of global health, as established by recent research emphasizing the need for an integrated approach to the treatment of skin disease (Callewaert et al., 2021; Greif et al., 2024) (Figure 6.1).

6.1. Understanding Eczema

Learning Outcome

1. Define the eczema
2. Describe the prevalence and demographics of eczema
3. Know the common symptoms and manifestations of eczema

Eczema, as is generally employed interchangeably with dermatitis, is a group of inflammatory dermatoses characterized by redness, itch, and dryness of the skin. Of all the types of eczema, the most prevalent is atopic dermatitis, which is characterized by chronicity and associations with other conditions such as asthma and allergic rhinitis. This state frequently occurs in infancy and can persist throughout life, requiring long-term management. Pathophysiology of atopic dermatitis includes a compromised skin barrier and aberrant immunity, emphasizing the importance of personalized therapeutic approaches. Treatment is usually focused on topical corticosteroids and emollients to decrease symptoms and enhance skin integrity, but the variability in patient response complicates repeated assessment of treatment effectiveness and adherence to management. Contact dermatitis, another major category of eczema, can be classified as irritant or allergic. Irritant contact dermatitis results from direct damage of the skin by chemicals or soaps, whereas allergic contact dermatitis is a result of an immune reaction to specific allergens. Because both have similar morphological appearances, they pose difficulties in diagnosis but are at times only identifiable upon the establishment of the causative agent. Clinical presentations can be extremely varied; therefore, the value of a thorough history and clinical examination lies in differentiating between such skin conditions and others. Accurate diagnosis not only provides symptom relief but also enables patients to avoid known offending agents, thereby enhancing overall quality of life. The complexity of contact dermatitis underscores the need for individualized management protocols and ongoing patient education on skin care practices. Seborrheic dermatitis, the third major type of eczema, occurs most commonly in areas of the body with abundant sebaceous glands, i.e., the scalp, face, and upper back. It is characteristically accompanied by greasy patches of scalp flakiness and redness.

Though the cause of seborrheic dermatitis remains unknown, it is routinely attributed to infestation with the yeast Malassezia, a fungus that resides on oily skin. Symptoms may be exacerbated by factors like hormonal imbalance, stress, and immune system imbalance. Treatment measures include antifungal medications, topical corticosteroids, and medicated shampoos. Diagnosis and treatment of seborrheic dermatitis are very important, not only for its physical appearance but also for its potential psychological effects, such as low self-esteem and social exclusion. Effective management will need to focus on symptom relief and flare-up prevention, thereby enhancing both functional outcomes and psychosocial well-being in those affected (Figure 6.2).

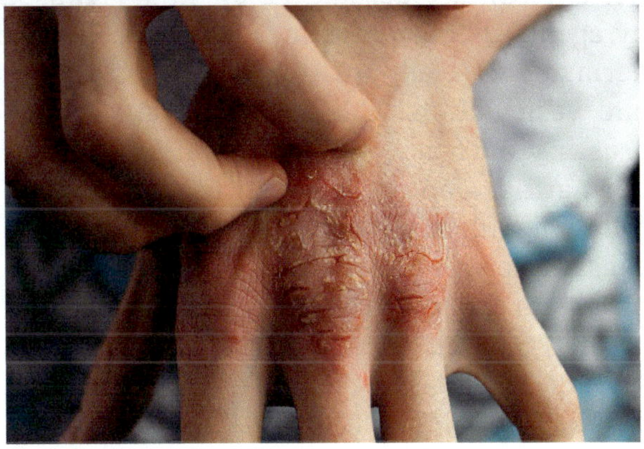

Figure 6.2. Eczema.

Source: https://images.squarespace-cdn.com/content/v1/59b85add3e00beef2521bbc4/1506626111887-ALZMLALGXZ0U88U57M1Q/Eczema+right+Pic++_137059687.jpeg.

6.1.1. Definition and General Characteristics

Eczema and dermatitis are inflammatory dermatoses with varied symptoms, including redness, swelling, and itching. Atopic dermatitis is itself chronic and tends to commence early in childhood. It is associated with a genetic predisposition to allergic illnesses and with environmental factors. Clinically, atopic dermatitis has diverse phenotypes, each with characteristic presentations and treatment responses. This heterogeneity makes it challenging to have one definition, as presentations as well as pathogenic processes are highly heterogeneous. Thus, an understanding of the characterization of atopic dermatitis is essential for clinicians seeking to personalize management strategies to meet the needs of individual patients (Abuabara et al., 2018). Contact dermatitis primarily results from external allergens or irritants that come into direct contact with the skin and induce local inflammatory reactions. It can occur either as allergic contact dermatitis, an immunologically mediated response to a particular allergen, or irritant contact dermatitis, an injury caused by agents that are caustic to the skin. Contact dermatitis typically presents by redness, edema, and vesiculation, which tends to evolve into crusting or scaling over time. Unlike atopic dermatitis, contact dermatitis will resolve following identification and removal of the causative agent, making its therapy avoidance-based. Its diagnosis relies on a detailed patient history, as well as, in some instances, patch testing to confirm sensitivities (Ascott et al., 2017). Seborrheic dermatitis involves an inflammatory response against *Malassezia yeast,* a fungus that occurs naturally on the skin. It prefers areas with a dense concentration of sebaceous glands, such as the scalp, face, and chest. Clinically, seborrheic dermatitis is seen as yellow or white oily, scaly lesions with concomitant pruritus. Although frequently seen in infants as cradle cap, it may be chronic or recur throughout life, sometimes exacerbated by stress and environmental factors. The clinical diagnosis of seborrheic dermatitis is one of distinguishing it from other dermatoses, most notably psoriasis. Therapy includes antifungal drugs, corticosteroids, or medicated shampoos, aimed at suppressing symptoms and inflammation (Abuabara et al., 2018).

6.1.2. Prevalence and Demographics

Eczema and dermatitis are prevalent across all demographics but vary substantially among them, suggesting a complex interplay of genetic, environmental, and socioeconomic factors. The most common eczema, atopic dermatitis, has been estimated to occur in 7%–20% of children and about 2%–10% of adults, with rising rates occurring in urban-dwelling populations. The inflammatory disease is most often found in confluence with other atopic conditions such as asthma and allergic rhinitis, characterizing the condition as multicentric. Furthermore, studies have shown that individuals with a family history of atopy carry an increased risk, suggesting a genetic factor for the condition. These population patterns underscore the need for vigorous public health interventions to effectively manage and curb the occurrence of atopic dermatitis. Seborrheic dermatitis, a common form of dermatitis, also exhibits varying patterns across the population. It is characterized by inflammatory lesions, predominantly on sebum-exuding areas of the skin. Its prevalence ranges from approximately 2%–5% of the global population, with the condition observed more often in men than in women. The research has shown that seborrheic dermatitis manifests in young adults and older adults, with age-related determinants dominant in its pathogenesis. The disease's relapsing and chronic character can lead to serious physical discomfort and emotional suffering, influencing the quality of patients' lives. According to recent studies, the emergence of seborrheic dermatitis is of special interest, and therefore it is essential to explore further its risk factors and best management strategies to prevent its growing impact across different populations (Khan et al., 2024). Demographics also play an important role in the development and presentation of contact dermatitis, which is usually preceded by exposure to irritants and allergens. Many studies have documented occupational exposure as a predominant cause, with health care workers, hairdressers, and manufacturing staff being particularly at risk. The increasing incidence of contact dermatitis among adults reflects changes in work environments and increased exposure to chemicals. Further, misuse of topical steroids, especially when in the situation of misdiagnosis of dermatoses, aggravates outcomes, as in the case of tinea incognito. This once more highlights the necessity of educating patients and healthcare professionals on proper treatment practices, as well as the importance of accurate diagnosis to reduce general incidence and improve patient outcomes across diverse demographic groups (Figure 6.3).

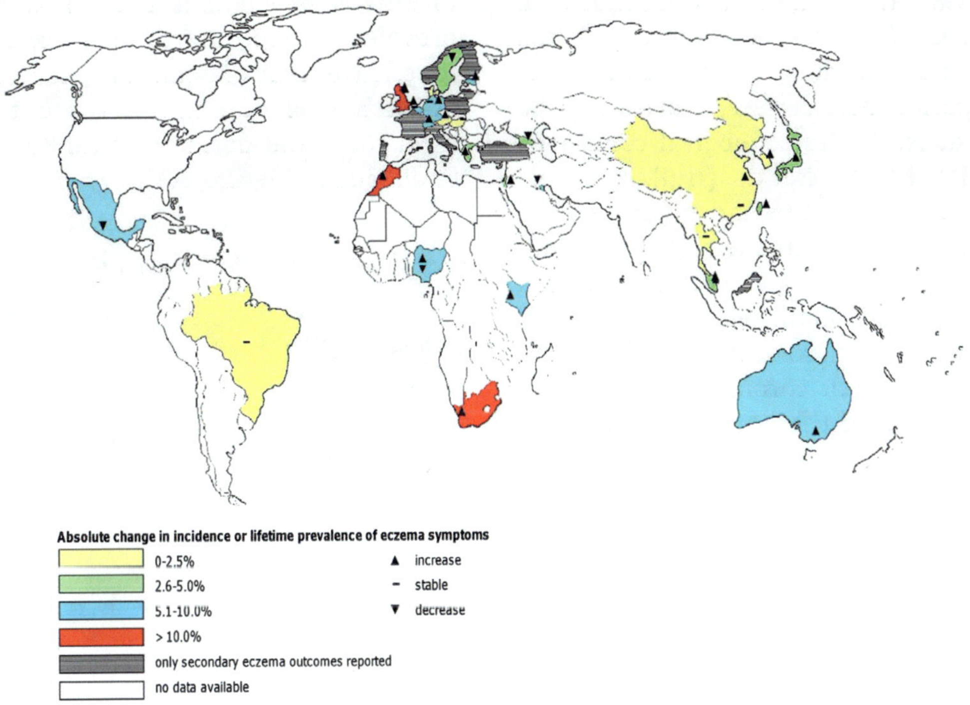

Figure 6.3. World map of the incidence and lifetime prevalence of atopic eczema symptoms (1990–2010). Overview of absolute changes in the incidence of atopic eczema and lifetime prevalence of atopic eczema symptoms between 1990 and 2010.

Source: https://www.researchgate.net/publication/229162109/figure/fig5/AS:341155851063300@1458349301412/World-map-of-the-incidence-and-lifetime-prevalence-of-atopic-eczema-symptoms.png.

6.1.3. Common Symptoms and Manifestations

Eczema and dermatitis, such as atopic, contact, and seborrheic types, share a common set of symptoms and manifestations that can significantly affect the quality of life of affected individuals. Typically characterized by skin inflammation, these diseases manifest as dryness, redness, pruritus, and scaling. Irritability of the skin typically causes scratching, intensifies symptoms, and can lead to secondary infection. For instance, atopic dermatitis, the most prevalent of all eczemas, frequently manifests in childhood, and its manifestations may significantly differ, leading to acute flare-ups that disrupt daily functioning. In addition, contact dermatitis is also caused by immediate external allergens or irritants and leads to localized signs and symptoms that can not only mimic but also drive the individual's overall skin hypersensitivity, thus the proper diagnosis and symptom control become essential (Aerts et al., 2024). Seborrheic dermatitis is another type that typically involves sebaceous gland-abundant areas of the scalp and face and leads to oily, yellowish scales with redness. This condition is most frequently seen in newborns as cradle cap and in adults as dandruff or redness of the face. The typical presentation of seborrheic dermatitis might, in some cases, overlap with other dermatitides, rendering them difficult to diagnose. Knowledge of the general symptoms is essential for healthcare professionals to appropriately identify these types of dermatitis. Research has also indicated that diseases such as seborrheic dermatitis can be associated with systemic health issues, including periodontal disease, illustrating the interdependence of dermatological conditions and broader health trends (Huilaja et al., 2023). Accurate definition and differentiation of symptoms of eczema and dermatitis are not academic exercises but have real implications for treatment and management strategies. Management of such conditions requires an understanding of their chronic nature and the precipitating events that result in flare-ups. For example, patients with atopic dermatitis typically benefit from the identification of offending irritants or allergens that exacerbate their skin condition, whereas those with contact dermatitis can be alleviated by avoidance of offending irritants. Furthermore, the ability to recognize overlapping signs, such as those seen in presentations of allergic and irritant contact dermatitis, can significantly enhance the effectiveness of therapeutic interventions. Therefore, healthcare professionals need to always be vigilant and familiar with the prevalent symptoms of such skin disorders to ensure that maximum intervention and assistance are administered to the patient throughout the dermatological process (Aerts et al., 2024) (Figure 6.4).

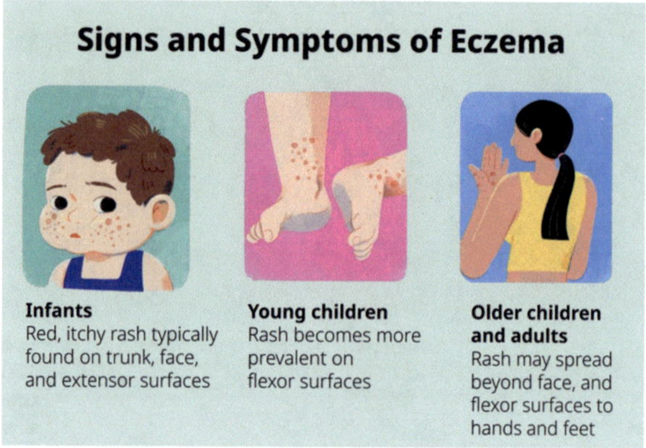

Figure 6.4. Symptoms of eczema.

Source: https://nursesrevisionuganda.com/wp-content/uploads/2024/02/Symptoms-of-atopic-eczema-vary-across-different-age-groups-1-1024x691.jpg.

Test Your Knowledge

1. What skin is eczema characterized by?
2. What are the signs and symptoms of eczema?

6.2. Atopic Dermatitis

Learning Outcome

1. Understand the causes of atopic dermatitis
2. Describe the risk factors and triggers of atopic dermatitis
3. Know the treatment options and management strategies for atopic dermatitis

The worldwide prevalence of atopic dermatitis (AD), particularly among children, has increased to alarming proportions, rendering it a significant public health concern. Research has established that not only do chronic inflammatory skin diseases affect the quality of life of patients and families, but also place a high socioeconomic burden. The multifactorial nature of atopic dermatitis is reinforced by genetic factors, environmental exposures, and immune system alterations. Dysfunction of the skin barrier has been highlighted as an important driver of disease onset in recent studies. Explaining and determining these mechanisms are crucial to the development of successful prevention strategies and treatments, as the increasing incidence necessitates state-of-the-art interventions to reduce the burden of the condition for both those affected and healthcare systems (Apfelbacher et al., 2014). In a welcome step forward, recent clinical trials have explored the therapeutic value of early intervention strategies aimed at improving skin barrier function. Of special note, a randomized controlled trial in high-risk neonates demonstrated significant preventive outcomes with daily application of emollients. In the intervention group, families who received the intervention had a 50% reduction in cumulative incidence of atopic dermatitis by six months compared with controls. These findings point to the potential for cheap, simple interventions that empower parents to initiate proactive behavior from birth. Also, the absence of adverse events associated with emollient use suggests that such treatments could be introduced safely at large-scale levels and therefore be an option for decreasing the rising prevalence of atopic dermatitis in various populations (Apfelbacher et al., 2014).

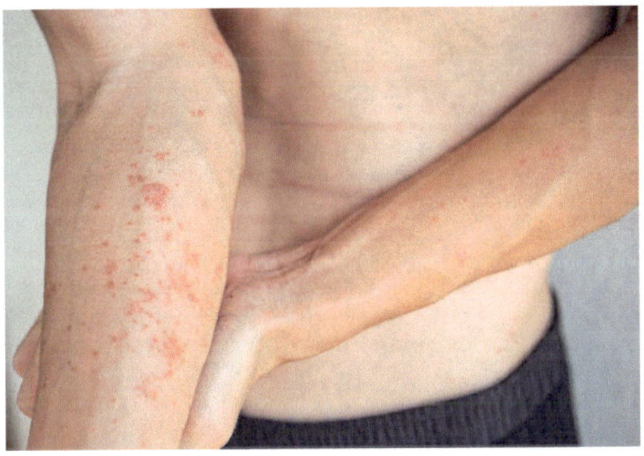

Figure 6.5. Atopic dermatitis.

Source: https://www.verywellhealth.com/thmb/Wc2d5mVzqp1m5qu8YcYQD6E3hKQ=/1500x0/filters:no_upscale():max_bytes(150000):strip_icc()/VWH-GettyImages-1311098421-6724b24f024c4055b8ad56c6cd2b12f2.jpg.

The diversified complexity of atopic dermatitis is also reflected through its comorbidities, which affect physical and psychological health. A retrospective study on adult and children populations reported that comorbidities like asthma and anxiety were common in patients with severe AD. This crosstalk with atopic dermatitis and the comorbidities complicates treatment, and treatment demands an integrated process to treat the patient. The medications involved include corticosteroids, immunosuppressants such as cyclosporine, and biologics, but the variation in their effectiveness underscores the need for further studies. An understanding of individuals' clinical profiles can guide individualized treatment pathways, optimizing treatment and possibly reducing the influence of allied health conditions (Figure 6.5).

6.2.1. Definition and Causes

Eczema, or dermatitis, refers to a group of skin conditions characterized by inflammation, itch, and irritation. Atopic dermatitis, contact dermatitis, and seborrheic dermatitis are some of the most prevalent forms, each with specific clinical presentation and etiology. Atopic dermatitis is defined by chronically dry and itchy skin, most commonly seen in children and in keeping with inherited tendencies and environmental stimuli, including allergens. Contact dermatitis occurs when the skin irritates or is allergic to something and evolves into a red rash with inflammation. Seborrheic dermatitis occurs primarily in oily areas of the body, including the scalp and face, and occurs with yeast overgrowth and excessive sebum. With these definitions, one can better understand the complexity of eczema and its varied presentations, underscoring the need for proper diagnosis and treatment. The pathophysiology of eczema differs across its presentations, with distinct genetic and environmental factors. For instance, atopic dermatitis is commonly associated with mutations in the gene that codes for filaggrin, which plays a critical role in the integrity of the skin barrier. When this barrier is broken, the skin becomes more susceptible to irritants, allergens, and microbial invasions. More significantly, environmental factors such as changes in temperature and humidity, as well as contact with some soaps or detergents, also worsen symptoms. Contact dermatitis is usually caused by specific substances, which may be identified through allergic patch testing. This type of dermatitis accentuates the importance of knowing a person's sensitivities to prevent breakouts. The multi-factorial pathophysiology of such conditions demands an integrative understanding of their etiology to allow effective management and treatment. The onset of eczema in infants and young children may be determined by either biological or environmental factors.

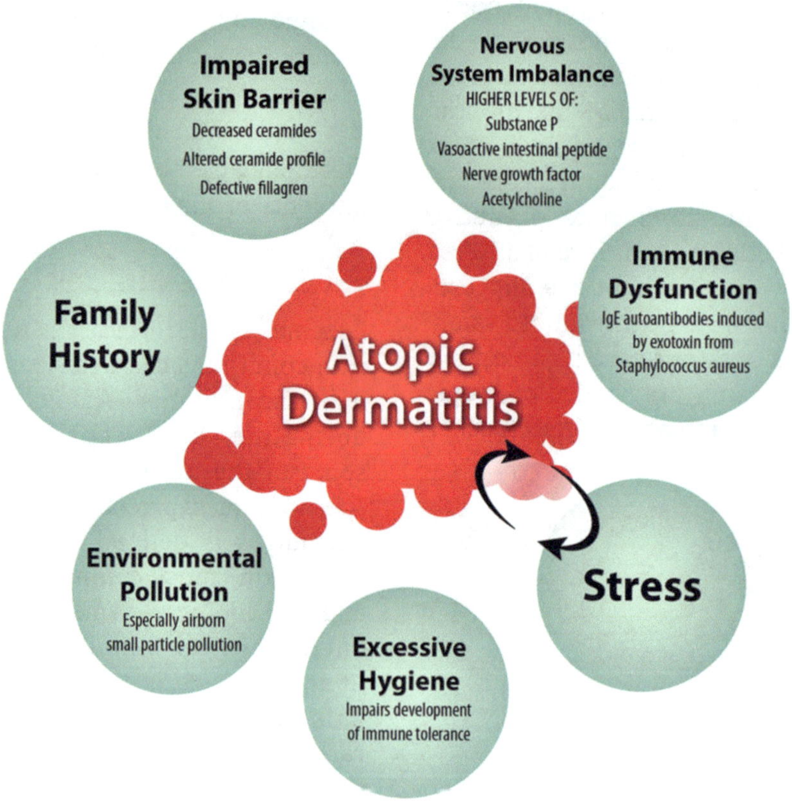

Figure 6.6. Causes of atopic dermatitis.

Source: https://hi-bliss.com/wp-content/uploads/2020/08/what-causes-atopic-dermatitis.jpg.

During this critical stage, the skin undergoes development and matures, becoming increasingly sensitive to stimuli. The underdeveloped immune system of the infant allows increased vulnerability to skin diseases like atopic dermatitis. Those with a family history of allergic illness, such as asthma or hay fever, are most at risk, suggesting a genetic link. Furthermore, the introduction of specific irritants and allergens during early life may provoke the onset of eczema-like symptoms. As has been discovered through research, the selection of products that are safe and suitable for skin care is important due to the susceptibility of infant skin to irritation. The use of products on infants without potentially offending ingredients reduces the likelihood of irritation and skin complications, thereby mitigating the enormity of the eczema challenge in such a vulnerable population (Jain et al., 2018) (Figure 6.6).

6.2.2. Risk Factors and Triggers

Identification of the triggers and risk factors for eczema and dermatitis is vital for effective management and prevention. Dermatitis, in particular, has a high genetic predisposition, and an atopic family history normally correlates with a greater chance of developing the disease. Environmental triggers also exist; detergents, soaps, and environmental allergens like pollen play a role in triggering the disease. In addition, weather conditions such as low humidity and high temperatures may contribute to flare-ups. Identification and avoidance of such triggers are paramount for those susceptible to the condition, as lifestyle modifications can effectively reduce exacerbation frequency and promote overall skin health. Outside of genetic and environmental contributory elements, psychosocial elements also come into play in the severity of eczema and dermatitis. Stress has also been identified as an important driver of flares, with psychological factors influencing immune function and skin barrier integrity. Psychological stressors can enhance scratching activity, further undermine the skin, and perpetuate the dermatitis cycle. Furthermore, nighttime disruptions characteristic of pruritus can exacerbate both physical and psychological stress, producing an additional burden on quality of life for the patient. Given these interlinked determinants, it is necessary that health practitioners consider the wider psychosocial environment when assessing and managing patients with eczema and dermatitis, and may incorporate stress management interventions into treatment plans. Individual allergic reactions also present important risk factors for contact dermatitis. Allergic contact dermatitis, an immune reaction to skin exposure with allergens such as nickel or perfume, relies on the patient's sensitivity to such chemicals. Allergen detection is important to prevention; therefore, patch testing to determine particular sensitivities in affected patients with dermatitis symptoms is advisable for doctors. A joint panel session of dermatological experts emphasized that medical practitioners should consider such allergic and immunologic stimuli in light of clinical characteristics and patient history, particularly the emergence of novel skin events (Ambrogio et al., 2024). Recognition of individualized triggers in each patient supports case-specific management and therapeutic response augmentation, underscoring the importance of tailored interventions in dermatitis management and related conditions (Figure 6.7).

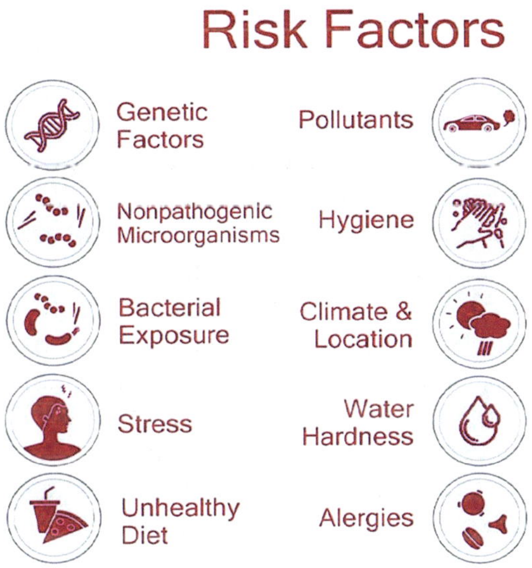

Figure 6.7. Eczema risk factors.

Source: https://remotederm.ca/blog/wp-content/uploads/2023/01/risk-factors-of-eczema.jpg.

6.2.3. Treatment Options and Management Strategies

Eczema and dermatitis treatment is a myriad of therapeutic approaches that are individually tailored to the specific type and severity of the condition. In atopic dermatitis, topical corticosteroids remain the pillar of treatment, providing symptomatic relief and reducing inflammatory reactions during flare-ups. Clinical consensus recognizes the need to balance efficacy against potential side effects, and attempts have been made to identify alternatives. Second-generation targeted topical therapies have emerged as potential non-corticosteroid substitutes, possessing promising safety and efficacy profiles. As dermatologists become more concerned with long-term management, the in-depth review highlights judicious use of corticosteroids while exploring newer options that can minimize the risks of traditional treatments (Burshtein et al., 2025). In addition to topical therapy, patient education is an important aspect of the treatment of eczema and dermatitis. Awareness of triggers, such as environmental factors and allergens, educates patients with the knowledge they need to prevent exacerbations. For instance, patients with contact dermatitis should be aware of potential irritants in their vicinity and learn how to avoid them. The joint conclave of experts has emphasized that clinicians need to accurately identify these triggers and educate patients on appropriate avoidance methods (Ambrogio et al., 2024). In addition, maintenance of proper skincare routines, including repeated moisturizing, also goes a long way in skin barrier function and therefore in reducing flare frequency and severity. Preventive measures also underscore the inseparable relationship between education and effective management of eczema and dermatitis. Finally, management of eczema and dermatitis often requires multidisciplinary treatment that incorporates dermatologic therapy, patient psychology, and, if necessary, pharmacologic therapy. Systemic therapy, including immunosuppressives, is an option in more severe cases, particularly if treatments applied topically are unsuccessful. With the psychosocial impact that chronic skin disease has, counseling for mental health is also invaluable; it helps the patient to cope with the emotional burden that eczema and dermatitis can impose. Furthermore, treatment regimens that consider these multifaceted factors will likely improve patient outcomes and quality of life. With the evolution of the field, an integrated approach to understanding eczema and dermatitis treatment will benefit both patients and clinicians in addressing the multifaceted nature of these conditions (Figure 6.8).

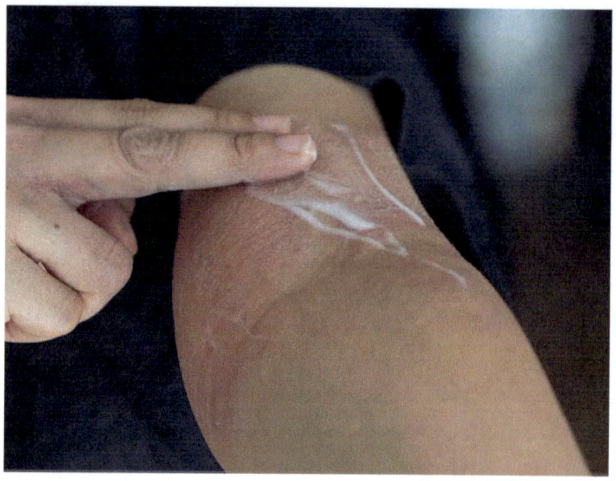

Figure 6.8. Eczema treatment options: Using cream on eczema.

Source: https://remotederm.ca/blog/wp-content/uploads/2023/01/Eczema-treatment-options.jpg.

Test Your Knowledge

1. What are the causes of atopic dermatitis?
2. What are the risk factors for atopic dermatitis?

6.3. Contact Dermatitis

Learning Outcome

1. Describe the types of contact dermatitis
2. Describe the common allergens and irritants
3. Understand the diagnosis and treatment approaches for contact dermatitis

Among the types of dermatitis, contact dermatitis is unique for its characteristic etiology and presentation. Contact dermatitis occurs when the skin comes in direct contact with an irritant or an allergen, which causes an inflammatory reaction. The symptoms occur mainly in the form of erythema, swelling, and vesiculation and have a measurable impact on the patient's quality of life. The condition can be classified into two significant forms: irritant contact dermatitis and allergic contact dermatitis. Irritant contact dermatitis occurs when substances such as detergents or strong chemicals break the skin barrier, whereas allergic contact dermatitis is an immunologic reaction to allergens such as nickel or scents. Identifying the precise form of contact dermatitis is necessary to provide effective treatment and management strategies that limit discomfort and prevent recurrence. The pathophysiology of contact dermatitis is a multifaceted interplay between extrinsic factors and the immune system. Exposure to an allergen provokes a sensitized T-cell response, which triggers a cascade of inflammatory responses resulting in characteristic symptoms. An immune reaction underscores the need to identify triggers to prevent flare-ups. Environmental triggers such as moisture and occlusion may also exacerbate the condition. Recent literature emphasizes the role of preventative therapy, including barrier creams and avoidance of the implicated allergen or irritant. Management of such problems can significantly enhance the patient's well-being and rate of occurrence of such episodes of dermatitis. As more information comes to light through research about such interactions, direct therapies and prophylactic approaches are set to evolve, offering hope to the parties involved. Furthermore, contact dermatitis has a psychosocial component that cannot be ignored. The distress resulting from visible lesions and pain can have serious psychological consequences, including depression and anxiety. Patients with chronic dermatitis themselves state a decrease in quality of life, both influenced by physical signs, stigma, and social isolation. This supports the necessity of intensive treatment of both medical and psychological history. Some studies suggest that integrating mental health services into dermatological treatment can improve outcomes for patients with debilitating skin conditions. The more we advance our knowledge of contact dermatitis, the more treating its physical manifestations, as well as the associated emotional toll, will be crucial in improving overall patient care and satisfaction (Figure 6.9).

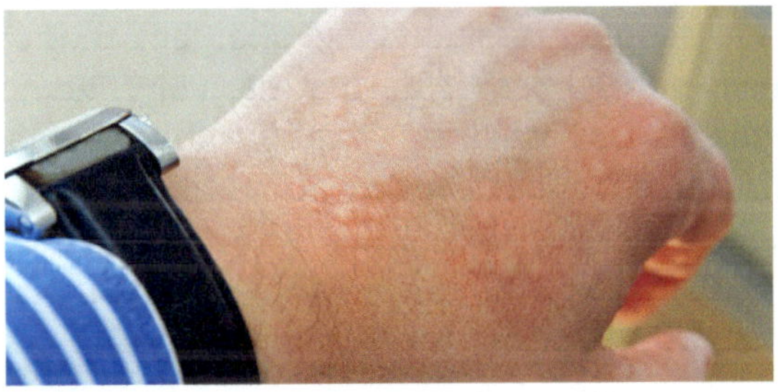

Figure 6.9. Contact dermatitis.

Source: https://dermskinhealth.com/wp-content/uploads/2022/05/contact-dermatitis-hero.jpeg.

6.3.1. Definition and Types (Irritant vs. Allergic)

It is crucial to understand the definition and types of dermatitis to ensure proper diagnosis and treatment of eczema. Dermatitis, or inflammation of the skin, can present in various forms, specifically irritant contact dermatitis and allergic contact dermatitis. Irritant contact dermatitis results from direct exposure to an irritant, leading to a local inflammatory response. This type is typically triggered by soaps, detergents, or chemicals and presents with redness, swelling, and itching. Allergic contact dermatitis occurs as a result of the skin developing a delayed hypersensitivity reaction against an allergen, occurring with the same symptoms on subsequent re-exposure. The distinction between these two types is significant because their treatment strategies differ widely, and accurate diagnosis is essential in clinical practice. In addition, the etiology and prevalence of irritant and allergic contact dermatitis provide valuable information for healthcare workers who are highly exposed. It has been reported in recent studies that more than 15% of the general population suffer from hand eczema in their lifetime, with healthcare workers being particularly at risk due to occupational exposures (Hamnerius et al., 2019). These include frequent handwashing and prolonged use of medical gloves, which expose these people to irritants and allergens that can cause both types of dermatitis. For instance, repeated exposure to soaps or disinfectants can cause irritant contact dermatitis, whereas allergic contact dermatitis is more likely due to sensitization to glove additives (Hamnerius et al., 2019). Given the chronic nature of such conditions, determining their causes is central to effective prevention and management strategies. Irritant and allergic contact dermatitides' influence does not simply extend to personal suffering but has far-reaching impacts on society at large. The infected typically endure a poor quality of life, putting them at risk for professional problems, especially for those working in close contact professions, such as those in a healthcare setting. The financial impact is also significant, as chronic dermatitis can lead to absenteeism, low productivity, and increased healthcare costs (Agner et al., 2022). Additionally, despite several preventive measures, the fact that these conditions are long-standing indicates a lack of effective intervention. As more recent data come to hand, it will be essential to understand the specific roles of irritant versus allergic forms of dermatitis in order to develop targeted management plans that minimize their effects on individuals and society (Figure 6.10).

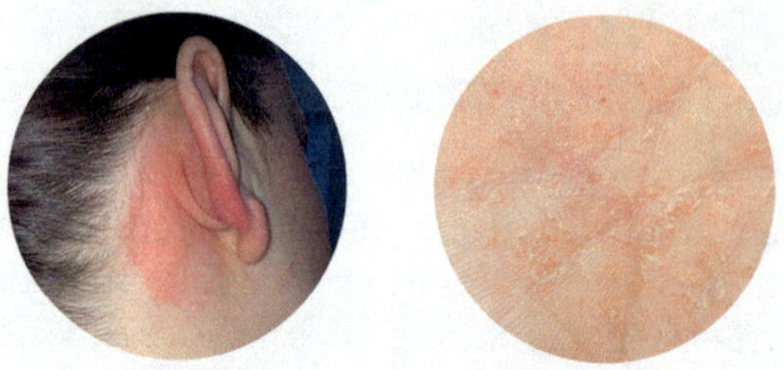

Figure 6.10. Types of contact dermatitis.

Source: https://cdn.shopify.com/s/files/1/2730/7792/files/Skin_Conditions_SC_Alleviates_IG_Stories_2048x2048.jpg?v=1599261439.

6.3.2. Common Allergens and Irritants

Dermatitis and eczema are inflammatory skin disorders that are exacerbated by exposure to common irritants and allergens. If the epidermal barrier is compromised, such as in atopic dermatitis, the skin becomes susceptible to environmental irritants. Common allergens are chemicals that may induce immune responses resulting in flare-ups, including pollen, dust mites, and animal dander. In addition, chemicals, soaps, and detergents are also irritants that contribute significantly to the pain that patients with this condition experience. The inflammation is the red, itchy kind and often leads to scratching, which worsens the condition and causes further damage and irritation to the skin. This cycle of scratching and inflammation highlights the importance of identifying and avoiding some of these allergens and irritants for proper control of eczema based on many clinical observations using patient response and environmental variables on skin conditions, based on many clinical studies. Contact dermatitis is a cutaneous reaction due to direct contact with allergens or irritants. The condition appears as red, erythematous lesions in areas of exposure to chemical or allergenic substances, such as nickel in ornamentation or perfumes in cosmetics. One surprising finding from recent research is that irritant contact dermatitis is among the most prevalent hand diseases, with a lifetime prevalence of 31.2% in the general population, according to a study of over 1,900 participants. This draws attention to the rising problem of occupational exposure, particularly in medical workers and those with frequent exposure to detergents.

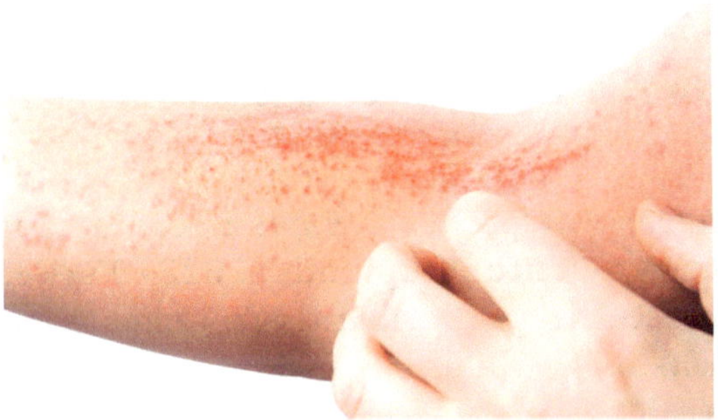

Figure 6.11. Allergic contact dermatitis.

Source: https://cdn.shopify.com/s/files/1/2730/7792/files/AdobeStock_181902053.jpeg?v=1599166004.

It is crucial that affected individuals understand their triggers and take preventive measures, such as wearing gloves and using mild, fragrance-free products, to ease symptoms and maintain the integrity of their skin. Management of common allergens and irritants is not only important for relieving eczema symptoms but also for improving overall quality of life. Eczema sufferers endure colossal psychological misery due to the prominence and chronicity of the disease, as well as a lack of education in society on skin diseases. The pruritus or chronic nature of itching is a key characteristic of the patient experience for skin disease sufferers (Briffa et al., 2009). In addition, hand eczema itself has been identified to disrupt personal relationships and activities of daily living for a significant proportion of patients. By raising awareness of allergens and irritants in everyday environments, public education can lead to improved management practices. These can help people control their skin condition, avoid flare-ups, and enhance their social and personal quality of life (Figure 6.11).

6.3.3. Diagnosis and Treatment Approaches

Effective diagnosis and treatment strategies for eczema and dermatitis require a comprehensive overview of the disease and its various subtypes, e.g., atopic, contact, and seborrheic dermatitis. The diagnosis is largely clinical, supported by an excellent patient history and objective findings, such as identification of primary lesions and some patterns characteristic of each dermatitis subtype. By classifying dermatitis on the basis of clinical presentation, clinicians can more clearly differentiate between irritant and allergic contact dermatitis, despite the two having differing pathogenesis but similar morphology and etiology. Differentiation is significant because a correct diagnosis may lead to certain management strategies that enhance symptoms and prevent deterioration. Therefore, determining diagnostic criteria and being familiar with the distinct characteristics of each subtype are the most important requirements for successful treatment (Abuabara et al., 2018). Individualized treatment protocols are required for atopic dermatitis, reflecting the heterogeneous nature of this condition. An attempt has been made to establish phenotypes of atopic dermatitis to learn about its etiology and to predict treatment success. Despite a multitude of suggested classifications in the literature, no consensus exists for the definition of these phenotypes. The multicomponent nature of atopic dermatitis often necessitates the use of combination topical therapy, systemic therapy, and lifestyle modifications. For example, emollients play a critical role in maintaining skin barrier function, while topical corticosteroids reduce inflammation during acute exacerbations. Moreover, novel treatments targeting specific inflammatory pathways highlight the ongoing evolution of eczema management strategies. Lastly, optimizing diagnosis and understanding the different phenotypes can reinforce the effectiveness of treatment approaches (Abuabara et al., 2018). Contact dermatitis remains a challenge because it is clinically heterogeneous and requires accurate diagnosis to avoid exposure to the causative factors. Irritant and allergic contact dermatitis need to be thoroughly examined since they may mimic other dermatoses, and presenting them makes it difficult to diagnose. The clinician must distinguish between such presentations in order to implement appropriate intervention. The occupational and socioeconomic impact of contact dermatitis further indicates the merit in early detection and management. Pivotal to effective management is identifying allergens and irritants through comprehensive patient history and patch testing, which can guide avoidance. A preventive approach, alongside certain treatments such as topical corticosteroids and immunomodulators, is essential for a person diagnosed with contact dermatitis to achieve long-term relief and minimize the condition's impact on their daily life (Aerts et al., 2024) (Figure 6.12).

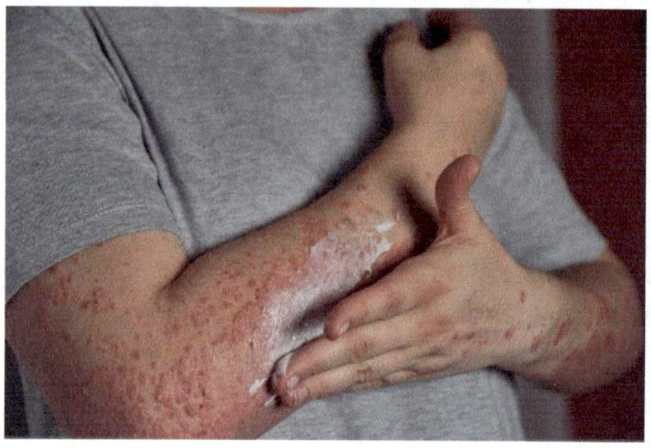

Figure 6.12. Contact allergic dermatitis treatment.

Source: https://www.oasisdermatology.com/wp-content/uploads/2023/03/Best-Contact-Allergic-Dermatitis-Treatment-Oasis-Dermatology-1000x658.jpg.

Test Your Knowledge

1. What are the types of contact dermatitis?
2. What are allergens and irritants?

6.4. Seborrheic Dermatitis

Learning Outcome

1. Define the seborrheic dermatitis
2. Describe the common areas affected and symptoms of seborrheic dermatitis
3. Know the treatment and management techniques for seborrheic dermatitis

Seborrheic dermatitis is a prevalent inflammatory skin condition with red, scaly patches and oily, greasy scales that mainly affect sebaceous gland-abundant regions such as the face, scalp, and upper back. It has a multifactorial pathogenesis involving genetic predisposition, environmental factors, and microbial colonization, especially by *Malassezia yeast*. This yeast cultures in sebaceous secretions, causing an inflammatory response that manifests as the clinical presentation of seborrheic dermatitis. Although the exact pathophysiology remains unclear, recent studies suggest that an overactive immune response, in association with changes in epidermal barrier function, can enhance the process. The chronicity of seborrheic dermatitis does, in fact, dramatically influence patients' quality of life, most frequently producing psychological distress as well as social stigma in its visible form. Epidemiologically, at all ages except infancy, seborrheic dermatitis appears in a heterogeneous population—primarily adult males—and the peak age is during adolescence and again in late adulthood. Stress, hormonal fluctuations, and comorbid medical conditions such as Parkinson's disease and HIV/AIDS have been associated with increased severity and prevalence of the condition. Significantly, the association between cutaneous inflammation and systemic disease has raised questions about how diseases such as immunosuppression affect the pathogenesis of seborrheic dermatitis. While immunocompromised individuals may develop more severe forms of the condition, it also serves to illustrate the importance of individualized management strategies. Treatment of the underlying cause and individualized treatment planning are both key to reducing symptoms and preventing flare-ups. Treatment for seborrheic dermatitis most often involves topical therapy, including antifungal agents, corticosteroids, and keratolytics. Antifungal shampoos containing active ingredients such as ketoconazole or selenium sulfide are commonly prescribed for their ability to reduce Malassezia colonization. Furthermore, corticosteroids can relieve symptoms of inflammation and itch, but must be used with caution to avoid long-term side effects. Other treatments, such as calcineurin inhibitors, offer an alternative without corticosteroid side effects, though more work is needed with larger numbers to ascertain their benefit. Overall, the management must be holistic, accounting for lifestyle adjustments and adherence to treatment, thereby cognizant of both the physical as well as the psychological components that are associated with seborrheic dermatitis as part of the broader subject matter of eczema and dermatitis, including atopic and contact dermatitis, within clinical practice (Figure 6.13).

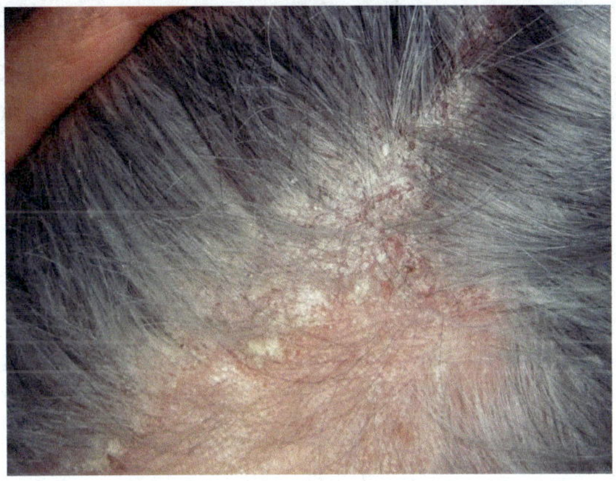

Figure 6.13. Seborrheic dermatitis.

Source: https://eczema.org/wp-content/uploads/sebderm6-compressed.jpg.

6.4.1. Definition and Distinguishing Features

It is necessary to understand the differential characteristics and definitions of eczema and dermatitis to ensure successful clinical practice and management. Loosely used synonymously with dermatitis, eczema is a term applied to a cluster of inflammatory dermatoses characterized by erythema, scaling, and pruritus. Of these, atopic dermatitis, contact dermatitis, and seborrheic dermatitis are distinct entities that vary in cause, clinical presentation, and treatment. Ateleiosis is most often restricted to individuals with a familial predisposition to allergy and is often accompanied by a personal or family history of atopy. Contact dermatitis, on the other hand, is an allergic response resulting from direct contact of the skin with allergens or irritants, whereas seborrheic dermatitis is most commonly induced by an overgrowth of yeast Malassezia, particularly in sebaceous areas of the skin. These differences in knowledge form the basis of correct diagnosis and targeted interventions. Clinical presentation and distribution distinguish among the various types of dermatitis. Pruritic, erythematous lesions, usually flexural, such as around the elbows and knees, in children, are characteristic of atopic dermatitis. Its chronic nature leads to phases of exacerbations and remissions, which can be precipitated by environmental stimuli or allergens. On the other hand, contact dermatitis is quite characteristic depending on whether it is irritant or allergic in nature. Irritant contact dermatitis is usually found to occur localized to the area of contact and can present with stinging, burning, or pruritic sensations, whereas allergic contact dermatitis presents with a more variable latency period, often vesicular in nature, with severe pruritus over involved areas.

The distribution of the lesions and their specificity within various parts of the body are important lead points during the diagnosis of such conditions (Aerts et al., 2024). Seborrheic dermatitis introduces an extra level of complexity into this paradigm, generally presenting as oily, yellow, scaled, erythematous plaques and usually found in locations with sebaceous glands, such as the scalp, face, and intertriginous zones. These distinctions are not merely important for diagnosis but also for management strategies, as each type of dermatitis mandates specific therapeutic approaches based on pathophysiologic mechanisms. Effective management of the conditions combines both pharmacologic therapy, including corticosteroids to suppress inflammation and emollients to repair the barrier, and non-pharmacologic therapy, including dietary modification to reduce triggers. With the rising prevalence of allergic and immunologic dermatoses in today's populations, as emphasized in recent discussions among dermatological specialists (Ambrogio et al., 2024), a clear understanding of the definitions and manifestations of eczema and dermatitis is vital for clinical practitioners to provide optimal patient care.

6.4.2. Common Areas Affected and Symptoms

Eczema and dermatitis also have characteristic signs that can significantly vary depending on the condition and the specific areas involved. For atopic dermatitis, classic sites involved include flexural regions such as the inner elbows and knees, and also the neck and face. Signs typically manifest as dry, itchy skin that may become red and inflamed. The intense itch is usually followed by scratching, leading to additional skin lesions and the potential to become an inflammation-irritation cycle. On children's cheeks, atopic dermatitis appears and causes distress to both the patient and caregiver. Chronicity of the aforementioned symptoms may affect quality of life, underscoring the importance of appropriate management techniques to alleviate distress and prevent subsequent exacerbations. Contact dermatitis, characterized by its occurrence following exposure to specific irritants or allergens, tends to affect areas that are directly exposed to them. Hands and face are frequently affected due to handling caustic substances or perfumes in personal care products, for instance. The symptoms are typically localized redness, swelling, and vesicles that weep or crust. Individuals may also experience a stinging or burning sensation together with itching. Identification of the causal agent is crucial since avoidance can result in significant improvement of symptoms. The ability to successfully treat contact dermatitis through lifestyle modifications and targeted treatments can minimize discomfort and prevent recurrence, underscoring the importance of patient education in dermatology. Seborrheic dermatitis, which is another common form of dermatitis, most often happens in regions that have high concentrations of sebaceous glands, such as the scalp, face, and upper back. Yellowish, oily scales and crusts, typically accompanied by itching, characterize it. On the scalp, it can manifest as dandruff, leading to flaking that may give rise to social discomfort for the individual. On the surface, seborrheic dermatitis appears on the nose, eyebrows, and ears, causing redness and inflammation. Its treatment relies on an understanding of the mechanisms underlying the skin's oil production, and its treatments range from medicated shampoos to topical steroids. Patients with seborrheic dermatitis may benefit from regular dermatological examinations to assess treatment efficacy and monitor any ensuing complications (Kompella et al., 2009). It is also crucial for health practitioners to recommend effective self-care practices for the successful management of disease (Nunns et al., 2017) (Figure 6.14).

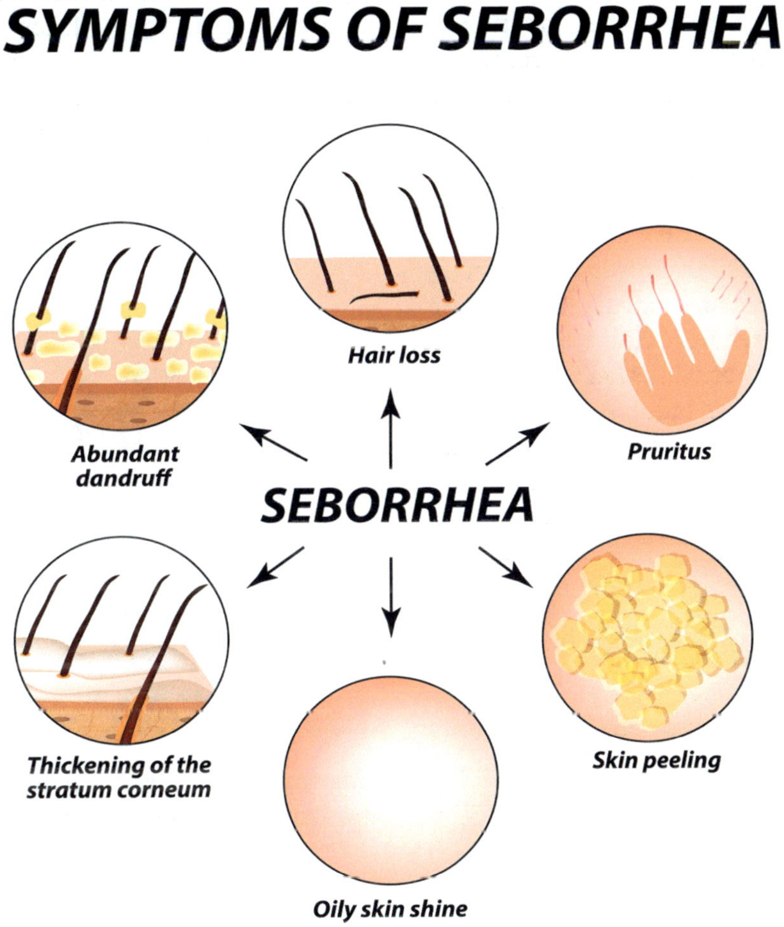

Figure 6.14. Symptoms of seborrheic dermatitis.

Source: https://www.hhclinics.co.uk/wp-content/uploads/2019/08/symptoms-of-Seborrheic-Dermatitis.jpg.

6.4.3. Treatment and Management Techniques

Right treatment and management options for eczema and dermatitis are crucial in relieving symptoms and improving the quality of life for patients. The therapy most often involves a blend of topical care, systemic medication, and lifestyle modification, depending on the type of dermatitis. For instance, topical corticosteroids are typically prescribed for atopic dermatitis and contact dermatitis, as they help reduce inflammation and suppress itching. Second, emollients play an important role in skin hydration and barrier function maintenance, which can be used to decrease the frequency and severity of flare-ups dramatically. Known triggers must also be identified and avoided by the patient, particularly in allergic contact dermatitis, and so thorough patient education forms part of the management plan (Aerts et al., 2024). Successful treatment for contact dermatitis depends on proper identification of the etiology—irritant or allergic. The treatment regimen may include corticosteroids, but also often includes implementing strict avoidance measures. Patch testing may be of great assistance in identifying specific allergens that elicited the reactions. When diagnosed, care must be taken to ensure the use of protective barriers, such as gloves or creams, particularly in the work environment, where irritant exposure is commonplace. Regular consultation with medical personnel can assist in modifying treatment regimens based on the patient's evolving state and reaction to treatment, emphasizing the importance of monitoring the patient's progress throughout management (Aerts et al., 2024). Seborrheic dermatitis, being common on sebum-plushed areas of the body, requires a special management plan, with antifungal and anti-inflammatory agents in combination. Over-the-counter and prescription-strength shampoos containing ingredients such as ketoconazole or zinc pyrithione may be useful for scaling reduction and inflammation control. In extensive cases, topical corticosteroids can be applied cautiously to minimize inflammation, but prolonged use should be avoided. Along with medical treatments, incorporating lifestyle modifications, e.g., regular shampooing and a proper diet, also improves symptom management. Therefore, an effective treatment approach that combines medical therapies and self-management interventions is critical for individuals with seborrheic dermatitis to successfully control flares and maintain their quality of life (Figure 6.15).

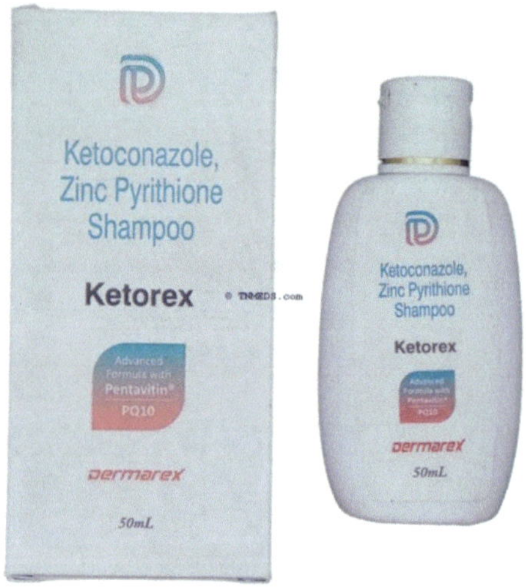

Figure 6.15. Ketorex shampoo.

Source: https://icdn.tnmeds.com/cache/data/tnimages/905549-500x500.jpg.

Test Your Knowledge

1. What are the features of seborrheic dermatitis?
2. What areas does seborrheic dermatitis affect?

6.5. Psychological and Social Impact

Learning Outcome

1. Know the emotional effects of living with eczema
2. Describe the social stigma and misconceptions surrounding eczema and dermatitis
3. Describe the coping strategies and support systems for patients dealing with eczema

The psychosocial impact of eczema and dermatitis cannot be exaggerated, particularly for atopic dermatitis (AD), the prevalence of which affects a significant percentage of children and adults. The patients of this chronic skin condition generally suffer intensely from emotional distress as a result of visible symptoms like lesions and inflammation. This visibility can result in stigma, social withdrawal, and decreased self-esteem, creating a cycle where psychological distress accentuates skin symptoms more. As noted, the multidimensional aspect of ADs pathology necessitates a unmonodimensional treatment protocol with multifaceted targets that is not solely dermatological but also manages the psychological effect of the disease. This holistic framework is essential for countering the emotional burden of conditions such as eczema and dermatitis, underscoring the need for integrative treatment modalities that consider both physiological and psychological responses to treatment (Abreu et al., 2020). Moreover, the social implications of having eczema and dermatitis extend beyond the patient, with significant and lasting ramifications on family dynamics and social interactions. Patients might struggle to engage in social activities because their condition provokes fears of appearance and sensitivity problems, leading to avoidance of interactions with people. Regular, and even intrusive, treatment could interfere with daily living and activities and bring additional stress to the patient and the family. This interpersonal conflict may also complicate social support networks, with family members feeling helpless or resentful toward attempts to provide care. In addressing these determinants, health professionals should focus on education and disease communication, which can empower families and patients to navigate social circumstances and build mutual resilience (Hita et al., 2020). Lastly, the interaction between eczema and dermatitis's social and psychological dimensions paints a clear cry for effective support systems. Healing interventions, like counseling and group support, can significantly improve patients' coping skills and life. Increased awareness of the psychological impact of skin illnesses can further lead to improved outcomes among patients through early intervention of mental illness. As research continues to bring into view the relationship between psychological distress and atopic dermatitis severity, it is increasingly apparent that treatment must be integrative in nature. The integration of both dermatological and psychological aspects into patient care will enhance the effectiveness of interventions, culminating in better health outcomes and improved quality of life for patients with eczema and dermatitis (Abreu et al., 2020) (Figure 6.16).

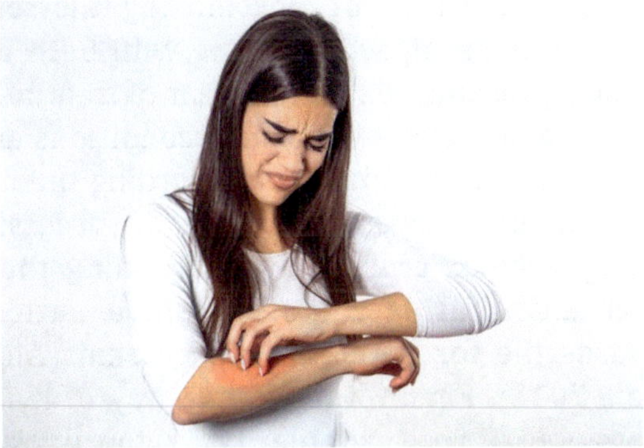

Figure 6.16. Psychological effects of eczema.

Source: https://images.onlymyhealth.com/imported/images/2023/July/17_Jul_2023/Ways-To-Prevent-Eczema-At-Home-During-Monsoon-Main.jpg.

6.5.1. Emotional Effects of Living with Eczema

The emotional consequence of having eczema is highly significant and complex, impacting individuals' self-esteem, mental well-being, and quality of life. Chronic skin conditions such as eczema have a tendency to induce embarrassment as well as social isolation, as individuals might feel stigmatized due to the appearance of their skin. This consciousness can disrupt interpersonal relationships, academic performance, and social activity, leading to feelings of isolation and anxiety. Evidence indicates that eczema patients are at increased risk of developing psychological comorbidities like depression and anxiety disorders. These affective challenges require an integrated treatment strategy, keeping in mind that managing the physical symptoms of eczema is only half the recipe for supporting patients' overall health. On top of that, the stress of eczema control may heighten these emotional issues. A number of patients experience a condition called topical steroid phobia, where fear of potential side effects from necessary treatments results in undertreatment. Avoidance, which worsens the condition and impacts emotional health even further, with the chronic skin flare-ups becoming a cause of unremitting distress. The combined impact of coping with both the physical presentation and the fear of treatment can create a cycle of worsening conditions and enhanced anxiety. Education regarding the use of topical steroids and their role in successful management is crucial to undermining these fears and infusing a more positive outlook towards life for patients with eczema (Anan et al., 2011). Finally, the eczema way of living is also beset with complexity, as the disease itself is chronic. With eczema prone to flare-ups, patients may feel uncertainty, leading to higher stress and annoyance. The abstract nature of pain and discomfort of eczema can make individuals feel undervalued by others who might not be able to assess the intensity of agony. Mental health interventions, such as cognitive-behavioral therapy, can potentially heal these emotional conditions. Support groups and other external sources are also of utmost importance in providing the validation and understanding individuals require to be able to open up and provide their experiences and management techniques for both eczema and its emotional consequences (Adaskevich et al., 2006).

6.5.2. Social Stigma and Misconceptions

The prevalence of social stigma and misconceptions relating to eczema and dermatitis is an immediate issue that has a severe impact on the lives of those suffering from the diseases. Most people have misconceptions about the etiology and nature of eczema and perceive it as nothing but a cosmetic problem and not as an unending skin disorder. Such a lack of knowledge fosters adverse judgments and attitudes toward individuals who are suffering from skin ailments. For instance, hand eczema patients frequently report a sense of not being understood, and stigmatization fosters a feeling of alienation from other people and society at large. Prejudices, in turn, create a vicious cycle by which sufferers socially withdraw as a reaction to negative impressions, thereby worsening their psychological and emotional suffering. Therefore, refuting these myths is critical to fostering empathy and sympathy among communities, thereby increasing the overall well-being of affected populations (Hertrich et al., 2014). Research has established that how eczema is perceived varies greatly among different populations and therefore leads to huge differences in attitude and stigmatization of the disease. Evidence shows that people with a dermatological history tend to be better informed about eczema, suggesting that well-educated people are less prone to negative stereotypes. It was found that women reported more knowledge and perception of eczema compared to men, which points towards the gender factor in social attitudes. This lack of knowledge among the general public leads to negative stigma that could discourage patients from seeking needed treatment or support. Thus, the impact of such myths extends beyond mere social awkwardness, influencing patient health outcomes and access to care (Hertrich et al., 2014). It is essential to appreciate these dynamics when formulating education programs capable of reversing stigma. Moreover, the psychosocial consequences of having eczema or dermatitis cannot be undervalued. Patients experience a blend of emotional difficulties that range from self-doubt and shame due to the visibility of their skin condition. Such stigmatization has the potential to produce very serious psychosocial issues, and in fact frequently leads to anxiety, depression, and lowered quality of life.

Investigating the relationship between perceived stigma and distress shows that those who perceive more stigmatization experience more emotional distress. Coping styles vary widely among individuals, with some managing the situation well and others being severely disadvantaged. Awareness of these coping mechanisms will inform therapeutic procedures, allowing healthcare workers to deliver improved care to patients managing the physical and psychological elements of eczema and dermatitis (Figure 6.17).

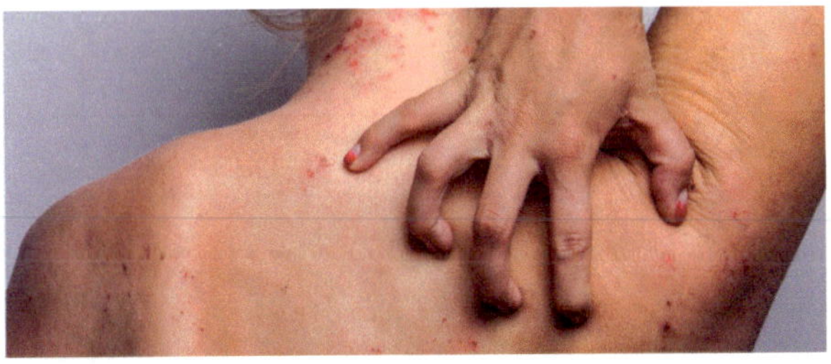

Figure 6.17. Eczema misconceptions.

Source: https://www.allergyuk.org/wp-content/uploads/2023/04/Copy-of-Copy-of-Copy-of-Banner.png.

6.5.3. Coping Strategies and Support Systems

Treatment of eczema, particularly atopic dermatitis, involves embracing effective coping mechanisms and robust support structures to manage the complexities of the condition. Eczema sufferers are likely to face not only physical discomfort but also psychological distress. The need for careful management is addressed in this situation by the critical role of educational intervention in enhancing treatment and self-management compliance. By incorporating psychological and educational facilitation, patients can be empowered to cope with the reality that eczema is a chronic condition. These treatments aim to reinforce the importance of regular topical therapy, ultimately maximizing overall disease control (Cowdell et al., 2014). In addition, patient education empowers individuals, encourages an active role in their skin care, and improves quality of life. Support systems are equally important for eczema patients, particularly for adolescents who face special social demands. Adolescence is the formative years that are characterized by social and identity development, both of which can be severely impacted by the visibility of skin disorders. Counseling and support groups from peers can offer a chance to openly discuss matters pertaining to eczema management, thereby reducing feelings of loneliness. These institutional environments provide a setting where patients feel safe discussing their experiences and coping mechanisms, leading to increased resilience and self-esteem. The literature indicates that successful interventions among adolescents involve training in the management of area therapy and participation in group discussions, enabling participants to learn and connect with one another (Hwang et al., 2017). Therefore, full systems of support are crucial for promoting emotional welfare and allowing effective disease control among younger populations. Additionally, clinicians play a central role in implementing these coping mechanisms and support systems. Physicians, physician assistants, and dermatologists should be aware of the psychosocial implications of eczema's effect on patients. This awareness is central to initiating the right referrals to support services or counseling when necessary. Continuing medical education for healthcare providers is needed to keep them up to date on the latest strategies that improve patient outcomes, especially among youth. By equipping clinicians with knowledge about psychological stress and treatment education, they are better positioned to assist patients in adapting to their condition and establishing effective coping mechanisms (Cowdell et al., 2014). Thus, a well-coordinated approach involving medical treatment, educational interventions, and strong support systems can significantly improve the quality of life for patients with eczema, ultimately leading to better long-term outcomes (Figure 6.18).

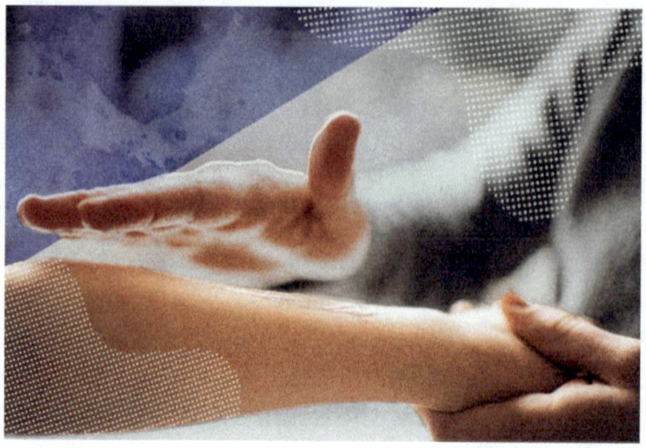

Figure 6.18. Navigating and coping with the unpredictable nature of atopic dermatitis.

Source: https://www.verywellmind.com/thmb/Z0Ct9tU6xsUPblONYHwD8ztKKQM=/4000x0/filters:no_upscale():max_bytes(150000):strip_icc()/vwm-Unpredictable-Nature1-58e4fd1f47d149eeaa77a9537a7aae2d.jpg.

Test Your Knowledge

1. How does eczema impact individuals' self-esteem and social interactions?
2. What misconceptions about eczema contribute to social stigma?

SUMMARY

Finally, the understanding of eczema and dermatitis conditions, such as atopic, contact, and seborrheic dermatitis, remains paramount to effective patient care. The conditions reflect the three-dimensional nature of skin, influenced by genetics, the environment, and immunology. Treatment must, as such, encompass an all-encompassing approach to the physical and psychological impacts of the conditions. Research indicates that the prevalence of seborrheic dermatitis is rising, possibly due to altering environmental and lifestyle factors that could serve as precipitants, which necessitate clinical practice being modified in accordance with evolving patient requirements (Khan et al., 2024). Holistic management calls for practitioners to remain informed about advances in the pathogenesis of these disorders and the effectiveness of management (Khan et al., 2024). Moreover, the therapeutic approach to dermatitis is shifting, and multiple modalities are available to address symptoms. Topical steroids have served as an anchor of first-line therapy, but their association with side effects requires careful choices by health professionals (Burshtein et al., 2025). Therefore, a quest for alternative types of therapy, such as innovative targeted topical therapies, can offer safer options in treating patients with inflammatory cutaneous disorders. This change in treatment focuses on the need for ongoing research and discussion among dermatologists for the risks versus benefits of each treatment approach. Patients are supported by a collaborative model that emphasizes individualized treatment based on specific symptomology and lifestyle. Lastly, advances in the pathophysiology of eczema and dermatitis will be important to guide future therapeutic strategies to maximize quality of life for patients. Insight into the complex nature of the diseases enables clinicians to tailor treatments to meet the physical and psychological needs of patients with skin disease. Ongoing education and study of the psychosocial impact of eczema and dermatitis will further emphasize the importance of comprehensive dermatologic care. Through the healthcare providers implementing evidence-based care for management, clinical outcomes will not only be improved, but patient empowerment to take an active part in their own skin health process, in spite of the adversity presented by these conditions, will also be maximized.

A detailed investigation of eczema and dermatitis, i.e., atopic, contact, and seborrheic dermatitis, summarizes key features relating to their incidence, signs, and treatment. Atopic dermatitis is the most common chronic skin condition, with a significant incidence among children from industrialized nations, which significantly impairs quality of life due to associated itching and skin lesions. Conversely, contact dermatitis results from direct skin contact with irritants or allergens, which provoke differing inflammatory responses according to duration of exposure and patient susceptibility. Seborrheic dermatitis, characterized by oily, scaly breakouts, typically occurs in regions of high sebaceous gland content, showing the interplay between environmental and endogenous factors in these inflammatory cutaneous disorders. Understanding these variations is essential to effective diagnosis and management strategies, enabling medical practitioners to tailor treatments in accordance with patient profiles while being sensitive to the emotional well-being of the suffering. Research highlights the importance of effective treatment regimens for managing the complex presentations of eczema and dermatitis. Topical corticosteroids, such as clobetasol propionate, have emerged as a go-to therapy due to their efficacy in blunting inflammation and controlling symptoms (Ojeda et al., 2024). In a more specific context, clobetasol propionate has been a dermatologist's favorite medication for treating scalp dermatoses, which can literally and figuratively affect a patient's lifestyle. Besides, more severe cases may require systemic therapy or adjunctive treatment, and often such cases require a multi-modal approach that includes pharmacological as well as non-pharmacological interventions. Such an integrated approach not only recognizes the biological basis of such disorders but also realizes the necessity of the reinforcement of psychological and emotional health in patients facing issues from their skin disorders. Furthermore, current epidemiological studies reveal notable differences in the prevalence and types of dermatitis, which vary with geography, economics, and exposure. To illustrate, in some regions, children exhibit a higher incidence of seborrheic dermatitis due to genetic and climatic variations, while the prevalence of atopic dermatitis is uniformly high in industrialized countries (Mahajan et al., 2019). Factors such as hygiene practices, environmental allergens, and genetics make it even more complex. Thus, health systems must introduce differential public health interventions based on these differences, with special focus on education regarding prevention measures and the availability of concerned healthcare facilities. Knowledge of the multifactorial aetiology of eczema and dermatitis, and of targeted interventions, can significantly enhance patient outcomes and public health in dermatology.

KEY TERMS FROM THIS CHAPTER

- Allergic rhinitis
- Atopic dermatitis
- Corticosteroids
- Dermatitis
- Eczema
- Itchiness
- Redness
- Asthma
- Contact dermatitis
- Cyclosporine
- Dysbiosis
- Immune dysregulation
- Microbial imbalance
- Sebaceous glands

CRITICAL THINKING QUESTIONS

1. **Which of the following is a hallmark feature of atopic dermatitis?**
   a. Vesicular lesions on the hands
   b. Chronic, relapsing itchy skin with a family history of atopy
   c. Yellow, greasy scales on the scalp and face
   d. Acute redness and swelling after exposure to an allergen
2. **What is the primary cause of contact dermatitis?**
   a. Genetic predisposition
   b. Immune response to environmental allergens or irritants
   c. Overactive sebaceous glands
   d. Systemic autoimmune disease
3. **Seborrheic dermatitis is commonly associated with which of the following microorganisms?**
   a. *Staphylococcus aureus*
   b. *Malassezia yeast*
   c. *Streptococcus pyogenes*
   d. *Candida albicans*
4. **Which of the following is a common trigger for atopic dermatitis?**
   a. Contact with poison ivy
   b. Stress, allergens, or cold weather
   c. Overgrowth of skin flora
   d. Direct physical trauma to the skin
5. **Which diagnostic test is most commonly used to confirm allergic contact dermatitis?**
   a. Biopsy
   b. Patch testing
   c. Dermoscopy
   d. Blood test for IgE levels

Short Answer Questions

1. What is eczema?
2. Define atopic dermatitis.
3. Define contact dermatitis.
4. What is seborrheic dermatitis?
5. What are the psychological effects of eczema?

Answer to Critical Thinking Questions

1. (b); 2. (b) ; 3. (b); 4. (b); 5. (b)

REFERENCES

1. Lopes, A., Sokolova, A., Abreu, C., & Lopes, C. (2019). Atopic Dermatitis Host and Environment Model: Revisiting Therapeutic options. *European Annals of Allergy and Clinical Immunology, 52*(01), 4. https://doi.org/10.23822/eurannaci.1764-1489.125Abuabara, K., Allen, V., Grindlay, D. J. C., Langan, S. M., et al. (2018). Classifying atopic dermatitis: Protocol for a systematic review of subtypes (phenotypes) and associated characteristics. https://core.ac.uk/download/161339171.pdf (accessed on 21st July 2025).
2. Adaskevich, V. P., Katina, M. A., & Valles-Kazlouskaya, V. V. (2006). *Practical Dermatology*. https://core.ac.uk/download/80150438.pdf (accessed on 21st July 2025).
3. Aerts, O., Ayala, F., Balato, A., Bizjak, M., et al. (2024). Differential diagnosis of contact dermatitis: A practical-approach review by the EADV Task Force on contact dermatitis. https://core.ac.uk/download/610613211.pdf (accessed on 21st July 2025).
4. Agner, T., & Ebbehøj, E. N. (2022). With focus on irritant contact dermatitis and prevention. https://core.ac.uk/download/620671369.pdf (accessed on 21st July 2025).
5. Ambrogio, F., Angilieri, L., Bonamonte, D., Boni, R., et al. (2024). A practical guide to recognize allergic and immunologic skin diseases: Diagnosis at first sight. https://core.ac.uk/download/636826782.pdf (accessed on 21st July 2025).
6. Amerio, P., Di Fino, S., Ferrucci, S. M., Galluzzo, M., Levi, A., Napolitano, M., Narcisi, A., et al. (2024). A multidisciplinary approach is beneficial in atopic dermatitis. https://core.ac.uk/download/621339749.pdf (accessed on 21st July 2025).
7. Anan, S., Aoki, V., Brunsting, A. L., Charman, C. R., Coca, C., Drake, L. A., et al. (2011). Current status of atopic dermatitis in Japan. https://core.ac.uk/download/pdf/8636983.pdf (accessed on 21st July 2025).
8. Apfelbacher, C., Blume-Peytavi, U., Boguniewicz, M., Brown, S. J., Danby, S. G., Darmstadt, G. L., et al. (2014). Emollient enhancement of the skin barrier from birth offers effective atopic dermatitis prevention. https://core.ac.uk/download/30662564.pdf (accessed on 21st July 2025).
9. Armario Hita, J. C., Baldrich, E. S., Herráez, L., Jáuregui, A., et al. (2020). Consensus on the clinical approach to moderate-to-severe atopic dermatitis in Spain: A Delphi survey. https://core.ac.uk/download/323288254.pdf (accessed on 21st July 2025).
10. Armario Hita, J. C., Navarro-Artieda, R., & Sicras-Mainar, A. (2019). Severe atopic dermatitis in Spain: A real-life observational study. https://core.ac.uk/download/288159225.pdf (accessed on 21st July 2025).
11. Ascott, A., Yu, A. M., Schmidt, M., Abuabara, K., et al. (2017). Association between eczema and major cardiovascular outcomes in population-based studies: A systematic review protocol. https://core.ac.uk/download/96628508.pdf (accessed on 21st July 2025).
12. Azad Khan, M. A. K., Begum, M., Happy Moon, R., Hasan, M., et al. (2024). Prevalence, risk factors and management approaches for seborrheic dermatitis. https://core.ac.uk/download/635338699.pdf (accessed on 21st July 2025).
13. Banks, J., Barrett, T. J., Baxter, H., Edwards, L., et al. (2019). Best emollients for eczema (BEE)–Comparing four types of emollients in children with eczema: Protocol for randomized trial and nested qualitative study. https://core.ac.uk/download/286135560.pdf (accessed on 21st July 2025).

14. Boekhout, T., Cafarchia, C., Gaitanis, G., Iatta, R., & Velegraki, A. (2015). *Malassezia* infections in humans and animals: Pathophysiology, detection and treatment. https://core.ac.uk/download/54137094.pdf (accessed on 21st July 2025).

15. Burshtein, J., Chovatiya, R., Golant, A., Lebwohl, M., et al. (2025). Risks of topical corticosteroid therapy and role for advanced targeted topical treatments for inflammatory skin diseases: An expert consensus panel. https://core.ac.uk/download/645980974.pdf (accessed on 21st July 2025).

16. Cabana, M. D. (2011). Early probiotic supplementation for the prevention of atopic disease in newborns—Probiotics and the hygiene hypothesis. https://core.ac.uk/download/323073583.pdf (accessed on 21st July 2025).

17. Callewaert, C., De Pessemier, B., Debaere, M., Grine, L., et al. (2021). Gut-skin axis: Current knowledge of the interrelationship between microbial dysbiosis and skin conditions. https://core.ac.uk/download/395605829.pdf (accessed on 21st July 2025).

18. Callewaert, C., Huang, S., Jing, G., Knight, R., et al. (2019). A microbiome-based index for assessing skin health and treatment effects for atopic dermatitis in children. https://core.ac.uk/download/323065351.pdf (accessed on 21st July 2025).

19. Cavaliere, G., Fava, P., Savoia, P., Veronese, F., et al. (2016). Inflammatory cutaneous diseases in renal transplant recipients. https://core.ac.uk/download/226199889.pdf (accessed on 21st July 2025).

20. Cowdell, F., Drury, A., Ersser, S. J., Farasat, H., et al. (2014). Psychological and educational interventions for atopic eczema in children. https://core.ac.uk/download/42142440.pdf (accessed on 21st July 2025).

21. Delgado Ojeda, J. G., Garcia-Patos Briones, V., Mir-Bonafé, J. F., Piquero Casals, J., et al. (2024). Use of topical corticosteroids in the treatment of noninfectious inflammatory dermatoses of the scalp: A survey of practicing dermatologists and dermatology residents using Delphi methodology. https://core.ac.uk/download/604467383.pdf (accessed on 21st July 2025).

22. Greif, C., Hivnor, C. M., Koopman, I. V., Mpunga, M., et al. (2024). Evaluating the effectiveness of ChatGPT4 in the diagnosis and workup of dermatologic conditions. https://core.ac.uk/download/617033339.pdf (accessed on 21st July 2025).

23. Hamnerius, N. (2019). Hand eczema and contact allergy in healthcare work. https://core.ac.uk/download/196251780.pdf (accessed on 21st July 2025).

24. Hertrich, F., Herzinger, T., Lange, D., Letule, A., et al. (2014). Chronic hand eczema: Perception and knowledge in non-affected individuals from general and dermatological practice. https://core.ac.uk/download/211701720.pdf (accessed on 21st July 2025).

25. Huilaja, L., Sinikumpu, S. P., Syrjälä, A. M., Tasanen, K., et al. (2023). Association between bleeding periodontal pockets and eczemas: Results of the Northern Finland Birth Cohort 1966. https://core.ac.uk/download/628857494.pdf (accessed on 21st July 2025).

26. Hwang, B. (2017). Educational interventions targeting adolescents with atopic dermatitis. https://open.bu.edu/bitstream/2144/26735/5/Hwang_bu_0017N_13190.pdf (accessed on 21st July 2025).

27. Imarenezor, O. (2020). Epidemiology and pathophysiology of common skin diseases in West Africa: An immunodermatological framework. https://core.ac.uk/download/395358179.pdf (accessed on 21st July 2025).

28. Jain, V., Sindhura, D. K., & Siri, A. (2018). Infant's skin and care needs with special consideration to formulation additives. https://core.ac.uk/download/477854665.pdf (accessed on 21st July 2025).
29. Kelman, L. V. (1999). Relationship between experience of stigmatization and coping styles: A comparison of individuals with eczema and psoriasis. https://core.ac.uk/download/429701114.pdf (accessed on 21st July 2025).
30. Kompella, A. (2009). Seborrheic dermatitis. https://core.ac.uk/download/62772153.pdf (accessed on 21st July 2025).
31. Mahajan, S. S. (2019). Clinic epidemiological profile of dermatological manifestations in preschool going children in a tertiary health care center. https://core.ac.uk/download/235670531.pdf (accessed on 21st July 2025).
32. Nunns, D., & Simpson, R. C. (2017). Skin diseases affecting the vulva. https://core.ac.uk/download/76975202.pdf (accessed on 21st July 2025).
33. Vella Briffa, D. (2009). Pruritus. https://core.ac.uk/download/83019812.pdf (accessed on 21st July 2025).

PSORIASIS AND PAPULOSQUAMOUS DISORDERS

7

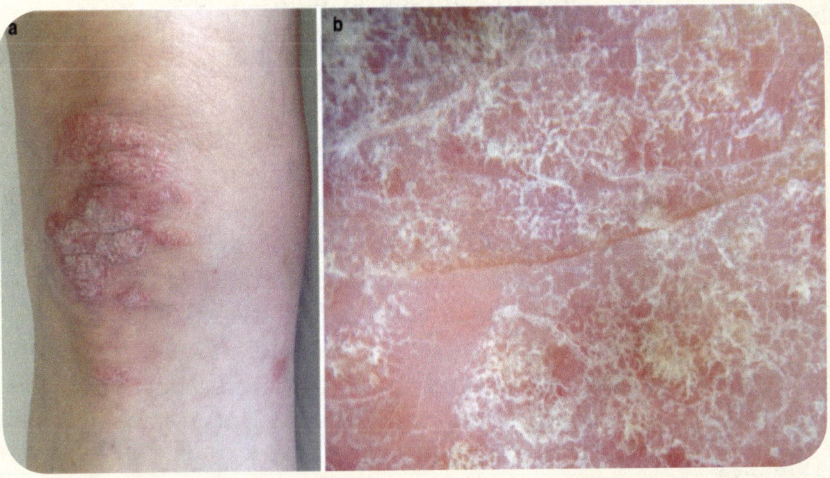

LEARNING OBJECTIVES

After studying this chapter, you will be able to:

1. Describe the types of psoriasis
2. Learn about symptoms and diagnosis of psoriasis
3 Understand the causes and risk factors associated with psoriasis and papulosquamous disorders
4 Know the treatment options for psoriasis and papulosquamous disorders
5 Understand the impact of psoriasis and papulosquamous disorders on quality of life

Introduction

Psoriasis, a papulosquamous autoimmune illness, is characterized by thick, silvery scales on erythematous patches. Prevalent in about 2-3% of the global population, psoriasis has widespread implications for the quality of life of individuals suffering from this condition, with physical discomfort and psychological morbidity as consequences. Psoriasis presents in many different manifestations, each with its own characteristics and clinical presentation. Among the forms, follicular psoriasis (FP) is a relatively rare subtype, underscoring the complex pathophysiology of psoriatic disorders. Understanding the heterogeneous appearance of psoriasis is significant for successful diagnosis and treatment, given variation across distinct patient factors, i.e., genetic predisposition and environmental factors (Tomar et al., 2024). Research has elucidated several key factors of psoriasis pathophysiology that is typified by immune dysregulation and deranged keratinocyte proliferation. Cytokines IL-17, IL-22, and TNF-α have been identified as key players in inflammatory pathways that drive the disease, fostering a setting that favors keratinocyte hyperactivity (Gaurav et al., 2024). The discovery of these processes has held the potential for targeted therapeutic approaches that can fine-tune the immune response and restore homeostasis. Therapies targeting these pathways could have a profound effect on psoriasis management, reducing the recurrent, often disabling symptoms of the disease. With greater insight into psoriasis, researchers have become increasingly interested in exploring novel treatment avenues, among them the role of S-phase kinase-associated protein 2 (Skp2). This protein has been identified based on its function in cell cycle regulation and its potential link to the inflammatory processes that characterize psoriasis (Tomar et al., 2024). Modulation of Skp2 activity could offer potent therapeutic approaches to treating the disease causally by targeting the root biological processes. Besides, dermoscopy advancement has enhanced diagnostic precision, particularly for rarer variants like FP, where visual inspection plays a vital role in the differentiation from other diseases (Gaurav et al., 2024). All these methods will enable dermatologists to better assess whether more personalized treatment is required in psoriasis patients, thereby addressing the complexity of the disorder and improving patient outcomes (Figure 7.1).

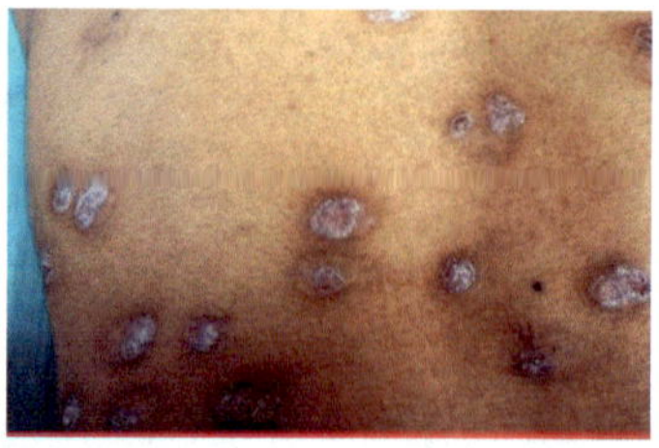

Figure 7.1. Distribution of papulosquamous disorders of skin.

Source: https://www.researchgate.net/profile/Shilpa-Narayankar/publication/322032061/figure/fig1/AS:574909374255104@1514080484872/Distribution-of-papulosquamous-disorders-of-skin-Out-of-42-cases-of-psoriasis-24.png.

Definition of Psoriasis

Psoriasis is a chronic inflammatory skin condition that includes the rapid proliferation of skin cells and the occurrence of red, thick, scaly patches on the skin's surface. Psoriasis is an autoimmune condition in which the immune system mistakenly attacks normal skin cells, triggering inflammation and an overactive response in the epidermis. There are many forms of psoriasis, with psoriasis vulgaris being the most widespread at approximately 80%-90% of all psoriasis. Psoriasis is a multifactorial disease involving the interconnection of genetic susceptibility, environmental elements, and immune dysregulation, making it a complex condition that remains a focal point of research for both dermatology and immunology. This condition not only affects the skin but also has systemic implications, underscoring the importance of understanding its etiology and presentation in detail. Various studies have enhanced awareness of psoriasis, clarifying its designation as an autoinflammatory keratinization disorder. This designation underscores the role of monogenic mutations and the innate immune system in the causation of the condition. Of particular interest, more recent findings have identified pathogenic mutations in CARD14 and IL36RN as linked to various forms of psoriasis, suggesting a genetic etiology of the disease's development. As suggested by more recent advances in medical genetics, our understanding of autoinflammatory keratinization disorders such as psoriasis has expanded incrementally, providing new insights into their etiology and clinical course (Blicharz et al., 2023). This finding underscores the importance of the development of treatment strategies for psoriasis pathophysiologic conditions in an effort to improve outcomes and quality of life in patients. Furthermore, psoriasis is an example of systemic inflammatory syndromes due to an overactive immune response secondary to as-yet-unidentified environmental stimuli. The concept of an environment-inadequacy status illustrates how the body may fail to handle various stresses, as evidenced by conditions such as psoriasis (Costache et al., 2022). Current therapies, particularly those aimed against cytokines such as TNF-α and IL-17, are designed to control this hyper-inflammatory state, so the central importance of cytokine balance in the management of disease. While such biologic therapies realize dramatic advances in disease control, they also risk inducing grave concern over the impact on immune surveillance for cancer. Thus, further research into the complex roles of cytokines in psoriasis is needed to understand both their therapeutic potential and their overall influence on patient health outcomes in managing papulosquamous disorders (Figure 7.2).

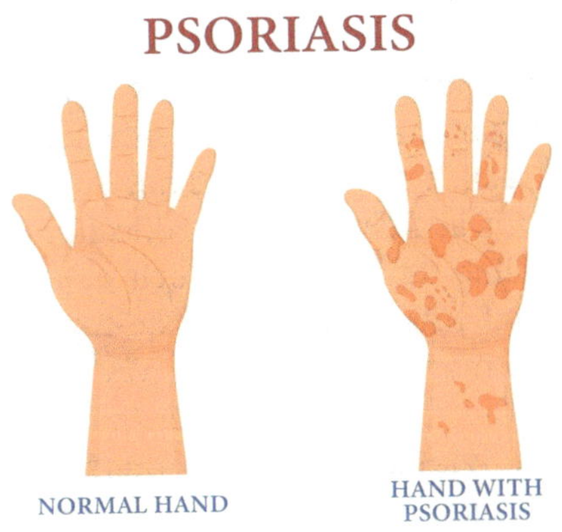

Figure 7.2. Understanding psoriasis.

Source: https://www.omcgahospitals.com/blog/storage/2024/10/frozenhand5-1536x1229.jpg.

Overview of Papulosquamous Disorders

Papulosquamous disorders are a group of skin conditions characterized by papules and scaling. Of these, the most prevalent is psoriasis, which affects millions of individuals worldwide. Psoriasis has many manifestations, and plaque psoriasis is the most prevalent, presenting as red, elevated plaques topped with silvery-white scales. There are also guttate, inverse, pustular, and erythrodermic psoriasis, each with distinct clinical features. These diseases not only constitute serious dermatological issues but also are linked to systemic disease, suggesting intricate interactions between skin and overall health. It is essential to be familiar with their pathophysiology, as they often involve immune dysregulation, inflammatory processes, and genetic factors. Their systemic impact, increasingly recognized, underscores the need for comprehensive management strategies that address skin manifestations and potential comorbidities. An important aspect of managing papulosquamous disease, particularly psoriasis, is incorporating both traditional and new therapeutic modalities. Conventional treatments include topical corticosteroids, vitamin D analogues, and phototherapy, which are used to alleviate symptoms and control flare-ups. However, as research continues, new treatments emerge, particularly biologics against known immune mechanisms. For instance, therapeutic research has further elucidated the roles that cytokines, such as tumor necrosis factor-alpha (TNF-α) and interleukins, play in exacerbating these conditions. The introduction of biologics holds greater promise for a cure and improved quality of life for those with severe disease. Furthermore, interest in the role of natural products in the management of skin disease is increasing, with certain studies suggesting an integrative model of care that combines conventional medicine and naturopathic treatment may yield better patient outcomes (Zaid et al., 2022). Apart from therapeutic problems, the psychosocial effects of papulosquamous disorders merit significant consideration. Patients are usually faced with problems in self-esteem, body image, and stigma due to easily observable manifestations like scaling and erythema. The psychological distress may further enhance the physical effects, making it a vicious cycle of stress and worsening. Psychiatric care is often a critical component of treatment for this complex disease process, underscoring the benefits of multidisciplinary management by psychologists, dermatologists, and patient support groups. Significantly, supportive therapy and patient education have been found in recent studies to alleviate some of the emotional distress associated with chronic skin diseases. Holistic management to treat both physical and psychosocial dimensions puts healthcare professionals in a unique position to encourage not just the well-being of the skin but also the general well-being of those who have papulosquamous disorders (Joosten et al., 2022) (Figure 7.3).

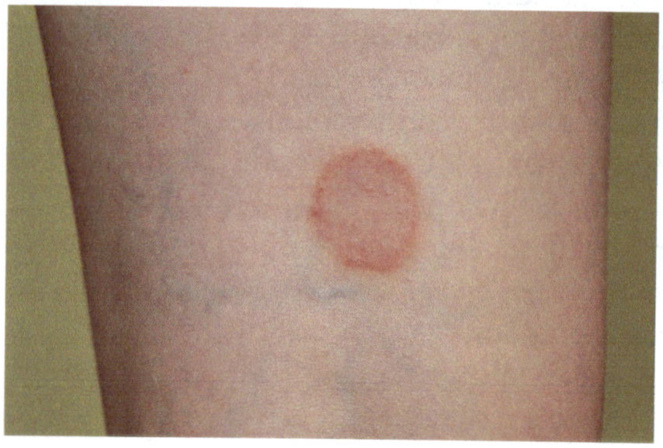

Figure 7.3. Papulosquamous disorders.

Source: https://www.verywellhealth.com/thmb/6Vaw62fSAwQUvRSMqDWmUT01MYY=/1500x0/filters:no_upscale():max_bytes(150000):strip_icc()/GettyImages-93486007-7cdef7ad674f4c78a7adf11d82d114df.jpg.

Importance of Understanding These Conditions

Awareness of psoriasis and papulosquamous disorders is valuable for several reasons, first of all due to their multifactorial etiology and the extensive impact they have on individuals' lives. These are not merely cosmetic issues; they are chronic inflammatory diseases that can cause significant psychological distress, physical discomfort, and social stigma. To develop an effective treatment strategy, medical professionals must understand the interactions among genetic, immunologic, and environmental factors in the pathogenesis of these diseases. As has been elucidated in recent research, dysregulation of immune cells, particularly T cells, is key to understanding psoriasis, and hence targeted therapies targeting these processes are warranted (Brănişteanu et al., 2022). A knowledge-informed perspective ensures better outcomes for patients due to tailored interventions, thereby enhancing the quality of life for patients. Aside from the patient implication, knowledge of such diseases contributes to a broader public health strategy. The increasing prevalence of psoriasis and related conditions underscores the necessity for increased awareness and education among medical professionals and the general public. By demystifying these conditions, experts can better assist with early detection, improve access to treatment, and reduce complications from poor management. Also, exploration of conditions such as lichen planus, which shares immunologic characteristics with psoriasis, is essential, especially since it is heterogeneous in presentation and can cause significant morbidity despite being self-limited (Boch et al., 2021). Educational interventions to de-mystify such conditions may be a valuable way to increase empathy and decrease stigma, thereby finally helping individuals deal with their conditions better and more supported. Moreover, a deeper understanding of psoriasis and papulosquamous diseases is required to advance research and treatment. With the evolution of medical science, new treatments are continuously surfacing, most of which are rooted in elucidating the pathogenic mechanisms of these disorders. The identification of new immunologic mechanisms, including the roles of antimicrobial peptides and interleukin-23, promises to unlock therapeutic strategies that selectively modulate disease manifestations (Brănişteanu et al., 2022). Thus, the blending of old-fashioned therapies with cutting-edge biologics and Janus kinase inhibitors offers new hope for patients. Through interdisciplinary research and collaboration, we are able to establish an environment that allows for continuous learning and development of the management of these disorders with complexity, which will translate to more effective and individualized treatment regimes.

7.1. Types of Psoriasis

Learning Outcome

1. Describe the plaque psoriasis
2. Understand the guttate psoriasis
3. Define the inverse psoriasis

Psoriasis has several forms, each with distinct characteristics and clinical significance. The most prevalent form, plaque psoriasis, manifests as thick, red skin lesions covered in thick, silvery scales on the elbows, knees, and lower back. The plaques arise from an overgrowth cycle of skin cells due to immune system dysfunction, generating inflammation and the condition's characteristic symptoms. In addition, guttate psoriasis is more common in younger patients and characterized by their small, drop-shaped lesions that follow an infection caused by a bacterium, such as strep throat. Such diverse presentations are indicative of the heterogeneous nature of psoriasis, and appropriate treatment methods are needed to address the individual pathophysiologic mechanisms of each subtype. In contrast to the above presentations, inverse psoriasis presents as red, smooth plaques in skin folds, such as the armpits, groin, and under the breast. This type presents particular challenges because the moist skin environment may even suppress the typical psoriasis scaling, thus making diagnosis and treatment more complicated. Also, pustular psoriasis is characterized by the development of white pustules with erythematous surrounding skin, often limited to the palms and soles or generalized, possibly associated with systemic findings, including fever and chills. These forms of psoriasis not only reflect the polymorphism of the disease but also highlight the necessity of an awareness of variation in presentation to improve patient outcomes more effectively. Nail psoriasis is also a very important sign that occurs in half of the disease patients, primarily affecting the toenails and fingernails. This type may lead to nail loss, discoloration, and pitting, and contributes even more to the patients' impaired quality of life and self-esteem. Psoriatic arthritis in certain patients makes it even more complicated, as it involves joint inflammation and creates significant mobility issues. Both nail psoriasis and psoriatic arthritis illustrate that psoriasis is more than just a skin condition, thereby highlighting the systemic nature of the disease. Due to the multifaceted nature of the conditions, further research into biomarkers—such as those identified in more recent research, i.e., SIGLEC8 and IL5RA—may be essential in continuing to drive diagnosis and therapeutic pathways for improving patient care in specific forms of psoriasis (Darvish et al., 2023; Alajroush et al., 2024) (Figure 7.4).

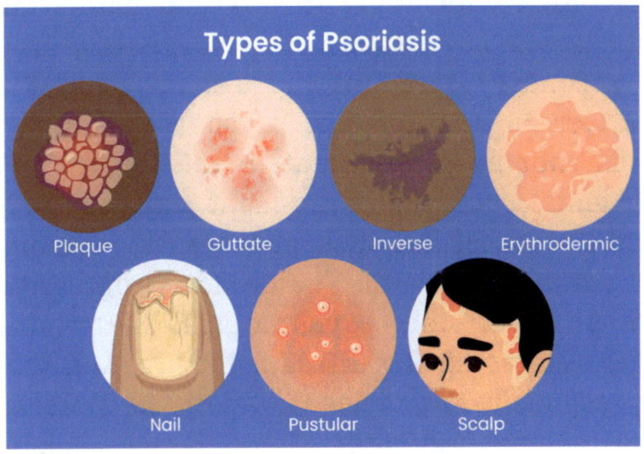

Figure 7.4. Types of psoriasis.

Source: https://images.ctfassets.net/yixw23k2v6vo/3V9ATGVPIQYuyuU0vCnCrN/95ffec0e9b899d706f1e9bfb7e19761c/GettyImages-2155294271-1306155463-872818970-psoriasis-types.jpg.

7.1.1. Plaque Psoriasis

Plaque psoriasis, the most common form of psoriasis, is characterized by well-defined, erythematous, scaling plaques that dominate on the extensor extremities and scalp. It is not a skin defect but a chronic inflammatory disease; it is an autoimmune condition with complex pathophysiology. The abnormal activation of the immune system leads to hyperproliferation of keratinocytes, resulting in thickened plaques characteristic of the disease. Furthermore, genetic susceptibility, environmental stimuli, and perturbations of the immune response significantly influence the development and occurrence of these conditions. Owing to the fact that chronic inflammation plays a central role in plaque psoriasis, understanding its immunopathogenesis is key to effective management and treatment, making ongoing research in this regard of vital significance. The disease has a significant impact on the quality of life of the patients, leading to physical discomfort, psychological distress, and social stigma. Plaque psoriasis is often associated with discomfort, including itching and pain from plaques. In severe cases, the disease may lead to secondary infections due to an impaired skin barrier. In addition, the psychosocial impact must not be overestimated; the majority of patients report embarrassment and poor self-esteem concerning their appearance, resulting in social withdrawal. The cyclical progression of physical and psychological symptoms necessitates having a treatment program that is responsive to the needs of both the material and nonmaterial costs of the disease, making more integrated models of care imperative. Research into the treatment of plaque psoriasis continues, with a focus on inflammatory disease mechanisms as targets for therapy. Traditional therapies include topical corticosteroids, phototherapy, and systemic therapies, but there is increasing interest in biologic drugs that target specific mediators of inflammation. More recent data have established the efficacy of interleukin inhibitors and other biologics in achieving important skin clearance and patient satisfaction. Similar to other papulosquamous diseases, the management of plaque psoriasis must be individualized to the patient, with consideration for their comorbid illnesses as well as any preconceptions or desires. Continued investigation into the pathogenesis of plaque psoriasis and the development of more specific therapies is promising for improved long-term outcomes and quality of life in patients, ushering in a new era in treatment development (Figure 7.5).

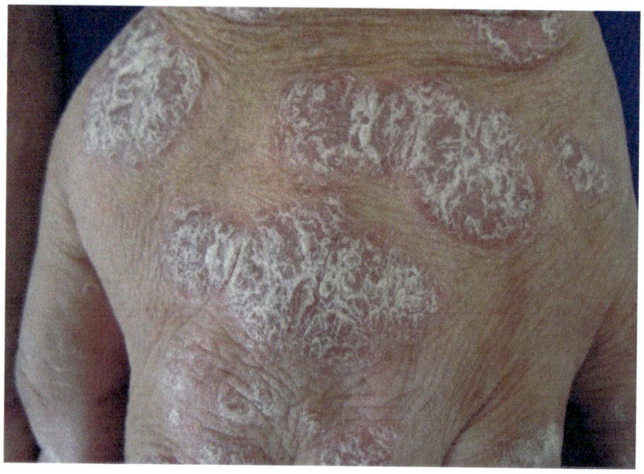

Figure 7.5. Plaque psoriasis.

Source: https://images.prismic.io/npf-website/6c538fed-39a1-40c0-94f0-1b33020eddb5_Plaque+Psoriasis+Hand.jpg.

7.1.2. Guttate Psoriasis

Guttate psoriasis is a clinical variant of psoriasis, with minuscule drop-shaped lesions with predominant distribution on the trunk and limbs. It follows streptococcal infection and thus presents as an unusual papulosquamous disease. The pathogenesis is thought to qualify as an autoimmune response to the etiologic infection, along with genetic predisposition, and thus this disorder is highly attractive to clinicians and researchers alike. Thus, the patient may experience sudden deterioration, greatly affecting quality of life. The visible nature of the lesions may be a source of worry, emphasizing the importance of appropriate treatment and diagnosis in reducing the disease burden. Guttate psoriasis is treated with a long-term strategy, often tailored to the patient's clinical presentation and lesion severity. Topical therapy, consisting of corticosteroids and vitamin D analogues, is typically employed for localized lesions, but more extensive disease can be treated with systemic therapy. Phototherapy, especially ultraviolet B light therapy, has also been found to be effective for symptom control and flare prevention. Given the risk of recurrent attacks following lower respiratory infections or stress, patient education is essential.

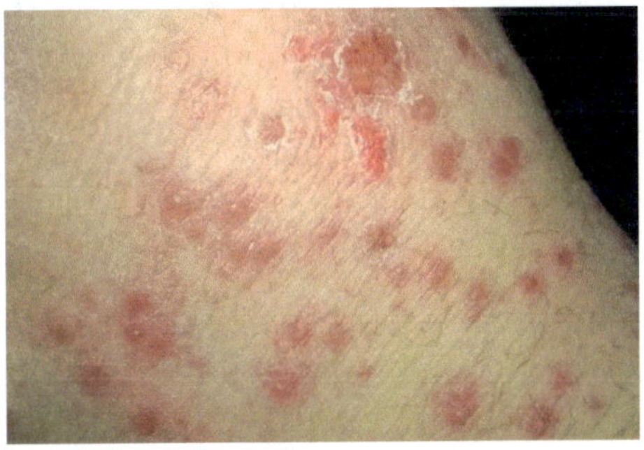

Figure 7.6. Guttate psoriasis.

Source: https://images.ctfassets.net/yixw23k2v6vo/6iW81gUFh8cVkeRqwLpqCe/fe58fd37ff2b523685cb44b0962c1993/05-guttate-psoriasis-PAMJ-17-273-g001.jpg?fm=webp&fit=thumb&q=65&w=824&h=549.

The patients must be aware of the relationship between streptococcal infection and exacerbation, and therefore it is necessary that health care professionals develop holistic management plans that include preventive and early therapeutic interventions. Additional research continues to further elucidate the pathophysiology of guttate psoriasis and its relation to other forms of psoriasis and papulosquamous disorders. As treated in recent literature, a systematic understanding of the general implications of guttate psoriasis, especially its relationship with infections, would enhance treatment models and patient outcomes. For instance, there is an urgent need for dermatology experts to be well-versed in recognizing the variations in skin diseases, as poor diagnostic agreement leads to delayed therapy and unfavorable outcomes (João Canedo et al., 2024). Furthermore, emerging research is identifying new therapeutic drugs and their long-term effects, emphasizing the necessity of ongoing education and training for medical practitioners treating psoriasis and its various forms, such as guttate psoriasis (Belmokhtar et al., 2024) (Figure 7.6).

7.1.3. Inverse Psoriasis

Inverse psoriasis is a form of psoriasis in which lesions typically occur in intertriginous regions, such as skin folds. This condition presents as smooth, red plaques that can be easily mistaken for other dermatoses, such as candidal infections or eczema, due to their location and appearance. Unlike the more common plaque-type psoriasis, inverse psoriasis does not include scaling, which is usually associated with the lesions of psoriasis, raising special diagnostic and treatment challenges. The inflammatory character of inverse psoriasis not only adds to the physical morbidity but also to the psychological distress of the patients, which is why it is essential to appreciate and treat this variant in the larger context of papulosquamous diseases properly. It is important to address the unique features of inverse psoriasis to improve patient outcomes and inform specific therapeutic interventions. Inverse psoriasis pathophysiology is identical to that of other forms of psoriasis, but has unique precipitating and worsening factors because of its location on the body. The condition can be provoked by moisture, sweating, and rubbing, suggesting the pivotal role of the skin's microenvironment in the production of the disease. The relationship between inverse psoriasis and systemic factors is complex; comorbidities such as obesity and metabolic syndrome typically coexist with this form, exacerbating cutaneous manifestations. Stress has also been thought to be a cause, perpetuating the cycles of flare-up and remission. Therefore, overall management should involve lifestyle changes, weight management, and stress reduction, as well as topical and systemic therapies to reduce inflammation and manage the disease effectively. Advances in the application of drugs in the management of inverse psoriasis have been encouraging but remain challenging to optimize in terms of getting the best patient outcomes. Traditional therapies, such as topical corticosteroids, have been widely used but are variable in their efficacy due to the delicate nature of the involved site. More recent treatment options, biologics and targeted therapies, potentially offer the advantage of targeting the cause of inflammation via a specific pathway without the side effects of conventional therapies. As in current studies, nanostructured lipid carriers (NLCs) have been noted to be a possible remedy to enhance drug delivery in the treatment of psoriasis with the benefits of improved penetrability in the skin and fewer side effects compared to regular ointments (Patil et al., 2023). This new approach emphasizes the necessity of ongoing research and inter-specialty communication within the medical community to optimize treatment regimens for inverse psoriasis, ultimately to enhance the quality of life of affected patients (Figure 7.7).

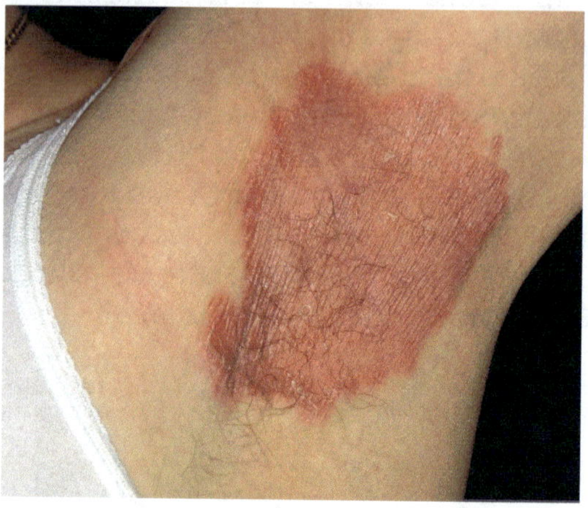

Figure 7.7. Inverse psoriasis.

Source: https://www.verywellhealth.com/thmb/Zo-lyR_rwkrqOsShpo_eIVHwD38=/1772x1464/filters:no_upscale():max_bytes(150000):strip_icc()/psorkai2-910d2d1a815244148012e1464001403c.jpg.

Test Your Knowledge

1. What is plaque psoriasis?
2. What is guttate psoriasis?

7.2. Symptoms and Diagnosis

Learning Outcome

1. Describe the common symptoms of psoriasis
2. Know the diagnostic procedures of psoriasis
3. Differentiate Psoriasis from Other Skin Conditions

The clinical presentation of psoriasis is most commonly described as a diverse range of signs, best characterized by the formation of papules and plaques on the skin's surface. The best-appearing skin lesions are silvery-white, scaly, and often seen on the elbows, knees, and scalp, with other sites, which corresponds to the condition's predilection for areas of trauma or friction. Moreover, patients with scalp psoriasis experience severe itching and irritation, which greatly affect their daily routines. As mentioned earlier, this characteristic presentation can result in diagnostic confusion with other skin conditions, such as seborrheic dermatitis, highlighting the need for precise diagnostic criteria. Worldwide awareness of the symptomatic spectrum is significant for establishing effective treatment plans, as the extent and severity of lesions may vary widely among patients and influence their overall quality of life (Bożena Podobińska, 2025). Diagnosing psoriasis requires acute clinical observation with the assistance of a detailed medical history, often incorporating the patient's self-reported symptoms and family history of dermatological disease. In children, the nuances in how these disorders present differently from those in adults are critical to grasp. This variation underscores the necessity of a separate diagnostic model that accommodates such variations, enabling timely and beneficial interventions. For example, one research on children with papulosquamous disorders identified the most common variant as psoriasis vulgaris, underscoring the importance of ascertaining its characteristic features to make a precise diagnosis. From the studied population, metabolic parameters were screened, and it was reported that while none of the children met the diagnosis criteria of metabolic syndrome, many of them reported abnormal serum levels, implying underlying pathological processes to be considered in the diagnosis process (Gurudev et al., 2023). Besides this, psychological effects of psoriasis and its manifestations cannot be overstated, particularly with the visibility and chronicity of the disease. Psychological distress is sometimes intensified by physical symptoms, leading to a vicious cycle of pain and anxiety for those affected. Accurate diagnosis not only involves identifying the physical manifestations but also the psychosocial determinants, enabling health professionals to deliver inclusive care. These patients, such as patients with scalp psoriasis, can feel embarrassed or have low self-esteem due to visible lesions and might, as a result, require holistic management strategies that address both their physical and psychological state. Successfully balancing this duality will optimize patient outcomes because proper diagnosis and treatment ultimately aim to alleviate symptoms and promote overall wellness, highlighting the importance of the interplay between symptom identification and efficient diagnosis in the management of psoriasis and papulosquamous dermatosis (Bożena Podobińska, 2025).

7.2.1. Common Symptoms of Psoriasis

Psoriasis has a clinical course comprising a range of symptoms that can significantly affect the quality of one's life. A characteristic sign of this papulosquamous condition is raised, red papules topped with silvery-white scales, typically appearing on the elbows, knees, scalp, and lower back. The lesions develop as a result of hyperproliferation of keratinocytes, often accompanied by inflammation, resulting in erythema. These presentation forms may vary in intensity, from minor types that may limit themselves to a few areas, to severe forms enveloping wide areas of the body. The notice should also be taken of the psychological effects of these external forms being entrenched as well, with the subjects typically exhibiting social withdrawal and reduced self-esteem, as was recorded in some research on dermatological disorders (Ramesan et al., 2025). Pruritus, or pruritic itching, is also a very common symptom of psoriasis and can worsen the condition. Itching in most patients is unrelenting and can lead to scratching, thereby aggravating skin lesions and increasing the risk of superinfection. Research has established a high correlation between the severity of itching and the psychological burden of patients, with findings indicating that patients suffering from intense itching experience high levels of anxiety and depression (Markevich et al., 2024). The symptom not only affects the physical status but can also disrupt routine activities and sleeping patterns, resulting in decreased quality of life. Thus, management of pruritus as part of psoriasis treatment becomes essential in maximizing dermatologic and, more significantly, psychological outcomes.

Aside from the primary signs of skin lesions and pruritus, patients may develop systemic manifestations that make treatment more difficult. Psoriasis is currently established as an immune-mediated disorder, in which patients may also manifest symptoms of arthritis, collectively referred to as psoriatic arthritis. This condition is associated with joint pain, swelling, and stiffness, causing mobility disability and affecting patients' functional status. Moreover, there is a high incidence of comorbid diseases such as cardiovascular disease and metabolic syndrome in patients with psoriasis, citing the nature of the condition as complex and multidimensional in its health impact (Ramesan et al., 2025). Thus, a combined treatment strategy that addresses both the cutaneous and extra-cutaneous psoriasis manifestations is needed to maximize patient care and overall quality of life (Figure 7.8).

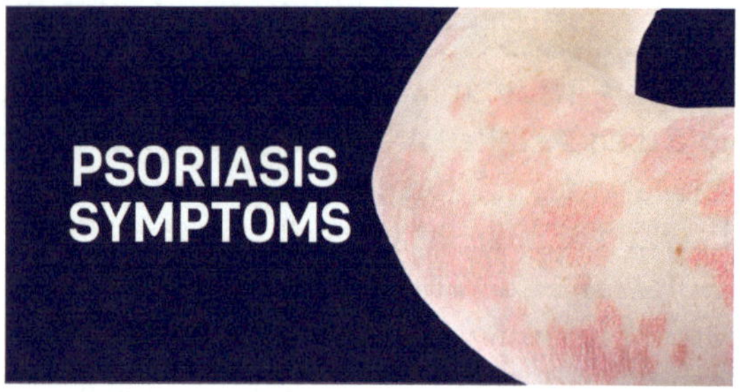

Figure 7.8. Symptoms of psoriasis.

Source: https://www.psoriasistreatmentbangalore.com/wp-content/uploads/2019/11/symptoms-of-Psoriasis.jpeg.

7.2.2. Diagnostic Procedures

Proper diagnosis is paramount for the treatment and management of psoriasis and other papulosquamous disorders. Clinical evaluation generally begins with the dermatologist analyzing skin lesions based on appearance, distribution, and associated symptoms. Since features that overlap among dermatological diseases may be present, clinical diagnosis may be inconclusive. In such situations, adjunct diagnostic tools become invaluable in fine-tuning and confirming the initial diagnosis. A case in point is dermoscopy (more onychoscopy), which provides high-resolution visualization of aberrant nails and can serve as an indicator of systemic psoriasis and other keratinization disorders. The use of this modality enables clinicians to visualize structural elements that the naked eye may miss and distinguish onychomycosis from psoriasis-related changes (Puri et al., 2024). The technique of onychoscopy has revolutionized the way that dermatologists approach nail disease, which in most instances is a portal to more extensive systemic diseases. Through systematic research of patients with various nail diseases, dermoscopy facilitated the detection of significant patterns specific to diseases such as psoriasis and onychomycosis. These features help dermatologists to make the right treatment decisions with a minimum of avoidable invasive procedures like biopsy, causing patient discomfort and psychological distress. For instance, some characteristic features observed under dermoscopy, e.g., onycholysis and notched margins, not only serve as diagnostic signs but also provide information about disease severity. With proper application of such methods, clinicians can enhance diagnostic precision, which leads to early treatment and improved patient outcomes (Puri et al., 2024). Except for a few such methods like onychoscopy, full diagnostic tests for psoriatic disease may vary from laboratory testing to imaging studies for comorbid evaluation. Evidence indicates that psoriatic patients are more intensively using health care services than other patients with mental illnesses, possibly because of the severity of their condition. One major study has found that patients with somatic symptoms and related disorders have greater healthcare expenditure and utilization prior to diagnosis, which follows the same pattern in psoriasis patients, where a delay in diagnosis results in more severe healthcare problems. Therefore, a multi-modal diagnostic strategy not only enables precise identification of psoriatic disorders but also underscores the importance of addressing underlying diseases that may complicate patient management. Utilizing different diagnostic modalities ensures that clinicians obtain a comprehensive picture of psoriasis and associated conditions (Figure 7.9).

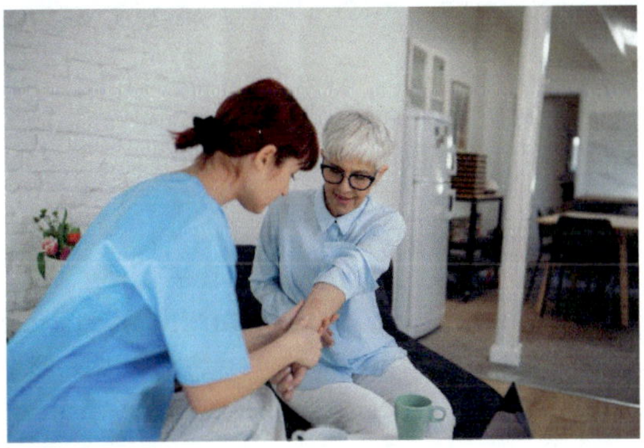

Figure 7.9. Diagnostic procedures for psoriasis.

Source: https://www.health.com/thmb/bYXlcBbF2ldt8XIVdEbjkDoejZ4=/1500x0/filters:no_upscale():max_bytes(150000):strip_icc()/psoriasis-diagnosis-GettyImages-1390339332-437734decaca4c8e8c4b23cceee7b5cf.jpg.

7.2.3. Differentiating Psoriasis from Other Skin Conditions

Psoriasis is distinguished from other papulosquamous diseases based on clear understanding of their pathophysiology and clinical presentations. Psoriasis is characterized primarily by erythematous plaques with overlying silvery-white scales, resulting from hyperproliferation of keratinocytes and migration of inflammatory cells. Hyperproliferation is secondary to a multifactorial process, including predisposing genetic factors and environmental stimulation. Other conditions such as seborrheic dermatitis or eczema have different scaling patterns and lesional distribution, which may influence the accuracy with which a diagnosis can be achieved. Thorough patient history, physical examination, and, occasionally, histological examination are crucial for distinguishing psoriasis from these differential diagnoses. For example, the absence of the typical silvery scale in eczema may prompt clinicians to consider an alternative diagnosis, given the more severe scaling in psoriasis. The immune system's involvement in psoriasis further complicates distinguishing it from other skin disorders.

Psoriasis has a very specific inflammatory profile, typically characterized by high levels of cytokines such as IL-17 and IL-23, which are key to its pathogenesis. These immunological alterations are responsible for the typical clinical manifestations of psoriasis, which usually culminate in well-demarcated plaque formation. In contrast, conditions like generalized pustular psoriasis (GPP) present with sterile pustules accompanied by systemic inflammatory signs, which may be confused with viral or bacterial infections due to overlapping findings. The clinical evaluation of the degree of disease in GPP is particularly challenging, as there are currently divergent diagnostic criteria that vary widely and may be disparate, making the exclusion of other inflammatory dermatoses challenging. Such an understanding of these immunologic differences is thus crucial for accurate diagnosis and effective treatment planning. In comparing the treatment of psoriasis with that of other dermatoses, the therapeutic distinctions underscore the importance of proper differentiation.

Psoriasis is typically managed with a combination of topical agents, phototherapy, and systemic medications targeting specific pathways involved in its pathogenesis, such as biologics that target key cytokines. The recent approval of the IL-36R antagonist spesolimab for GPP highlights the specificity of pustular psoriasis and the requirement for individually tailored treatments targeting the distinctive inflammatory pathways involved in its pathogenesis (Rivera-Díaz et al., 2023). Conversely, eczema and seborrheic dermatitis respond better to emollients and corticosteroids, highlighting the importance of correct diagnosis. The specificity of the therapy is an indicator of the clinical importance of misdiagnosis and underscores healthcare workers' responsibility to distinguish these complex skin diseases based on their varying features and pathogenetic mechanisms (Pondeljak et al., 2023).

Test Your Knowledge

1. What are symptoms of psoriasis?
2. What is the diagnostic procedure for psoriasis?

7.3. Causes and Risk Factors

Learning Outcome

1. Understand the genetic predisposition in psoriasis and other papulosquamous disorders
2. Describe the role of environmental factors in the exacerbation and triggering of psoriasis
3. Understand the role of the immune system in maintaining the body's homeostasis

An understanding of causes and risk factors in psoriasis and papulosquamous diseases requires consideration of both genetic and environmental factors. Research has shown that certain alleles are associated with a greater propensity to develop psoriasis. These genetic markers usually manifest as immune dysregulation that leads to keratinocyte proliferation and inflammation, typically seen in the condition. Environmental triggers, such as stress, infection, and skin injury, can also cause the illness to manifest in genetically susceptible persons. It is this intricate interaction that necessitates an integrated strategy for the research of the multi-factorial etiology of psoriasis, as understanding both genetic and environmental aspects will enable more targeted prevention and treatment strategies. In addition to genetic predisposition, lifestyle factors also contribute significantly to the development and exacerbation of psoriasis. For instance, obesity has been found to be an important risk factor; excessive body weight may lead to systemic inflammation, thus exacerbating the disease severity. Furthermore, cigarette smoking and alcohol consumption have also been implicated in increasing the risk of psoriasis. The inflammatory pathways induced by these lifestyle factors can further complicate the management of the disorder. Additionally, patients with psychological disorders, such as depression and anxiety, are susceptible to more aggressive psoriatic disease, which characterizes the interrelationship between psychological status and psoriatic disease. Hence, control of these lifestyle factors is essential in holistic prevention and management. Some chronic medical conditions also serve as significant risk factors for psoriasis and papulosquamous diseases, which must be taken into account in clinical settings. For instance, diseases like diabetes, cardiovascular conditions, and autoimmune disease are commonly co-morbid with psoriasis, creating a complex relationship that requires specific management. Recent research has shown an association between these diseases and more frequent psoriatic flare-ups, suggesting that the inflammatory processes underlying these conditions may contribute to psoriasis pathology. Furthermore, chronic inflammation underlying these comorbidities could exacerbate psoriasis manifestations. Thus, recognition and management of these interacting health conditions must be a key component of an integrated care plan for patients with psoriasis and papulosquamous disorders (Steinmann et al., 2024; Vlasova et al., 2024) (Figure 7.10).

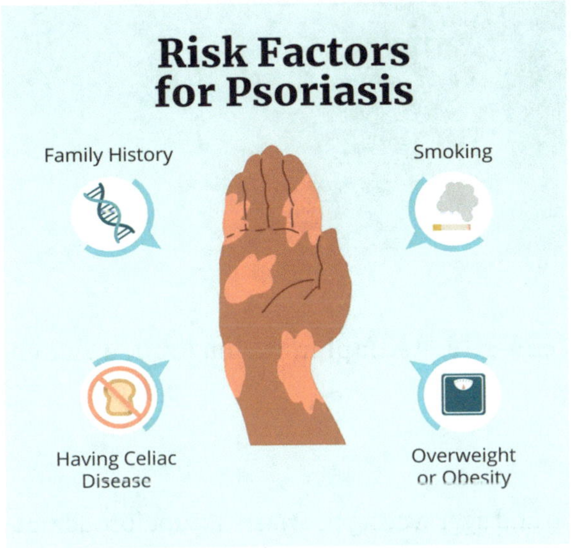

Figure 7.10. Risk factors for psoriasis.

Source: https://images.everydayhealth.com/images/seo-graphic-content-initiative/eh-risk-factors-for-psoriasis-seo-graphics.png?w=1110.

7.3.1. Genetic Predisposition

The concept of genetic predisposition lies at the heart of our understanding of psoriasis and other papulosquamous diseases. Recent research has elucidated the genetic mechanisms underlying psoriasis, indicating a multifactorial interplay between genetic and environmental factors. Importantly, the HLA-Cw6 antigen has been identified as a powerful genetic marker with an increased risk of getting psoriasis. The above connection underlines the significance of genetic testing and family history in the clinical assessment of high-risk patients. Besides, recent research on epigenetic variation, such as DNA methylation and histone modification, indicates that genetic predisposition materializes only under particular environmental conditions. Thus, a thorough understanding of genetic factors is essential in developing targeted interventions and maximizing patient benefits in treating psoriasis (Roszkiewicz et al., 2019). Beyond identifying genetic markers, researchers are increasingly interested in environmental factors that interact with genetic susceptibilities to cause psoriasis. Physical trauma, lifestyle, and infections are several factors that can increase the genetic susceptibility. For example, the Koebner phenomenon is a classic example of how skin trauma can cause psoriasis in patients with a genetic predisposition. It is critically important to educate patients on how to manage these environmental stimuli, as they significantly contribute to disease progression and exacerbation.

The intricate interplay between genetic susceptibility and the environment enables clinicians to create more individualized and effective treatment plans, ultimately improving the quality of life for those afflicted with psoriasis and its associated diseases (Roszkiewicz et al., 2019). Furthermore, the progress of psoriasis therapeutic management has been greatly influenced by what is understood about genetic predisposition. Biological therapies have emerged as a revolutionary class of agents, with high efficacy in immune-mediated conditions, such as psoriasis.

Despite this, these medications are not without side effects; paradoxical reactions, such as the development of psoriasis while on therapy, have been reported in those receiving these biologics. Evidence indicates that specific genetic backgrounds may influence the risk of such reactions, and genetic predisposition plays a crucial role in the induction of psoriasis and its response to treatment modalities. Therefore, the incorporation of genetic profiling into clinical practice would provide insight into one's risk for such reactions, enabling more appropriate decision-making within treatment strategies and general management plans for patients with psoriasis (Figure 7.11).

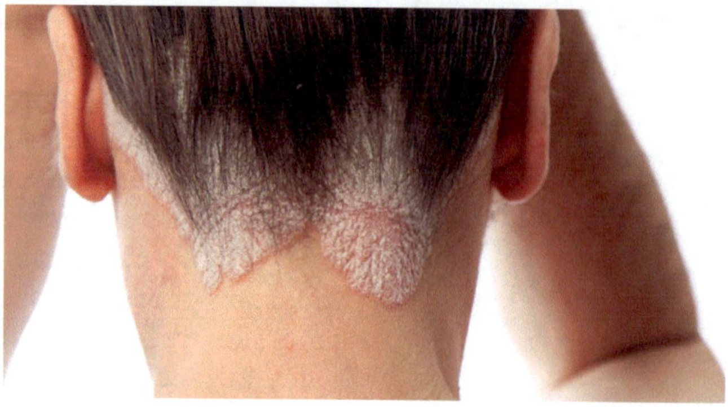

Figure 7.11. Genetic basis of psoriasis.

Source: https://s3.eu-north-1.amazonaws.com/cdn-site.mediaplanet.com/app/uploads/sites/112/2023/03/07220712/CDA-HEADERS.png.

7.3.2. Environmental Triggers

Environmental factors are critically involved in triggering and aggravating psoriasis, a papulosquamous disorder involving immune-mediated skin inflammation. Stress, for instance, is generally known to be an aggressive trigger for worsening of psoriasis. Emotional distress can initiate the release of pro-inflammatory mediators, which augment the underlying pathogenic mechanisms associated with the disease. Similarly, physical trauma to the skin, or Koebner phenomenon, is known to cause the onset of psoriatic lesions in vulnerable subjects. Environmental stimuli, therefore, not only initiate disease development but also cause chronicity by perpetuating a cycle of inflammation and lesion recurrence, and hence the necessity of controlling these extrinsic stimuli in the treatment of psoriasis. One fascinating interaction between environmental stimuli and psoriasis is that of the effect of infections, particularly viral. Hepatitis C, for example, was mentioned as a potential trigger for the concurrent presentation of autoimmune diseases such as bullous pemphigoid and psoriasis vulgaris in certain cases. Such concurrent presentation suggests that long-standing infections may trigger immune responses that unwittingly result in skin features characteristic of psoriatic conditions. Moreover, recent research has revealed the role of environmental determinants in regulating the immune response responsible for psoriasis by activating tissue-resident memory T cells (TRMs). The interaction of such immune cells with environmental determinants may lead to enhanced inflammatory responses, underscoring the need to understand these adaptive interactions when planning psoriasis management. Evidence suggests that molecular scarring, a consequence of the complex cross-talk between psoriatic keratinocytes and immune cells, can be augmented by environmental cues and, in turn, influence psoriasis disease relapse. Environmental cues may reactivate TRMs, leading to the production of inflammatory cytokines that cause the resurgence of psoriatic lesions. Moreover, evidence indicates that scarring patterns at the molecular level are not completely resolved even after successful therapy, indicating the need for therapies that take into account such residual actions. Therapies directly inhibiting TRM activation might significantly impact disease remission duration and lesion recurrence. Further research must elucidate the mechanisms by which environmental stimuli initiate and sustain these immune responses and enhance personalized treatment regimens for patients with psoriasis and other papulosquamous disorders (Figure 7.12).

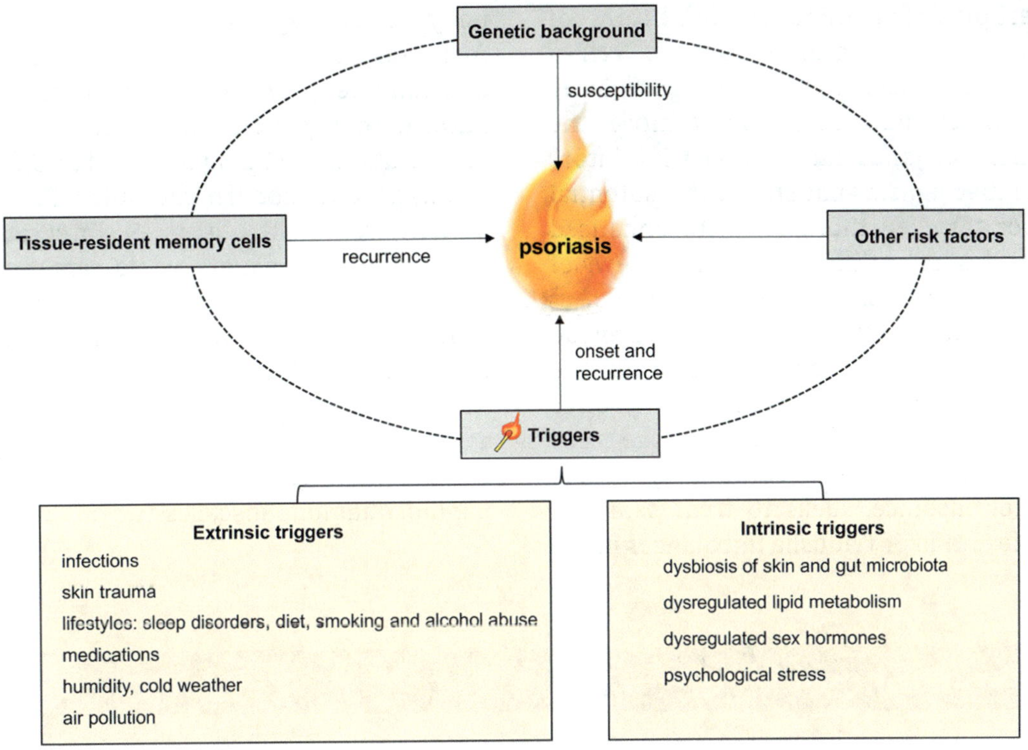

Figure 7.12. The extrinsic and intrinsic triggers for the onset and recurrence of psoriasis. Psoriasis can be induced by these triggers under a genetic predisposition. The recurrence of psoriasis also involves the role of tissue-resident memory cells.

Source: https://media.springernature.com/full/springer-static/image/art%3A10.1186%2Fs12964-023-01381-0/MediaObjects/12964_2023_1381_Fig1_HTML.png?as=webp.

7.3.3. Immune System Dysfunction

The immune system is a very important part of the body that helps maintain homeostasis, and its dysfunction can lead to a variety of pathological conditions, including psoriasis. Psoriasis is an abnormal immune reaction that manifests as overgrowth of skin cells and inflammation. It is not simply a product of external factors; rather, it is the result of a multifaceted interplay among immunological, environmental, and genetic factors. When the immune system becomes deregulated, particularly in T cells and cytokine production, inflammatory responses are amplified. This results in the development of the typical skin lesions of psoriasis, i.e., thickened scaly red lesions, which impair the quality of life of the patients by causing pain and emotional distress. Knowledge of these mechanisms underscores the need for targeted therapy that addresses immune dysfunction per se. In the last decade or so, the management of psoriasis has undergone a dramatic shift, with advancements in both traditional and modern medical interventions. The traditional treatment options broadly include topical corticosteroids and systemic immunosuppressants with the goal of managing the immune system and alleviating symptoms. These treatments carry inherent disadvantages, including side effects and the need for ongoing administration, which compromise patient compliance. More novel biologic agents, targeted at molecular mechanisms of immune dysregulation, are promising new therapies. For instance, inhibitors of pro-inflammatory cytokines such as TNF-α and IL-17 have been shown to significantly improve clinical outcomes. Furthermore, the development of Janus kinase (JAK) inhibitors is a novel mechanism that shows the potential for further targeted therapies with enhanced safety profiles, as outlined in recent reviews of autoimmune dermatologic conditions (Godse et al., 2024). While novel medical therapies provide immediate relief from psoriasis symptoms, the inclusion of integrative modalities may offer long-term benefits by addressing the root causes of immune dysregulation. Ayurvedic therapy, for instance, seeks to treat psoriasis as a manifestation of Tridosha imbalances in the body's energy system. Psoriasis treatments in Ayurvedic therapy are based on detoxification and immune system balance restoration through natural therapies, such as diet and lifestyle modifications. Blending these old traditions with sophisticated modern therapies can improve patient treatment outcomes. Integrative care theory advocates a more whole-person approach to treating psoriasis, not just for symptom relief but also for remission of immune system dysfunctions. These integrative interventions require ongoing clinical practice to achieve a more efficient and sustainable process for the management of psoriasis and other papulosquamous diseases (Goyal, 2025).

Test Your Knowledge

1. Which genetic marker has been strongly associated with an increased risk of psoriasis?
2. What type of immune cells are implicated in the inflammatory response exacerbated by environmental triggers in psoriasis?

7.4. Treatment Options

Learning Outcome

1. Describe the topical treatments of psoriasis
2. Understand the role of systemic medications in the management of psoriasis and other papulosquamous disorders
3. Describe the phototherapy for the management of psoriasis and other papulosquamous disorders

Effective treatments for psoriasis and papulosquamous disorders include a multi-modal therapy that includes topical medications, systemic drugs, and novel natural therapies. Topical medications, such as corticosteroids and vitamin D analogues, remain the first-line therapy for moderate disease. These medications work by reducing inflammation and slowing the rate of skin cell growth, a characteristic of psoriasis. Nonetheless, long-term corticosteroid administration is associated with skin thinning and other unwanted effects, which are concerns for both clinicians and patients. Natural products, including Rosa × damascena Mill., have been of interest due to their anti inflammatory properties, offering a different mechanism of action from conventional treatments and reducing some side effects. Thus, the resultant mix of these options would provide significant improvement in patient quality of life, particularly in cases that are resistant to traditional therapy (Gavra et al., 2024). With dermatology continuing to evolve, systemic therapies have been the standard of care for moderate-to-severe psoriasis. Biologic agents, by targeting selective immune mechanisms, have revolutionized treatment by targeting the abnormal immune dysregulation seen in psoriasis. These biologics, such as TNF-alpha inhibitors and IL-17 inhibitors, have been clinically efficacious and have improved patient outcomes. They also carry their own risks, including susceptibility to infection and the need for regular monitoring. These drugs have elevated the status of personalized medicine, enabling doctors to tailor treatments depending on the severity of an individual patient's condition and his overall profile. The challenge remains to balance efficacy, safety, and patient preference in choosing the most appropriate therapeutic regimen (Baboun et al., 2023). Alternative and complementary therapies are gaining popularity for the treatment of psoriasis, with most patients preferring natural therapies alongside conventional therapies. A number of natural foods and dietary interventions have shown promise in initial studies, suggesting potential for alleviating symptoms.

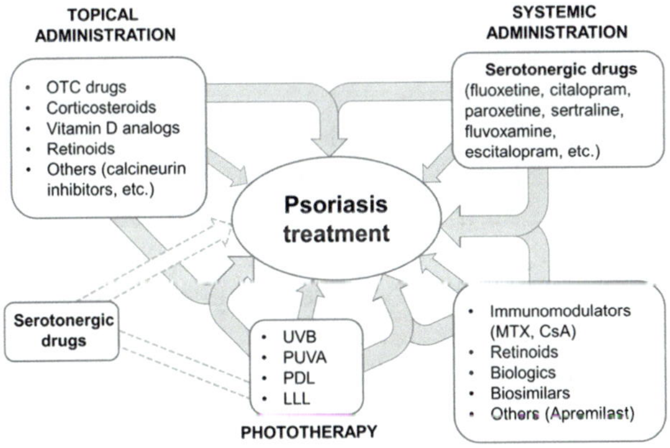

Figure 7.13. Psoriasis treatment.

Source: https://www.researchgate.net/publication/339294074/figure/fig1/AS:962718249013254@1606541325147/of-current-therapies-for-psoriasis-These-include-systemic-therapies-using-small.png.

For instance, local application of Rosa × damascena Mill. Extract has produced a reduction in psoriatic lesions in line with a reduction in the Psoriasis Area and Severity Index (PASI) and quality of life in patients. However, the lack of sufficient scientific evidence for most alternative therapies requires healthcare clinicians to approach them with caution. Clinicians must inform patients of such alternatives so they can distinguish between evidence-based treatment and hearsay. Using interactive dialogue, caregivers can guide patients through the complexities of therapeutic options, thereby enhancing the treatment process and facilitating safe management of psoriasis and associated disorders (Gavra et al., 2024) (Figure 7.13).

7.4.1. Topical Treatments

Management of psoriasis, a long-standing skin condition characterized by inflammatory plaques, typically includes topical therapies as first-line therapy. These treatments are effective due to their topical use, avoiding systemic absorption and side effects. Topical corticosteroids remain a staple in treatment, with anti-inflammatory action that leads to thinning of the plaque, erythema, and scaling. However, the possibility of long-term adverse effects, such as skin atrophy and tachyphylaxis, necessitates other topical options to be sought after. These alternatives involve vitamin D analogs, which have proven effective in controlling skin cell development and optimizing clinical outcomes. Also, the development of innovative drug delivery platforms, e.g., bioadhesive nanoparticles (BNPs), enhances the efficacy of such drugs by facilitating deeper penetration of therapeutic agents into the layers of the skin, thereby improving patient response in diseases such as psoriasis (Almuqbil et al., 2025). Increasingly, research encourages the use of natural alternatives in the treatment of psoriasis, preferring bioactive compounds with healing and anti-inflammatory properties. Plant-based compounds such as these have become such promising alternatives since patients would like to opt for safer therapeutic paths with fewer adverse effects compared to conventional synthetic drugs. Rosa × damascena Mill. is such a remarkable agent, a plant with a high content of bioactive constituents. Recent studies have demonstrated this plant's ability to alleviate psoriasis symptoms, as evidenced by reduced self-assessment scores on the Psoriasis Area and Severity Index (PASI) and the Dermatology Life Quality Index (DLQI). The rich phytochemical profile of Rosa × damascena Mill. justifies its application in external preparations, and evidence suggests that natural products can be employed as adjuvant therapy in the management of psoriatic disorders at large, complementing standard practices (Gavra et al., 2024). The use of state-of-the-art formulations and innovative delivery systems in topical psoriasis treatments reflects advances in dermatological therapeutics.

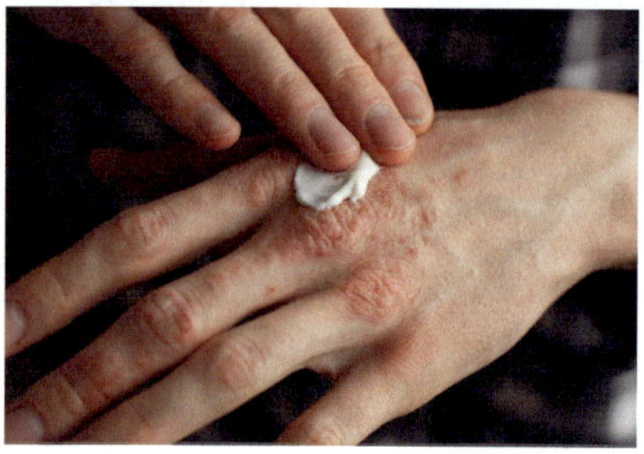

Figure 7.14. Topical treatments of psoriasis.

Source: https://plymouthmeetingdermatology.com/wp-content/uploads/2023/02/AdobeStock_132611271-1024x683.jpeg.

The use of bioadhesive nanoparticles (BNPs) not only enhances the bioavailability and potency of therapeutic agents but also facilitates patient compliance by improving the cosmetic acceptability and handlability of treatments. BNPs leverage their inherent characteristics, including extended skin residence and targeted delivery, to optimize therapeutic effects while reducing side effects. With further research exploring the interactions between these new delivery systems and conventional topical treatments, individualized treatment regimens tailored to a patient's needs are increasingly becoming a reality. This multidimensional approach represents a paradigm shift in the management of psoriasis and related disorders, with the potential to improve quality of life for patients with these chronic diseases (Almuqbil et al., 2025) (Figure 7.14).

7.4.2. Systemic Medications

Systemic medications play a crucial role in the management of psoriasis and other papulosquamous disorders, particularly in cases of resistance to topical management. These treatments act by modulating the immune response and targeting the pathophysiology of psoriasis, based on an abnormal immune response that leads to chronic inflammation and dysregulated skin cell turnover. Systemic drugs include the traditional immunosuppressants methotrexate and cyclosporine, as well as biologic targeted therapies targeting the inflammatory pathway. All of these medications have distinct profiles of benefits and drawbacks that clinicians need to consider carefully when developing a comprehensive treatment plan for patients. The efficacy of these systemic agents is established, but further study will further maximize their application, particularly in the setting of greater environmental influences that also complicate the clinical picture of psoriasis (Seirafianpour et al., 2020). Above all, the advent of biologic drugs has dramatically altered therapeutic strategies for managing moderate-to-severe psoriasis. Unlike traditional systemic medications, biologics are engineered to target specific components of the immune system, creating a more targeted approach to treatment. For instance, medications that inhibit tumor necrosis factor-alpha (TNF-alpha) or interleukin pathways have been particularly effective in reducing disease severity and improving patients' quality of life. Furthermore, these therapies have demonstrated a great safety profile, eluding most side effects of conventional systemic drugs. However, as with all immunomodulatory treatment, the emergence of infections, in particular during the COVID-19 period, merits close monitoring and possible adjustment of treatment plans according to the individual risk factors of patients and recent health status (Seirafianpour et al., 2020). With advancements in knowledge about psoriasis, the integration of systemic treatment into a holistic treatment plan also changes. Although efficacy naturally takes precedence, patient quality of life, patient compliance, and potential drug interactions are also factors to consider when making clinical choices. With the introduction of epigenetic determinants and environmental influences comes the exigency for personalization of treatment, which may include lifestyle modification in addition to pharmacotherapy. Health professionals are also tasked with educating patients about the importance of adherence to systemic drug treatment while concurrently promoting healthy lifestyle choices. This multi-faceted approach not only manages the physical characteristics of psoriasis but also empowers patients to take responsibility for their care and management, ultimately leading to better long-term outcomes and patient satisfaction with treatment (Roszkiewicz et al., 2019) (Figure 7.15).

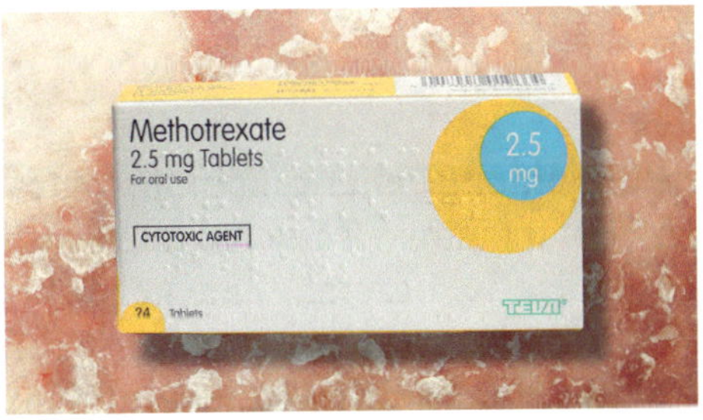

Figure 7.15. Systemic medications of psoriasis.

Source: https://assets.medpagetoday.net/media/images/97xxx/97943.jpg?width=0.8.

7.4.3. Phototherapy

Phototherapy is a significant therapeutic approach to the management of psoriasis and other papulosquamous diseases using light to induce biologic changes in the skin. Treatment is effected by ultraviolet (UV) light, using UVB and UVA, targeting inflamed skin and inhibiting the hyperplasia of keratinocytes evident in psoriasis. The mechanism of action involves downregulation of proinflammatory cytokines, namely those implicated in the Th17 immune response, which plays a central role in psoriasis pathology. By unmasking the immunological substrate underlying the psoriatic lesion, phototherapy can effectively reduce chronic inflammation and facilitate remission maintenance. As patients are prone to relapse after treatment, systemic application of phototherapy becomes absolutely essential for achieving long-term therapeutic response and minimizing the effect of molecular scarring, which otherwise will cause complex management of the disorder (Zhiltsova et al., 2025). In planning phototherapy, it goes without saying that some protocols and doses need to be standardized on a patient-by-patient basis to ensure maximum treatment efficacy. There is increasing evidence that a combination of phototherapy with newer biologic agents, including those targeting interleukins, like IL-17, will enhance clinical response. The mechanism by which phototherapy modulates immune cell function, particularly in the dermis, helps explain its effectiveness in managing residual lesions and psoriasis recurrences. Evidence indicates that phototherapy can induce changes in cutaneous tissue-resident memory T cells (TRMs), a key driver of chronic inflammation and reactivation of psoriatic skin lesions (Hatami et al., 2024). Not only does phototherapy treat short-term symptoms, but by increasing the treatment options against psoriasis, it also has the possible benefit of reducing the long-term possibility of relapse. With evolving knowledge in the management of psoriasis, phototherapy continues to be a significant contributor to the management of this multifactorial disease. Its established safety profile and ability to provide quick results make it highly appealing to patients, particularly those with systemic agent resistance. The ongoing investigations into new phototherapeutic methods, including narrowband UVB and targeted lasers, underscore the need for continued research in this area. Individualizing phototherapy treatment regimens for enhanced effectiveness with less side effects is crucial, to allow easier patient compliance and overall treatment success. By understanding more about the interaction of phototherapy with immune mechanisms, dxclinicians can better tailor complete treatment regimens that address sustained remission and improved quality of life in patients with psoriasis and papulosquamous disorders (Zhiltsova et al., 2025) (Figure 7.16).

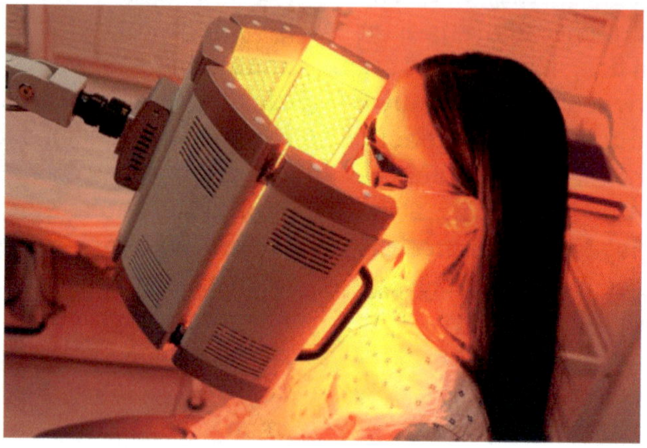

Figure 7.16. Phototherapy for psoriasis.

Source: https://metropolisdermatology.com/wp-content/uploads/2024/08/image1-1024x673.jpg.

Test Your Knowledge

1. Which is a traditional systemic medication used to manage psoriasis?
2. What type of light is primarily used in phototherapy for psoriasis?

7.5. Papulosquamous Disorders Overview

Learning Outcome

1. Understand the definition and characteristics of papulosquamous disorders
2. Describe the common types of papulosquamous disorders
3. Know the relationship between psoriasis and various papulosquamous disorders

Papulosquamous conditions are a category of skin diseases characterized by the development of papules and scales, often resulting from interactions among genetic, immunological, and environmental factors. They include conditions such as psoriasis, eczema, and lichen planus, each with characteristic features. Psoriasis, for example, is characterized by erythematous, elevated plaques with silvery scales, often localized to the elbows, knees, and scalp, and is associated with an overactive immune response and increased skin cell turnover. The pathogenesis of these disorders involves a deep examination of the interplay between genetic susceptibility and environmental exposures. The multifactorial pathogenesis of such conditions underscores the need for an individualized diagnostic and therapeutic approach that considers both endogenous and exogenous factors when establishing therapeutic interventions. Progress in ongoing studies has enhanced our understanding of the molecular pathomechanisms of papulosquamous diseases, particularly by identifying potential biomarkers and therapeutic targets. Studies on psoriasis have, for instance, identified the role of genes such as SIGLEC8, IL5RA, and CCR3 in immune control, making them potential candidates for diagnosis and treatment.

These findings are derived from weighted gene co-expression network analysis, which pinpoints the complex interactions among molecular pathways of the disease process. In addition, research on gene modules in psoriasis has indicated that some biological processes and pathways are profoundly altered in patients. Not only does this advance the understanding of the pathophysiology of disease, but it also enables the development of new therapies that can effectively target the underlying mechanisms rather than merely relieve symptoms (Darvish et al., 2023). The therapeutic practice for papulosquamous disorders continues to evolve to incorporate traditional treatment modalities and other practices, including herbal treatments. Recent literature demonstrates the potential anti-inflammatory benefits of herbs such as calendula and aloe vera in the management of conditions like eczema and psoriasis. The popularity of integrative therapies is indicative of a broader movement towards holistic patient care, with greater focus on individual responses to each intervention. However, the differential efficacy and safety of herbal therapy must be carefully considered and communicated to healthcare providers to avoid inappropriate use. By integrating established medical practice with complementary practices, patients can receive more personalized and effective treatment plans tailored to their specific cases, leading to improved outcomes in papulosquamous disorders (Chandy, 2023) (Figure 7.17).

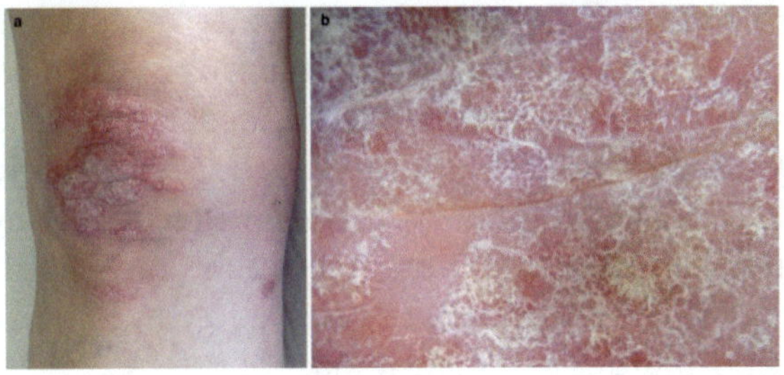

Figure 7.17. Common papulosquamous disorders.

Source: https://media.springernature.com/lw685/springer-static/image/chp%3A10.1007%2F978-3-031-19688-1_2/MediaObjects/517117_1_En_2_Fig1_HTML.png.

7.5.1. Definition and Characteristics

The origin of psoriasis, as a papulosquamous condition, is characterized by a chronic inflammatory process with high skin cell turnover. This results in the generation of lesions which are typified by red plaques covered with silvery scales, usually on extensor surfaces, scalp, and lower back. Psoriasis may present in various forms, viz., plaque, guttate, inverse, pustular, and erythrodermic, with varying characteristics. Among these, generalized pustular psoriasis (GPP) is a dangerous subtype that needs to be approached seriously due to its life-threatening nature and systemic inflammation, necessitating hospitalization and complex treatment modalities (Chen et al., 2025). The variability in the presentation of psoriasis therefore provides a reason for stringent definitions and classification, so that it may be properly handled and therapeutic management offered. Psoriasis's characteristics extend beyond its visible skin eruptions to include a range of systemic symptoms and comorbidities. Symptoms, including itching, pain, and a significant reduction in quality of life, are prevalent among patients (Tang et al., 2025). Psoriasis has also been linked with other clinical conditions like psoriatic arthritis, metabolic syndrome, and cardiovascular diseases, which increase the degree of complexity entailed in patient care. Across varied pediatric populations, pustular psoriasis is often associated with systemic manifestations such as fever and elevated inflammatory markers, necessitating an integrative treatment approach (Tang et al., 2025). The clinician must also determine these comorbidities and their impact on overall health to guide integrated treatment regimens involving both systemic and dermatological manifestations of the disease. Furthermore, treatment regimens for psoriasis reflect an understanding of its multi-factorial nature. Topical corticosteroids and systemic immunosuppressants have been the mainstay of traditional therapies, but since the advent of biologics, treatment paradigms have changed, especially in severe conditions like GPP (Chen et al., 2025).

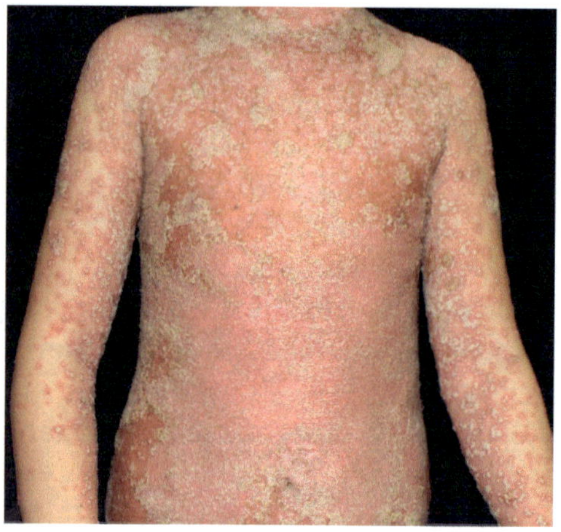

Figure 7.18. The clinical presentation of generalized pustular psoriasis.

Source: https://www.researchgate.net/publication/374057142/figure/fig1/AS:11431281190226768@1695257052978/The-clinical-presentation-of-generalized-pustular-psoriasis.jpg.

The use of inpatient teledermatology has emerged as a valuable tool, optimizing care delivery in settings with limited dermatologic expertise. Secondarily, characterization of treatment response, as seen in studies of acitretin and combination therapies in children with pustular psoriasis, emphasizes tailoring treatment by phenotype and patient population (Tang et al., 2025). Lastly, an educated, patient-centered approach to treatment is indispensable for managing the complexity of psoriasis and its multifaceted presentations in papulosquamous disease (Figure 7.18).

7.5.2. Common Types of Papulosquamous Disorders

Papulosquamous disorders are a leading category of skin conditions characterized by characteristic lesions, predominantly erythematous papules capped with variable amounts of scaling. Some of the most common ones are psoriasis, lichen planus, and pityriasis rosea. Psoriasis is characterized by discrete plaques covered with silvery scales due to increased keratinocyte proliferation. Lichen planus, on the other hand, is characterized by flat-topped, purple papules that are typically smooth in appearance and very pruritic. Pityriasis rosea typically starts with a herald patch and a pattern of smaller lesions clearing spontaneously over weeks to months. The overlap in clinical presentations requires accurate differentiation, as misdiagnosis will lead to inappropriate management plans; hence, a thorough understanding of such disorders is essential to facilitate correct treatment and patient care (Errichetti et al., 2016). Seborrheic dermatitis is also a common papulosquamous condition that favors sites rich in sebaceous glands, such as the face and scalp. It presents as oily-looking red plaques with yellowish-white scales. Contrary to psoriasis, seborrheic dermatitis tends to be scaly plaques rather than the bordered form of psoriasis. It is chronic in character and is liable to flare with stress and hormonal upset, so it is harder to manage. Similarly, pityriasis rubra pilaris (PRP) is a rare type characterized by orange-red plaques with a typical distribution, with the scalp, elbows, and knees involved. All these diseases, though sharing the features of erythema and scaling, possess specific morphological features that need to be assessed clinically to ascertain the true diagnosis and treatment (Errichetti et al., 2016). Parapsoriasis is also a crucial entity involved in papulosquamous diseases. It consists classically of patches of psoriasis without the plaques seen in psoriasis, which can lead to confusion in clinical diagnosis. Clinicians need to recognize these types separately so that they do not perform unjustifiable treatment for what may be mere imitation of classical psoriasis. Drug eruptions and secondary infections like tinea corporis can exhibit differing papulosquamous morphology and thus, on top of mimicking classic psoriasis, diagnosis is further complicated. With the above in consideration, a multidisciplinary approach encompassing clinical evaluation and perhaps histopathology is essential for making a correct diagnosis and management plan. In practice, understanding the subtle differences among papulosquamous disorders is crucial for effective treatment and improved patient satisfaction (Narayankar et al., 2017) (Figure 7.19).

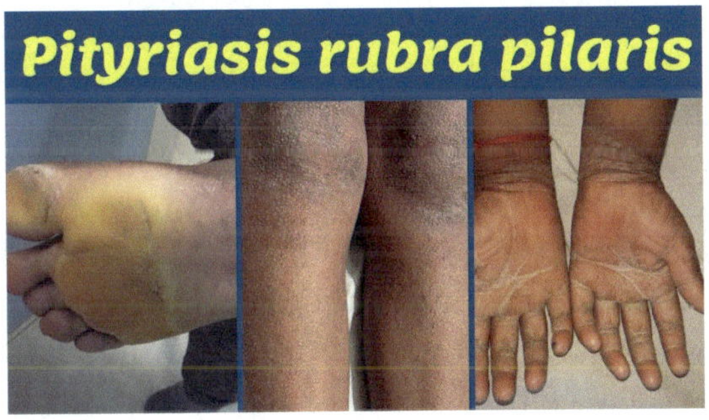

Figure 7.19. Pityriasis rubra pilaris.

Source: https://i.ytimg.com/vi/-112c8iiGhQ/maxresdefault.jpg.

7.5.3. Relationship to Psoriasis

The association between psoriasis and other papulosquamous disorders has significant implications for the complex interplay between immunological and genetic factors in skin pathology. Psoriasis manifests as a chronic inflammatory condition with predominantly hyperproliferative keratinocytes and marked immune cell infiltrate, particularly T cells and dendritic cells. It offers a unique biological environment that sheds light on the pathogenesis of psoriasis and related disorders, suggesting that common mechanisms are accountable for their pathogenesis. The effort highlights the disruption of immune responses in the skin, as seen in conditions such as psoriatic arthritis and other papulosquamous disorders. Thus, the study of these comorbid disorders provides valuable insights into psoriasis treatment, suggesting the need to target inflammatory pathways to improve symptom relief and outcomes for patients (Joosten et al., 2022). Furthermore, advances in the pathogenesis of ichthyosis, a disease characterized by a spectrum of skin disorders of keratinization, underscore therapeutic potential in psoriasis and related diseases. Recent developments in gene therapy and protein replacement therapy offer the prospect of a paradigm shift in the management of inherited skin disorders, with implications extending beyond immune-mediated diseases such as psoriasis. Effective treatments for ichthyosis involving biological therapeutics are of potential benefit to individuals afflicted with these specific genetic disorders and those with psoriasis as well. The ongoing search for new therapeutic methods, especially those based on the pathogenic principles shared by these disorders, underscores the importance of an integrative treatment plan that harnesses advances in dermatology research to improve psoriasis control (Joosten et al., 2022). In exploring the roles of newly identified immune mediators, it is evident that psoriasis pathology necessitates a complex understanding of its pathogenic mechanisms. Central actors such as antimicrobial peptides, interleukins, and tissue-resident memory T cells are now central to disease pathogenesis. Evidence proposes that T-cell dysregulation—and the unique functional roles of such immune cells—may be important in chronic inflammation in psoriasis. As studies continue to elucidate the pathogenetic role of such immune constituents, it becomes increasingly clear that targeted therapy, specifically against the IL-23/IL-17 axis, can transform treatment strategies for psoriasis and other papulosquamous disorders. It is crucial to integrate such information into therapeutic strategies to optimize patient care and advance the field of dermatology (Brănişteanu et al., 2022).

Test Your Knowledge

1. Which form of psoriasis is considered life-threatening and often requires hospitalization?
2. Which disorder is marked by a "herald patch" followed by smaller lesions?

7.6. Impact on Quality of Life

Learning Outcome

1. Describe the physical effects of psoriasis
2. Know the psychological effects of psoriasis and other papulosquamous disorders
3. Understand the social implications of psoriasis and papulosquamous disorders

Psoriasis and other papulosquamous diseases are prevalent conditions and also have a direct impact on the overall quality of life of the affected patients, both physically and mentally. It subjects patients to a range of symptoms, including pain, itching, and discomfort, which ultimately impair their day-to-day activities. Research indicates that the symptoms not only compromise physical functioning but also result in social isolation and emotional distress. Psoriasis and other disorders have been linked with various comorbidities such as depression and anxiety, further contributing to their negative effect on quality of life. Additionally, the fact that it presents itself in the form of skin lesions makes it vulnerable to stigmatization, which leads to low self-esteem and isolation. Understanding the multifaceted consequences of such diseases, medical professionals can address patients' more holistic needs and implement targeted interventions to improve their quality of life. Psychosocial concerns are of the highest priority in the quality of life of psoriasis and other papulosquamous disease sufferers. Helplessness and frustration feelings are often stated by patients due to the chronic nature of these diseases and the consequent vicious circle of emotional suffering. Research has found that the long-term inflammation of such disorders has the ability not only to affect skin health but also to induce psychological states such as depression and anxiety. For instance, patients may struggle to maintain social relationships or engage in activities they previously enjoyed due to fears of being judged or exacerbating symptoms. This negative effect is most pronounced in oral health-related quality of life (OHRQoL) in disorders that occur concomitantly with compound health states. Management of the psychiatric aspect is instrumental in achieving total control of psoriasis and can have a significant impact on the overall patient's quality of life. Therapies to improve quality of life in patients with psoriasis need to adopt a multi-dimensional approach that combines both medical management and psychiatric support. Evidence has shown that well-managed psoriasis via dermatological care can relieve physical symptoms, thereby improving the overall well-being of patients. Incorporation of a mental health component, such as counseling and support groups, also improves the effectiveness of management by giving patients coping mechanisms as well as a sense of belongingness. Lifestyle modifications, such as coping with stress and optimal skin care routines, also have a significant impact on patients' experiences. Evaluating quality of life outcomes, like monitoring health-related quality of life following ICU discharge in patients with COVID-19, emphasizes that physical and mental aspects of health are to be treated in long-term diseases like psoriasis (Deana et al., 2023; Liberton et al., 2024). So, an integrated treatment plan can lead to significant improvement in the quality of life among patients with papulosquamous disorders.

7.6.1. Physical Effects

The physical symptoms of psoriasis extend beyond surface-level expression, with widespread effects on the individual's overall quality of life. The condition is characterized by inflammatory lesions that typically present as red, scaly patches on the skin, often appearing on the elbows, knees, scalp, and lower back. These plaques can turn into a vicious cycle of distress because the physical discomfort involved in psoriasis has a tendency to exacerbate the psychological problems of the patients. Studies have established that psoriasis patients usually experience burning and itching, which can lead to issues in day-to-day functioning and severe disturbances in sleep patterns. This somatic unease is further augmented by other systemic effects, showing that psoriasis also presents as both an aggravation of physical health and an issue that challenges the overall well-being of the sufferer. Further, the effects of psoriasis are actualized in affected populations, particularly children, with the physical effects influencing growth and development. Childhood psoriasis has been correlated with increased psychosocial dysfunction, putting them at risk for emotional disturbance in the form of depression and anxiety. Psoriatic children have been reported to exhibit higher rates of suicidal thoughts as well as addiction tendencies due to the fact that their disease is visible and, in many cases, stigmatizing. The weight of coping with physical signs leads to a sense of isolation and vulnerability, making the emotional setting in which affected children live challenging (Shah et al., 2024). From this, it is necessary to recognize the full spectrum of physical effects associated with psoriasis in children to develop appropriate management strategies for both the perceived symptoms and their psychosocial consequences. The physical signs of psoriasis may also be gender-specific, depending on hormonal changes at various stages of life. The history of women with psoriasis and psoriatic arthritis is significantly influenced by hormonal changes occurring in menstruation, pregnancy, postpartum, and menopause. Estrogen, among other hormones, has been shown to affect immune mechanisms and can modulate the severity of the disease, thus making how women cope with physical symptoms unique. Lesions of the skin tend to lead to psychosocial challenges, since outside circumstances affect self-esteem, interpersonal relationships, and even fertility planning in women. Such gender-related data emphasizes the need for a tailored approach in treatment procedures that address body treatments with mental support, highlighting the need for an in-depth understanding of the way body manifestation of psoriasis specifically affects women (Cassalia et al., 2024) (Figure 7.20).

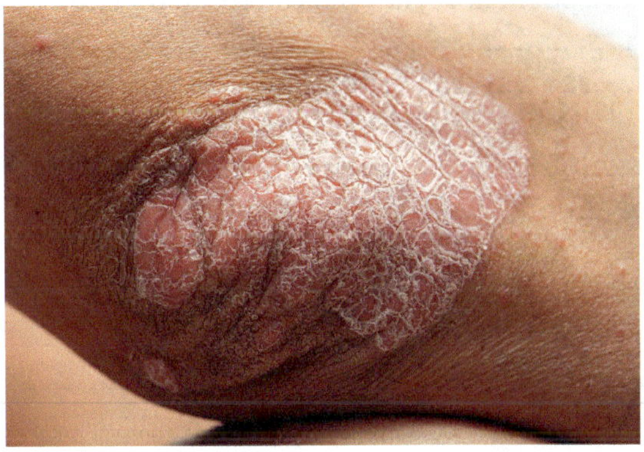

Figure 7.20. Physical effects of psoriasis.

Source: https://images.ctfassets.net/yixw23k2v6vo/4rW7E95KIGB22krxefHZNw/3db983f3cfa455811f4bdfea39e9b6e2/large-GettyImages-1409632955-3000x2000.jpg.

7.6.2. Psychological Effects

The psychological effects of psoriasis and other papulosquamous conditions extend far beyond the condition's physical appearance. Patients frequently remark on a diminished quality of life because of the visibility of skin lesions, and this produces extreme anxiety and depression. Psoriasis diagnosis generates loss, inasmuch as individuals grapple with the shame and stigma of visible disease on the skin and associated social isolation. It has been established that the greater the severity and perceived impact on daily social interactions, the greater the resultant level of psychological distress. The psychological effect of the disease—stemming from both body manifestations and social perceptions—indicates the necessity of mental health contributions in treatment protocols for patients who are experiencing such conditions (Isdianto et al., 2025). The relationship between psoriasis and mental diseases, like depression and anxiety, becomes more important with the consideration of chronic stress. Psychological stress not only aggravates symptoms of the skin but may also play a role in the deterioration of mental health disorders in those afflicted. Studies have shown that the distress generated by psoriasis potentially creates a vicious cycle, where poor skin symptoms increase psychological stress, and this exacerbates the condition. This two-way interaction makes one realize the importance of recognizing the bidirectional interdependence between physical disease and mental well-being. It is thus prudent to tackle mental health needs to effectively handle patients, as unchecked psychological conditions can be deleterious to treatment adherence and disease control in general (Isdianto et al., 2025). To properly reverse the psychological impact of psoriasis, an integrated model of care that includes dermatology and psychology is called for. Interventions such as Cognitive Behavioral Therapy (CBT) and support groups are available to avoid body image issues and overcome social stigma. Yet the use of these interventions in day-to-day practice remains limited, indicating a gap in comprehensive patient care. Interestingly, studies highlight the crucial function played by mental health interventions in enhancing the quality of life in psoriasis patients. There is a pressing need for further research to explore comprehensive care models that capture both the physical and psychological aspects of living with psoriasis, thereby promoting general well-being (Figure 7.21).

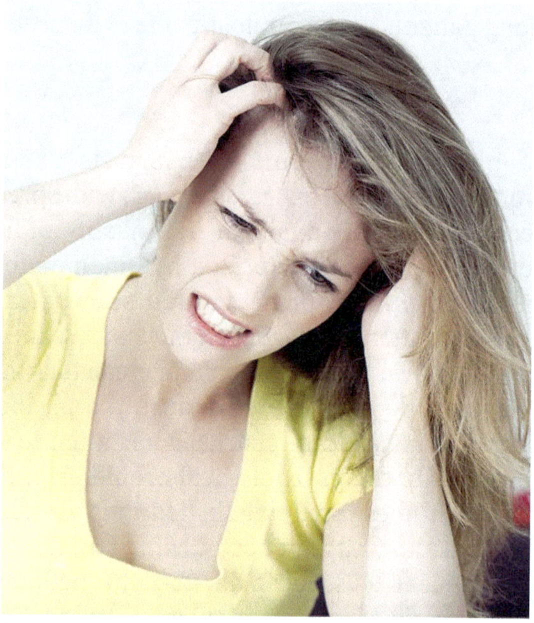

Figure 7.21. Psychological effects of scalp psoriasis.

Source: https://cdn2.stylecraze.com/wp-content/uploads/2013/11/15-Best-Home-Remedies-To-Get-Rid-Of-Scalp-Psoriasis-Effectively-1.jpg.webp.

7.6.3. Social Implications

The social implications of psoriasis and papulosquamous disorders extend far beyond their physical manifestations. The affected individuals usually experience significant psychosocial distress due to the high visibility of their skin conditions, becoming withdrawn, stigmatized, and experiencing a lower quality of life. For adolescents in particular, the struggle against skin conditions might coincide with years of peak growth, so they feel vulnerable and low in self-esteem. One study that highlighted the prevalence of skin conditions among adolescents found that almost three-quarters reported adverse impacts on the quality of their lives related to their skin issues (Oyedepo et al., 2023). This illustrates how cultural perceptions of beauty and normality can significantly affect the emotional well-being of individuals and carry long-term psychological implications that extend into adulthood. Besides, there is no downplaying the impact of these disorders on social relations. On some occasions, victims of psoriasis and other related disorders become victims of discrimination, either in society, schools, or at work. The appearance-driven aspect of such disorders has a tendency to elicit excessive scrutiny from people and looks that may discourage individuals from pursuing social relationships or even career development. The far-reaching dermatological effect on self-concept can contribute to social anxiety, particularly in young adults, since they have body-focused thoughts. According to research, skin illness can significantly lower overall well-being, reinforcing the fact that societal attitudes toward visible illnesses significantly affect the lives of victims (Oyedepo et al., 2023). This leads to a cycle of social exclusion, further making the management and treatment of these disorders more challenging. Treatment options also have social consequences, as individuals might have to face disclosure of their condition, particularly when undergoing therapies that reduce their overt symptoms or require lifestyle changes. For instance, the use of biologic therapies in conditions like Psoriasis has been shown to achieve clinical remission in cases that are resistant, linking physical health to social reintegration. However, the persistent need for treatment, together with its side effects, can lead to economic burden and social implications, with the affected person being pushed into having to prioritize healthcare against other personal or social interests. Understanding these dynamics is crucial not only to healthcare providers but to society as a whole, as reducing stigma and the provision of supportive environments will go a long way toward improving the quality of life for papulosquamous disorder sufferers.

Test Your Knowledge

1. Which areas of the body are commonly affected by psoriatic plaques?
2. How do psoriasis and papulosquamous disorders affect adolescents?

SUMMARY

In conclusion, it is important to to best understand psoriasis and related papulosquamous disorders to ensure optimal treatment of these advanced skin diseases. Psoriasis's multigenic and multifactorial pattern of disease, with both genetic background and environment playing roles, requires a comprehensive treatment approach. Recent advances in immunology have revealed the intricate pathogenesis of psoriasis. Of special interest, the roles of some immune cells and pathways identify targets for new therapies. More research on these mechanisms is needed since it forms the foundation for more precise and effective therapies, thereby improving patient outcomes and quality of life. In addition, emerging therapies based on pathophysiological understanding, such as those targeting T cells and cytokine interference, have the potential to revolutionize the treatment of psoriasis. The recent discovery of antimicrobial peptides (AMPs) and their relevance to the disease map is a great breakthrough. There has been success in disorders such as Netherton syndrome and congenital ichthyosis due to improvements in biological therapeutics, and this is anticipated to continue with psoriasis, where new advancements will continue to unfold (Joosten et al., 2022). Maintaining the pace of clinical trials will expand drug options and enable personalized medicine initiatives. As the field evolves, synergistic integration of new therapeutic modalities and traditional approaches is vital. The present study, which compares the effectiveness of new immunotherapies, indicates the evolving character of psoriasis treatment. Building on knowledge of immune cell behavior, such as that of TRMs, in relation to skin tissue provides a more accurate picture of disease pathogenesis (Brănişteanu et al., 2022). By committing to interdisciplinary collaboration among patients, clinicians, and researchers, the medical profession can enhance outcomes and foster a better understanding of psoriatic disease, thereby improving treatment settings and reducing the burden on those suffering.

The complexity of psoriasis and papulosquamous diseases reveals a knotty landscape of interdependent disease states. Psoriasis, given its chronic inflammatory state and systemic disease, encompasses a wide range of comorbidities, including metabolic syndrome, cardiovascular complications, and diabetes mellitus. Inflammation intrinsic to psoriasis not only affects the skin but also systemic health, suggesting the need for an integrative therapy approach. Psoriatic disease's interconnectedness with metabolic derangement makes surveillance of associated risks even more pertinent, thereby enabling healthcare professionals to provide more integrated care. Increased cardiovascular risks associated with psoriasis require a cautious approach to patient counselling and lifestyle modification as these factors can play significant roles in the overall disease outcome. In the treatment of psoriasis, significant advances have been achieved over the last few years to enhance therapeutic efficacy and patient outcomes. Agents such as statins and fibrates, traditionally used for lipid disorder management, have been shown to mitigate some of the systemic manifestations of psoriasis. The pleiotropic effects of statins, including their anti-inflammatory, antioxidant, and antiproliferative properties, represent a dual benefit: managing psoriasis and addressing cardiovascular threats. More recently developed medications, such as pioglitazone and GLP-1 receptor agonists, are also promising; not only do these drugs improve lipid profiles, but they also enable better metabolic control in patients with psoriasis (Sadeghi et al., 2023). These medications highlight the need for individualized treatment based on patients' individual health profiles and the incorporation of diverse therapies to address not just psoriasis but the plethora of comorbid conditions that accompany it. Further, the effects of autoimmune diseases during the COVID-19 pandemic revealed persistent knowledge gaps regarding how autoimmune diseases affect vulnerable groups. Despite children with autoimmune diseases, like psoriasis, being part of the high-risk groups during the pandemic, their relatively low occurrence in research has raised many questions regarding their particular health outcomes (Sadeghi et al., 2023). This lack of directed research underscores the imperative to continue investigating how treatment and autoimmune diseases can influence the course of viral diseases, such as COVID-19. Through efforts to fill these knowledge gaps and render findings relevant through clinical application, the medical field as a whole can better prepare to meet the challenges posed by the complexities of both underlying autoimmune disease and intermittent infection, ultimately delivering improved care to affected communities.

KEY TERMS FROM THIS CHAPTER

- Candida infections
- Environmental triggers
- Follicular psoriasis
- Guttate psoriasis
- Immune response
- Papulosquamous disorders
- Protein
- Cytokine balance
- Erythrodermic psoriasis
- Genetic predispositions
- Immune dysregulation
- Inverse psoriasis
- Plaque psoriasis
- Psoriasis

CRITICAL THINKING QUESTIONS

1. **Which of the following is the most common type of psoriasis?**
   a. Guttate psoriasis
   b. Plaque psoriasis
   c. Pustular psoriasis
   d. Erythrodermic psoriasis
2. **What is the Koebner phenomenon in psoriasis?**
   a. Scaling of the scalp
   b. Lesions triggered by trauma to the skin
   c. Appearance of pustules on the palms and soles
   d. Nail pitting associated with psoriasis
3. **Which papulosquamous disorder is strongly associated with the herald patch?**
   a. Psoriasis
   b. Pityriasis rosea
   c. Lichen planus
   d. Seborrheic dermatitis
4. **Which of the following is a hallmark histopathological feature of psoriasis?**
   a. Acanthosis and parakeratosis
   b. Basal cell hyperplasia
   c. Subepidermal blistering
   d. Hypergranulosis and interface dermatitis
5. **Nail involvement in psoriasis is often characterized by:**
   a. Yellow discoloration
   b. Beau's lines
   c. Pitting, onycholysis, and oil spots
   d. Thickened, brittle nails

Short Answer Questions

1. Define psoriasis.
2. What is a papulosquamous disorder?
3. List the types of psoriasis.
4. Which environmental triggers are known to exacerbate psoriasis?
5. What treatment options are available for psoriasis?

Answer to Critical Thinking Questions

1. (b); 2. (b) ; 3. (b); 4. (a); 5. (c)

REFERENCES

1. Alajroush, W. A., Alrshid, A. I., Alajlan, A. H., Alsalamah, Y. B., Alhumaidan, M. I., Alhoumedan, A. I., Alrasheed, M. I., Alowairdhi, Y. A., Alowirdi, F., Aljoufi, A. Z., Alsubaie, D. S., & Alarfaj, N. H. (2024). Psoriasis and Metabolic Disorders: A Comprehensive Meta-Analysis of Million Adults worldwide. *Cureus, 16*(1), e52099. https://doi.org/10.7759/cureus.52099Almuqbil, R. M., & Aldhubiab, B. E. (2025). Bio adhesive nanoparticles in topical drug delivery: Advances, applications, and potential for skin disorder treatments. *Pharmaceutics, 17*. https://www.semanticscholar.org/paper/8752b5eccf0b2cc9e3c31c05525832bae5b22201 (accessed on 21st July 2025).
2. Baboun, D., Yaghi, M., Keri, J., & Morrison, B. W. (2023). Natural treatment options for nail disorders. *Skin Appendage Disorders, 10*, 83–91. https://www.semanticscholar.org/paper/81924652fe4620bb694e3cdd491e3beb3eef159e (accessed on 21st July 2025).
3. Belmokhtar, Z., Djaroud, S., Matmour, D., & Merad, Y. (2024). Atypical and unpredictable superficial mycosis presentations: A narrative review. *Journal of Fungi, 10*, 295–295. https://doi.org/10.3390/jof10040295 (accessed on 21st July 2025).
4. Blicharz, L., Czuwara, J., Rudnicka, L., & Torrelo, A. (2023). Autoinflammatory keratinization diseases—The concept, pathophysiology, and clinical implications. *Clinical Reviews in Allergy & Immunology, 65*, 377–402. https://doi.org/10.1007/s12016-023-08971-3 (accessed on 21st July 2025).
5. Boch, K., Langan, E. A., Kridin, K., Zillikens, D., Ludwig, R. J., & Bieber, K. (2021). *Lichen planus. Frontiers in Medicine, 8*. https://doi.org/10.3389/fmed.2021.737813 (accessed on 21st July 2025).
6. Brănişteanu, D., Cojocaru, C., Diaconu, R., Porumb-Andrese, E., Alexa, A. I., Nicolescu, A. C., Brihan, I., et al. (2022). Update on the etiopathogenesis of psoriasis (Review). *Experimental and Therapeutic Medicine, 23*. https://doi.org/10.3892/etm.2022.11124 (accessed on 21st July 2025).
7. Canedo, J. V. R., Mello, J. L. da S., Rodrigues, A. S., Santana, L. M. S., Kagohara, G. T., Morikawa, M., & Diogo, A. B. (2024). Main dermatological diseases treated in Children's Emergency Room: A systematic review. *International Journal of Health Science, 4*, 2–14. https://doi.org/10.22533/at.ed.1594152405011 (accessed on 21st July 2025).
8. Cassalia, F., & Fortina, A. B. (2024). Psoriasis in women with psoriatic arthritis: Hormonal effects, fertility, and considerations for management at different stages of life. *Reumatismo, 76*(3). https://www.semanticscholar.org/paper/2fbe8720f990f43202086b21bf43ecfa252c7f2e (accessed on 21st July 2025).
9. Chandy, A. (2023). Comprehensive overview of medicinal plants utilized for treatment of skin disorders. *Pharmaceutical and Biosciences Journal*. https://www.semanticscholar.org/paper/c3570f861b41504c7809198366984c8463cc4800 (accessed on 21st July 2025).
10. Chen, J., & English, J. C. (2025). Characteristics and outcomes of generalized pustular psoriasis patients managed through inpatient asynchronous teledermatology: A retrospective study. *Telemedicine Reports, 6*, 23–26. https://www.semanticscholar.org/paper/ac4b642dbb32024653ac4beded907cea10264a37 (accessed on 21st July 2025).

11. Costache, D. O., Feroiu, O., Ghilencea, A., Georgescu, M., Căruntu, A., Căruntu, C., Țiplica, S. G., et al. (2022). Skin inflammation modulation via TNF-α, IL-17, and IL-12 family inhibitors therapy and cancer control in patients with psoriasis. *International Journal of Molecular Sciences, 23*, 5198–5198. https://doi.org/10.3390/ijms23095198 (accessed on 21st July 2025).

12. Darvish, Z., Ghanbari, S., Afshar, S., Tapak, L., & Amini, P. (2023). Psoriasis associated hub genes revealed by weighted gene co-expression network analysis. *Cell Journal (Yakhteh), 25*, 418–426. https://www.semanticscholar.org/paper/567b4a19942131603fa0706527fa8f009a268e3b (accessed on 21st July 2025).

13. Deana, C., Vetrugno, L., Cortegiani, A., Mongodi, S., Salve, G., Mangiagalli, M., Boscolo, A., et al. (2023). Quality of life in COVID-related ARDS patients one year after intensive care discharge (ODISSEA study): A multicenter observational study. *Journal of Clinical Medicine, 12*. https://www.semanticscholar.org/paper/6cf8ce186af524698be547e7670a190e297fff77 (accessed on 21st July 2025).

14. Errichetti, E., & Stinco, G. (2016). Dermoscopy in general dermatology: A practical overview. https://core.ac.uk/download/80135885.pdf (accessed on 21st July 2025).

15. Garcovich, S., De Simone, C., Genovese, G., Berti, E., Cugno, M., & Marzano, A. V. (2019). Paradoxical skin reactions to biologics in patients with rheumatologic disorders. *Frontiers in Pharmacology, 10*. https://doi.org/10.3389/fphar.2019.00282 (accessed on 21st July 2025).

16. Gaurav, V., Anand, G. R. P., & Grover, C. (2024). Follicular psoriasis: A case report and review of literature. *Skin Appendage Disorders, 10*, 148–155. https://www.semanticscholar.org/paper/1f1f774abb24da78c80ef8023b929311c8ebc1d7 (accessed on 21st July 2025).

17. Gavra, D. I., Kósa, D., Pető, Á., Józsa, L., Ujhelyi, Z., Fehér, P., Pallag, A., et al. (2024). Exploring the correlation between the PASI and DLQI scores in psoriasis treatment with topical ointments containing *Rosa × damascena* Mill. extract. *Pharmaceuticals, 17*. https://www.semanticscholar.org/paper/946c920b14a0f2e5e6dd795defcc3198fa4d5bbe (accessed on 21st July 2025).

18. Godse, K., Girdhar, M., Jagadeesan, S., & Laiker, R. (2024). Role of topical tofacitinib in autoimmune skin disorders: An expert opinion. *IP Indian Journal of Clinical and Experimental Dermatology*. https://www.semanticscholar.org/paper/7389a73116a700056372f3107802d8391d70b32d (accessed on 21st July 2025).

19. Goyal, G. (2025). *Eka Kustha (Psoriasis)*–A comprehensive review of Ayurvedic and modern approaches. *AYUSHDHARA*. https://www.semanticscholar.org/paper/e6912db760fb3675a5572fd97dffde624e1978e9 (accessed on 21st July 2025).

20. Gurudev, S., Pise, G. A., Manohar, N., Sanagoudar, V., Rao, K., & Patil, M. N. (2023). Clinico-epidemiological study of papulosquamous disorders in childhood at a tertiary care hospital in South India. *Indian Journal of Pediatric Dermatology, 24*, 121–128. https://www.semanticscholar.org/paper/bcff89ad0bce6096136296ed98db59cb9f6db693 (accessed on 21st July 2025).

21. Hatami, P., Nicknam Asl, H., Aryanian, Z., Hatami, D., Homayouni, M., & Khayyat, A. (2024). Molecular scarring in relapsing psoriasis: Crosstalk of keratinocytes and immune cells. *American Journal of Clinical Pathology*. https://www.semanticscholar.org/paper/316fb55c521cf5e520cdbb2e86b1965979b03788 (accessed on 21st July 2025).

22. Isdianto, A., Al Indunissy, N., & Fitrianti, N. (2025). The impact of mental health disorders on physical disease risks: A comprehensive review. *Multidisciplinary Indonesian Center Journal*

(MICJO). https://www.semanticscholar.org/paper/8911daee373d776bcdd31a097c49bc0f6ed2c99d (accessed on 21st July 2025).

23. Joosten, M. D. W., Clabbers, J. M. K., Jonca, N., Mazereeuw-Hautier, J., & Gostyński, A. (2022). New developments in the molecular treatment of ichthyosis: Review of the literature. *Orphanet Journal of Rare Diseases, 17*. https://doi.org/10.1186/s13023-022-02430-6 (accessed on 21st July 2025).

24. Keser, G., & Namdar Pekiner, F. (2023). *Artificial Intelligence Applications in Dentistry*. Özgür Yayınları eBooks. https://doi.org/10.58830/ozgur.pub91.c383 (accessed on 21st July 2025).

25. Liberton, D., Almpani, K., Mishra, R., Bassim, C., Van Ryzin, C., Moebius Syndrome Research Consort, Webb, B., et al. (2024). Oral health-related quality of life in rare disorders of congenital facial weakness. *International Journal of Environmental Research and Public Health, 21*. https://www.semanticscholar.org/paper/45910f00af34b863158b0cee87eb98c9ee1de4af (accessed on 21st July 2025).

26. Markevich, E. B., Khvorik, D., & Stanko, E. P. (2024). Characteristics of pruritus and some neuropeptides in psoriasis associated with mental disorders. *Journal of the Grodno State Medical University*. https://www.semanticscholar.org/paper/6bcbc3ab721fc59f0e7d61652455c7df78318140 (accessed on 21st July 2025).

27. Matwiejuk, M., Myśliwiec, H., Jakubowicz-Zalewska, O., Chabowski, A., & Flisiak, I. (2023). Effects of hypolipidemic drugs on psoriasis. *Metabolites, 13*, 493–493. https://doi.org/10.3390/metabo13040493 (accessed on 21st July 2025).

28. Mohd Zaid, N. A., Sekar, M., Bonam, S. R., Gan, S. H., Lum, P. T., Begum, M. Y., Mat Rani, N. N. I., et al. (2022). Promising natural products in new drug design, development, and therapy for skin disorders: An overview of scientific evidence and understanding their mechanism of action. *Drug Design Development and Therapy, 16*, 23–66. https://doi.org/10.2147/dddt.s326332 (accessed on 21st July 2025).

29. Narayankar, S. L., & Pandit, G. A. (2017). Papulosquamous: Clinicopathological. https://core.ac.uk/download/543135106.pdf (accessed on 21st July 2025).

30. Oyedepo, J. T., Katibi, O. S., & Adedoyin, O. T. (2023). Dermatological disorders and dermatology-specific quality of life among secondary students in public and private schools in Kwara State, Nigeria. *Nigerian Journal of Pediatrics, 49*. https://doi.org/10.4314/njp.v49i4.2 (accessed on 21st July 2025).

31. Patil, T. S., Gujarathi, N. A., Aher, A. A., Pachpande, H. E., Sharma, C., Ojha, S., Goyal, S. N., et al. (2023). Recent advancements in topical anti-psoriatic nanostructured lipid carrier-based drug delivery. *International Journal of Molecular Sciences, 24*, 2978–2978. https://doi.org/10.3390/ijms24032978 (accessed on 21st July 2025).

32. Podobińska, B. (2025). The role of trichological interviewing and imaging in the diagnosis and treatment of scalp psoriasis. *Aesthetic Cosmetology and Medicine*. https://www.semanticscholar.org/paper/92bedc965796076efde0c1ae473ab2f3589470da (accessed on 21st July 2025).

33. Pondeljak, N., Lugović-Mihić, L., Tomić, L., Parać, E., Pedić, L., & Lazić-Mosler, E. (2023). Key factors in the complex and coordinated network of skin keratinization: Their significance and involvement in common skin conditions. *International Journal of Molecular Sciences, 25*. https://www.semanticscholar.org/paper/5765692a08faad012fee566009aa77849c250cc3 (accessed on 21st July 2025).

34. Puri, N., Brar, B., Goyal, S., & Kumar, S. (2024). A study on onychoscopic findings of various benign nail disorders. *Malaysian Journal of Dermatology*. https://www.semanticscholar.org/paper/ca2345ee73618e2850216cb9e2a3c3b7a4618b4c (accessed on 21st July 2025).

35. Raef, H. S., & Elmariah, S. B. (2021). Vulvar pruritus: A review of clinical associations, pathophysiology and therapeutic management. *Frontiers in Medicine, 8*. https://doi.org/10.3389/fmed.2021.649402 (accessed on 21st July 2025).

36. Ramesan, G. K., & Madhu, P. M. (2025). Ayurvedic management of Sidhma Kushta: An evidence-based case report. *International Journal of Ayurveda and Pharma Research*. https://www.semanticscholar.org/paper/75d193df0a047d8faf34a2bec10e5eea8493e6ce (accessed on 21st July 2025).

37. Rivera-Díaz, R., Daudén, E., Carrascosa, J., Cueva, P., & Puig, L. (2023). Generalized pustular psoriasis: A review on clinical characteristics, diagnosis, and treatment. *Dermatology and Therapy, 13*, 673–688. https://www.semanticscholar.org/paper/f407fcb906205e8a8e7bd2b7a2a275aa4ac1b2ae (accessed on 21st July 2025).

38. Roszkiewicz, M., Dopytalska, K., Szymańska, E., Jakimiuk, A., & Walecka, I. (2019). Environmental risk factors and epigenetic alternations in psoriasis. *Annals of Agricultural and Environmental Medicine, 27*, 335–342. https://doi.org/10.26444/aaem/112107 (accessed on 21st July 2025).

39. Sadeghi, P., Pezeshki, P. S., & Rezaei, N. (2023). Coronavirus disease 2019 (COVID-19) in pediatric patients with autoimmune disorders. *European Journal of Pediatrics, 182*, 2967–2988. https://doi.org/10.1007/s00431-023-04958-6 (accessed on 21st July 2025).

40. Seirafianpour, F., Sodagar, S., Pour Mohammad, A., Panahi, P., Mozafarpoor, S., Almasi, S., & Goodarzi, A. (2020). Cutaneous manifestations and considerations in COVID-19 pandemic: A systematic review. *Dermatologic Therapy, 33*. https://doi.org/10.1111/dth.13986 (accessed on 21st July 2025).

41. Seo, J., Han, M., Kang, S., Kim, S. J., Jung, I., & Kang, J. I. (2024). Healthcare utilization and costs in patients with somatic symptom and related disorders compared with those with depression and healthy controls: A nationwide cohort study. *Depression and Anxiety, 2024*. https://www.semanticscholar.org/paper/f60a87a5e5588efd8edaa229b17812aa6692eb6f (accessed on 21st July 2025).

42. Shah, V., Larson, A., & Jafferany, M. (2024). Exploring the psychological impact of childhood-onset psoriasis: A systematic review. *Clinical and Experimental Dermatology*. https://www.semanticscholar.org/paper/86f2415e50cdfe716573ac1b24cf22cd7b084bca (accessed on 21st July 2025).

43. Steinmann, M., Lampe, D., Grosser, J., Schmidt, J., Hohoff, M. L., Fischer, A., & Greiner, W. (2024). Risk factors for herpes zoster infections: A systematic review and meta-analysis unveiling common trends and heterogeneity patterns. *Infection, 52*, 1009–1026. https://www.semanticscholar.org/paper/668bd9dcc1a4a8aab0c49b8033efe0bbe559d929 (accessed on 21st July 2025).

44. Tang, J., Hou, Z., Liao, W., Wang, Y., Zhang, G., Luo, Y., Gao, X., et al. (2025). Pediatric pustular psoriasis in Southern China: A 12-year retrospective analysis of 41 cases focusing on clinical characteristics and treatment outcomes. *Psoriasis: Targets and Therapy, 15*, 185–195. https://www.semanticscholar.org/paper/b53dbb77adad19704ec9ff1db5487f19cc0de5c1 (accessed on 21st July 2025).

45. Timofte, M. A., Căruntu, C., Bălăceanu-Gurău, B., Mărgăritescu, I., Giurcaneanu, C., & Mihai, M. (2025). Bullous pemphigoid overlapping psoriasis vulgaris: A rare case report and literature review. *Clinics and Practice, 15*. https://www.semanticscholar.org/paper/d7933c788b810e96a00c033522ec71b401e0945a (accessed on 21st July 2025).

46. Tomar, Y., Baidya, M., Chadokiya, J., Bhatt, S., & Singhvi, G. (2024). An overview of Skp2: A promising new therapeutic target of psoriasis. *Expert Opinion on Therapeutic Targets, 28*, 689–700. https://www.semanticscholar.org/paper/f6703f1fe066eceecd3a7ab6440b32952a49fed3 (accessed on 21st July 2025).

47. Vlasova, N. V., Masyagutova, L. M., Stepanov, E., Rafikova, L., Sadrtdinova, G., & Gizatullina, L. G. (2024). Risk factors and integrated assessment of health disorders in teachers of rural comprehensive schools. *Health Risk Analysis*. https://www.semanticscholar.org/paper/b0a9e9fe7ea9695d67df034bd87706215d6cb402 (accessed on 21st July 2025).

48. Zhiltsova, E., Shilin, R. R., Sonin, D. B., Bakovetskaya, O. V., & Filchkova, A. E. (2025). Targeted therapy for psoriasis: Pathogenetic aspects and effectiveness. *Meditsinskiy sovet=Medical Council*. https://www.semanticscholar.org/paper/25d359f0c4cf909fdb0d5beb28bc952a357ff765 (accessed on 21st July 2025).

URTICARIA, ANGIOEDEMA, AND MASTOCYTOSIS

8

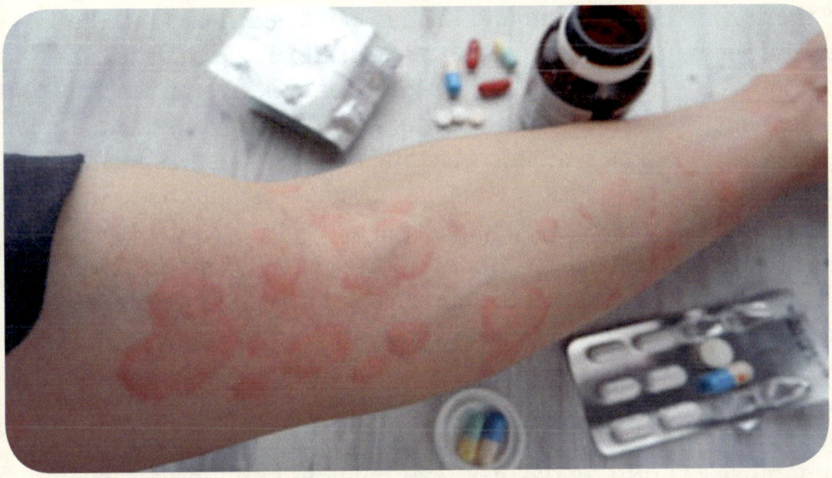

Introduction

The relationship among urticaria, angioedema, and mastocytosis creates a confusing landscape in the study of allergic and inflammatory disorders in humans. Urticaria, characterized by wheals and pruritus, is typically caused by mast-cell activation and degranulation, resulting in the release of inflammatory mediators such as histamine. This disease, particularly chronic spontaneous urticaria (CSU), has been of significant interest in clinical science in recent times due to its seriously debilitating effect on the quality of life of patient sufferers. At the same time, angioedema, manifested as potentially life-threatening edema of the dermis and subcutaneous tissue, adds another layer of complexity to the clinical picture, as in hereditary angioedema (HAE), in which bradykinin plays a pivotal role. Awareness of these related conditions obliges investigation into their pathophysiologic mechanisms and clinical presentations. New knowledge about serum biomarkers sheds light on the relationship between mast-cell degranulation and angioedema. A fine example is the upregulation of human

LEARNING OBJECTIVES

After studying this chapter, you will be able to:

1. Understand the pathophysiology of urticaria, angioedema, and mastocytosis
2. Describe the types of urticaria and angioedema
3. Give an overview of mastocytosis
4. Know the treatment options for urticaria, angioedema, and mastocytosis

β-defensin 2 (HBD2) in CSU patients, which has been correlated with the severity of concomitant symptoms such as angioedema. In a study, there was a positive correlation of the concentration of serum HBD2 with translationally controlled tumor protein (TCTP) levels and a reverse correlation with values such as basophils' peripheral percentages and vitamin D levels (Cao et al., 2021). Identification of these biomarkers not only sheds light on the underlying pathophysiology but also enhances the therapeutic prospects for targeted therapy. Translation of these findings into the clinic is utilized to minimize acute symptoms and improve outcomes in patients. Additionally, management of angioedema, particularly in patients with hereditary forms, has been transformed by the existence of targeted treatments. Having such therapies as human C1 inhibitor concentrate brings hope to patients with life-threatening attacks caused by angioedema. There have been reports documenting cases in which early application has made a significant difference to patients, especially in the case of acute attacks (Gavrilović et al., 2023). As more and more patients are exposed to such sophisticated care, it becomes important to unravel the long-term consequences for mortality and morbidity of such conditions. By aligning treatment regimens with emerging science, health care providers can optimize therapy for patients with urticaria, angioedema, and mastocytosis.

Definition of Urticaria

Urticaria, or hives, is a cutaneous condition characterized by the acute appearance of pruritic, elevated welts on the skin as a result of the release of inflammatory mediators from mast cells. These responses may vary in duration, acute urticaria lasting less than six weeks and chronic urticaria lasting longer to clear. The pathogenesis of urticaria is multifactorial, involving allergic response, drug sensitivity, infection, and even stress reactions. Above all, the mast cell's role in urticaria pathogenesis is central, as their activation initiates the release of histamine and other pro-inflammatory mediators that elicit the presenting symptoms in individuals affected by urticaria. Both the type and cause distinctions in urticaria are crucial for successful management and intervention. The clinical picture of urticaria can range from mild irritation to severe distress, with a profound effect on the quality of life in patients. Its appearance is usually accompanied by angioedema, which is a more profound swelling of the skin and tissues, particularly around the eyes and lips. The relationship between urticaria and angioedema is integral to the overall picture of mast cell disorders. Studies have indicated that systemic mastocytosis has been reported to cause urticaria as well as angioedema, presenting particular challenges in the diagnosis and management of the same. Practitioners thus have the onus of identifying the causes of the conditions and differentiating urticaria from other similar skin conditions to ensure that interventions for symptom reduction and control are appropriately conducted. Also, the differential diagnosis includes chronic urticaria, where a complete history and laboratory evaluation may identify underlying mast cell activation syndromes (MCAS). This condition is characterized by characteristic symptoms of mast cell degranulation and may have a different treatment algorithm, particularly if standard antihistamines fail. With further development of investigations in mast cell biology and its relevance to diseases such as urticaria, the incorporation of updated criteria and classification systems for MCAS becomes pertinent. This is underscored by an appreciation of the possibility of misdiagnosis under nonspecific criteria, leading to patient frustration and delays in the diagnosis of more severe underlying illnesses (Theo Gülen et al., 2021). Therefore, researching the definitions and classification of urticaria not only clarifies its complications but also improves clinical outcomes for victims (Figure 8.1).

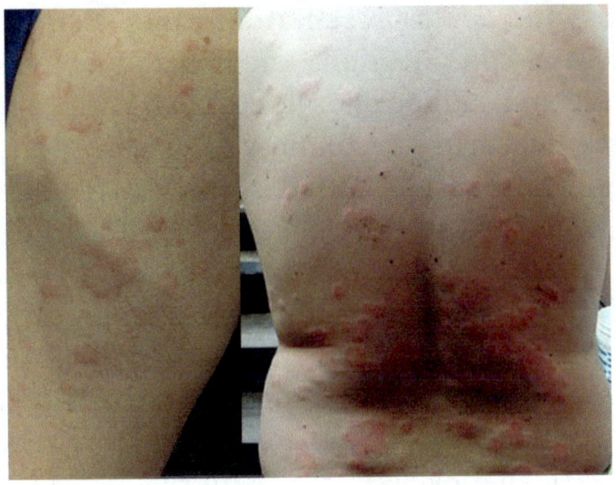

Figure 8.1. Urticaria (hives).

Source: https://media.springernature.com/full/springer-static/image/art%3A10.1186%2Fs13223-018-0288-z/MediaObjects/13223_2018_288_Fig1_HTML.jpg?as=webp.

Definition of Angioedema

Angioedema is defined as an edematous swelling that occurs beneath the skin, primarily in the dermis and subcutaneous tissues. This condition is traditionally defined by the acute onset of edema and can be caused by numerous different inducing factors, including allergens, medications, or disease. Angioedema, in the majority of cases, occurs with urticaria, when the two conditions occur in combination, or one follows the other. The most common areas to become swollen are the eyelids, lips, and extremities, and they are very painful and can impair function. Knowledge of the etiology of angioedema is crucial since it differs based on its classification—either hereditary or acquired—and both have unique pathophysiologic mechanisms that require special therapeutic interventions. The pathophysiology of angioedema is closely related to mast cell activation and subsequent histamine release, as with mechanisms in urticaria. Traditionally, this condition has been divided into two main forms: acute and chronic. Acute angioedema is typically an allergic response that occurs acutely, frequently secondary to food allergens or arthropod exposure, whereas chronic angioedema may be extended secondary to autoimmune conditions or idiopathic reasons. In mastocytosis, a condition with an excess of mast cells, angioedema may be particularly severe and disabling. The complexity of the interaction between mast cells and angioedema demands large clinical guidelines to enable diagnosis and treatment (Zuberbier et al., 2021). Effective treatment of angioedema requires a multidisciplinary approach, based on an adequate understanding of its potential causes, the patient's clinical presentation, and the patient's history. Some diagnostic tests for hereditary angioedema may include skin testing, serum tryptase measurement, and genetic testing to identify C1-inhibitor deficiency. Treatment plans commonly include antihistamines and corticosteroids, but in cases of severe angioedema or recurrent episodes, more advanced treatments, such as C1-inhibitor replacement therapy, may be required. Recent guidelines emphasize the importance of alertness among healthcare professionals, as angioedema can present similarly to other acute conditions and may be included in the differential diagnosis (Ujiie et al., 2022). With continued research, the hope is to enhance both treatment outcome and accuracy in the diagnosis of patients with this disabling disease (Figure 8.2).

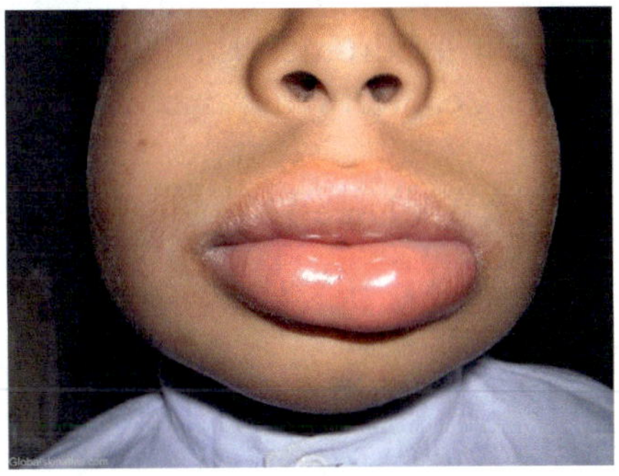

Figure 8.2. Angioedema.

Source: https://i0.wp.com/coreem.net/content/uploads/2016/06/Angioedema-Lip-Swelling.jpg?fit=1024%2C768&ssl=1.

Definition of Mastocytosis

Mastocytosis is a rare hematologic disorder characterized by the abnormal accumulation of mast cells in multiple tissues, particularly the skin, bone marrow, and gastrointestinal tract. These cells, which are a part of the body's immune response, become central to modulating allergy and infection by secreting mediators such as histamine and tryptase upon stimulation. In mastocytosis, excessive proliferation and degranulation of mast cells lead to a range of symptoms, including cutaneous manifestations such as urticaria and angioedema. It is further divided into two large categories: cutaneous mastocytosis, primarily involving the skin, and systemic mastocytosis, in which mast cell proliferation occurs in more than one organ system. The presentation is very heterogeneous, and hence there is a need for knowledge of its pathophysiology and patient management subtleties as outlined in current literature. Diagnosis of mastocytosis involves careful evaluation of the clinical history, physical examination, and laboratory testing, including measurement of serum tryptase levels, which reflect the mast cell burden. A significantly elevated serum tryptase level, especially during symptom periods, confirms the diagnosis of mast cell activation, whereas a baseline elevation points towards systemic disease. Beyond common criteria, novel definitions, such as those of mast cell activation syndromes (MCAS), emphasize understanding clinical symptoms and responses to targeted therapy. Discrete differentiation of mastocytosis from MCAS is necessary, since misdiagnosis may delay appropriate treatment and management. For instance, individuals diagnosed with MCAS inappropriately may be subjected to inappropriate treatment that fails to address underlying conditions pertaining to mast cell abnormalities, exemplifying the difficulty in diagnosing mastocytosis given its resemblance in clinical presentations, as evidenced by recent MCAS literature (Theo Gülen et al., 2021). The effects of mastocytosis go beyond acute presentations; they also cover potential complications such as anaphylaxis, a severe and sudden allergic reaction with a rapid onset, featuring systemic vascular responses. Anaphylaxis results from the release of mediators from activated mast cells, which induce increased vascular permeability, vasodilation, and cardiovascular instability (Nuñez-Borque et al., 2022). Vascular response in anaphylaxis is directly related to knowledge of dysregulation in mastocytosis, where elevated levels of mast cells increase anaphylactic risk. With rising incidence and awareness of mastocytosis and related syndromes, more education on the vascular and immune processes that underlie this disease will strengthen clinical approaches to prevent adverse outcomes. Thus, there is a need for an integrated approach to adequate diagnosis, treatment, and management of mastocytosis and its life-threatening aspects (Figure 8.3).

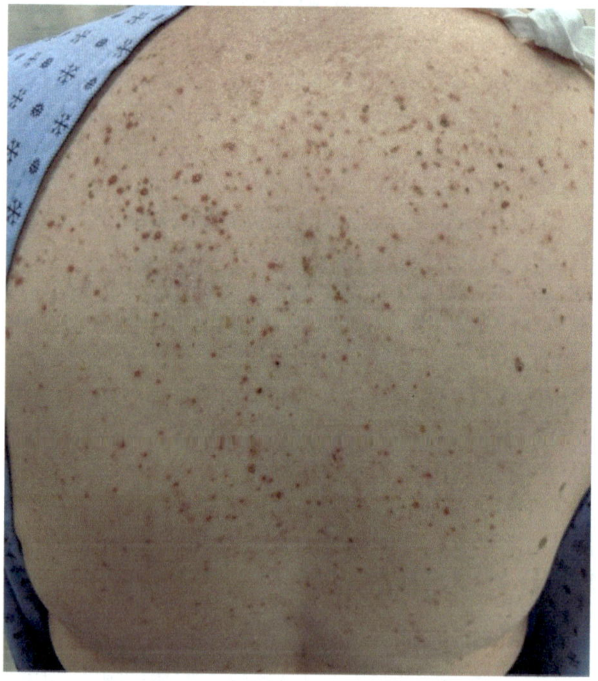

Figure 8.3. Mastocytosis.

Source: https://upload.wikimedia.org/wikipedia/commons/thumb/c/c8/Mastocytosis2019.jpg/800px-Mastocytosis2019.jpg.

8.1. Pathophysiology

Learning Outcome

1. Understand the role of the immune systemin the pathophysiology of urticaria, angioedema, and mastocytosis
2. Describe the role of mast cells in the pathophysiology of urticaria, angioedema, and mastocytosis
3. Describe the histamine release mechanisms in the pathophysiology of various allergic conditions

The underlying pathophysiology of urticaria, angioedema, and mastocytosis is complex and multifaceted and involves both non-immunological and immunological factors. Mast cell degranulation and release of histamine and other inflammatory mediators lead to urticaria or hives. Any one of a multitude of stimuli, including allergens, medications, or physical stimuli, can trigger degranulation, resulting in vasodilation and increased vascular permeability. Thus, the patients acquire pruritic wheals and local swelling that characterize the disease. Notably, chronic spontaneous urticaria has also been linked to autoimmune mechanisms, in which autoantibodies target high-affinity IgE receptors on mast cells, leading to an inflammatory vicious cycle. It is essential to decipher these pathways for the development of targeted treatments, as chronic skin inflammation remains prevalent and refractory to effective treatment (Ujiie et al., 2022). Angioedema, often with urticaria, is caused by deeper swelling of the dermal and subcutaneous tissue, particularly around the eyes, lips, and throat. The pathophysiology is similar to that of urticaria, and the most common cause is mast cell degranulation, releasing vasoactive substances. However, angioedema can also be caused by bradykinin-mediated mechanisms, such as hereditary angioedema, in which C1-inhibitor deficiency leads to uncontrolled bradykinin levels, producing severe edema. Differential diagnosis is very important because treatment varies with the causative agent: antihistamines are effective in mast cell-mediated angioedema, while replacement with C1-inhibitor is necessary in hereditary cases. Elucidation of the specific mechanisms of angioedema facilitates appropriate management and improves quality of life in affected patients (Ring et al., 2021). Mastocytosis, a condition characterized by mast cell proliferation in the skin, bone marrow, and other organs, poses a special challenge in its pathophysiology. The disease can present in many forms, ranging from cutaneous mastocytosis, with clinical features of brown macules, to systemic mastocytosis, in which mast cells infiltrate multiple organ systems. In most cases, genetic mutations, particularly of the KIT gene, are implicated, leading to constitutive activation of mast cells and hyperresponsiveness to stimuli. The relationship between mast cells and other immune cells further complicates the pathophysiological background, as these cells release mediators that can influence the behavior of surrounding immune cells. With ongoing research, it becomes crucial to understand these pathways to formulate targeted therapy, particularly in systemic mastocytosis, where traditional antihistamines may be insufficient (Ujiie et al., 2022).

8.1.1. Immune System Involvement

The immune system plays a central role in urticaria, angioedema, and mastocytosis pathophysiology, with particular emphasis on the function of mast cells and their mediators. They are components of the immune system and are found in virtually all connective tissues. In conditions such as chronic spontaneous urticaria (CSU), mast cell degranulation releases inflammatory mediators, including histamine, which directly causes symptoms such as itching and swelling. In experiments, it has been demonstrated that inappropriate activation of mast cells is one of the most important points in CSU patients that links the immune system with disease manifestations. Higher levels of human β-defensin 2 (HBD2), a protein involved in immune modulation, were found in CSU patients and have been suggested to reflect a link among mast cell activation, immune dysregulation, and the disease process itself (Maja Štrajtenberger et al., 2024). Similarly, even in angioedema, the immune system's role can be significant, particularly in conditions associated with chronic urticaria. Understanding the mechanisms of localized edema involves research into the interactions between various immune factors, such as plasma proteins and cytokines. Notably, research has identified that patients with angioedema have very high salivary levels of HBD2 compared to healthy controls, highlighting its potential as a biomarker of disease activity. The association between increased HBD2 levels and mast cell activity supports the hypothesis that these immune mediators can be a central pathogenic factor in angioedema, namely by engaging vascular permeability and promoting further tissue edema (Maja Štrajtenberger et al., 2024). Such an observation raises the question of targeted therapies that aim to correct the fundamental immune dysfunction rather than simply mask symptoms.

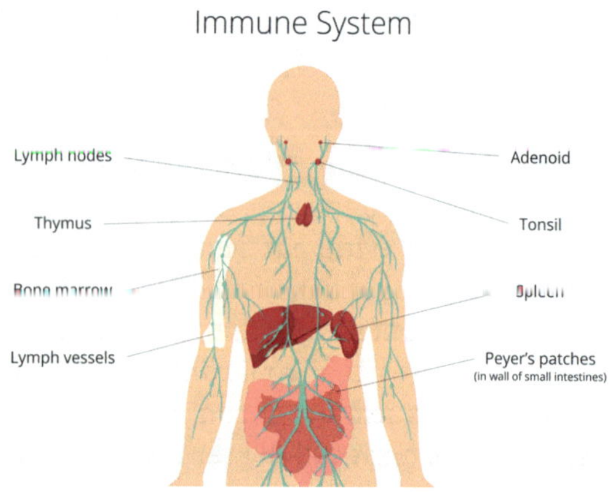

Figure 8.4. Immune system.

Source: https://cdn.shopify.com/s/files/1/0257/1046/0991/files/Immune_system_infographic.jpg?v=1674650552.

Mastocytosis is a second term for mast cell involvement in the immune system, characterized by abnormal mast cell proliferation in many tissues. Mastocytosis may be associated with overexpression of mediators, leading to a wide range of manifestations and signs, from skin lesions to systemic ones. The interaction between the mast cell and the immune environment is similar to a prolonged pathological process that affects skin health and general well-being. Studies have indicated the significance of skin immunity in various allergic diseases, such as mastocytosis, highlighting the skin's dual roles as both a barrier and an immunological actor in the body's immune response to external stimuli. Such an understanding of the immunological basis of mastocytosis can inform the most effective interventions and improve the quality of life for individuals with the condition (Figure 8.4).

8.1.2. Role of Mast Cells

The role of mast cells in the pathopharmacology of urticaria, angioedema, and mastocytosis is central, given that these cells are major mediators of inflammatory responses. Mast cells are best positioned in areas of barrier function, such as the skin and mucosa surfaces, and play a crucial role in the body's defense against environmental pathogens. Upon activation, these cells release a spectrum of mediators, including histamine, leukotrienes, and cytokines, that induce immediate hypersensitivity reactions. Mast cell degranulation in urticaria, for instance, results in capillary leakage and vasodilation, which manifest as the welts and rashes of the disease. Chronic conditions such as chronic spontaneous urticaria may feature ongoing mast cell activation, which significantly affects patients' quality of life and must be addressed with therapeutic interventions aimed at stabilizing these cells or inhibiting their activity (Zuberbier et al., 2021). Mastocytosis, a systemic disorder characterized by an abnormal overgrowth of mast cells in several tissues, is another example of their pivotal role in allergic and inflammatory disorders. Patients with mastocytosis may have a wide range of presentations, ranging from mild flushing and pruritus to severe anaphylactic attack. Both mast cell activation and mediator release contribute to the symptoms. In particular, quantification of serum tryptase levels has proven to be a crucial biomarker for diagnosing and monitoring mast cell activation in patients with systemic mastocytosis, as reflected by elevated tryptase levels. Above all, the interaction between mast cells and other components of the immune system highlights their contribution to the overall pathophysiology of mastocytosis, where the dynamic interplay typically complicates clinical management (Sheldon et al., 2014). The growing consensus on the definitive role of mast cells underscores the need for ongoing research to elucidate their multifaceted functions in health and disease. Therapeutic strategies targeting mast cells hold the potential to suppress symptoms of urticaria, angioedema, and mastocytosis. For instance, antihistamines are most commonly used to address symptoms resulting from mast cell degranulation, while newer therapies, such as monoclonal antibodies that modulate mast cell function, are under development. As researchers gain a deeper understanding of the intricate biology of mast cells, it becomes increasingly clear that unraveling their roles will ultimately lead to improved treatments and patient outcomes in diseases driven by these ubiquitous immune cells (Sheldon et al., 2014; Zuberbier et al., 2021) (Figure 8.5).

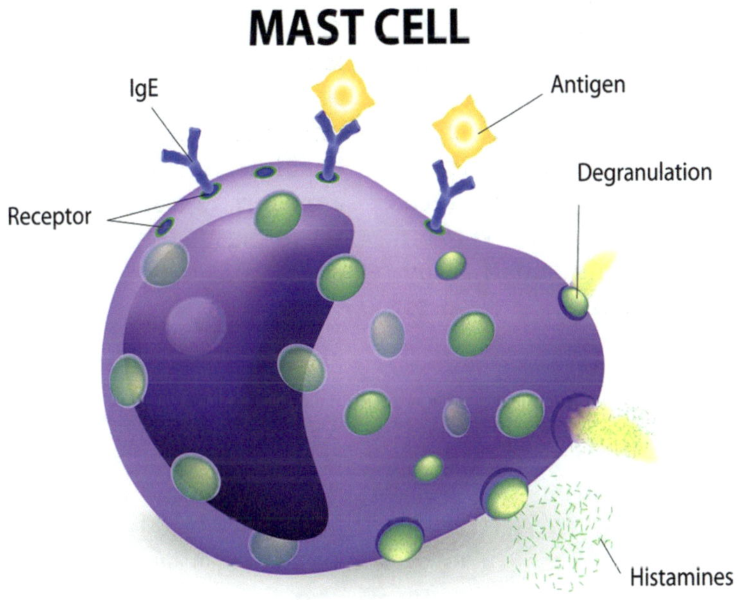

Figure 8.5. Mast cells.

Source: https://www.bkallergy.com/wp-content/uploads/2021/04/Depositphotos_43804211_s-2019-1-768x666.jpg.

8.1.3. Histamine Release Mechanisms

Mechanisms of histamine release play a central role in the pathophysiology of many allergic conditions, such as urticaria, angioedema, and mastocytosis. Histamine, primarily stored in mast cells and basophils, is released after various stimuli like allergens, physical stimuli, and certain drugs. Upon stimulation, mast cells degranulate and release histamine into the surrounding tissue, triggering an inflammatory cascade. This process is at the heart of urticaria, in which vasodilation, increased vascular permeability, and smooth muscle contraction, expressed as wheals and angioedema, are triggered by histamine release. In addition, chronic mast cell stimulation can result in significant impairment of quality of life, making it crucial that a profound understanding of histamine's role in such diseases informs appropriate therapeutic and management strategies for the affected (Zuberbier et al., 2021). Apart from allergic stimuli, histamine release may be influenced by other factors in conditions such as chronic spontaneous urticaria and mastocytosis. In mastocytosis, which is a condition with abnormal mast cell accumulation, these cells are predisposed to hyperreactivity and to over-release of histamine irrespective of the presence of the characteristic stimuli. This uncontrolled degranulation can result in episodic urticaria and angioedema, and incapacitating symptoms for the patients. Furthermore, various external factors, such as stress, temperature changes, and certain foods, can stimulate mast cells and thereby trigger histamine release. There is a need to evaluate patients' individual triggers and tailor treatment protocols accordingly, as this can lead to improved patient outcomes and quality of life (Zuberbier et al., 2018). Understanding the mechanisms of signaling pathways that mediate histamine release illuminates the plan for targeted treatments for urticaria and its associated diseases. Surprisingly, the interaction between immunoglobulin E (IgE) antibodies and their corresponding receptors on mast cells is essential for histamine release. With allergen binding to IgE, a conformational change occurs, leading to mast cell activation and degranulation. There has been recent research exploring potential therapeutic interventions to prevent this allergic cascade from occurring, including monoclonal antibodies that have an inhibitory effect on IgEs binding capacity. This line of study is significant because the successful management of urticaria and mastocytosis depends on our understanding of these mechanisms, which enables clinicians to offer more precise and appropriate treatment options to patients with these mast cell-related conditions (Zuberbier et al., 2021).

Test Your Knowledge

1. What is the primary immune cell involved in the pathophysiology of urticaria, angioedema, and mastocytosis?
2. Which mediator released from mast cells is primarily responsible for itching and swelling in chronic spontaneous urticaria (CSU)?

8.2. Types of Urticaria

Learning Outcome

1. Describe the acute vs. chronic urticaria
2. Understand the physical urticaria
3. Learn about allergic urticaria

Urticaria or hives describes a number of types categorized based on various etiologic factors. The most common type is acute urticaria, which typically occurs within six weeks of an inciting agent such as an allergen, drug, or infection. Its rapid onset can be very troubling and make people seek quick treatment. Chronic urticaria persists for six weeks or longer and is either idiopathic or secondary to other disorders like autoimmune diseases. Chronic spontaneous urticaria is a condition in which hives appear without a discernible cause, significantly impacting the patient's quality of life. It is essential to understand the nature of such groups so that treatment and management can be properly implemented, as each group may require a varied treatment protocol depending on the case. Physical urticaria is another applicable categorization, caused by varied physical stimuli. This category includes dermographic urticaria, in which local hives appear following skin pressure or friction; cholinergic urticaria, which is triggered by heat, exercise, or stress; and cold urticaria, which follows exposure to cold or cold substances. All of these subtypes underscore the importance of recognizing precipitating factors that induce mast cell activation. As the mast cell activation pathophysiology and its relationship to urticaria have expanded with the latest research, the need for utilizing proper criteria in the diagnosis of these variants becomes evident. Misdiagnosis would lead to improper treatment modalities, hence leading to additional distress to patients, according to debate about mast cell activation syndromes (Theo Gülen et al., 2021). Hence, identifying these distinctive physical stimulants is pivotal to establishing appropriate treatment protocols. Mastocytosis is a complex disorder most frequently associated with urticarial rashes and underscores the significance of careful classification. The link between mastocytosis and urticaria is critical in the treatment of chronic urticaria, where mast cell degranulation plays a crucial role. In patients with mastocytosis, uncontrolled growth of mast cells may induce spasmodic urticaria-like manifestations, along with potential systemic reactions. Recent developments in understanding mast cell activation mechanisms emphasize the use of rigorous diagnostic criteria to differentiate mastocytosis from urticaria caused by other mechanisms (Ring et al., 2021). While the health community continues to explore such correlations, accurate classification is expected to not only improve symptom management but also yield improved patient outcomes by preventing misdiagnosis and enabling early treatment (Figure 8.6).

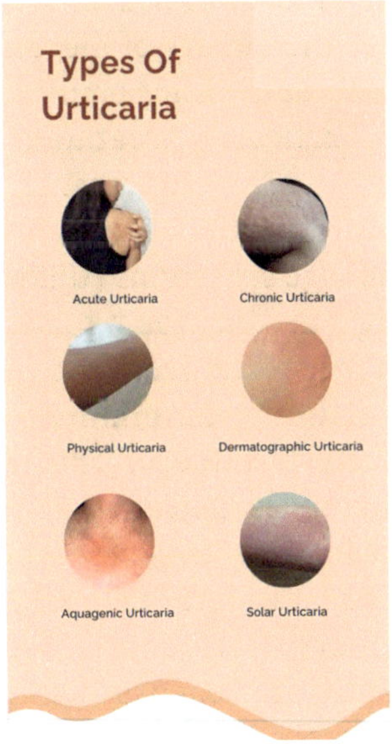

Figure 8.6. Types of urticaria.

Source: https://urbanskinhairclinic.com/wp-content/uploads/2023/08/Types-Of-Urticaria-1-768x1422.webp.

8.2.1. Acute vs. Chronic Urticaria

The distinction between acute and chronic urticaria is crucial in understanding the pathogenic mechanisms and appropriate management. Acute urticaria typically presents as fleeting wheals and angioedema that are self-limiting within 6 weeks and can generally be ascribed to identifiable stimuli, such as infections, drugs, or food allergy. Notably, acute urticaria has a lifetime prevalence of approximately 20%, making it a common condition. Patients typically experience intermittent episodes of hives that resolve spontaneously. This type is usually manageable with antihistamines or by avoiding precipitating factors, emphasizing a pragmatic, focused treatment regimen for clinicians working with the affected. Chronic urticaria, however, persists beyond six weeks and can be chronic spontaneous urticaria or chronic inducible urticaria. The former is spontaneous with no discernible cause, while the latter is provoked by specific stimuli, such as heat or pressure. Chronic urticaria has a significant impairment of the quality of life, affecting daily activity as well as causing emotional distress. Unlike acute urticaria, treatment of chronic urticaria may involve long-term antihistamine, corticosteroid, or other immunosuppressive therapy to manage symptoms (Ujiie et al., 2022). The difficulty in diagnosing and managing this condition stems from its multifarious etiologies, including autoimmune responses that complicate treatment. The management of acute and chronic urticaria has evolved over time, reflecting ongoing research and new guidelines. The latest international guideline for urticaria supported evidence-based diagnostic and therapeutic approaches distinct to every form of urticaria (Zuberbier et al., 2021). While acute urticaria typically responds well to simple interventions, chronic forms may require a more comprehensive approach given their persistent nature. As our understanding of urticaria advances, particularly regarding its relationship with underlying mast cell biology, future research will likely focus on developing targeted therapies. This reflects a broader tendency towards personalized medicine in urticarial dermatological conditions, addressing the patient-specific needs of both acute and chronic urticaria (Figure 8.7).

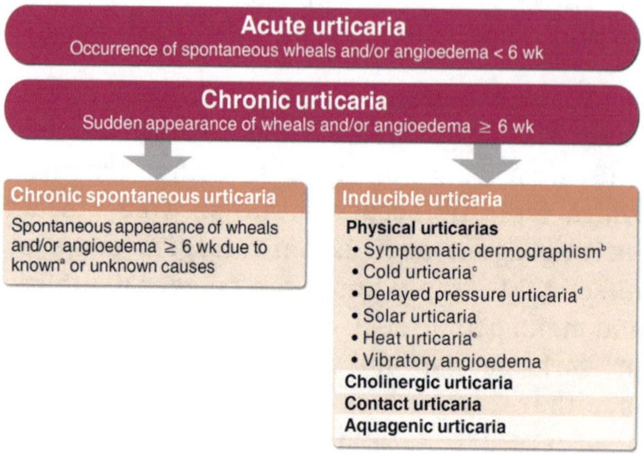

Figure 8.7. Acute and chronic urticaria.

Source: https://www.researchgate.net/publication/337361732/figure/fig3/AS:826951203844097@1574171939058/Acute-and-chronic-urticaria.ppm.

8.2.2. Physical Urticaria

Physical urticaria is a distinct subgroup of urticaria in which wheals are provoked by specific physical stimuli. This condition includes several forms, including cold urticaria, heat urticaria, pressure urticaria, and dermographic urticaria, each differentiated by the nature of the stimulus. In patients with physical urticaria, symptoms in the majority of cases appear within minutes following stimulation, inducing extreme distress and potential disruption of activities of daily living. The development of wheals and accompanying pruritus is primarily a result of mast cell degranulation, which releases histamine and other mediators into the tissue. These pathophysiological mechanisms are relevant to the process of diagnosis and management because physical urticaria requires patient-specific treatment plans that consider the individual patient's specific precipitating factors and lifestyle. Physical urticaria is treated by identifying and, where possible, avoiding the precipitant, as well as pharmacotherapeutic intervention. Antihistamines remain the treatment of choice, effectively suppressing the symptoms by blocking the action of histamine. Still, certain patients may require more advanced treatment if standard dosages fail to provide relief. Some evidence also suggests that higher doses of antihistamines may be warranted in certain subtypes, particularly in chronic cases where symptoms could be prolonged and intense. In addition to drug treatment, lifestyle modification, such as wearing protective clothing or altering the environment to limit exposure to causal factors, is useful.

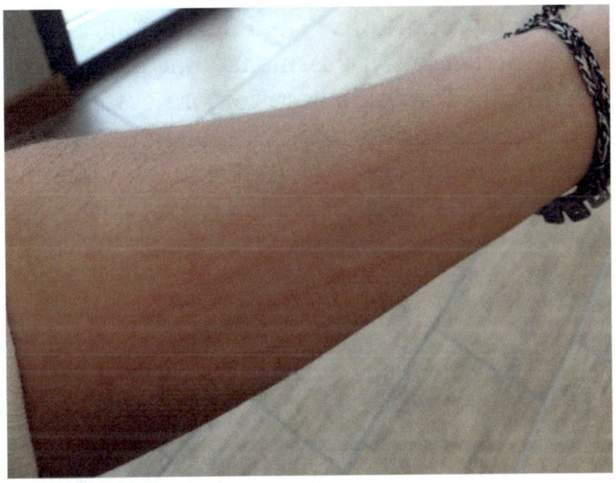

Figure 8.8. Physical urticaria.

Source: https://upload.wikimedia.org/wikipedia/commons/5/56/Physical_Urticaria_.jpg.

The combination of these practices highlights the importance of a multidimensional approach to the management of physical urticaria, particularly regarding the psychological and social associations of chronic illness. Furthermore, the intersection between physical urticaria and mental health cannot be overlooked; emotional aspects of suffering from a chronic skin condition usually increase symptoms and lower quality of life. The narrative theory of medicine, as expounded in classical Chinese medicine, underscores the significance of acknowledging both the body and the mind in relation to health. This unifying perspective supplements the understanding that patients with urticaria are usually stressed and anxious due to their unpredictable presentation and visible skin lesions. Through concepts in narrative medicine, practitioners can better understand patients' lives, thereby enhancing clinical practice to be more effective and compassionate. This kind of strategy builds a stronger clinician-patient relationship, enabling a better management plan for those facing the dilemma of physical urticaria (Liu et al., 2024; Young et al., 2025) (Figure 8.8).

8.2.3. Allergic Urticaria

Allergic urticaria is an immunmediated disease with the acute onset of pruritic, raised welts on the skin. When allergens such as certain foods, drugs, or insect stings are encountered, the body releases histamines and other inflammatory mediators. This produces vasodilation and increased vascular permeability, resulting in the characteristic urticarial lesions. Unlike in chronic urticaria, allergic urticaria tends to resolve quickly following elimination of the offending allergen. Gain an appreciation for the pathophysiology of mast cell activation (MCA) in understanding why such allergic responses are generated. Current studies have highlighted the importance of appropriate diagnostic criteria in MCA syndromes, particularly for distinguishing between true allergic reactions and pseudo-allergic reactions, the latter of which can present with the same clinical findings but with variable mechanisms (Theo Gülen et al., 2021). Allergic urticaria can also be treated with antihistamines, which counteract histamine release by activating mast cells. When antihistamines are inadequate, clinicians can resort to corticosteroids to minimize inflammation and achieve rapid symptom relief. Also critical is the identification of and avoidance of known causatives to avert future attacks. Patient education cannot be overemphasized, especially in developing an active coping strategy for allergic urticaria. Individuals are also instructed to maintain an allergy diary in which they record symptoms related to dietary intake or environmental exposure.

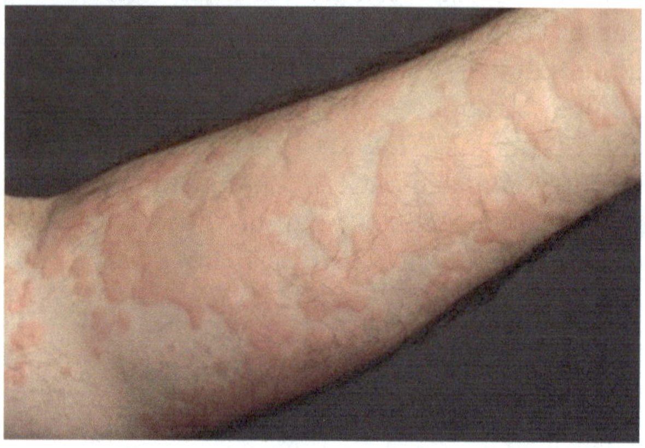

Figure 8.9. Allergic urticaria.

Source: https://www.dermatology.org.sg/wp-content/uploads/2019/12/0b3245405367fa17c8dad441f4408496.png.

The record can reveal patterns that help provide early recognition of elicitors and ultimately save unnecessary misery and misdiagnosis, which are prevalent in the absence of clear diagnostic criteria (Ring et al., 2021). Furthermore, the convergence of systemic factors with allergic urticaria underscores the subtlety of its management. Underlying disease: patients with mast cell disease may have increased symptoms, and differentiating allergic urticaria from other mast cell syndromes can be challenging. With progress, there is a requirement for an immediate standard consensus set of criteria to reliably diagnose mast cell activation syndromes. Misdiagnosis of MCAS due to nonspecific symptoms may lead to frustration and confusion among both patients and physicians, resulting in unwarranted delays in the proper treatment of underlying conditions (Theo Gülen et al., 2021). Hence, meticulous assessment of the patient and interdisciplinary collaboration are essential to achieve an accurate diagnosis and personalized therapeutic approaches that enhance patient outcomes and quality of life (Figure 8.9).

Test Your Knowledge

1. What is the difference between acute and chronic urticaria?
2. What is a physical urticaria?

8.3. Types of Angioedema

Learning Outcome

1. Learn about hereditary angioedema
2. Describe the acquired angioedema
3. Understand the drug-induced angioedema

Angioedema, a condition that presents with localized swelling of the skin in deeper layers, on the face and in the mouth, can be divided into various types based on causes and mechanisms. The most frequent form is allergic angioedema, most often secondary to an immunologic response to allergens such as foods, medications, or insect stings. It commonly accompanies urticaria (hives) and arises secondary to histamine and other inflammatory mediators released from mast cells. Mast cells are activated when exposed to these allergens and degranulate, leading to increased vascular permeability and, hence, extreme swelling. Separation of allergic and non-allergic angioedema is important for therapeutic management, especially because the incidence of such reactions continues to increase in at-risk populations, necessitating the development of targeted therapeutic approaches. Non-allergic angioedema, on the other hand, is a complex problem that occurs in two typical forms: hereditary and acquired. Hereditary angioedema (HAE) is a hereditary disorder characterized by recurrent attacks of swelling caused by mutations in the C1 inhibitor gene, which compromise the normal regulation of bradykinin, a peptide that increases vascular permeability. Acquired angioedema may occur with other systemic diseases such as autoimmune diseases or secondary to the side effect of ACE inhibitors, a common medication given for hypertension and other cardiovascular diseases. Research identifies that autoimmune responses can also be the underlying condition of acquired cases of angioedema, as in the case of ASIA syndrome, which occurs with a complex of autoimmune signs, including recurrent angioedema (Fomina et al., 2025). These need to be differentiated, since HAE may require long-term treatment, whereas acquired forms generally require treatment of the inciting disease or the medication causing the symptoms. Chronic spontaneous angioedema, distinguished from both allergic and hereditary subtypes, is another significant subtype with symptoms occurring in the absence of identifiable causative agents. It is increasingly recognized as a variant of chronic spontaneous urticaria (CSU) and is hypothesized to involve mast cell activation and autoimmunity. Elevated serum IgE against autoantigens, such as tissue transglutaminase, has been associated with CSU, which also emphasizes how immunological mechanisms are to blame for this form of angioedema (Su et al., 2023). More research is underway to identify specific biomarkers and therapeutic targets for CSU and to enhance management outcomes for patients experiencing involuntary, recurrent swelling. By understanding the interaction between autoantibodies and mast cells in this context, clinicians are able to learn more about the pathophysiology, as well as design individualized interventions, thus improving patients' quality of life (Figure 8.10).

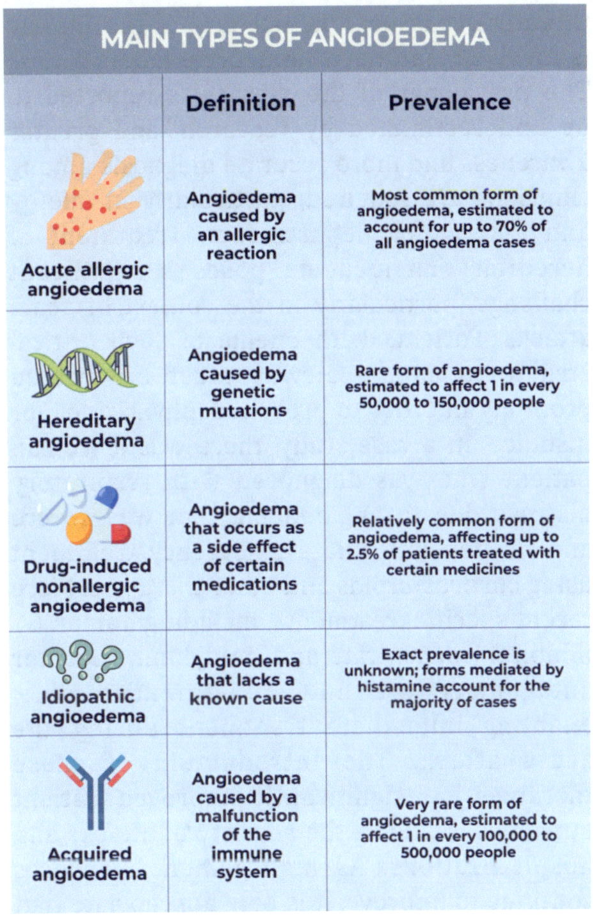

MAIN TYPES OF ANGIOEDEMA

	Definition	Prevalence
Acute allergic angioedema	Angioedema caused by an allergic reaction	Most common form of angioedema, estimated to account for up to 70% of all angioedema cases
Hereditary angioedema	Angioedema caused by genetic mutations	Rare form of angioedema, estimated to affect 1 in every 50,000 to 150,000 people
Drug-induced nonallergic angioedema	Angioedema that occurs as a side effect of certain medications	Relatively common form of angioedema, affecting up to 2.5% of patients treated with certain medicines
Idiopathic angioedema	Angioedema that lacks a known cause	Exact prevalence is unknown; forms mediated by histamine account for the majority of cases
Acquired angioedema	Angioedema caused by a malfunction of the immune system	Very rare form of angioedema, estimated to affect 1 in every 100,000 to 500,000 people

Figure 8.10. Types of angioedema.

Source: https://angioedemanews.com/wp-content/uploads/2025/03/MAIN-TYPES-OF-ANGIOE-768x1152.png.

8.3.1. Hereditary Angioedema (HAE)

HAE is an inherited disorder with recurrent episodes of severe swelling, usually of the extremities, the gastrointestinal tract, and the airway. This disorder is primarily the result of a deficiency or dysfunction of the C1 inhibitor, a protein that plays a critical role in regulating the complement and contact activation pathways. Deficiency or dysfunction of this inhibitor results in elevated bradykinin concentrations, a peptide that causes much of the vascular permeability and edema defining the disorder. Patients with HAE often have life-threatening issues, particularly if the airway is involved, and need immediate medical care. The prevalence of the disease is reported to be underestimated by research, and greater awareness and more accurate diagnosis among clinicians are required, particularly in allergy and emergency departments. Treatment of hereditary angioedema poses a significant challenge, particularly in the context of acute attacks. Patients with edema of such critical structures as the airway must be treated promptly in order to prevent asphyxiation. For instance, in a case study, there was a woman patient who was diagnosed with respiratory distress due to angioedema that was severe and needed immediate emergency treatment using corticosteroids and other therapies. More recent specific treatments, including human C1 inhibitor concentrate and bradykinin receptor antagonists, are now self-administerable, enabling immediate treatment during the acute attack. The introduction of these therapies has significantly improved patient outcomes, reducing the severity of attacks and hospitalizations. As management measures continue to improve, it is only appropriate that patients and doctors remain informed about new therapies and procedures for HAE. The pathophysiology of hereditary angioedema is closely linked to the immune system and, in particular, involves molecular mechanisms related to mast cell activation. There is recent evidence pointing to an overlap between HAE and CSU, namely through the expression of human β-defensin 2 (HBD2). HBD2 levels have been greater in CSU patients, and ongoing research is examining whether it can serve as a biomarker for isolated angioedema. This indicates that HBD2 is significant in mast cell degranulation and subsequent symptoms in HAE. Investigation of these molecular mechanisms will enhance the pathophysiology of hereditary angioedema and potentially lead to novel therapeutic approaches. Combined, this avenue of research could provide critical answers to the etiology of angioedema, further elucidating the pathophysiologic connections between each of the mast cell-related disorders, as well as optimizing treatment paradigms in the clinical setting (Figure 8.11).

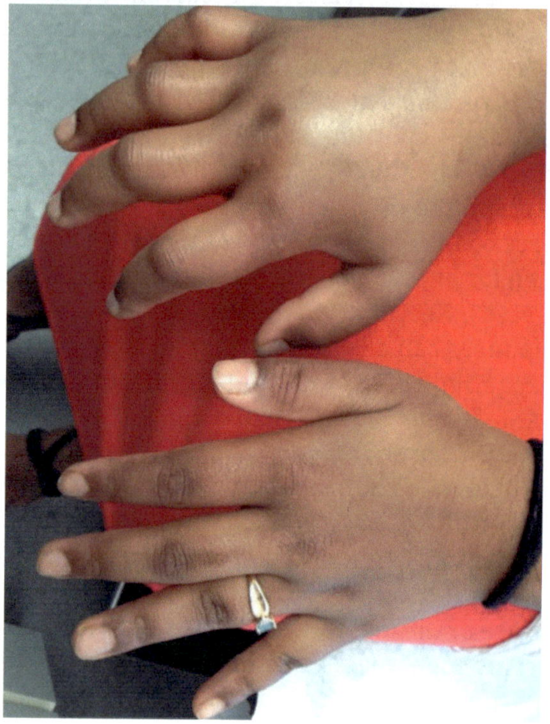

Figure 8.11. Hereditary angioedema (HAE).

Source: https://media.springernature.com/full/springer-static/image/art%3A10.1186%2Fs13223-018-0288-z/MediaObjects/13223_2018_288_Fig4_HTML.jpg?as=webp.

8.3.2. Acquired Angioedema

Acquired angioedema is a significant subgroup of angioedema, characterized by edema of the superficial layers of the skin, typically without associated urticaria. In contrast to hereditary angioedema, which is due to a predisposing genetic component, acquired angioedema typically results from other causative conditions or environmental exposures, such as certain drugs, infections, or autoimmune disease. This condition may arise acutely in adulthood, producing painful attacks that significantly impair quality of life. The pathogenesis of the condition is usually mast cell activation and the release of vasoactive mediators, as well as multifaceted interactions between the immune system and the environment, leading to the development of acquired angioedema symptoms. Understanding these mechanisms is essential for proper diagnosis and treatment of this multicausal disorder in the context of mast cell disorders. Proper classification of acquired angioedema directs treatment. Clinically, the condition can be divided by its causes, the most common of which are medication-induced angioedema, most commonly due to angiotensin-converting enzyme (ACE) inhibitors, and autoimmune diseases, in which excessive immune activity may trigger tissue swelling episodes. Different triggers necessitate different therapies; for instance, patients with angioedema as a side effect of an ACE inhibitor may require a different antihypertensive drug. The emergent nature of some episodes, especially those with laryngeal edema, necessitates careful knowledge of patient histories for effective diagnosis and intervention. By acknowledging the varied etiologies of acquired angioedema, healthcare providers are better able to apply treatment protocols that address the symptoms and etiologies to achieve the best patient outcomes. Treatment of acquired angioedema is generally multidisciplinary and involves allergists, immunologists, and primary care physicians. Combination of various therapeutic modalities is central to the treatment of the multifactorial nature of the disorder. The treatments range from the administration of antihistamines and corticosteroids to more complex therapy like the employment of monoclonal antibodies targeting certain immune mechanisms. Further, patient education about potential precipitants, such as food or drug-related precipitants, raises awareness and allows the individual to manage the condition successfully. Since acquired angioedema remains common in the population, additional effort to advance its pathophysiology and optimal management is warranted. Use of treatment options as per the latest clinical guidelines gives practitioners the best information to treat patients effectively and avoid the negative side effects associated with this complex disorder. The updated worldwide guidelines for urticaria and angioedema provide a platform to address the challenges posed by these disorders, thereby helping clinicians deliver high-quality care to affected individuals (Zuberbier et al., 2021) (Figure 8.12).

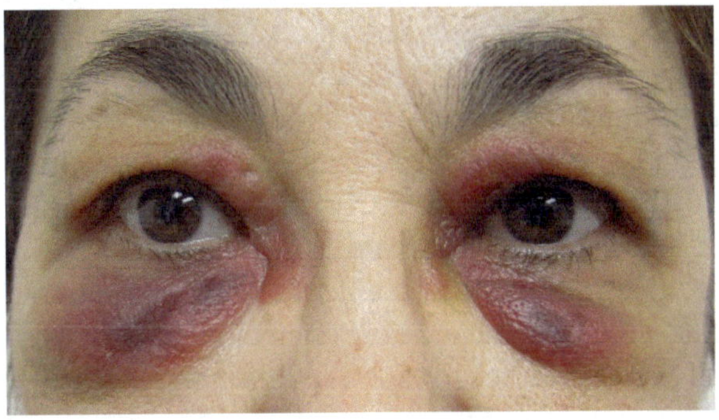

Figure 8.12. Acquired angioedema.

Source: https://www.google.com/url?sa=i&url=https%3A%2F%2Fcommunity.the-hospitalist.org%2Fcontent%2Fatypical-presentation-acquired-angioedema&psig=AOvVaw2QNi0vy2zvFRiK0qpNFqRm&ust=1751196861337000&source=images&cd=vfe&opi=89978449&ved=0CBQQjRxqFwoTCNiFz6iJlI4DFQAAAAAdAAAAABAE.

8.3.3. Drug-Induced Angioedema

In drug-induced angioedema, knowledge of the mechanisms and potential causes is essential for effective management of patients. Angioedema, which is associated with the rapid swelling of the deeper skin layers, is often associated with the consumption of some drugs. ACE inhibitors, non-steroidal anti-inflammatory drugs (NSAIDs), and penicillin are some of the culprits. Pharmacological activity of the drug may induce allergic reactions or inflammatory processes, leading to the release of bradykinin and histamine, both being key mediators of the syndrome of angioedema. History of allergic or genetic predisposition, such as certain patient-related genetic polymorphisms, may predispose to drug-induced angioedema. These cases underscore the importance of health care providers remaining vigilant for early signs and conducting thorough drug history intake in affected individuals. Drug-induced angioedema's causal link with autoimmune conditions also increases the difficulty in diagnosis and treatment. A recent study emphasizes the association between drug-induced angioedema and autoimmune/inflammatory syndrome induced by adjuvants (ASIA), which can follow certain vaccines or implants, particularly in women (Fomina et al., 2025). This condition can exist in the form of intermittent episodes of angioedema necessitating a check for environmental as well as genetic factors responsible for predisposing the patient to such an event. Clinicians must bear in mind the possibility of polypharmacy while treating patients with autoimmune disorders since multiple medications can predispose to angioedema. It is important to understand drug induction-autoimmunity interaction to develop treatment regimens that minimize patient risk and manage symptoms effectively. Because of the subtlety of drug induced angioedema, effective management methods need to be employed so as to prevent severe reactions. Patients experiencing recurrent angioedema should be instructed about potential precipitating factors and the avoidance of specific medications. A combination of antihistamines and, if needed, corticosteroids would be the usual first-line management to treat acute symptoms. According to more recent literature, chronic urticaria and angioedema have been reported to overlap, so diagnosing with caution is key to distinguishing between these disorders and guiding appropriate therapeutic approaches (Ensina et al., 2022). Moreover, other therapies, including monoclonal antibodies, have shown to be effective treatments in refractory cases. These developments underscore the importance of continued research to refine management guidelines and improve outcomes in drug-induced angioedema (Figure 8.13).

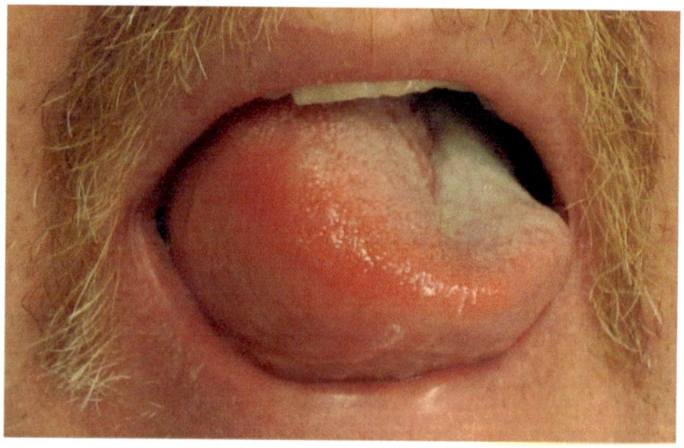

Figure 8.13. Angiotensin-converting enzyme (ACE) inhibitor-induced angioedema.

Source: https://emottawablog.com/wp-content/uploads/2022/11/Angioedema2013-1080x675.jpg.

Test Your Knowledge

1. What Is Hereditary Angioedema (HAE)?
2. Which class of medication is commonly used as a first-line treatment for acquired angioedema?

8.4. Mastocytosis Overview

Learning Outcome

1. Understand the definition and classification of mastocytosis
2. Know the symptoms and clinical presentation of mastocytosis
3. Describe the diagnosis and testing methods for mastocytosis

Mastocytosis is a rare hematological disorder characterized by an abnormal increase and accumulation of mast cells in numerous tissues, including the skin, bone marrow, and gastrointestinal tract. It creates serious clinical challenges because mast cells play a major role in allergic reactions following the release of histamine and other mediators. Patients with mastocytosis may present with a range of symptoms, from skin involvement such as urticaria pigmentosa to systemic involvement such as anaphylaxis. Mastocytosis is classified into cutaneous and systemic forms, with systemic being more severe due to its potential for involvement of multiple organ systems. Understanding the mechanisms of mast cell activation and regulation is not only critical for the diagnosis of mastocytosis but also for the development of effective therapy tailored to individual patient needs to improve their quality of life. The significance of allergic skin conditions was made apparent in the recent past, and mastocytosis is one such disorder that is used to illustrate the finesse of mast cell activity versus more universal immunological reactions. As defined, the skin is the largest organ and an important moderator of many physiological functions; malfunction of mast cells can lead to significant breakdowns in skin integrity and overall health (Wedi, 2021). Mastocytosis becomes crucial to address since it has the capacity to escalate allergic disorders. For instance, the presence of mast cells in the skin can cause chronic urticaria and angioedema to cause recurring manifestations that significantly compromise a patient's quality of life. The distinctive pathophysiology present in mastocytosis provides the possibility for new therapeutic strategies that include monoclonal antibodies and small molecules that target specific pathways utilized in the proliferation and activation of the mast cells. In addition, emerging evidence indicates a complex interrelationship between parasitic infections, including helminth infections, and mast cell responses. The immune response to infection with, for example, Taenia solium has been associated with elevated levels of IgE and tissue eosinophilia, which may, in turn, affect mast cell activity (Minciullo et al., 2016). Such interaction can potentially explain the mechanisms underlying mastocytosis and allergic disease. Unraveling these interactions has the potential to offer important insights into the etiology of allergic reactions, thereby helping to clarify the intricate interplay among mastocytosis, urticaria, and angioedema. By further unraveling this dynamic interaction, researchers can create knowledge gaps visible and bring forward new therapeutic maneuvers aimed at both the pathologic origins of mastocytosis and its resulting allergic aftermath (Figure 8.14).

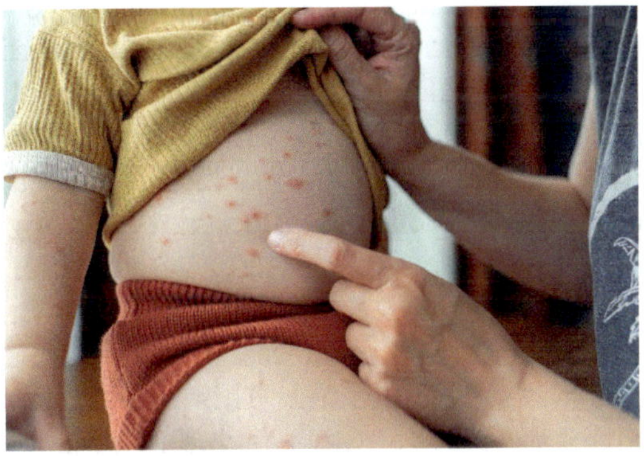

Figure 8.14. Understanding mastocytosis.

Source: https://www.health.com/thmb/yyDs486proYxnT3RbTftVAnOvNE=/6000x0/filters:no_upscale():max_bytes(150000):strip_icc()/mastocytosis-GettyImages-1478102214-6f06a30042304819bb7530b0a4530dfa.jpg.

8.4.1. Definition and Classification

Urticaria, or hives, is a frequent dermatologic condition defined as an acute onset of wheals, which are itchy, raised welts on the skin. The condition occurs in patients of any age, and its classification is important in understanding its various presentations. Urticaria is also broadly classified as acute or chronic, the former lasting less than six weeks and the latter six weeks or more. Chronic urticaria can again be divided into spontaneous and inducible, the former being triggered by some stimuli such as pressure, temperature, or physical exertion. Being aware of these subtypes is important for effective diagnosis and management, as the pathophysiology and clinical considerations can differ across urticaria subtypes (Brehler et al., 2023). Angioedema, usually associated with urticaria, is also an important component of these mast cell-related disorders. It is characterized by edema of the deeper tissues of the skin and can affect any area, such as the face, neck, and gastrointestinal tract. Correct classification of angioedema is important because it can be caused due to allergic reactions, hereditary factors, or acquired factors. Allergic angioedema versus non-allergic conditions must be differentiated as this determines the outcome of treatment directly. The intervention by international consensus bodies, including the European Academy of Allergology and Clinical Immunology, emphasizes the need to understand the classification and etiology of angioedema to guide treatment (Zuberbier et al., 2021). Besides this, mastocytosis, which refers to abnormal mast cell growth, also has issues with classification. This condition can occur in a variety of ways, including cutaneous mastocytosis, which is primarily limited to the skin, and systemic mastocytosis, in which mast cells have spread all over the body. The difference between the two forms is essential, especially in children, where they may have a milder form or be misdiagnosed as other conditions like urticaria. For example, maculopapular mastocytosis may mimic chronic urticaria, but important distinguishing features include the longevity of macules versus the fleeting nature of urticarial wheals. Accurate classification and awareness of mastocytosis enable appropriate management strategies and improved patient outcomes (Brehler et al., 2023) (Figure 8.15).

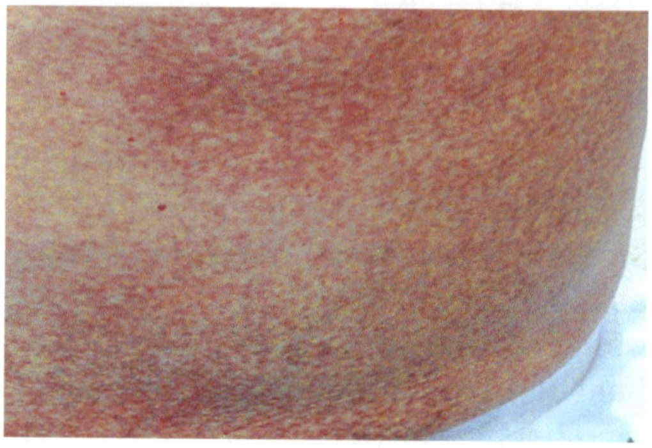

Figure 8.15. Systemic mastocytosis.

Source: https://my.clevelandclinic.org/-/scassets/Images/org/health/articles/24386-systemic-mastocytosis.

8.4.2. Symptoms and Clinical Presentation

Urticaria, or hives, are pruritic, elevated welts on the skin that are typically acute or chronic in duration. The lesions are typically of variable size and may change shape and position over hours. In most cases, urticaria is secondary to mast cell degranulation that results in the release of histamine and other pro-inflammatory mediators. The patients will not only have the physical symptoms but also, in most instances, the psychological impact of frequent recurrence, such as that for anxiety or sleep. Moreover, the distinction between spontaneous chronic urticaria and chronic inducible urticaria—due to stimuli such as pressure, heat, or exercise—complicates the clinical situation. Because urticaria can be an overlapping symptom, a detailed patient history is critically important for identifying specific triggers and shaping appropriate management protocols. Angioedema, characterized by severe swelling in the deeper dermis of the skin, typically occurs concomitantly with urticaria but can also occur independently. The condition most commonly manifests in the face, lips, tongue, and airways, potentially resulting in obstruction of the airway, a life-threatening situation. The etiology ranges from allergic responses to hereditary angioedema (HAE), in which patients experience periodic, profound edema due to an inherited deficiency of C1 esterase inhibitor. Interestingly, symptom burden in hereditary instances has unique features, with attacks potentially being without prior urticaria and often indistinguishable from other presentations of angioedema, and diagnosis is further made difficult. Recognition of these nuances in presentation helps doctors to ideally individualize treatment regimens and enhance patient outcomes, particularly in emergency department settings where timely assessment is critical (Kamran et al., 2024). Mastocytosis, a rare overabundance disease of mast cells, can manifest in various ways based on the extent of mast cell infiltration in organs. Flush, abdominal cramp, and anaphylactic attack have been reported to occur as symptoms, typically due to the discharge of mediators from mast cells. The patient with mastocytosis is also likely to show signs that coincide with urticaria and angioedema, thus posing a challenge in differential diagnosis. Furthermore, indolent and aggressive forms of the disease can present differently, affecting treatment. For instance, patients with indolent mastocytosis can present with spontaneous urticaria or angioedema, and this will require a multidisciplinary management plan. Innovations in treatment, including the use of corticosteroids and antihistamines during acute episodes, have been promising, highlighting the importance of comprehensive clinical evaluations to identify the most effective treatment strategies (Radojicic et al., 2024) (Figure 8.16).

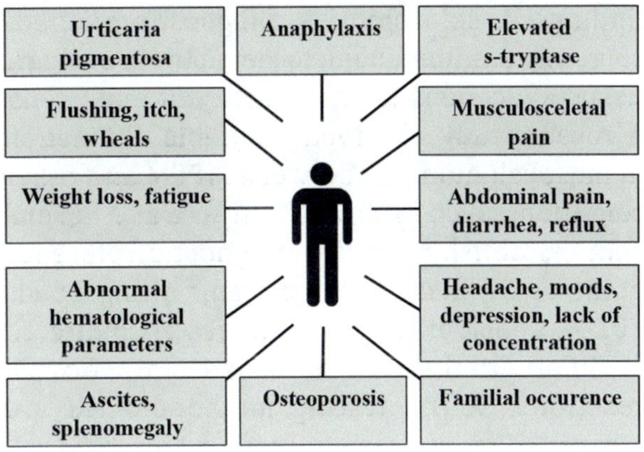

Figure 8.16. Various clinical presentations of mastocytosis.

Source: https://www.medicaljournals.se/acta/content_files/files/web/4613-web-resources/image/10705.png.

8.4.3. Diagnosis and Testing Methods

Diagnosis of urticaria, angioedema, and mastocytosis is accurate when integrating clinical assessment with targeted testing strategies. The first clinical assessment typically includes a comprehensive patient history of the onset, duration, and precipitants of the symptoms. In chronic urticaria, physicians tend to differentiate between chronic idiopathic urticaria (CIU) and chronic inducible urticaria (CIndU) based on symptomatology and triggers. The presence of angioedema can complicate diagnosis, where an enquiry into possible underlying causes or allergy is indicated. Additionally, based on a study of children whose laboratory evaluations did not reveal any significant clinical differences between the patient groups with positive and negative SPT results, the utility of such tests must be questioned. A more individualized diagnostic approach is required, integrating findings with presentation for better patient management (Erbay et al., 2025). Diagnosis in mastocytosis, particularly maculopapular cutaneous mastocytosis (MPCM), is also hampered by the subtlety of the histologic findings in skin biopsies. Diagnostic methods currently use immunohistochemistry to evaluate tissue specimens for the density of mast cells. A recent study observed a notable distinction in mast cell numbers between MPCM and other conditions, such as chronic urticaria and normal skin, establishing a key diagnostic reference point of 66 mast cells per mm^2 (King et al., 2024). Considering the subtleties encountered in differentiating mastocytosis from urticarial reactions, sound testing methodologies are essential. Use of digital microscopy for mast cell counting enhances diagnostic accuracy and may streamline clinical decision-making. As research continues, the possibility of computer-aided computations of cellular density may further refine diagnostic criteria and their application in clinical practice. Effective management of urticaria, angioedema, and mastocytosis necessitates the use of a multifaceted system of diagnosis. This approach integrates clinical assessment, cutaneous testing, and laboratory testing, all appropriate to the patient's history and presentation. For instance, while SPTs may not be feasible for all presentations of children with chronic urticaria, incorporating serologic testing, such as immunoglobulin E levels and thyroid function tests, can provide valuable information regarding atopic conditions underlying chronic urticaria (Erbay et al., 2025). In addition, the presence of co-morbid disorders, including infections or allergies, can reveal patterns to assist in designing successful treatment regimens. Lastly, encouraging collaborative discussion between allergy and immunology specialties will enhance diagnostic acuity, potentially leading to more accurate therapeutic modalities that address the subtleties of these disorders (Figure 8.17).

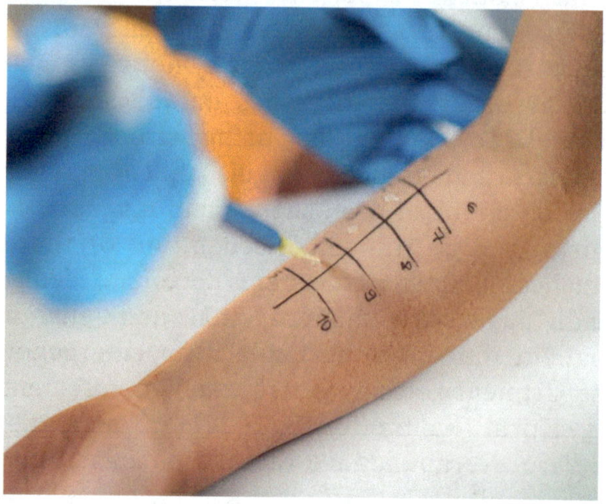

Figure 8.17. Skin prick testing.

Source: https://www.imc-healthcare.com/wp-content/uploads/2022/12/imc-skin-prick-allergy-testing.jpg.

Test Your Knowledge

1. Indolent mastocytosis is most commonly managed using which treatment?
2. What threshold of mast cells per mm^2 has been established as a diagnostic benchmark for MPCM?

8.5. Treatment Options

Learning Outcome

1. Utilize the antihistamines and corticosteroids for the management of urticaria and angioedema
2. Avoid triggers in managing urticaria, angioedema, and mastocytosis
3. Emerging therapies and research for various allergic conditions

The management of urticaria, angioedema, and mastocytosis typically involves a multidimensional approach to address both symptoms and underlying causes. Antihistamines are the initial treatment of choice in the majority of chronic urticaria patients. Non-sedating antihistamines such as cetirizine or loratadine relieve swelling and itching without causing sleepiness and thus can be used long-term. In severe cases, if antihistamines fail, dermatologists consider corticosteroids or omalizumab, a monoclonal antibody. Omalizumab acts by blocking the IgE-mediated pathways, providing huge relief to patients with chronic spontaneous urticaria, particularly when other traditional therapies have failed. The autoimmune pathophysiology of the disease, as explained by such research as that by ASIA, mirrors the complexity of treatment approaches, in particular, that some patients are able to benefit from a personalized immunomodulatory therapy (Fomina et al., 2025). Treatment protocols for angioedema are determined by the disease's pathophysiology. Allergic angioedema patients must avoid known precipitating factors, with the use of antihistamines to manage acute attacks. In hereditary angioedema, precipitating drugs such as C1-inhibitor concentrates or bradykinin receptor antagonists can safely be used to prevent attacks. Identification of precipitating factors should precipitate the use of prophylactic therapy in patients with frequent angioedema attacks. The intricate relationship between genetic propensities and angioedema underscores the importance of tailored treatment measures, which may also include genetic testing to anticipate potential autoimmune responses (Fomina et al., 2025). This is a shift from prophylactic to reactive management in treating angioedema.

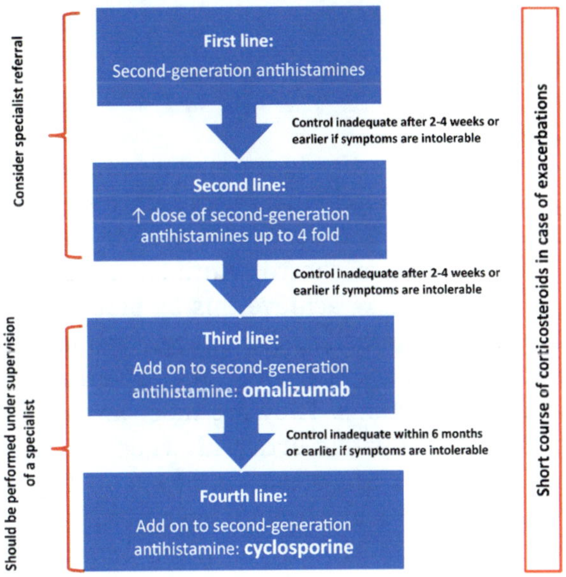

Figure 8.18. Simplified stepwise algorithm for the treatment of urticaria.

Source: https://media.springernature.com/full/springer-static/image/art%3A10.1186%2Fs13223-018-0288-z/MediaObjects/13223_2018_288_Fig3_HTML.png?as=webp.

Mastocytosis treatment is also highly individualized, as the conditions manifest differently. Antihistamine therapy may be utilized in the treatment of patients, as in the case of angioedema and urticaria, for symptom control resulting from mast cell degranulation. Moreover, new therapies such as tyrosine kinase inhibitors can be explored in patients with severe presentation of systemic mastocytosis. Omalizumab has recently been established to be useful, with its potential role in preventing symptoms of mastocytosis through interference with the complex signaling pathway of mast cell function. The application of genetic screening to identify susceptibility to autoimmune syndromes has begun to pave the way for novel therapeutic strategies. This brings into focus an integrated treatment plan that not only provides relief from symptoms but also personalizes interventions based on the patient's genetic profile and clinical presentation (Figure 8.18).

8.5.1. Antihistamines and Corticosteroids

Management of urticaria and angioedema usually involves a multidisciplinary approach, using both antihistamines and corticosteroids to achieve optimal symptom control. Antihistamines, the preferred therapy, achieve this by blocking H1 receptors responsible for allergic responses, thus abolishing the itch and swelling of urticarial reactions. They are most impressive in chronic idiopathic urticaria, when standard antihistamines are often employed in higher doses to achieve adequate symptom relief. Corticosteroids are useful when immediate management of severe symptoms is warranted. These anti-inflammatory agents can very quickly dampen the enormous inflammatory response that occurs in acute urticaria and angioedema, thereby becoming invaluable in emergency cases. The timely and correct use of these drugs can significantly improve the patient's quality of life. Present-day clinical experience favors a combination regimen of antihistamines and corticosteroids to achieve optimal results in acute urticaria and angioedema. In a comparison of treatment outcomes in patients treated with antihistamines alone with those in patients treated with antihistamines and corticosteroids, a notable difference in symptom resolution time was found. In particular, the group receiving the combination therapy improved in symptom resolution, with an average of 3.6 hours, compared with 5.1 hours for the group receiving only antihistamines (Kamran et al., 2024). This finding underscores that corticosteroids not only hasten symptom improvement but also result in fewer instances of relapse and fewer requirements for hospitalization, marking them as an important adjunct to treatment regimens for severe urticaria and angioedema manifestations. The manner in which these agents interact with patient variables, including those of surgical intervention, is also critical to consider. For instance, a 44-year-old female patient with chronic idiopathic urticaria post-surgery demonstrated the complex interactions between hormonal changes and urticarial exacerbations (Al-Saedy et al., 2025). This case demonstrates the imperative of an adaptable treatment protocol that exposes patients to varying doses or regimens of antihistamines and corticosteroids as they navigate the complexity of their illnesses. The therapeutic decisions in such cases should also be guided by ongoing investigation into hormonal and immunological factors that may influence treatment efficacy. Therefore, a thorough understanding of the pharmacodynamics of antihistamines and corticosteroids can lead to improved patient care and management of urticaria, angioedema, and mastocytosis in humans (Figure 8.19).

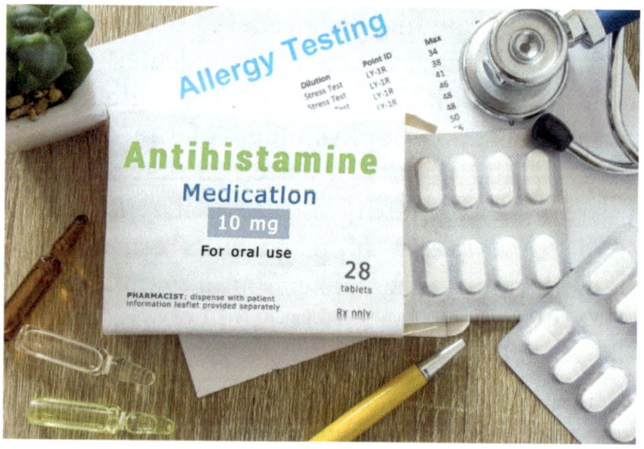

Figure 8.19. Antihistamine medicine.

Source: https://www.pharmathirdpartymanufacturer.com/wp-content/uploads/2020/07/Antihistamine-Medicine-Manufacturers-in-India-1024x683-1.jpg.

8.5.2. Avoidance of Triggers

Triggers avoidance is the core of the management of urticaria, angioedema, and mastocytosis, as exposure to some stimuli may worsen the symptoms and lead to life-threatening reactions. In most instances, patients need to develop a very cautious approach to identifying and avoiding potential triggers, including allergens, environmental exposures, and certain drugs. In mastocytosis, for instance, individuals are particularly susceptible to numerous causative agents due to the dysregulation of mast cell proliferation. In treating such individuals, avoidance of known allergens, e.g., shellfish, nuts, and insect bites, as are characteristically associated with allergic reactions, may be among the interventions. Environmental provocation, such as alterations in temperature, stress, and even certain forms of physical activity, may also act as causative factors in exacerbation. Therefore, it is very important to have a clear understanding of personal triggers to manage the disease appropriately and prevent symptom exacerbation (Marchaj et al., 2024). In diseases like aquagenic urticaria, avoidance is an even greater challenge because the trigger is intrinsic: exposure to water. The patients with this extremely rare form of urticaria need to be cautious when performing routine tasks since even brief exposure to water results in marked discomfort. Treatment strategies for aquagenic urticaria involve symptomatic management, such as antihistamines and the application of barrier creams prior to water exposure, but avoidance is the keystone of treatment. Good management by healthcare professionals is essential in such cases to individualize treatment plans, considering the patient's lifestyle and the inevitable nature of some triggers, such as water. Thus, symptom management and trigger avoidance need to be balanced to enhance the quality of life for patients with this condition (Jaabouti et al., 2023). Trigger-specific educational programs are essential in maximizing patient education and self-management interventions. Knowledge of what precipitates symptoms gives patients power, enabling them to take preventive action that leads to improved health. Health care providers need to help patients develop individualized avoidance plans so that individuals know their specific triggers and take action to avoid them. With a partnership model, patients can learn to navigate their environment safely, avoid triggers, and manage conditions more effectively. As research continues to uncover the complexities of conditions such as mastocytosis, ongoing education on trigger avoidance can be a valuable approach to reducing symptoms and enhancing overall health in patients (Marchaj et al., 2024).

8.5.3. Emerging Therapies and Research

Recent therapies and research are rapidly transforming the treatment landscape for conditions such as urticaria, angioedema, and mastocytosis. Biologic medications constitute a key advancement in the therapeutic management of severe allergic diseases. They target specific immune processes, namely type 2 inflammation-promoting mechanisms, which are mediated by the IL-4, IL-5, and IL-13 cytokines. Recent advances have focused on biologics that inhibit alarmins such as TSLP and IL-33. While these agents offer considerable benefits to nonresponsive patients, their high costs and potential long-term safety concerns are major barriers to wide use. Advances in ultra-long-acting treatments, bispecific antibodies, and digital health technologies to support home monitoring also foretell a future in which personalized care can be made more accessible and effective (Alska et al., 2025). Chronic spontaneous urticaria (CSU) is the best example of the need for new treatments, particularly in those patients who do not adequately respond to second-generation H1-antihistamines. According to current guidelines, one of the first-step strategies is increasing antihistamine dosing, but this is not effective for everyone. Therefore, omalizumab has been established as a cornerstone of CSU treatment, as it is definitively effective in the majority of affected patients. But still, there remains a subpopulation of patients who remain refractory, which has led scientists to look for alternative therapies. New drugs targeting Bruton's tyrosine kinase (BTK), such as remibrutinib, and those that target the Mas-related G protein-coupled receptor X2 (MRGPRX2) have the potential to reverse mast cell activation. These novel strategies represent a paradigm shift in how CSU can be addressed, emphasizing the need for targeted treatments that target underlying pathophysiologic processes (Asero et al., 2024). Further research into therapeutic options for mastocytosis also highlights the widening reach of available treatment. The rare condition, in which mast cells aggregate within tissues, often leads to highly debilitating symptoms like flushing, pruritus, and gastrointestinal distress. Ongoing research is investigating inhibitors of the tyrosine kinase receptor Kit, holding the promise of a patient-specific treatment for patients with significant symptoms. Additionally, the application of biologics like dupilumab that target the IL-4 and IL-13 pathways is investigated to determine if they can potentially decrease symptoms of mastocytosis. As studies progress, knowledge of the diverse roles of mast cells in mastocytosis and urticaria will become critical to the development of targeted therapies that improve patient outcomes. Collectively, these new treatments promise greater efficient measures in the field of allergic and mast cell disorders, with the potential for future treatment breakthroughs (Asero et al., 2024) (Figure 8.20).

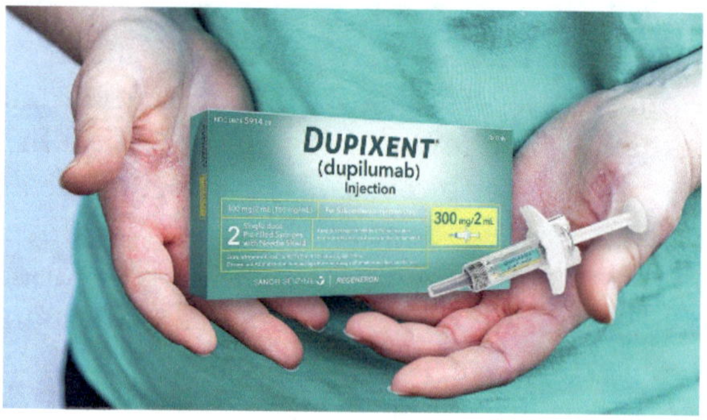

Figure 8.20. Biologic therapy Dupixent (dupilumab) approved for urticaria and mastocytosis.

Source: https://assets.medpagetoday.net/media/images/103xxx/103088.jpg.

Test Your Knowledge

1. What is the primary mechanism of action for antihistamines in the treatment of urticaria?
2. Which environmental factor is a common trigger for mastocytosis?

8.6. Impact on Quality of Life

Learning Outcome

1. Know the psychological effects of various allergic conditions
2. Understand the social implications of urticaria, angioedema, and mastocytosis
3. Describe the management strategies for urticaria, angioedema, and mastocytosis

The effect of conditions like urticaria, angioedema, and mastocytosis on a patient's quality of life is immense and complex. Patients with these mast cell disorders often have not only physical complaints but also vast emotional and psychological burdens. Repeated, chronic symptoms such as skin lesions, discomfort, and unpredictable bouts may result in social withdrawal and restrictions in engaging in daily life activities. Research indicates that chronic urticaria possesses the disabling ability to compromise quality of life as well as work or school performance. This concern about potential breaks significantly detracts from overall well-being for most patients, making control over such conditions essential for boosting life satisfaction. In addition, psychological effects that accompany chronic skin disorders should not be downplayed. These patients experience increased anxiety and depression compared to the overall population. The visible external signs and sometimes warning features of their illnesses, i.e., wheals and swelling, trigger concern and result in self-consciousness and stigmatization. This social suffering combines with the challenge of physical signs and creates a vicious cycle that compromises mental well-being. Importantly, the treatment of such conditions could be multisided in nature, and not only the alleviation of physical symptoms, but also ensuring psychological support (Ujiie et al., 2022). Current evidence is in favor of introducing psychological care into treatment planning that can significantly enhance patients' overall quality of life and help in dealing with emotional distress. Lastly, the type of treatment for these conditions may even exacerbate the effect on quality of life. Along with the developments in the treatments, the patients are bombarded with side effects from these treatments, which may include systemic immunosuppression, which leads to other complications (Ujiie et al., 2022). This creates a scenario where possible relief of the symptoms has the potential of leading to more health issues, amounting to a humongous treatment burden." Additionally, the uncertainty about the development of symptoms and reactions to treatments leads to further frustration and helplessness in patients. Therefore, it is necessary to promote cooperation between patients and healthcare professionals through customized management plans and consistent communication. It not only hinders more effective treatment options but also empowers the patient to a great extent, greatly enhancing their quality of life despite the problems caused by their conditions.

8.6.1. Psychological Effects

The psychological effects of conditions such as urticaria, angioedema, and mastocytosis go well beyond the physical aspects typically associated with these conditions. Patients often experience intense psychological distress, which may be manifest in the forms of depression, anxiety, and social withdrawal. The physical signs, like skin rashes and swelling, can lead to body image problems and detract from self-esteem, also complicating mental health. Some of this psychological burden may be alleviated through treatments for the physical symptoms, but the emotional and mental health aspects require the same amount of attention as well. By understanding the bidirectional impact of such diseases on mental and physical well-being, medical professionals can adopt a more holistic approach to treatment. Research indicates that patients with mastocytosis, for instance, undergo a plethora of changes in cognition and neuropsychiatry. A systematic review indicated that a significant proportion of mastocytosis patients are faced with issues such as cognitive impairment, anxiety, and excessive stress, which affect their lifestyles to a significant degree. Specifically, studies have shown that between 68% and 75% of the patients are depressed, and approximately 27%–54% report anxiety or irritability. These psychological issues can interfere not only with the emotional recovery of patients but also with their social adaptation and vocational performance.

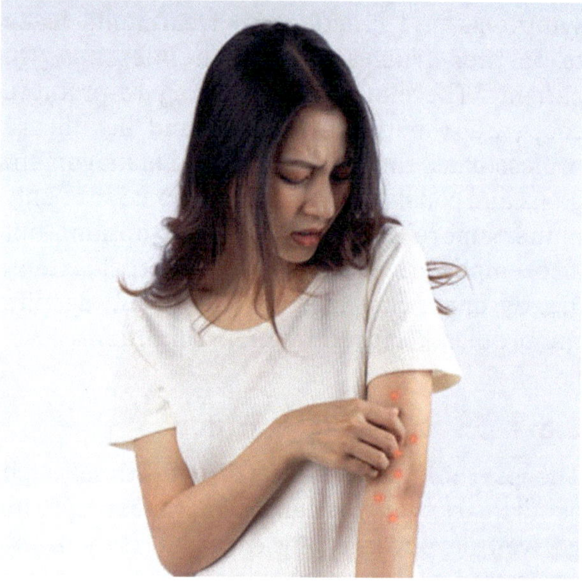

Figure 8.21. Psychological effects of urticaria.

Source: https://24-7medcare.com.au/wp-content/uploads/2021/06/iStock-1324674436-724x400.jpg.

Hence, provision for mental health care should be included in treatment programs to make up for these universal psychological issues. Moreover, the impact of chronic diseases like urticaria and mastocytosis might involve complexities in psychological functioning that require further investigation. Neuroimaging studies show that certain cognitive and attention issues could be related to underlying neurological changes in such patients. There has also been a reported incidence of neurodevelopmental disorders, particularly in children, which is clearly reflective of the importance of early recognition and intervention. The findings highlight the need for comprehensive healthcare practices that include both psychological and neurological evaluations. Efficient management of these psychological effects not only enhances patients' quality of life but also fosters resilience, thereby strengthening coping mechanisms among people with such chronic ailments (Sagües-Sesé et al., 2023; Kou et al., 2024) (Figure 8.21).

8.6.2. Social Implications

The social consequences of urticaria, angioedema, and mastocytosis are wide-ranging, affecting the lives of affected individuals at personal, familial, and societal levels. These patients become withdrawn and anxious due to the reasons of their unpredictability and risk of severity. The fear of an acute attack at any moment, similar to anaphylaxis, which may arise suddenly and prove to be life-threatening, is responsible for social withdrawal. They get disturbed in their everyday life. When individuals are unable to engage in social activities such as family meetings or social gatherings due to fear of allergic reactions, this compromises their sense of belonging and connection. Exclusion of this type not only affects mental health but also tends to strain interpersonal relationships, with friends and family members at times unable to understand the gravity or severity of such conditions, leading to a need for increased public awareness and education about the lived experience of chronic suffering from allergic conditions. Furthermore, the increasing prevalence of food allergies, in particular those that lead to anaphylactic reactions, is a significant social trend that needs serious consideration. Food allergies are a very serious public health concern, with rising incidence rates affecting not only the misery of affected individuals but also broader societal institutions, such as schools, the workplace, and restaurants. In school settings, food allergies necessitate strict practices to protect affected students, typically resulting in modifications to cafeteria lunches and classroom celebrations. These adaptations, being protective though, can be tensing for students and lead to a culture of exclusion for individuals with dietary needs. Considering that anxiety tends to be a comorbid condition, the need for systemic modifications that adapt to affected individuals arises, requiring social efforts to foster inclusivity through education and policy changes in matters pertaining to food safety and allergy control (Valentina D'Aiuto et al., 2024). Healthcare systems are also strained by the social effects of urticaria, angioedema, and mastocytosis. The increasing incidence of the disorders contributes to the increasing cost of healthcare because of the necessity for repeated medical attention and therapy. The cost of diagnostic workups and prompt treatment for anaphylactic episodes can be a barrier to access, particularly among vulnerable populations. This financial cost not only burdens individuals but also stretches public health resources to the point that policymakers must take into account the allocation of funds and services targeted at improving allergic disease management. Additionally, public health efforts must focus on education regarding the prevention of allergies, the identification of allergens, and management approaches to empower patients. Lastly, creating a community that lives with these social impacts will enhance overall health outcomes and quality of life for patients with urticaria, angioedema, and mastocytosis (DuToit et al., 2024).

8.6.3. Management Strategies

Effective management strategies for urticaria, angioedema, and mastocytosis are critical in minimizing symptoms and preventing life-threatening complications. One of the most frequent approaches is the use of antihistamines to counteract the release of histamine in these conditions. Antihistamines can considerably diminish symptoms such as itching and swelling by blocking histamine's action on target cells. Systemic corticosteroids may also be used in acute urticaria or angioedema to reduce inflammation and provide relief quickly. But for those with chronic symptoms, the treatment plan needs to be integrated and incorporate both pharmacologic and non-pharmacologic interventions. This may include the avoidance of established allergens and irritants and lifestyle modifications aimed at stress reduction and overall health well-being. Multi-modal approaches such as these are key in optimizing the quality of life for those suffering from these conditions. Monitoring and patient education are included in comprehensive management plans for mastocytosis, urticaria, and angioedema. Patients must be empowered to recognize the signs and symptoms of their disease, thereby enabling timely interventions and reducing the risk of catastrophic events. Education programs about understanding triggers can enhance patient compliance and encourage proactive interventions. For instance, patients with mastocytosis can be assisted through education on how diet and the environment may exacerbate their condition. Ongoing follow-up with physicians may also enable changes in treatment modalities to address evolving patient needs. According to recent research, validated quality-of-life questionnaires can provide a strong assessment of the impact of these conditions on daily life and guide patients and clinicians alike on optimal management to ensure the highest possible patient satisfaction and outcomes (Agosta et al., 2021). In the case of severe or acute urticaria and angioedema, especially compromising airway stability, emergency treatment is the priority. Expedient therapies such as epinephrine infusion are necessary to prevent anaphylactic attacks. In combination with these treatments, traditional Persian Medicine methods, including bloodletting and hijama, have been explored as complementary treatments. These would seem to alleviate symptoms by restoring balance to the body's inner humors, addressing root system issues that conventional treatments might overlook (Shirazi et al., 2022). The addition of such strategies not only broadens the therapeutic arsenal available to clinicians but also appeals to patients who seek complete and culturally competent alternatives for management. Finally, an individualized and comprehensive management plan involving several modalities is essential for the management of mastocytosis, urticaria, and angioedema (Figure 8.22).

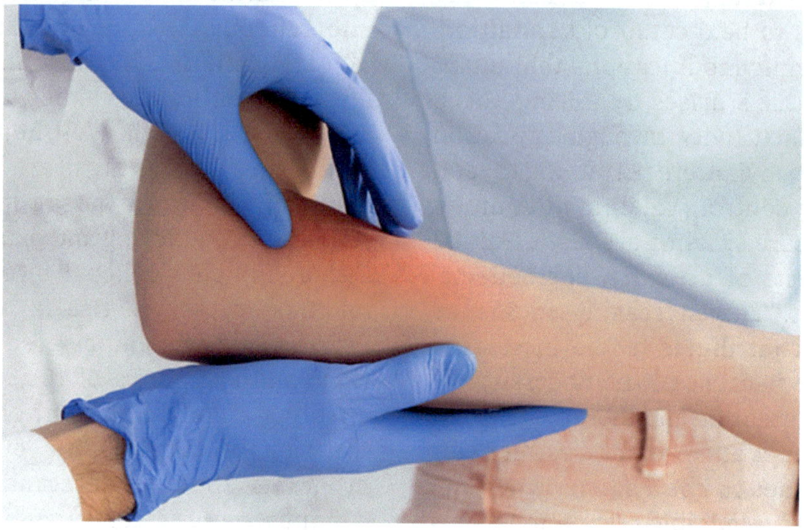

Figure 8.22. Managing chronic urticaria: Treatment strategies.

Source: https://static.wixstatic.com/media/8de7d4_aa8eeaa4b7974fe3afe5403088039533~mv2.png/v1/fill/w_568,h_356,al_c,q_85,usm_0.66_1.00_0.01,enc_avif,quality_auto/8de7d4_aa8eeaa4b7974fe3afe5403088039533~mv2.png.

Test Your Knowledge

1. What are common psychological effects associated with urticaria, angioedema, and mastocytosis?
2. What is a common social consequence experienced by individuals living with urticaria, angioedema, and mastocytosis?

SUMMARY

Generally, studies on urticaria, angioedema, and mastocytosis in human subjects highlight the complex and heterogeneous nature of these diseases at both the physiological level and in patient experience. Chronic spontaneous urticaria (CSU) is also a significant quality of life affector for patients because the majority of patients state that they still have symptoms despite treatment, which creates mental and emotional distress. This highlights the demand for a better understanding of what patients have experienced as evidenced by studies exploring their experiences with these illnesses. Research verifies that there is often a diagnostic delay, which suggests the need for more awareness and education of medical professionals, which can enhance early intervention strategies and management of the disease in general, resulting in better patient outcomes (Migliarino et al., 2025). Furthermore, findings from idiopathic histaminergic angioedema (IH-AAE) research are useful in understanding the natural history of the condition. The retrospective review points to improvement in the majority of patients toward remission in the long term, with a decrease in the frequency of attacks. This means that even though angioedema may be chronic and troublesome, it is largely a self-limiting, benign condition for the majority, with the majority of patients exhibiting a return to normal in a given time frame. Because the intensity of the initial symptoms does not appear to adversely affect long-term results, treatment can be made less sensational, prioritizing symptom relief and quality-of-life enhancement over fear of continued recurrence (Migliarino et al., 2025). While researchers continue to investigate mechanisms and treatment efficacy for these disorders, future research must prioritize patient-centered approaches. Focusing on the necessity of general care that recognizes the physiological and psychosocial characteristics of individuals with urticaria, angioedema, and mastocytosis to tailor interventions is likely to result in effective therapies. Ongoing interaction with patients will shed light on their experiences and needs, promoting creative treatment that augments not only physical well-being but also general well-being. By combining clinical understanding and patient experience, healthcare practitioners can best improve health outcomes for those suffering from these complex disorders and reduce the burden created by delayed diagnosis and ineffective treatment (Weller et al., 2025).

The pathophysiology of urticaria, angioedema, and mastocytosis is defined by complicated interactions between immune cells, histamine release, and innate genetic vulnerabilities. Urticaria, or hives, results when histamine is released from mast cells and produces swelling and inflammation on the skin surface. The reaction is caused by many different factors, such as allergens, drugs, and temperature extremes. Angioedema is a deeper edema of the dermis or subcutaneous tissue that typically accompanies urticaria but can occur on its own. The overlap between mast cell activation and the release of pro-inflammatory mediators is critical to their pathogenesis. While the conditions themselves are normally benign, they have the potential to cause serious morbidity and hence require rigorous understanding and targeted therapy. Mastocytosis, an abnormal accumulation of mast cells in tissues, poses particular challenges for clinical management. This condition may present as either a juvenile or an adult form, depending on the number and activation of mast cells. Symptoms depend on the number and activation of mast cells and include frequent flushing, itching, and secondary anaphylaxis due to histamine hypersecretion, both of which have a marked effect on quality of life. The literature also suggests relevant genetic contributions to the pathogenesis of mastocytosis, including mutations of the KIT gene. Knowledge of the overlap in symptoms with the other mast cell disorders, including urticaria and angioedema, is relevant in the development of appropriate diagnostic criteria. This recognition of the current complex nature of such disorders underscores the need for an interdisciplinary approach, marrying patient history and advanced diagnostic techniques to individualize therapeutic interventions. Treatment of urticaria, angioedema, and mastocytosis often involves the use of histamine receptor antagonists, which relieve symptoms by blocking histamine action. Application of H1 and H2 receptor antagonists has become a standard treatment for these histamine-mediated conditions and leads to marked symptomatic relief. Clinical evidence suggests that combining these antagonists may enhance therapeutic efficacy over monotherapy, especially in multifaceted cases with multiple presentations. Yet, literature demonstrates the existence of a gap for systematic reviews that would better clarify the clinical impact and possible side effects of such combined treatment. As the body of evidence grows, upcoming studies must tackle the process of optimizing treatment regimens without side effects and, finally, produce improved outcomes for the patient in the treatment of urticaria, angioedema, and mastocytosis in human subjects (Kou et al., 2024; Nashrudin et al., 2025).

KEY TERMS FROM THIS CHAPTER

- Acute angioedema
- Bone marrow
- Cytokines
- Genetic mutations
- Hereditary angioedema
- Mast cells
- Plasma proteins
- Angioedema
- Chronic spontaneous urticaria
- Gastrointestinal tract
- Genetic testing
- Histamine
- Mastocytosis
- Serum biomarkers

CRITICAL THINKING QUESTIONS

1. What is the primary feature of urticaria?

a. Persistent scaling plaques

b. Transient wheals or hives associated with pruritus

c. Thickened, lichenified skin

d. Vesicular eruptions on the hands and feet

2. Angioedema typically affects which of the following areas?

a. Epidermis only

b. Deep dermis and subcutaneous tissues

c. Stratum corneum

d. Hair follicles

3. Which of the following is the most common cause of acute urticaria?

a. Autoimmune disorders

b. Viral or bacterial infections

c. Chronic systemic diseases

d. Drug-induced hypersensitivity

4. Chronic urticaria is defined as urticaria lasting for:

a. Less than one week

b. More than six weeks

c. Three months or longer

d. Over a year

5. Which of the following is a hallmark symptom of mastocytosis?

a. Hyperpigmentation

b. Frequent episodes of wheals and flushing

c. Rapid onset of angioedema

d. Persistent scaling lesions

Short Answer Questions

1. What is urticaria?
2. Define angioedema.
3. What is mastocytosis?
4. List the types of urticaria.
5. Name the types of angioedema.

Answer to Critical Thinking Questions

1. (b); 2. (b) ; 3. (b); 4. (b); 5. (b)

REFERENCES

1. Al-Saedy, M., Al-Saedy, S., & Robinson, D. (2025). Recurrent chronic idiopathic urticaria post-hysterectomy and loss of xolair effectiveness: a case report. *Cureus, 17*(4), e81624. https://doi.org/10.7759/cureus.81624Alska, E., Łaszczych, D., Napiórkowska-Baran, K., Szymczak, B., Rajewska, A., Rubisz, A. E., Romaniuk, P., et al. (2025). Advances in biologic therapies for allergic diseases: Current trends, emerging agents, and future perspectives. *Journal of Clinical Medicine, 14*. https://www.semanticscholar.org/paper/136e99243b50a5b838644eb306411a2005ab36e1 (accessed on 21st July 2025).
2. Asero, R., Calzari, P., Vaienti, S., & Cugno, M. (2024). Therapies for chronic spontaneous urticaria: Present and future developments. *Pharmaceuticals, 17*. https://www.semanticscholar.org/paper/71c18c76b263d5673e22ef4f81975cb088dd3bb2 (accessed on 21st July 2025).
3. Brehler, A. C. E., Bauer, A., & Wedi, B. (2023). Urticaria in childhood—What's new? *Allergo Journal International, 32*, 318–325. https://www.semanticscholar.org/paper/95ca5156c8cc4ce11a62c19550c819b97e7d4cf4 (accessed on 21st July 2025).
4. Cao, T. B. T., Cha, H. Y., Yang, E. M., Choi, B., Park, H. S., & Ye, Y. (2021). Serum human β-defensin 2 is increased in angioedema accompanying chronic spontaneous urticaria. *International Archives of Allergy and Immunology, 182*, 1066–1071. https://www.semanticscholar.org/paper/bb1adb826c69b5e8188d1adcdff21c7cbbd75c25 (accessed on 21st July 2025).
5. D'Aiuto, V., Mormile, I., Granata, F., Napolitano, F., Lamagna, L., Della Casa, F., de Paulis, A., et al. (2024). Worldwide heterogeneity of food allergy: Focus on peach allergy in Southern Italy. *Journal of Clinical Medicine, 13*, 3259–3259. https://doi.org/10.3390/jcm13113259 (accessed on 21st July 2025).
6. Di Agosta, E., Salvati, L., Corazza, M., Baiardini, I., Ambrogio, F., Angileri, L., Antonelli, E., et al. (2021). Quality of life in patients with allergic and immunologic skin diseases: In the eye of the beholder. *Clinical and Molecular Allergy: CMA, 19*. https://www.semanticscholar.org/paper/62beb86b99221b69221d29cab5703900b77a6964 (accessed on 21st July 2025).
7. DuToit, G., Smith, P., Muraro, A., Fox, A., Roberts, G., Ring, J., & Worm, M. (2024). Identifying patients at risk of anaphylaxis. *World Allergy Organization Journal, 17*, 100904–100904. https://doi.org/10.1016/j.waojou.2024.100904 (accessed on 21st July 2025).
8. Ensina, L., Brandão, L. S., Neto, H. C., & Ben-Shoshan, M. (2022). Urticaria and angioedema in children and adolescents: Diagnostic challenge. *Allergologia et Immunopathologia, 50*(S Pt 1), 17–29. https://www.semanticscholar.org/paper/3586039ce17246d15d2cb3e47c20500bf3e75190 (accessed on 21st July 2025).
9. Erbay, M. F., Kökçü Karadağ, Ş. İ., Üstün, T., Çalışkan, N., Yıldırım, G., Bologur, H., Güngör, H., et al. (2025). Is routine skin prick testing essential in managing pediatric chronic urticaria? *Pediatric Allergy, Immunology, and Pulmonology*. https://www.semanticscholar.org/paper/dfaaec457a620414da878d2600e0c6097c844c16 (accessed on 21st July 2025).
10. Fomina, D., Lebedkina, M., Nikitina, E., Kovalkova, E. V., Andrenova, G., Kruglova, T. S., Bobrikova, E., et al. (2025). ASIA syndrome masked as recurrent angioedema: Can development be predicted by genetic screening. *Russian Journal of Allergy*. https://www.semanticscholar.org/paper/b33098e11472d0ef566e109ccfd5f11a39296cd4 (accessed on 21st July 2025).

11. Gavrilović, N., Momirović-Stojković, M., & Budimski-Soldat, M. (2023). A case of angioedema of hereditary origin in a rural clinic near Subotica. *ABC–Časopis Urgentne Medicine*. https://www.semanticscholar.org/paper/721d1534fc158dd92bb8908e3ed2fa8d62e6178f (accessed on 21st July 2025).

12. Gülen, T., Akin, C., Bonadonna, P., Siebenhaar, F., Broesby-Olsen, S., Brockow, K., Niedoszytko, M., et al. (2021). Selecting the right criteria and proper classification to diagnose mast cell activation syndromes: A critical review. *The Journal of Allergy and Clinical Immunology: In Practice, 9*, 3918–3928. https://doi.org/10.1016/j.jaip.2021.06.011 (accessed on 21st July 2025).

13. Jaabouti, G., Benchidmi, S., Hafidi, N., Bencchakroun, S., & Mahraoui, C. (2023). A case report on aquagenic urticaria. *Asian Journal of Medicine and Health*. https://www.semanticscholar.org/paper/a754d66038494fee6213f3c3f403bb295ac4c521 (accessed on 21st July 2025).

14. Kamran, H., Khan, H. K., Ayub, N., Youas, M., Ullah, R., Ur Rahman, A., Khan, M. S., et al. (2024). Comparative analysis of treatment protocols and clinical outcomes in the management of acute urticaria and angioedema in the emergency department. *World Journal of Advanced Research and Reviews*. https://www.semanticscholar.org/paper/89c8331c22582208492891ac9459e45889d82927 (accessed on 21st July 2025).

15. King, A. L., Montagnon, C. M., Todd, A., Agrawal, S., Wieland, C., Lehman, J. S., & Johnson, E. F. (2024). Quantifying mast cell and eosinophil cellular density in skin biopsy tissue from adults with maculopapular cutaneous mastocytosis as compared with urticaria and normal skin: A retrospective histopathologic study. *The American Journal of Dermatopathology, 47*, 105–109. https://www.semanticscholar.org/paper/7e8e614363affe40772ff3708047749d9ec2fe19 (accessed on 21st July 2025).

16. Kou, E., Zhang, X., Dong, B., Wang, B., & Zhu, Y. (2024). Combination of H1 and H2 histamine receptor antagonists: Current knowledge and perspectives of a classic treatment strategy. *Life, 14*, 164–164. https://doi.org/10.3390/life14020164 (accessed on 21st July 2025).

17. Liu, S., Ren, T., Yaqoob, M. D., & Zhou, R. (2024). Clinical humanistic needs of Chinese medicine treatment for patients with chronic urticaria from the perspective of narrative medicine. *Chinese Medicine and Culture*. https://www.semanticscholar.org/paper/d92e0b378b9a5a8dcfb4481ec970e9f4f4af6ff2 (accessed on 21st July 2025).

18. Marchaj, M., Basiaga, B., Żądecka-Kobiałka, K., Putra, A., Bednarz, K., Nowicka-Jasińska, M., Frączyk, P., et al. (2024). Comprehensive review of mastocytosis from pathophysiology to management strategies. *Journal of Education, Health and Sport*. https://www.semanticscholar.org/paper/047d5e58a99411ffea2a47552cd5874b816a2b3a (accessed on 21st July 2025).

19. Migliarino, V., Zago, A., Martelossi, C., Barbi, E., Giangreco, M., Berti, I., & Badina, L. (2025). Natural history of pediatric idiopathic histaminergic angioedema: A retrospective monocentric study. *Children, 12*. https://www.semanticscholar.org/paper/e3360779528eab7335c0c4f9b5a43794573ee4ea (accessed on 21st July 2025).

20. Minciullo, P., Cascio, A., Isola, S., & Gangemi, S. (2016). Different clinical allergological features of *Taenia solium* infestation. *Clinical and Molecular Allergy: CMA, 14*. https://www.semanticscholar.org/paper/3f3417ed4b7897bd8dfd985e4140e4e4495c9144 (accessed on 21st July 2025).

21. Mohamed Nashrudin, K. N., Zainal Abidin, M. A., Ng, S., Razali, H., Jawin, V., Zakaria, A. F., Mohd Ali, R., et al. (2025). RASGRP1 deficiency associated with diffuse mesangial sclerosis infantile nephrotic syndrome and Epstein–Barr virus-induced Hodgkin's lymphoma. *Pediatric Allergy Immunology and Pulmonology*. https://doi.org/10.1089/ped.2024.0062 (accessed on 21st July 2025).

22. Nuñez-Borque, E., Fernández-Bravo, S., Yuste-Montalvo, A., & Esteban, V. (2022). Pathophysiological, cellular, and molecular events of the vascular system in anaphylaxis. *Frontiers in Immunology, 13*. https://doi.org/10.3389/fimmu.2022.836222 (accessed on 21st July 2025).

23. Radojicic, C., & Anderson, J. (2024). Hereditary angioedema with normal C1 esterase inhibitor: Current paradigms and clinical dilemmas. *Allergy and Asthma Proceedings, 45*(3), 147–157. https://www.semanticscholar.org/paper/fc828870937955eba4e664e62a889013987659b4 (accessed on 21st July 2025).

24. Ring, J., Beyer, K., Biedermann, T., Bircher, A. J., Fischer, M., Fuchs, T., Heller, A. R., et al. (2021). Guideline (S2k) on acute therapy and management of anaphylaxis: 2021 update. *Allergo Journal International, 30*, 1–25. https://doi.org/10.1007/s40629-020-00158-y (accessed on 21st July 2025).

25. Sagües-Sesé, E., García-Casares, N., & Álvarez-Twöse, I. (2023). Cognitive, neuropsychiatric and neurological alterations in mastocytosis: A systematic review. *Clinical and Translational Allergy, 13*. https://doi.org/10.1002/clt2.12319 (accessed on 21st July 2025).

26. Senol, M., & Kutlu, A. (2016). Postural tremor due to use of omalizumab. *Medicine Science | International Medical Journal, 5*, 171. https://www.semanticscholar.org/paper/4ee3c0fec63050fd930d7ca05e1990ae8c57745a (accessed on 21st July 2025).

27. Sheldon, J. M., & Philips, B. J. (2014). Laboratory investigation of anaphylaxis: Not as easy as it seems. *Anaesthesia, 70*, 1–5. https://doi.org/10.1111/anae.12926 (accessed on 21st July 2025).

28. Štrajtenberger, M., Lugović-Mihić, L., Stipić-Marković, A., Artuković, M., Glavina, A., Pravica, N. B., Hanžek, M., et al. (2024). Assessment of salivary and serum levels of HBD2 in patients with chronic angioedema. *Journal of Clinical Medicine, 13*. https://www.semanticscholar.org/paper/f76adb3d6d18e9d14b193de212027e2a96bca431 (accessed on 21st July 2025).

29. Su, H., Kolkhir, P., Scheffel, J., Xiang, Y., Yao, X., Maurer, M., & Altrichter, S. (2023). One in five patients with chronic spontaneous urticaria has IgE to tissue transglutaminase 2. *Allergy, 78*. https://www.semanticscholar.org/paper/b0c8ee3efcdc058d522227754cce485ab7a54c8e (accessed on 21st July 2025).

30. Taghavi Shirazi, M., Kenari, H. M., & Eghbalian, F. (2022). The role of bloodletting and cupping in severe acute urticaria and angioedema as skin emergencies in Persian medicine. *Journal of Pharmacopuncture, 25*, 7–14. https://www.semanticscholar.org/paper/41c5ea9d0524c560d8450e877a1c2b4a0470584f (accessed on 21st July 2025).

31. Ujiie, H., Rosmarin, D., Schön, M. P., Ständer, S., Boch, K., Metz, M., Maurer, M., et al. (2022). Unmet medical needs in chronic, non-communicable inflammatory skin diseases. *Frontiers in Medicine, 9*. https://doi.org/10.3389/fmed.2022.875492 (accessed on 21st July 2025).

32. Wedi, B. (2021). Contemporary grand challenges and opportunities in skin allergies. *Frontiers in Allergy, 2*. https://www.semanticscholar.org/paper/9ae22990dff5dcde663eeb5162b58bea6850eb54 (accessed on 21st July 2025).

33. Weller, K., Winders, T., Mccarthy, J., Raftery, T., Saraswat, P., Constantinescu, C., Balp, M., et al. (2025). Urticaria Voices: Real-world experience of patients living with chronic spontaneous urticaria. *Dermatology and Therapy, 15*, 747–761. https://www.semanticscholar.org/paper/08d4c5fdfd34547eee07d920285b5e9f5cce5161 (accessed on 21st July 2025).

34. Young, M. C., & Banerji, A. (2025). Angioedema without urticaria: Diagnosis and management. *Allergy and Asthma Proceedings, 46*(3), 185–191. https://www.semanticscholar.org/paper/fdde2845bea54717c0a3e07818cac42e4f752894 (accessed on 21st July 2025).

35. Zuberbier, T., Abdul Latiff, A. H., Abuzakouk, M., Aquilina, S., Asero, R., Baker, D. R., Ballmer-Weber, B., et al. (2021). The international EAACI/GA^{2}LEN/EuroGuiDerm/APAAACI guideline for the definition, classification, diagnosis, and management of urticaria. *Allergy, 77*, 734–766. https://doi.org/10.1111/all.15090 (accessed on 21st July 2025).

36. Zuberbier, T., Aberer, W., Asero, R., Abdul Latiff, A. H., Baker, D. R., Ballmer-Weber, B., Bernstein, J. A., et al. (2018). The EAACI/GA^{2}LEN/EDF/WAO guideline for the definition, classification, diagnosis and management of urticaria. *Allergy, 73*, 1393–1414. https://doi.org/10.1111/all.13397 (accessed on 21st July 2025).

LICHEN PLANUS AND RELATED CONDITIONS

9

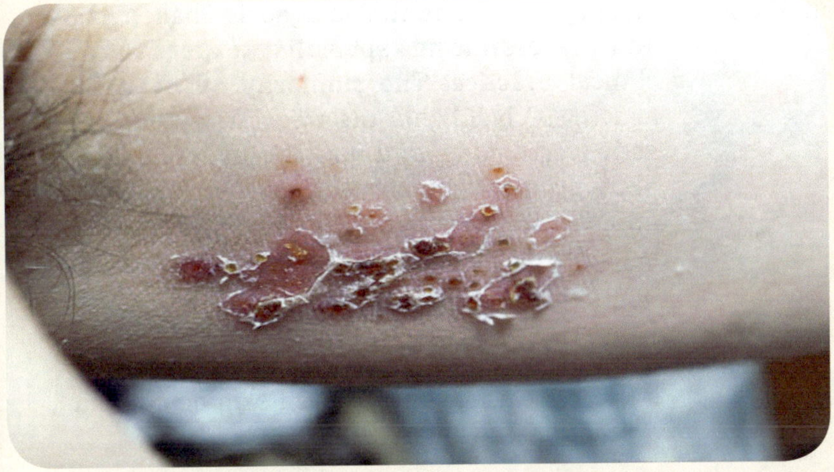

LEARNING OBJECTIVES

After studying this chapter, you will be able to:

1. Examine the clinical presentation of lichen planus
2. Describe the treatment options for lichen planus
3. Know the lichen planus and its psychological impact
4. Describe the related conditions of lichen planus

Introduction

Lichen Planus (LP) is a multifactorial dermatological condition characterized by typical papules and plaques that most often involve the mucous membranes and the skin. LP is an idiopathic inflammatory disease characterized by pruritic lesions that follow a symmetric distribution. The pathogenesis of LP remains obscure; however, it is theorized that LP arises from an abnormal immune reaction attributable to environmental factors and genetic factors, including stress and certain drugs. The significance of early diagnosis and management cannot be overstressed as LP is linked to morbidity and complications of secondary infection. Further, the psychosocial value of this condition is great as patients' quality of life and self-esteem are usually compromised. Identification of this condition's underlying mechanisms is valuable for developing targeted therapies and improving patient outcomes. The relationship between lichen planus and other dermatologic conditions presents a fascinating set of research avenues. For instance, LP has been infrequently associated with other autoimmune diseases, such as hepatitis C infections and lichen simplex chronicus, creating a perplexing interaction between cutaneous presentation and systemic health. More contemporary studies indicate that LP can have geographically variable prevalence, suggesting potential environmental determinants or regulatory differences in immune function between populations. Investigation of such associations assists in delineating the pathophysiology of LP and perhaps explaining common biological pathways towards developing a number of autoimmune diseases.

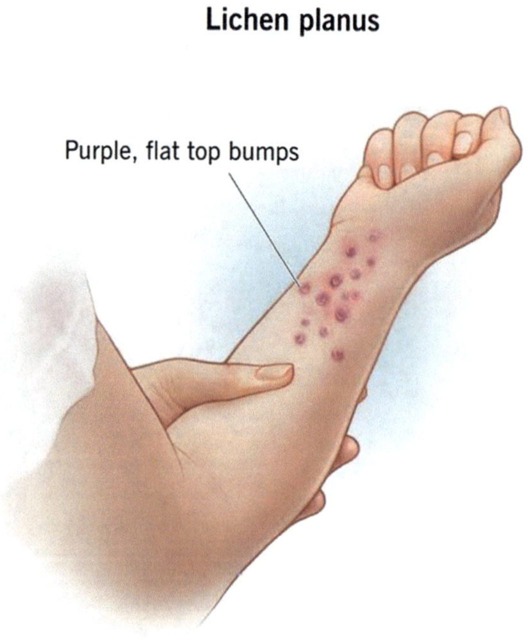

Figure 9.1. Lichen planus (LP) causes a rash with small, discolored dots on your skin. These dots are typically less than 1 cm wide.

Source: https://my.clevelandclinic.org/-/scassets/images/org/health/articles/17723-lichen-planus.

Such research is critical to formulating an integrated perception of lichen planus, thereby enabling clinicians to develop balanced treatment regimens that address both skin and overall health concerns. Within the broader context of dermatological disorders, familiarity with lichen planus is the gateway to the nuances of cutaneous disorders affecting human health. Interestingly, LP patients have a higher risk of developing non-melanoma skin cancers (NMSC), including basal cell carcinoma and squamous cell carcinoma, underscoring the importance of caution during dermatological examination and skin observation in these patients. The histopathological presentations of these malignancies overlap with those of LP, making the differential diagnosis challenging and necessitating specialist expertise in clinical practice. The similarity between LP and NMSC highlights the imperative need for active screening and patient education on photoprotective measures as well as early intervention strategies to prevent potential malignancies. By taking an integrative approach to the study of lichen planus and its associations with other illnesses, we not only enrich clinical practice but also further knowledge of the intricate relationship between skin health and overall health (Figure 9.1).

Definition of Lichen Planus (LP)

LP is an inflammatory, chronic disease primarily of the skin and mucous membranes, characterized by the occurrence of purplish, pruritic lesions. LP dermatosis is thought to be an autoimmune process in which the body's immune system attacks its own skin cells by mistake. While the etiology of LP is unclear, certain precipitants such as stress, certain drugs, and hepatitis C infection have been suggested as potential triggers. Clinically, lichen planus occurs in numerous manifestations involving the cutaneous, oral, and genital forms, with each presenting special diagnostic and treatment challenges. The ability to differentiate between lichen planus and other closely related disorders, such as psoriasis, is key to effective management, underscoring the need for a complete understanding of its definition and presentation in patients. The lichen planus lesions are highly variable in severity and appearance, making them difficult to diagnose and treat. Lesions are most often flat-topped papules or plaques with a typical lace-like pattern known as Wickham's striae. Oral lichen planus, in particular, is of significant clinical importance due to its potential association with dysplasia and oral squamous cell carcinoma, although corticoid treatment and patient education can establish effective management strategies. Evidence has shown that oral lichen planus can mimic other intraoral lesions, such that differential diagnosis must be conducted sensitively to preclude unnecessary interventions. The more one becomes aware, the more ongoing research into the precise mechanisms and potential treatment options for lichen planus remains critical to improving patient outcomes and managing this complex disease.

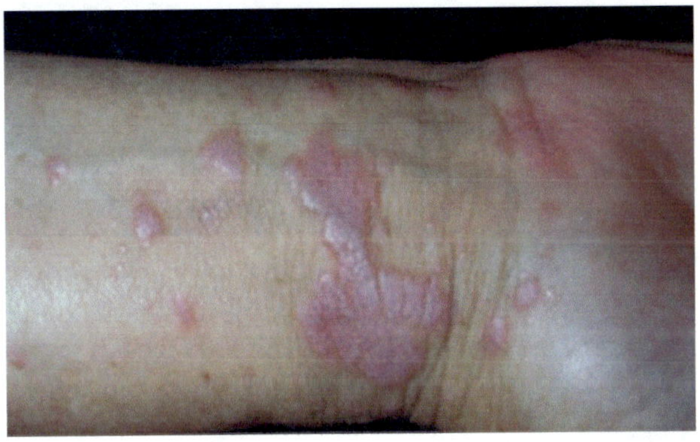

Figure 9.2. Lichen planus (LP).

Source: https://appnhs24wp41a8c38064.blob.core.windows.net/blobappnhs24wp41a8c38064/wp-content/uploads/2023/05/lichen-planus-1.jpg.

Beyond the intrinsic implications of lichen planus, the correlation with other illnesses further emphasizes the importance of proper identification and understanding of its definition. For instance, lichen planus patients are usually at risk for the development of other autoimmune disorders, such as thyroid disease or alopecia areata, which complicates their clinical presentation. Moreover, studies on the impact of comorbid conditions, such as those resulting from infectious diseases, reveal an interplay that must be monitored closely. The identification of such interactions also might enable better patient education and preventive strategies to avoid complications. As lichen planus continues to challenge health practitioners, it remains crucial to investigate its pathophysiology and associated risk factors, paving the way for new therapeutic interventions and greater awareness of this multifaceted disease (Figure 9.2).

Importance of Studying Lichen Planus (LP)

LP is worthy of study because it has several implications for both patients and health workers. Being a chronic inflammatory condition that may affect the skin, oral mucosa, and nails, LP has greater than presentation importance. The pathophysiology of LP is a complex interaction of immunologic processes, with special activation of mast cells and their mediators. Studies have indicated that mast cells in the oral tissues are involved in inflammatory reactions to be a part of LP, assisting in leukocyte infiltration and exacerbation of symptoms (Walsh et al., 2003). While researchers continue to search for such mechanisms, they can reveal therapeutic targets that may help modulate chronic inflammation, ultimately improving the quality of life for those afflicted. Also, the Lichen Planus study is essential because of its potential associations with other systemic diseases. The pathogenesis of LP still remains unclear, but it is well established that the disease may have a similar origin to autoimmune diseases and may even antedate malignancy. For instance, a recent analysis of oral candidiasis underscores the importance of understanding how various infections, such as those caused by Candida species, may affect conditions like LP (Vikholt et al., 2014). This underscores the importance of healthcare providers adopting a holistic perspective in diagnosing and treating patients with LP, as they may present with symptoms or underlying issues that should be addressed simultaneously.

Apart from its clinical implications, research on Lichen Planus also offers a better understanding of dermatologic and immunologic diseases as a whole. LP is a chronic inflammatory model that will illuminate therapeutic options for associated diseases. As a result of technical developments in molecular biology and immunotherapy, researchers can increasingly investigate the involvement of cytokines and other mediators in LP pathogenesis, particularly the contribution of mast cells to immune reactions (Walsh et al., 2003). Greater knowledge of LP may eventually enable additional uses, paving the way for new treatments not only for LP but also for related inflammatory diseases.

9.1. Clinical Presentation

Learning Outcome

1. Describe the common symptoms of lichen planus
2. Describe the variants of lichen planus
3. Know the diagnosis criteria of lichen planus

Regarding the clinical presentation of lichen planus, it should be noted that this disease is characterized by a wide range of distinctive symptoms that vary significantly from person to person. Typically pruritic, flat-topped, polygonal papules, lichen planus tends to occur on skin, mucous membranes, and nails. The lesions are typically violaceous in color, with a shiny, reflective appearance that may assist in diagnosis. In oral disease, of especial importance to the disease's comprehension, patients present frequently with white striations or reticular patterns of the buccal mucosa, tongue, and gums. The disease calls for cautious clinical evaluation, as it can present as other mucosal and dermatological conditions, thereby necessitating effective diagnosis and relevant management strategies. Lichen planus does not present solely with a dermatological picture but has a multisystemic presentation that suggests its association with systemic components and other autoimmune diseases. Their presence in salivary and crevicular fluid specimens explains the pathophysiology and clinical behavior of the disease. Specifically, the presence of HBD-2 can also be used as a potential marker of activity, but with implications for clinical monitoring as well as therapeutic treatment. This evolving knowledge underscores the interplay between lichen planus and local and systemic health, requiring an integrated approach to patient management to effectively treat disease manifestations and their overall impact on health (Azzi et al., 2016).

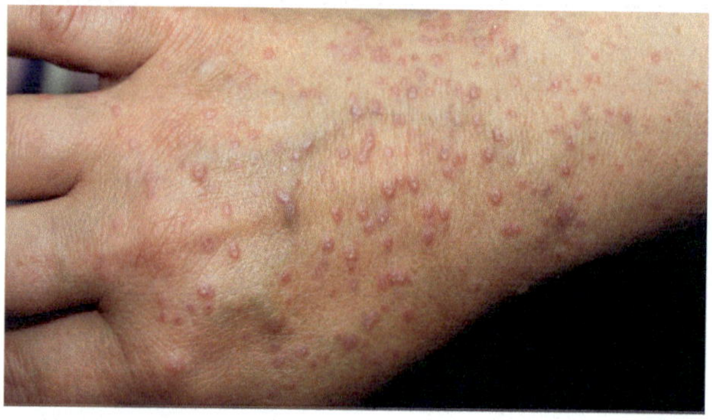

Figure 9.3. Lichen planus clinical presentation.

Source: https://dermskinhealth.com/wp-content/uploads/2022/05/lichen-planus-hero.jpeg.

Saliva as a diagnostic tool to assist in the management of lichen planus is gaining prominence, underscoring the importance of comprehensive clinical assessment. Salivary analysis has been shown to be of significant diagnostic value in a variety of oral diseases, including lichen planus, as saliva is an elaborate fluid in close association with systemic health. The study of salivary biomarkers can provide deeper insight into disease behavior, opening up possibilities for non-invasive monitoring techniques. Through researchers now laying down these connections, the convoluted interplay between oral health, systemic illness, and immunological reaction becomes more transparent. These findings attest to the important role of advanced diagnostic methods in clinical practice, potentially leading to more knowledge-based treatment plans and better patient outcomes in lichen planus and related diseases (Eid et al., 2022) (Figure 9.3).

9.1.1. Common Symptoms

Clinical presentations of lichen planus and related conditions often manifest a variety of common symptoms, with a considerable impact on patients' quality of life. The most frequent symptom is pruritus, or intense itching, which is incapacitating. Pruritus is not only a minor annoyance; it is a physiological response to irritants such as cutaneous parasites. This sensation typically prompts individuals to scratch, often leading to further skin inflammation and secondary infection. Thus, pruritus treatment is most important in lichen planus and other skin diseases, since remission of the symptom would yield significant relief and overall improvement in patients' quality of life (Briffa et al., 2009). In addition to pruritus, the lichen planus patient also usually features characteristic cutaneous lesions that are required for diagnosis. These lesions usually appear as flat-topped, polygonal papules that predominate on the extremities and mucous membranes. The normal morphology and distribution of these lesions form a significant component of the clinical evaluation. Further, patients may develop pigmentation changes, including hyperpigmentation and hypopigmentation, during the post-inflammatory stage of the disease. In addition to physical appearance, these visible manifestations can be a source of emotional distress, highlighting the importance of comprehensive care that addresses both the dermatologic and emotional aspects of lichen planus (Tüting et al., 2008). In addition to skin lesions, lichen planus can involve the mucous membranes, causing oral lichen planus, which has special challenges. Symptoms may include painful erosions and white striations on the oral mucosa, which can make everyday activities such as eating and talking more difficult. Such mucosal involvement may be even more problematic, since oral lesions may be harder to treat and can be longer-lasting than their cutaneous counterparts. In recognizing these diverse symptoms, clinicians are forced to adopt a multidisciplinary treatment strategy, modifying interventions not just to address dermatological symptoms but also to address their impact on daily functioning. This is not simply a physical management technique but one that includes patient education and psychotherapy to enhance patient outcomes more generally (Figure 9.4).

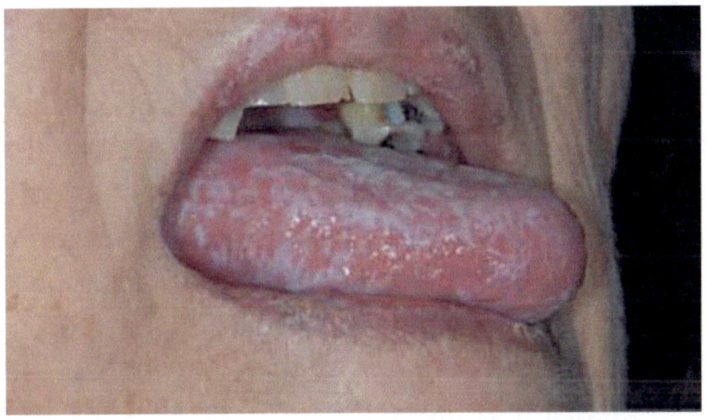

Figure 9.4. Symptoms of oral lichen planus.

Source: https://i0.wp.com/images-prod.healthline.com/hlcmsresource/images/642x361_Oral_Lichen_Planus.jpg?w=1155&h=758.

9.1.2. Variants of Lichen Planus

The clinical presentation of lichen planus can be highly variable, and as such, multiple variants have been included in classification systems. Oral lichen planus (OLP), cutaneous lichen planus, and hypertrophic lichen planus are the most commonly recognized forms, all with distinct features and complications. OLP is particularly important since it has been associated with lesions of the oral mucosa that predispose to dysplastic change. Literature has shown that a wide prevalence of human papillomavirus (HPV) exists in patients with oral lesions, and the most prevalent detection of HPV infection occurs in OLP among those using other OPMDs (Antonelli et al., 2016). This raises a concern about the evolution of OLP to squamous cell carcinoma, necessitating a determination of the significance of follow-up for patients with this variant to avoid potential malignant changes. A second notable variant, hypertrophic lichen planus, is characterized by thickened, elevated lesions, typically on the lower legs. Hypertrophic lichen planus is potentially very refractory to treatment due to the potential for severe itching and pain. While less common than the non-hypertrophic lesion, hypertrophic lesions may require both local and systemic treatment to reduce symptoms and inflammation.

There is evidence that the risk of secondary infection is possibly heightened in hypertrophic lesions and should be handled with special care during treatment. Moreover, the cosmetic impact of hypertrophic lichen planus can cause psychological distress, underscoring the widespread effects of this variant beyond its appearance. Lichen planus is present in a number of other less common variants, such as follicular lichen planus and erosive lichen planus. Follicular lichen planus mainly affects hair follicles in the form of hair loss in affected areas, with the possibility of scarring alopecia.

The erosive form, which is very common in the oral cavity, is characterized by painful ulcers and can significantly affect a patient's quality of life. Research has shown that whether parakeratosis or hyperkeratosis is present can influence the detectability of HPV in these variants, making it even harder to discern their potential malignancy (Campisi et al., 2017). Through knowledge of these variations, clinicians and researchers gain valuable information on the pathophysiology of lichen planus, which increases the accuracy and likelihood of diagnosis by enabling more effective therapeutic interventions tailored to each variant's presentation and risks.

9.1.3. Diagnosis Criteria

Multidisciplinary treatment is needed for accurate diagnosis of Lichen Planus (LP) and related disorders. Clinical examination is generally used in diagnosis, where clinicians assess lesions with a characteristic lacy white texture, particularly on mucous membranes. The recognition of reticular or erosive forms of oral lichen planus differentiates the condition from other mucosal lesions. A full medical history is also crucial, allowing clinicians to explore potential precipitates or associations with systemic illnesses, optimizing diagnostic sensitivity. The variable presentation and the capacity of lesions to mimic other illnesses mean that clinicians must bear in mind a differential diagnosis — including oral candidiasis and aphthous ulcers — in a bid to diagnose and treat these cases appropriately. Histopathological examination remains a cornerstone of the diagnostic features of lichen planus, particularly in atypical cases. Microscopic examination of a lesion biopsy may reveal typical features such as liquefactive degeneration of the basal cell layer and a characteristic band-like lymphocytic infiltrate at the dermal-epidermal junction. This microscopic analysis not only augments the clinical presentation but also helps exclude malignancy or other lip lesions that may simulate it. Clinical and histopathological parameters, together, play a crucial role in the absolute diagnosis of LP, thereby enabling appropriate treatment and management options tailored to individual patient needs, such as medication aimed at symptom alleviation and inflammation control. Apart from clinical and histopathological investigations, serological investigations can be a doorway to the diagnosis of related conditions secondary to Lichen Planus. For instance, studies have reported a high incidence of zinc deficiency among patients with oral mucosal disease, including lichen planus, suggesting that systemic nutritional status may influence disease pathology. Such deficiencies may guide therapeutic management, as zinc supplementation has been reported to alleviate symptoms in many mucosal conditions of the oral cavity. This multiaxial evaluation process, including clinical assessment, histological assessment, and serological testing, underscores the complexity of diagnosing Lichen Planus and related conditions and ultimately guides a more effective management approach (Bao et al., 2016; Amadori et al., 2017) (Figure 9.5).

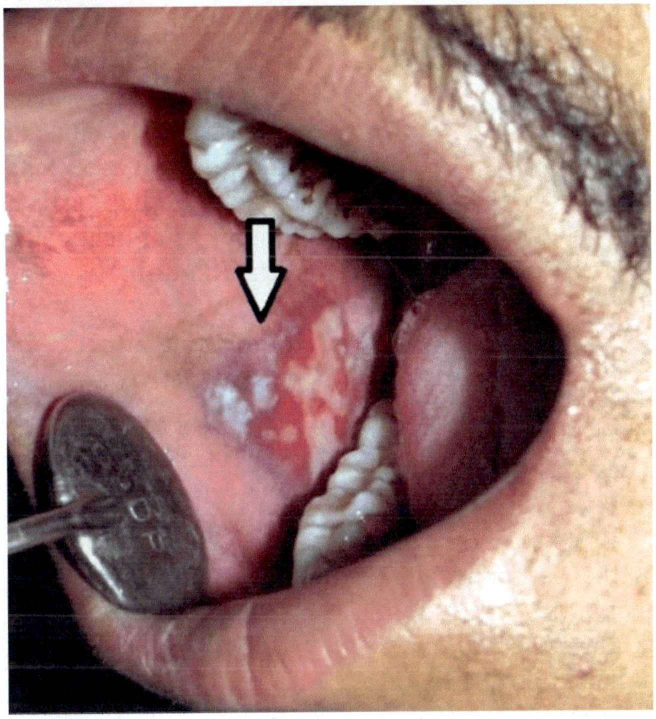

Figure 9.5. Intraoral examination of the patient showing mixed red and white lesion in the right buccal mucosa suggestive of erosive lichen planus.

Source: https://assets.cureus.com/uploads/figure/file/1032307/article_river_829afed01f0811ef9e8879dc7cc7294c-Figure_1.png.

Test Your Knowledge

1. What is a common symptom associated with lichen planus?
2. What are the variants of lichen planus?

9.2. Treatment Options

Learning Outcome

1. Understand the role of topical therapies in the management of lichen planus
2. Describe the systemic medications for lichen planus
3. Know the alternative treatments for lichen planus

Lichen planus is most commonly treated with a multidimensional approach that targets both symptomatic relief and immunological processes responsible for the condition. Topical corticosteroids remain a cornerstone of therapy, delivering local anti-inflammatory properties that can readily alleviate discomfort and inflammation associated with the disease. For moderate-to-severe lesions, intralesional corticosteroid injections may be used to more effectively treat individual lesions. However, as our understanding of the pathophysiology of lichen planus advances, other treatments are evolving. Systemic therapies, such as corticosteroids and immunosuppressants, are reserved for generalized or recalcitrant disease, particularly if topical treatment fails. Patient-based treatment must balance the benefit of prompt symptom relief against the potential side effects of systemic treatment, such that proper clinician assessment and continued patient communication are essential. Incubating evidence also suggested the potential of Janus kinase inhibitors (JAKi) as a new treatment for lichen planus, based on what is known about similar autoimmune cutaneous diseases. JAKi, acting on intracellular signaling pathways, have the potential to regulate well-inflammatory processes and are being considered for possible dermatologic uses. The efficacy of JAK inhibitors in treating other conditions, such as atopic dermatitis and psoriasis, presents a hopeful model for their use in lichen planus. Suppression of the JAK/STAT pathway with these medications may provide a double dividend: a lack of inflammation and a lack of chronic systemic corticosteroids, which have severe side effects. As clinical trials advance, JAKi may revolutionize the development of more effective and safer drugs to manage lichen planus and related disorders (Ghoreschi et al., 2019). In addition, research into other treatment modalities, such as phototherapy and emerging biologic drugs, has opened new avenues for patients who are not responding to conventional therapies. Phototherapy, especially narrowband ultraviolet B (nbUVB), has proven useful in reducing the symptoms of lichen planus by modulating skin inflammation. In a similar manner, studies on biologics targeting individual cytokines implicated in the pathogenesis of lichen planus are becoming popular. In particular, the identification of immune cell infiltrates, such as FoxP3+ regulatory T cells and IL17+ cells, suggests that treatments targeting these pathways may improve prognosis (Anderson et al., 2020). As the scientific community continues to untangle the complex immunological landscape of lichen planus, one may suspect that new treatment strategies will be identified, eventually resulting in personalized, more effective care for those affected.

9.2.1. Topical Therapies

Topical therapies are an important component of the management of lichen planus, particularly for controlling inflammation and symptoms of this chronic condition. Topical therapies are commonly used for their local action, which spares systemic side effects and delivers a potent anti-inflammatory effect directly to the involved tissue. Corticosteroids are most commonly used as topical drugs and are very effective in reducing erythema, pruritus, and lesions due to their immunosuppressive effects. The variety of preparation forms, including ointment, cream, and gel, allows for customized treatment that may accommodate patient-specific needs and comfort. Because symptomatic relief is the defining feature of quality of life in symptomatic patients, such local treatment emerges as a fundamental aspect of total lichen planus therapy, often used in combination with other therapies. In addition to corticosteroids, other agents, such as calcineurin inhibitors, have gained wider recognition as therapeutic modalities for lichen planus, primarily in refractory cases. Tacrolimus and pimecrolimus are two such potent immunomodulators that work on the subpathophysiology of lichen planus by inhibiting T-cell activation and resultant inflammatory responses.

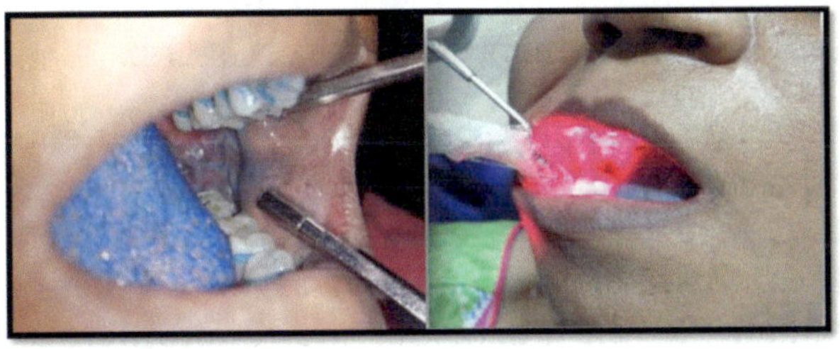

Figure 9.6. Photo-dynamic therapy (PDT).

Source: https://www.researchgate.net/publication/373950199/figure/fig3/AS:11431281188945939@1694823449629/Photo-dynamic-therapy-PDT-Methylene-blue-001-was-applied-onto-the-lesional-areas-and.tif.

These are especially useful to employ in sensitive areas, such as the oral mucosa or genitalia, where the risk of cutaneous atrophy may limit the safety of corticosteroid therapy. Clinical experience indicates these agents generally offer significant relief from symptoms and generally enjoy an excellent safety profile. With ongoing research into the relative efficacy of these agents, topical calcineurin inhibitors represent a very appealing avenue to enhance treatment regimens for patients with lichen planus-related conditions. Newer technologies for photodynamic therapy (PDT) have uncovered a novel approach to treating topically involved lichen planus. PDT uses photosensitizing medications activated by specific light wavelengths to induce a localized inflammatory response that may deter lesion progression. As highlighted by recent research, PDT is a less invasive option with great potential for patients with severe or refractory lichen planus, particularly those with erosive lesions. This new treatment not only conforms to existing dermatological therapy but also supplements the therapeutic arsenal of practitioners. In general, the chronology of topical therapy, both traditional and new, mirrors the unceasing push to improve outcomes in lichen planus treatment (Briffa et al., 2009; Georgescu et al., 2019) (Figure 9.6).

9.2.2. Systemic Medications

Treatment of lichen planus frequently requires systemic therapy, especially in resistant cases to topical therapy. Systemic therapy with corticosteroids and immunosuppressive drugs is important for controlling inflammation and modulating the immune response, which is necessary given the autoimmune pathogenesis of lichen planus. Corticosteroids, such as prednisone, are frequently employed due to their immediate anti-inflammatory action, but long-term use is potentially to produce significant side effects, including osteoporosis and hypertension. The above findings underscore the narrow margin that health care professionals must navigate to alleviate symptoms with the least potential for complications. In desperate cases, other systemic medications such as azathioprine and mycophenolate mofetil may be effective alternative therapeutic agents to manage chronic inflammation effectively. Aside from corticosteroids and immunosuppressants, systemic retinoids such as acitretin can also be employed as a therapeutic measure for lichen planus. Retinoids exert their action by regulating photoregulated growth and differentiation of epithelial cells to cure photodamage to the affected skin. Because of the chronic nature of the disease, lichen planus, it is necessary that the therapies should be capable of effectively treating long-term patient outcomes. However, the use of systemic retinoids must be closely monitored for their potential harmful effects, which can include teratogenicity and risk of hyperlipidemia. The complexity of systemic treatment regimens underscores the necessity of patient-tailored therapy that considers patient factors such as comorbidities, age, and preferences. Hence, the role of systemic drugs is essential for long-term management of the disease and for improving the quality of life in patients with lichen planus. Along with this, it is not possible to overlook the interaction between the environment and systemic drugs in managing lichen planus. Patients on systemic immunosuppressants are at increased risk of infection, and proper caution must be exercised when handling them. Certain phototoxic agents may induce a reaction in patients on systemic therapy, complicating the patient's skin (Zammit et al., 2010). These factors highlight the importance of proper patient education on lifestyle modification and avoidance of known offending agents that may worsen the disease. Periodic follow-ups are essential for ensuring evaluation of both efficacy of treatment and evolving side effects. An integrated model that brings together systemic drug treatment and educational support is needed to optimize patient outcomes in lichen planus and related conditions (Agarwala et al., 2017) (Figure 9.7).

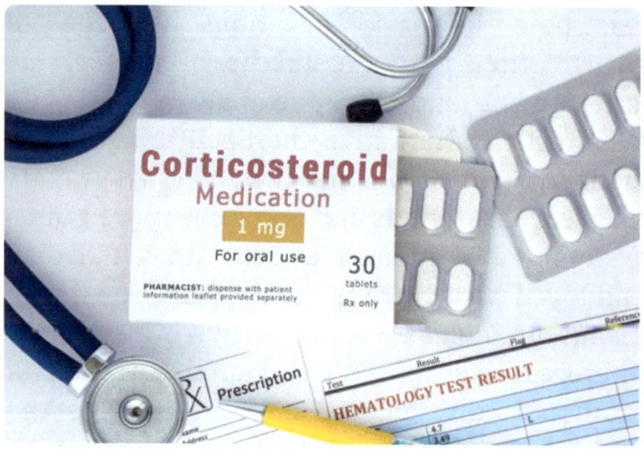

Figure 9.7. Corticosteroid medication.

Source: https://www.news-medical.net/image-handler/ts/20200929082107/ri/673/picture/2020/9/shutterstock_1380391247.jpg.

9.2.3. Alternative Treatments

Alternative treatments of lichen planus have gained prominence as patients opt for alternative medicine outside of conventional medical treatment. Alternative treatments include topical, systemic, and phototherapy, all targeting symptom reduction and improvement in skin lesions. Herbal medicine, such as the use of natural oils like tea tree oil or coconut oil, has also shown promise in reducing inflammation and promoting healing, but more research is needed to substantiate these claims. Dietary interventions that promote an anti-inflammatory diet can also benefit overall skin health.

These novel approaches not only offer patients the hope for symptomatic improvement but potentially enable them to be actively involved in their treatment regimens, hence enhancing the quality of life. Phototherapy, such as narrowband ultraviolet B (NB-UVB), has been a prominent alternative treatment for lichen planus. The non-surgical treatment is effective by suppressing immune-mediated processes leading to skin lesions. Phototherapy is particularly beneficial in cases where topical agents have failed, as it offers a focused approach to managing symptoms. As mentioned under related conditions, the judicious use of UV radiation has been extensively researched for its effectiveness as a therapy for many skin disorders and for its associated safety profile when used appropriately. With favorable results noted in pruritus treatment and skin integrity re-establishment, phototherapy offers a promising alternative for individuals seeking non-conventional approaches to conventional therapy.

Ongoing investigation into phototherapy continues to solidify its potential to revolutionize treatment paradigms for lichen planus and other skin conditions. The association of complementary modalities like acupuncture and mindfulness exercises with the treatment of lichen planus is not uncommon. Acupuncture, originating from traditional Chinese medicine, aims to modulate the body's immune system and improve skin conditions through the precise placement of needles. Others experience increased relaxation and reduced stress, further promoting overall relief from symptoms. Similarly, elements of mindfulness, including yoga and meditation, help with the psychological management of chronic skin disease and developing emotional resilience.

By lessening the tension that tends to exacerbate lichen planus, these lifestyle patterns can help benefit the treatment process. Although scientific proof of the effectiveness of these techniques remains the focus of ongoing research, their incorporation into a comprehensive treatment plan represents a major step toward managing not only the body but also the emotional and psychological components of lichen planus (Figure 9.8).

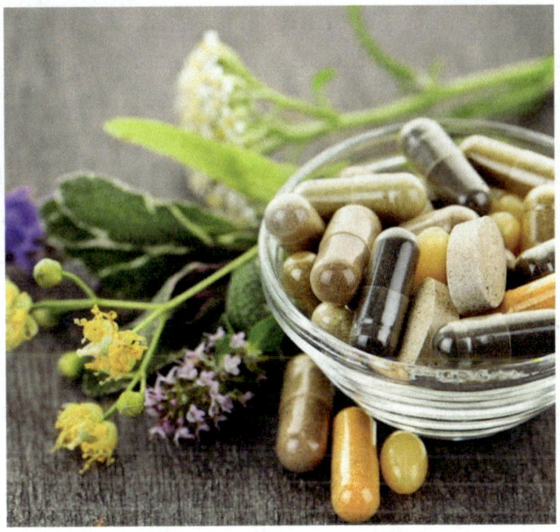

Figure 9.8. Lichen planus ayurvedic treatment.

Source: https://www.ayurclinic.com.au/wp-content/webpc-passthru.php?src=https://www.ayurclinic.com.au/wp-content/uploads/2018/10/Best_Ayurvedic_Medicine_for_weight_loss.jpg&nocache=1.

Test Your Knowledge

1. What topical medication is used for lichen planus?
2. Which is the best medicine for lichen planus?

9.3. Lichen Planus and Its Psychological Impact

Learning Outcome

1. Understand the emotional effects of lichen planus on patients
2. Describe the role of coping strategies in managing the psychological and emotional impacts of lichen planus
3. Understand the importance of mental health support in managing chronic skin conditions

The convergence of psychological health and chronic dermatological conditions, such as lichen planus, is a key area of study since the physical manifestations of this autoimmune disease have the potential to cause severe emotional and psychological distress. Lichen planus patients have been found to develop alterations in their body image due to lesions that disrupt the look of the skin, resulting in low self-esteem and heightened anxiety levels. The psychosocial burden of coping with an uncertain state could lead to irritability and hopelessness, confirming that chronic illnesses are not only physical blockages but also psychosocial barriers. This condition necessitates a good grasp of the impact of lichen planus on mental health because the psychological impact can influence treatment adherence and the overall quality of life, making well-integrated care strategies to heal both physical and psychological dimensions equally crucial.

Moreover, the psychological impact of lichen planus is compounded by the stigma typically associated with visible skin conditions, which can provoke social withdrawal and loneliness. The common view of dermatological illness can regulate the behavior of individuals with lichen planus in regard to their surroundings, sometimes causing the avoidance of social situations or activities once visited. A study concerned with general psychosomatics in oral illnesses indicates that emotional issues regulate oral conditions and, therefore, oral lichen planus manifestations, suggesting a two-way interdependence of psychosocial stress and illness (Azzi et al., 2016). This exchange reflects the necessity for psychological elements to be added to treatment plans in order to increase the efficiency of medical intervention, pointing to health awareness among practitioners in relation to the intricate connection between physical symptoms and mental health. The necessity for a multidisciplinary team in treating lichen planus is also justified by the identification of the disorders' psychological components. Current research highlights that psychiatric treatment can have a significant role to play in helping patients navigate the psychological complexities of the illness, assisting coping mechanisms and education as a counteractive measure against stress and anxiety. Offering treatment interventions, such as psychological care and stress management, can lead to improved patient outcomes. By fostering open communication about mental health, healthcare professionals can increase awareness of the psychosocial impact of lichen planus, ultimately improving patient care and quality of life. Establishing a step for including psychological care in the treatment of lichen planus enables a more holistic practice of medicine that addresses both the outwardly visible symptoms and the internalized emotional load of this chronic disease (Figure 9.9).

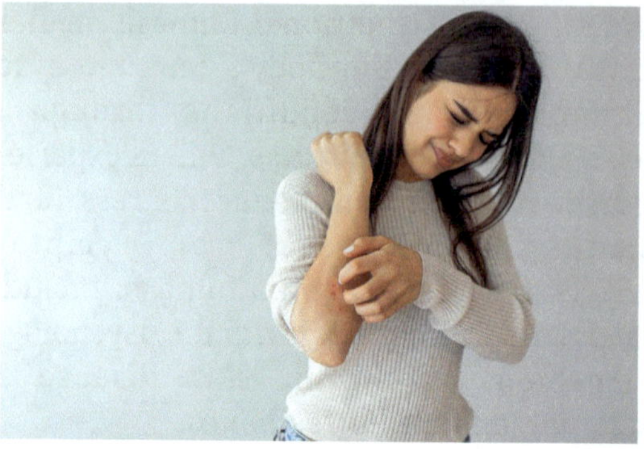

Figure 9.9. Psychological effects of lichen planus.

Source: https://images.ctfassets.net/iqo3fk8od6t9/ZZCLO1WSdNobWMUbjHAJs/4d13227673df3e029e36136d4e76ced3/Rash.jpg.

9.3.1. Emotional Effects on Patients

It is essential to understand the emotional effects of lichen planus and related conditions to provide holistic patient care. Lichen planus's chronic nature can lead to excessive psychological distress because patients have symptoms that are persistent as well as distressing. For most, the onset of lesions—both cutaneous and mucosal—may cause embarrassment and self-consciousness. This emotional discomfort is compounded by the unpredictable nature of the flares and remissions of the condition, subjecting patients to continuous fear of their appearance and discomfort. Such psychoemotional distress can interfere with everyday functioning, affecting social interactions and general quality of life, and therefore necessitating comprehensive emotional care in treatment therapies. The impact of pruritus, or itch, is particularly relevant to emotional well-being in patients with lichen planus. Described, pruritus is so much more than just an annoying physical sensation; it really impacts psychological well-being by creating frustration and powerlessness (Briffa et al., 2009). As the repetitive sensation of itching can make individuals itch compulsively, which will in turn create potentially worsening skin lesions and cause additional embarrassment.

This cycle of distress can create worsening psychological well-being, like anxiety and depression. Identifying these emotional effects is crucial for healthcare providers because they can significantly affect treatment compliance. Therefore, addressing these psychological factors is crucial for improving overall health in patients with lichen planus. Furthermore, treatments such as topical therapy have been investigated to determine their efficacy not only in lessening physical pain but also in potentially enhancing emotional states. In a study of the impact of topical tocopherol acetate on oral pain in patients with reticular oral lichen planus (ROLP), the findings showed significant symptom alleviation, which can be attributed to improved emotional well-being (Bacci et al., 2016). Relief of discomfort most likely translates to relief of psychological tension, enabling the patients to engage more fully with social and professional possibilities. This transdisciplinary model that unites physical comfort with emotional care underscores the importance of a multidimensional approach to patient care, wherein emotional wellness is accorded equal status alongside physical symptoms (Figure 9.10).

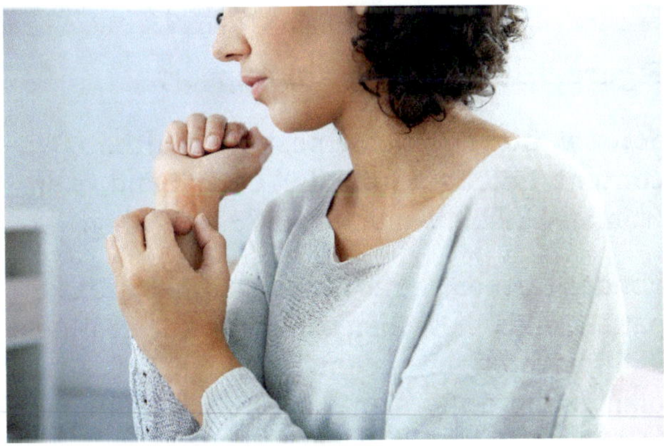

Figure 9.10. Emotional effects of lichen planus.

Source: https://ucmscdn.healthgrades.com/8b/e5/13009d8f4b32ac2932fb387a5520/gettyimages-697567367.jpg.

9.3.2. Coping Strategies

Coping strategies are at the core of dealing with psychological and emotional sequelae of lichen planus and related disorders. These chronic skin conditions may cause significant distress and discomfort for patients, and the demand for effective adaptive mechanisms is enormous. Psychological resilience, the ability to adapt to stressful situations and recover from adversity, has been linked to better health in individuals with skin diseases. Cognitive-behavioral coping strategies, such as reframing negative attitudes and positive outlook, can empower patients to cope with the psychosocial challenges of lichen planus. These coping strategies, apart from enhancing emotional well-being, also contribute to compliance with medical treatment, thereby improving disease control. Mechanisms of social support are also of great significance in coping with the challenges presented by lichen planus and other dermatologic disorders. Individuals who actively seek support from family, friends, or support groups also report less loneliness and greater emotional stability. Discussion with others who share a similar understanding of what it means to have a chronic skin condition may be an important way of establishing a sense of belonging and acceptance. Face-to-face or online support groups are additional forums in which individuals can exchange coping strategies, receive support, and learn from each other's experiences. This social interaction can go a long way in lessening the psychological strain of skin diseases, fostering resilience, and encouraging healthy coping behaviors. In addition to psychological and social coping styles, lifestyle modification may also increase an individual's capacity for coping with lichen planus. Taking up stress-reduction techniques such as mindfulness meditation or yoga can be helpful immediately, given that stress is a disease flare-up trigger. Further, a healthy diet in practice with plenty of antioxidants might play a supporting role in the condition's healing and demineralization. Similarly, phototherapy has been positioned for its dual role of safeguarding the body and calming the psyche in that it reduces evident lesions in association with dermatological diseases, thereby helping decrease self-consciousness and stigma. By combining psychological, social, and lifestyle approaches, individuals with lichen planus are better able to work within a solid structure of coping tools that address the physical and emotional concerns of the condition, thereby enhancing quality of life.

9.3.3. Importance of Mental Health Support

There is an important role contributed by mental health care to dealing with chronic skin conditions, like lichen planus, inasmuch as such illnesses have a high level of psychological morbidity. Patients also tend to have difficulty with the visible and most often stigmatizing nature of skin disease, leading to depression, anxiety, and an impaired quality of life. Research indicates that skin disease has the ability to induce a heavy psychological burden, which is not often treated in traditional biomedical models of care, which are primarily concerned with physical symptoms and not mental well-being.

Poor mental health treatment may thus exacerbate the emotional toll that chronic illnesses such as lichen planus can inflict, threatening a cycle of worsening symptoms and worsening mental health. An awareness of the interdependence of psychological and physical well-being highlights the necessity for a more integrated healthcare model that recognizes not only medical treatment but mental health. The emergence of digital technology is a promising avenue for innovation in mental health treatment for patients with skin disorders. A recent study was conducted to coproduce a complex digital behavior-change intervention specifically for adults with skin issues, with a focus on the need for a platform that offers psychosocial support alongside physical therapy. Given that patients complained in questionnaires and interviews about an insufficiency of available psychological resources for coping with their illnesses, there is a direct need for other mechanisms of support. Thus, interventions such as smartphone applications can offer reliable resources with informational, emotional, behavioral, and peer support elements tailored to the particular challenges of this population. This model aims to empower the patient through self-management skills alongside routine medical therapy, addressing the lack of readily available psychotherapeutic support in conventional medical settings.

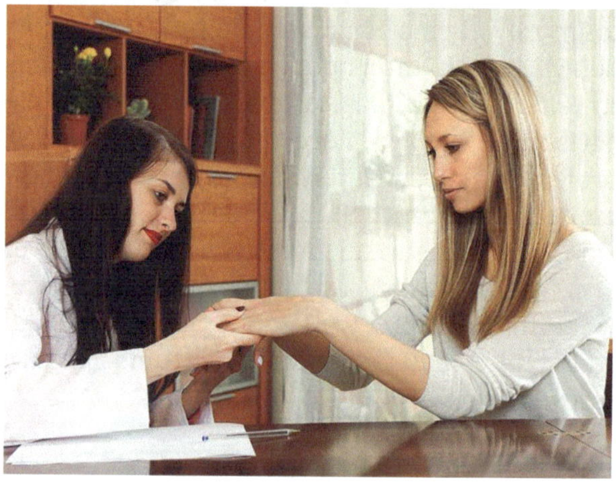

Figure 9.11. Mental health support.

Source: https://media.post.rvohealth.io/wp-content/uploads/2020/09/6408-hand_exam_woman-732x549-thumbnail-732x549.jpg.

Ponder further on the broader implications for patient outcomes when mental health treatment is integrated in the management of lichen planus and other skin diseases. Mental health treatment not only occurs at the psychological level but can also positively influence treatment adherence and outcomes. With reduced anxiety and improved self-esteem, patients will tend to be more active in adhering to recommended treatment timelines. Such a holistic approach justifies the need to incorporate mental health centers into dermatological treatment, citing that emotional well-being can directly impact physical health. Integration of psychological support as part of an overall treatment plan has been shown to provide greater control over chronic conditions, thereby offering a two-way advantage that optimizes the emotional and physical aspects of patient care (Hewitt et al., 2025; Kerr et al., 2012) (Figure 9.11).

Test Your Knowledge

1. What are coping strategies for managing emotions?
2. What is the importance of mental health support?

9.4. Related Conditions

Learning Outcome

1. Understand the oral lichen planus
2. Describe the lichen planopilaris
3. Define the Lichen Sclerosus

Lichen planus, an inflammatory chronic disease of the mucous membranes and the skin, can also be associated with many other ailments that are difficult to diagnose and treat. Pruritus, a very unpleasant sensation that induces scratching, is one of the frequent ailments that can occur in association with lichen planus. The development of pruritus, a common dermatological issue, can even worsen the discomfort of lichen planus because patients may find themselves trapped in a vicious cycle of inflammation and damage to previously sensitive lesions. This connection brings to mind that healthcare providers need to manage pruritus not only as such but also as a key underlying contributor to lichen planus' overall clinical picture (Briffa et al., 2009). Understanding such concomitant signs helps formulate an effective management plan and improves patients' quality of life. Another condition linked to lichen planus is psoriasis, an autoimmune disorder characterized by chronic skin inflammation and scaly plaques. Psoriasis shares several immunopathological features with lichen planus, such as T-cell activity and hyperproliferation of the skin. The etiologic overlap between lichen planus and psoriasis suggests that individuals with one disease are at risk of developing the other. The overlap between the conditions complicates the diagnosis, as healthcare practitioners must identify both conditions to treat them properly (Bhaswanth et al., 2023). Proper differentiation between the conditions is essential because treatment for one condition is quite different from that for the other; hence, detailed patient evaluations are necessary to understand their overall dermatological condition. Furthermore, other associated conditions, such as autoimmune diseases and liver diseases, have been reported with lichen planus. For instance, lichen planus has been reported to have a documented association with chronic liver diseases, particularly hepatitis C. Shared underlying pathomechanisms in liver diseases and autoimmune processes can increase the incidence of lichen planus in patients with liver disease. This connection highlights the importance of employing a multidisciplinary approach in lichen planus patients, as addressing potential underlying medical issues may help manage the skin condition as well. With knowledge of the intricate nature of lichen planus and related conditions, medical practitioners can develop a more effective treatment strategy tailored to their patients' specific needs, thereby addressing both dermatological concerns and overall well-being.

9.4.1. Oral Lichen Planus (OLP)

OLP is a subacute to chronic inflammatory mucosal disorder characterized by oral mucosal lesions and usually presents as white striations, plaques, or ulcerations. Its etiology remains multifactorial, with the interplay of genetic, immunologic, and environmental factors. Clinically, the presentation of OLP is variable from individual to individual, with some individuals having asymptomatic lesions and others reporting severe discomfort. Because of its chronic duration, patients may undergo recurrent attacks, with extensive impairment of quality of life. Diagnosis is crucial because OLP tends to be mimicked by other oral diseases, and thus requires a proper evaluation to determine an appropriate treatment plan. Current literature suggests that understanding the complex nature of the condition is a cornerstone for effective treatment, thereby assisting clinicians in offering appropriate therapeutic measures tailored to patient needs (Srivastava et al., 2017). New data present a strong association between oral lichen planus and cutaneous lichen planus with lesions in both locations in some individuals. In a clinical study of patients with OLP diagnoses, 18.2% exhibited concomitant cutaneous lesions, underscoring the frequency of involvement and the need for broader diagnostic evaluation in affected individuals (Koberová Ivančaková et al., 2021). Furthermore, patients with cutaneous forms had a higher prevalence of ulcerative OLP, which contributed to more severe symptoms and greater need for systemic treatment, e.g., corticosteroids. These findings underscore the need for greater health professional awareness of the possible greater overall health impact of OLP, as a high suspicion followed by early detection and intervention can greatly improve patient outcomes. Treatment of OLP is difficult on several fronts, with its chronicity and potential to worsen. Treatment modalities typically focus on symptom reduction and inflammation control, with options ranging from topical corticosteroids to systemic therapy in more widespread cases. Effective treatment includes continuous monitoring and titration of therapy, as the disease can be relapsing-remitting. Education of the patient is also critical, as the patient may be taught to make lifestyle modifications that can reduce flare-ups, such as improved oral hygiene and avoidance of known irritants. Knowledge of the psychosocial impacts of OLP is also necessary because the condition could provoke anxiety and distress due to its visibility and unpleasantness. Therefore, an integrated approach that considers both medical and psychological interventions is necessary to optimize care in such complicated cases (Srivastava et al., 2017) (Figure 9.12).

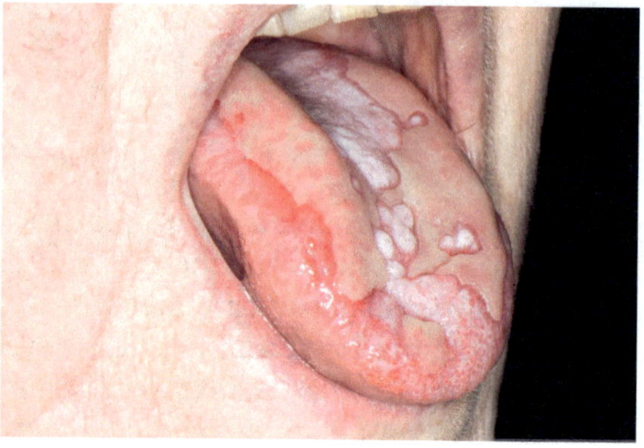

Figure 9.12. Oral lichen planus (OLP).

Source: https://img.lb.wbmdstatic.com/vim/live/webmd/consumer_assets/site_images/article_thumbnails/SEEDs/oral-lichen-planus-seeds/1800x1200-oral-lichen-planus-seeds-alt.jpg

9.4.2. Lichen Planopilaris (LPP)

LPP is a distinctive type of lichen planus that primarily affects hair follicles, leading to scarring alopecia. It is characterized by an inflammatory infiltrate that encircles and destroys hair follicles, leading to massive hair loss, primarily on the scalp. In contrast to other types of lichen planus, which may occur only on the skin or mucosae, LPP affects the hairy regions only. This condition will cause psychological distress and social impact in impacted individuals, and therefore, there is a need for early diagnosis and treatment. LPP has the potential to cause chronic inflammation that can lead to permanent hair loss; therefore, it is important for doctors to diagnose its clinical symptoms and signs promptly to implement corrective management aimed at preventing inflammation and preserving existing hair. Histopathological examination of LPP reveals several notable features that distinguish it from other conditions. Of particular mention is liquefactive degeneration of the epithelial interface, with a lichenoid tissue reaction, often accompanied by an inflammatory infiltrate comprising lymphocytes. Involvement of cytokeratin 15 (CK15) of the hair follicles inner and outer root sheath holds a special place in the pathology of LPP. Research has indicated that CK15 expression is altered in LPP, with decreased expression found near inflammatory infiltrates (Cauce et al., 2016). In addition, the apoptotic index in LPP is significantly increased, suggesting that cell apoptosis may contribute to the pathogenesis of LPP. These findings emphasize the importance of continued research to determine the molecular mechanisms of LPP and to establish a stronger basis for targeted therapy. Furthermore, lichen planopilaris frequently co-exists with other hair conditions, such as frontal fibrosing alopecia (FFA), to illustrate their related status within dermatological literature. FFA is a form of LPP that predominantly affects postmenopausal females and is clinically characterized by progressive hair loss that can extend to eyebrows and facial hair. Genome-wide association studies have also identified robust loci genetically linked to FFA, underscoring the genetic determinacy of inflammatory conditions like these (Rayinda et al., 2023). Such a connection suggests shared pathophysiology, which can better explain LPP. Genetic risk factor identification may not only aid in the identification and early diagnosis of LPP but can also lead to new personalized therapeutic approaches based on patient genetics, highlighting the need for multidisciplinary research in this direction (Figure 9.13).

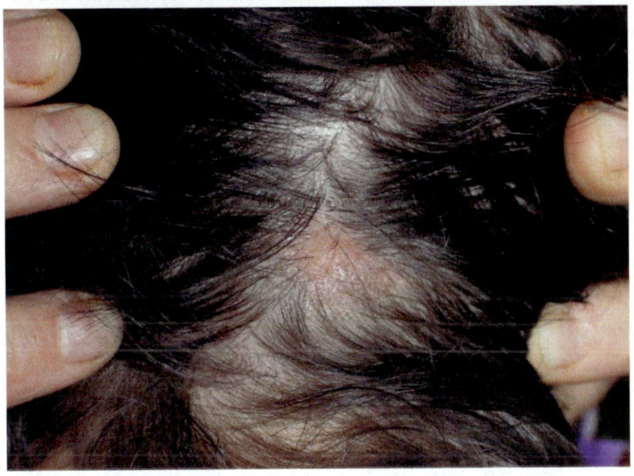

Figure 9.13. Lichen planopilaris (LPP).

Source: https://thedermdigest.com/wp-content/uploads/2023/01/LPP-shutterstock_1338490475.jpg.

9.4.3. Lichen Sclerosus

Lichen sclerosus is a type of inflammatory skin condition that affects the genital and anal regions, though it can affect other parts of the body. It is a condition characterized by whiteatrophic patches that can cause significant pain and disability through their effects of itch, pain, and scarring. It occurs most frequently in prepubertal females and postmenopausal women, suggesting a potential hormonal influence on etiology. Despite an unknown etiology, autoimmune mechanisms are suspected to play a major role, and an association between lichen sclerosus and other autoimmune illnesses has been described. Early, precise diagnosis and treatment are necessary to prevent complications, including the development of squamous cell carcinoma over affected tissue. Therefore, further research into the pathophysiology and treatment of lichen sclerosus is imperative to improve the patient's course and alleviate the psychological consequences of this distressing condition. Therapy for lichen sclerosus is typically symptomatic relief and disease prevention from worsening. Therapy is initially initiated with topical corticosteroids, which have proven effective in combating inflammation and improving symptoms. Emollients are similarly useful, providing wetness and improving skin integrity. These are in addition to these general interventions. Care needs to be individualized because many patients will likely have comorbidities that affect response to treatment. For instance, lichen sclerosus usually appears together with other dermatologic conditions, and an emphasis on thorough examinations and individualized management approaches is necessary. Knowledge of the patient's broader health history supports the clinician in optimizing care plans, including the timing of referrals to specialist care. Follow-up visits and monitoring treatment efficacy are crucial to managing this chronic condition and ensuring the patient achieves a reasonable quality of life (Nunns et al., 2017). This overlap is evident in studies comparing lichen sclerosus and lichen planus, particularly regarding histopathological features and clinical presentations. In a cross-sectional study assessing the frequency of genital involvement in women with oral lichen planus, many subjects had vulval lichen sclerosus or genital lichen planus, suggesting these conditions are associated. The difficulty of such correlations highlights the importance of comprehensive exams, including both oral and genital assessments. Besides, it was determined that the majority of women presented with asymptomatic lichen involvement, a silent form of the disease in females that requires frequent gynecologic examination in individuals with diagnosed oral lichen planus. This cross-linking underscores that clinicians must adopt a holistic approach to the management of lichen sclerosus and related conditions and ensure that treatment regimens are proactive and address potential complications (Belfiore et al., 2006) (Figure 9.14).

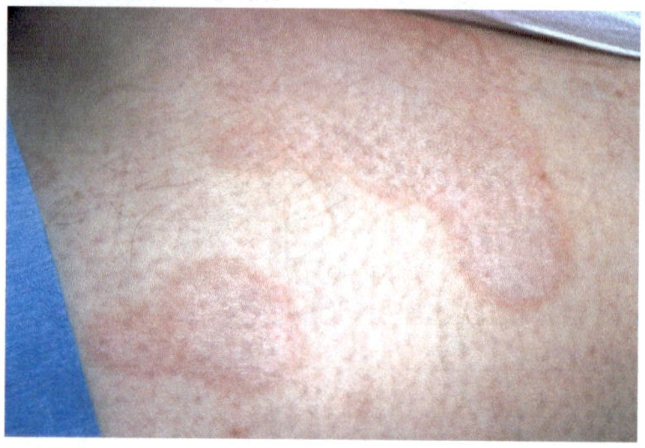

Figure 9.14. Lichen sclerosus.

Source: https://img.lb.wbmdstatic.com/vim/live/webmd/consumer_assets/site_images/article_thumbnails/BigBead/lichen_sclerosis_bigbead/1800x1200_lichen_sclerosis_bigbead.jpg.

Test Your Knowledge

1. What is oral lichen planus?
2. What is lichen planopilaris?

SUMMARY

In synthesizing studies on lichen planus and its comorbidities, the reader should remember the complexity of diagnosis and treatment. Lichen planus is more than a specific dermatological disease; it is a multifaceted disease that affects various body systems. Where genetics and environment meet is a strong focus of recent studies. Research on the efficacy of putative therapeutics, such as topical tocopherol acetate, has shown some benefit in alleviating symptoms of oral lichen planus, notably pain relief and overall patient quality of life (Bacci et al., 2016). With growing information on lichen planus, the significance of targeted therapeutic approaches becomes more critical, moving dermatological practice toward personalized medicine. Furthermore, insights from other inflammatory diseases underscore the need to understand immune response pathways in the treatment of lichen planus. Research on mesenchymal stem cells (MSCs) recognizes their potential to modulate immune responses as therapeutic avenues. First, recent findings confirm that adipose-derived mesenchymal stem cells have been found to treat oral mucosal inflammation, such as that occurring in oral lichen planus, effectively. Successful translation of MSCs into veterinary medicine, particularly in feline gingivostomatitis, has the potential to impact human therapeutic interventions (Arzi et al., 2020). Such transspecies knowledge transfer opens the door to new treatment modalities that correct the immune dysregulation observed in lichen planus and its homologs. In summary, although there are barriers to efficient treatment of lichen planus and its variants, advancing research promises improved therapeutic interventions. Research into targeted therapy, conventional therapy, and novel methods such as MSCs is an active response to treatment needs observed in current practice. As embraced in novel clinical research, continued advances in understanding immune responses are essential for optimizing therapeutic paradigms. The need for further longitudinal studies remains paramount to validate these findings and optimize treatment algorithms, with the aim of improving patient outcomes in patients with lichen planus and other inflammatory conditions. Through cooperation by means of research and clinical observation, a better comprehension of lichen planus will lead to novel therapeutic strategies that are attuned to the particular needs of each patient.

In summary, LP is an autoimmune disease with multiple facets that can significantly affect multiple organ systems, particularly the skin and mucous membranes. The pathogenesis of LP remains unclear, but it has been inferred to result from an inappropriate immune response against epithelial cells. One of the distinguishing features of LP is its association with stress and other psychosomatic disorders, which highlights the intricate interaction between the immune system and psychological factors. This interaction underscores the importance of multimodal strategies in treating LP, whereby both medical and psychosocial treatments need to be integrated to improve patient outcomes. Secondly, understanding the multifactorial etiology of LP is crucial for effective treatment and management strategies, suggesting that future research will need to explore these underlying mechanisms more deeply to develop better therapeutic approaches. The role of salivary and crevicular fluid in the diagnosis and monitoring of LP has been of great interest in the recent past. Saliva as a complex biological fluid reflects systemic biological events and may potentially be a good tool in reflecting oral manifestations of LP. One such study recently conducted in Oral Lichen Planus patients investigated whether and how Human β-defensin 2 (HBD-2), an antimicrobial peptide, was expressed. HBD-2 plays a central role in immunity. Findings indicated that HBD-2 levels may serve as biomarkers of aggressive disease activity and progression, thereby opening a new pathway for monitoring this autoimmune disease. These advances underscore the need to integrate biochemical analysis into clinical practice to manage LP and related diseases more effectively (Azzi et al., 2016). Further, the correlations of LP with systemic disease underscore the necessity of a multi-disciplinary management approach for the patient with this disorder. Research has established strong correlations between LP and systemic illnesses, including Hepatitis C and autoimmune diseases, which could complicate treatment and diagnosis. Awareness of these correlations is necessary because they have therapeutic implications and long-term treatment planning considerations. As evidence of the association between oral health and systemic diseases grows, incorporating dental assessment into treatment for LP can enhance overall patient care. Future research should examine these correlations in more detail, including how comorbidities present in patients may influence the therapeutic environment for Lichen Planus (Gow et al., 2016).

KEY TERMS FROM THIS CHAPTER

- Autoimmune diseases
- Hyperpigmentation
- Immunological markers
- Lichen planopilaris
- Lichen sclerosus
- Oral health
- Oral mucosa
- Flat-topped papules
- Hypopigmentation
- Immunotherapy
- Lichen planus
- Molecular biology
- Oral lichen planus
- Pruritus

CRITICAL THINKING QUESTIONS

1. **What is the primary characteristic of lichen planus lesions?**
   a. Yellow, greasy scales
   b. Purple, polygonal, pruritic papules
   c. Red, scaly plaques with silver scales
   d. Vesicles with clear fluid
2. **Which body parts are most commonly affected by lichen planus?**
   a. Scalp and face
   b. Palms and soles
   c. Flexor surfaces of the wrists, lower back, and oral mucosa
   d. Elbows and knees
3. **What is the name of the fine, white, lace-like lines often observed on lichen planus lesions?**
   a. Koebner phenomenon
   b. Wickham striae
   c. Darier's sign
   d. Nikolsky's sign
4. **Lichen planus is commonly associated with which of the following conditions?**
   a. Hepatitis C infection
   b. Tuberculosis
   c. Syphilis
   d. HIV infection
5. **Which of the following is a common symptom of oral lichen planus?**
   a. Painful ulcerations in the mouth
   b. Thickened plaques on the tongue
   c. Persistent dryness in the mouth
   d. White, reticulated patterns on the buccal mucosa

Short Answer Questions

1. Define the lichen planus.
2. Where are oral manifestations of lichen planus most commonly observed?
3. What is the best treatment for lichen planus?
4. What is a common psychological consequence of living with visible skin conditions like lichen planus?
5. What is lichen sclerosus?

Answer to Critical Thinking Questions

1. (b); 2. (c) ; 3. (b); 4. (a); 5. (d)

REFERENCES

1. Bose, A., Teh, M., Mackenzie, I., & Waseem, A. (2013). Keratin K15 as a biomarker of epidermal stem cells. *International Journal of Molecular Sciences, 14*(10), 19385–19398. https://doi.org/10.3390/ijms141019385Abu Eid, R., Cruickshank, M., Hijazi, K., McGee, J., et al. (2022). Disease severity scoring systems in mucosal lichen planus: A systematic review. https://core.ac.uk/download/590971285.pdf (accessed on 21st July 2025).
2. Agarwala, S. S., Burgess, J., Cade, J. E., Lynch, T. J., et al. (2017). *Hairy Leukoplakia*. https://core.ac.uk/download/213072866.pdf (accessed on 21st July 2025).
3. Amadori, F., Bardellini, E., Conti, G., Majorana, A., et al. (2017). Oral mucosal lesions in teenagers: A cross-sectional study. https://core.ac.uk/download/84586186.pdf (accessed on 21st July 2025).
4. Anderson, J. G., Bizikova, P., Ford, K., Jimenez, D. A., et al. (2020). Immunopathogenesis of canine chronic ulcerative stomatitis. https://core.ac.uk/download/286728806.pdf (accessed on 21st July 2025).
5. Antonelli, G., Cannella, F., Ciolfi, C., Gentile, L., et al. (2016). Frequent detection of high human papillomavirus DNA loads in oral potentially malignant disorders. https://core.ac.uk/download/54524230.pdf (accessed on 21st July 2025).
6. Arzi, B., Battig, J., Borjesson, D. L., Clark, D. G., et al. (2020). A multicenter experience using adipose-derived mesenchymal stem cell therapy for cats with chronic, non-responsive gingivostomatitis. https://core.ac.uk/download/323069092.pdf (accessed on 21st July 2025).
7. Azzi, L. (2016). *Oral Fluids and Auxiliary Diagnostic Techniques in Autoimmune and Neuropathic Disorders of The Oral Cavity. Local and Systemic Implications. Fluidi Orali E Tecniche Ausiliarie Diagnostiche Nei Disordini Autoimmuni E Neuropatici Del Cavo Orale. Implicazioni Locali E Sistemiche*. https://core.ac.uk/download/322777872.pdf (accessed on 21st July 2025).
8. Bacci, C., Frigo, A. C., Sbricoli, L., Stellini, E., et al. (2016). Topical tocopherol for treatment of reticular oral lichen planus: Randomized, double-blind, crossover study. https://core.ac.uk/download/53531315.pdf (accessed on 21st July 2025).
9. Balaha, H. M., & El-Sayed Hassan, A. (2022). Skin cancer diagnosis based on deep transfer learning and sparrow search algorithm. *Neural Computing and Applications, 35*, 815–853. https://doi.org/10.1007/s00521-022-07762-9 (accessed on 21st July 2025).
10. Bao, Z. X., Liu, L. X., Shi, J., Yang, X., et al. (2016). Serum zinc levels in 368 patients with oral mucosal diseases: A preliminary study. https://core.ac.uk/download/71060443.pdf (accessed on 21st July 2025).
11. Belfiore, P., Cabibi, D., Campisi, G., De Cantis, S., et al. (2006). Unexpected high frequency of genital involvement in women with clinical and histological features of oral lichen planus. https://core.ac.uk/download/53220022.pdf (accessed on 21st July 2025).
12. Bhaswanth, N., Reddy, M. P., & Sekhar, D. V. (2023). Psoriasis skin disease classification based on clinical images. https://core.ac.uk/download/588567846.pdf (accessed on 21st July 2025).
13. Bianchini, D., Calvieri, S., Cantisani, C., Cantoresi, F., et al. (2014). Overview on topical 5-ALA photodynamic therapy use for non-melanoma skin cancers. https://core.ac.uk/download/188827444.pdf (accessed on 21st July 2025).

14. Bigby, M., Khan, A., Savage, N. W., Seymour, G. J., et al. (2002). The pathogenesis of oral lichen planus. https://core.ac.uk/download/14998554.pdf (accessed on 21st July 2025).

15. Borgia, F., Li Pomi, F., Vaccaro, M., Alessandrello, C., Papa, V., & Gangemi, S. (2022). Oxidative stress and phototherapy in atopic dermatitis: Mechanisms, role, and future perspectives. *Biomolecules, 12*, 1904–1904. https://doi.org/10.3390/biom12121904 (accessed on 21st July 2025).

16. Bruni, F., Cedirian, S., Pampaloni, F., Piraccini, B. M., Quadrelli, F., Rapparini, L., & Starace, M. (2024). Enhanced insights into frontal fibrosing alopecia: Advancements in pathogenesis understanding and management strategies. https://core.ac.uk/download/620486966.pdf (accessed on 21st July 2025).

17. Campisi, G., Capra, G., Giovannelli, L., & Panzarella, V. (2017). Human papillomavirus (HPV) detection in keratotic variants of oral lichen planus: Negative results in a preliminary open study. https://core.ac.uk/download/153520551.pdf (accessed on 21st July 2025).

18. Cantisani, C., Didona, D., Donati, M., Mercuri, S. R., et al. (2017). Histology of non-melanoma skin cancers: An update. https://core.ac.uk/download/153368938.pdf (accessed on 21st July 2025).

19. Cauce, V., Groma, V., Skuja, S., Upeniece, I., et al. (2016). Eradication of damaged keratinocytes in cutaneous lichen planus forms demonstrated by evaluation of epidermal and follicular expression of CK15, indices of apoptosis and regulatory protein S100. https://core.ac.uk/download/429953050.pdf (accessed on 21st July 2025).

20. d'Apuzzo, F., Grazia, M., Minervini, G., Moccia, S., Nucci, L., & Spagnuolo, C. (2020). Polyphenols as potential agents in the management of temporomandibular disorders. https://core.ac.uk/download/521168944.pdf (accessed on 21st July 2025).

21. Georgescu, S. R., Mitran, C. I., Mitran, M. I., Popa, G. L., et al. (2019). Photodynamic therapy as a new therapeutic approach of oral lichen planus. https://core.ac.uk/download/216811053.pdf (accessed on 21st July 2025).

22. Ghoreschi, K., Meier, K., & Solimani, F. (2019). Emerging topical and systemic JAK inhibitors in dermatology. https://core.ac.uk/download/286097357.pdf (accessed on 21st July 2025).

23. Gow, N. A. R., Lilic, D., Moorhouse, A. J., Raza, A., et al. (2016). Clonal strain persistence of *Candida albicans* isolates from chronic mucocutaneous candidiasis patients. https://core.ac.uk/download/77050515.pdf (accessed on 21st July 2025).

24. Hewitt, R. (2025). The MiDerm App: A mixed methods approach to developing a complex digital behavior change intervention for adults living with skin conditions. https://core.ac.uk/download/613173442.pdf (accessed on 21st July 2025).

25. Kerr, O. A. (2012). An analysis of patients presenting to primary and secondary care with dermatological conditions in south-east Scotland with reference to the dermatological training of general practitioners. https://core.ac.uk/download/429705995.pdf (accessed on 21st July 2025).

26. Koberová Ivančaková, R., Radochová, V., & Slezák, R. (2021). Analysis of coexistence of oral and cutaneous lesions in 253 patients with lichen planus–Single-center retrospective analysis. https://core.ac.uk/download/493042921.pdf (accessed on 21st July 2025).

27. Nunns, D., & Simpson, R. C. (2017). Skin diseases affecting the vulva. https://core.ac.uk/download/76975202.pdf (accessed on 21st July 2025).

28. Rautava, J., & Tuominen, H. (2021). Oral microbiota and cancer development. https://core.ac.uk/download/554075586.pdf (accessed on 21st July 2025).

29. Rayinda, T. (2023). Molecular genetic exploration of frontal fibrosing alopecia and uncharacterized hair disorders. https://core.ac.uk/download/595954650.pdf (accessed on 21st July 2025).

30. Rodrigues, V. (1998). Oral cancer in the UK: To screen or not to screen. https://core.ac.uk/download/2778984.pdf (accessed on 21st July 2025).

31. Srivastava, S. (2017). Oral lichen planus: A case report. https://core.ac.uk/download/354382239.pdf (accessed on 21st July 2025).

32. Tüting, T., & Wenzel, J. (2008). An IFN-associated cytotoxic cellular immune response against viral, self-, or tumor antigens is a common pathogenetic feature in "interface dermatitis". https://core.ac.uk/download/pdf/82402560.pdf (accessed on 21st July 2025).

33. Vella Briffa, D. (2009). *Pruritus*. https://core.ac.uk/download/83019812.pdf (accessed on 21st July 2025).

34. Vikholt, K. J. (2014). Oral candidiasis and molecular epidemiology of *Candida glabrata*. https://core.ac.uk/download/30907335.pdf (accessed on 21st July 2025).

35. Walsh, L. J. (2003). Mast cells and oral inflammation. https://core.ac.uk/download/15000714.pdf (accessed on 21st July 2025).

36. Zammit, M. L. (2010). *Photosensitivity: Light, Sun and Pharmacy*. https://core.ac.uk/download/83019863.pdf (accessed on 21st July 2025).

ACNE VULGARIS AND ROSACEA

10

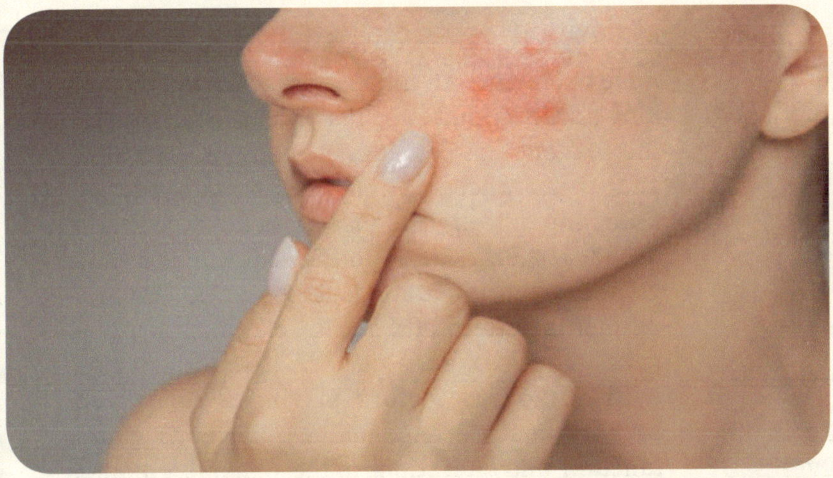

LEARNING OBJECTIVES

After studying this chapter, you will be able to:

1. Understand the causes of acne vulgaris
2. Understand the causes of rosacea
3. Know the symptoms of acne vulgaris
4. Know the symptoms of rosacea
5. Describe the treatment options for acne vulgaris
6. Describe the treatment options for rosacea

Introduction

Acne vulgaris and rosacea are two of the most common skin conditions worldwide, especially among adolescents and adults. Both conditions are characterized by inflammatory processes that manifest as varied skin lesions, ranging from comedones and pustules in acne to erythema and telangiectasia in rosacea. Prevalence of these conditions not only impacts body appearance but also significantly impacts victims' psychological well-being, in most instances leading to low self-esteem as well as increased social anxiety. Knowledge of the epidemiology and pathophysiology of these conditions is essential for planning effective intervention measures. More research has only increased understanding of the molecular mechanisms underlying the occurrence and severity of these skin diseases, strengthening the necessity of pathogen-specific therapy. These therapies would aim to meet the specific needs of patients with acne vulgaris and rosacea. The pathologies of acne vulgaris and rosacea are not merely the tip of the iceberg; they encompass the intricate relationship between host immune responses and skin microbiota. Skin, as the biggest organ, is a key element of overall health and plays a barrier role to pathogens, and is densely populated with commensal microbes that influence skin pathology. Dysbiosis of the skin microbiota has been implicated in various inflammatory cutaneous diseases, including acne and rosacea, as alterations in the microbial community favor inflammation and impair homeostasis. New perspectives on the skin microbiome have opened new avenues for future treatment.

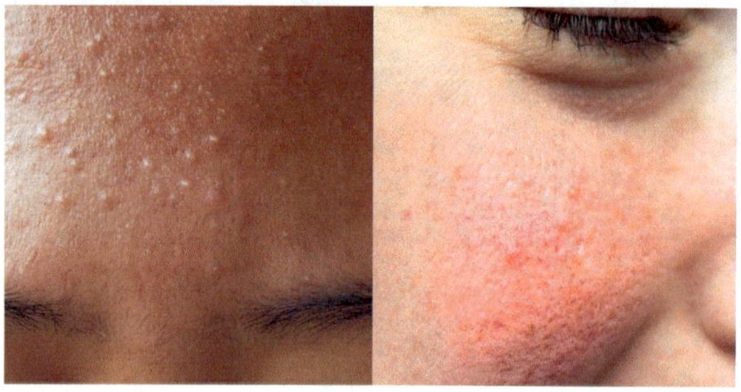

Figure 10.1. Acne vulgaris and rosacea.

Source: https://encrypted-tbn0.gstatic.com/images?q=tbn:ANd9GcTqBm9CjSPLIEbT2ygHE2OwVI6S2OONdzeFXg&s.

New therapeutic strategies that restore and modulate the skin microbiota can offer promising avenues for easing the physiological derangements experienced in both acne vulgaris and rosacea, with improved prospects for healthy skin (Yang et al., 2022). Other than microbial factors, the innate role of inflammation in the pathogenesis of acne and rosacea cannot be denied. Chronic inflammation is a hallmark feature of both conditions and is caused by a range of factors, including hormonal imbalances, environmental stress, and dietary habits. Exaggerated inflammatory responses provoke the release of various pro-inflammatory mediators, leading to tissue injury and exacerbation of clinical manifestations of the diseases. Emerging research into dietary phenolic compounds' function has indicated their potential in influencing inflammatory pathways in such skin ailments. These compounds could potentially neutralize the negative effects of chronic inflammation by targeting inflammatory mediators and pathways, such as cyclooxygenase and nuclear factor-κB. This can ultimately help control acne vulgaris and rosacea (Rahman et al., 2021). Thus, identifying microbial as well as inflammatory contributions provides a unifying paradigm for understanding and treating these prevalent skin disorders (Figure 10.1).

Definition of Acne Vulgaris

Acne vulgaris is an inflammatory dermatosis of long duration that is primarily characterized by the presence of comedones, papules, pustules, and, in advanced lesions, cysts and nodules. Epidemiologically, the disease is most common in adolescents and young adults and has gained attention due to its potential impact on mental health and social relationships. The pathogenesis of acne vulgaris is multifactorial, with numerous factors playing a role, such as hormonal derangements, sebaceous gland function, and alterations in the skin microbiome. In particular, androgens stimulate the sebaceous glands to secrete sebum, and the proliferation of *Propionibacterium acnes* contributes to the inflammatory response that manifests as acne lesions. Such sophistication of interaction places emphasis on why the condition has to be seen in intricate detail so that treatment protocols can be properly altered, aimed at reducing symptoms as much as eliminating causative agents. The management of acne vulgaris requires a multi-level approach, combining topical and systemic therapies with advances in dermocosmetics. Recent work highlights the evolving role of dermocosmetics in the treatment of acne, with a focus on their active ingredients that can bolster conventional therapy. These products are designed to combat acne while preserving the integrity of the skin's lipid barrier and minimizing irritation, thereby ensuring improved curative results. The use of soft, non-comedogenic ingredients in dermocosmetics has the potential to prevent or diminish the signs of acne vulgaris without compromising healthy skin, a consideration given that the condition tends to worsen when aggressively treated. This combination of dermatological science and cosmetic technology represents a paradigm shift in the management of acne vulgaris, meeting the skin's need for both therapeutic and restorative care (Borkowska et al., 2024). Skin microbiome dysbiosis has also been found to play a significant role in the pathophysiology of acne vulgaris.

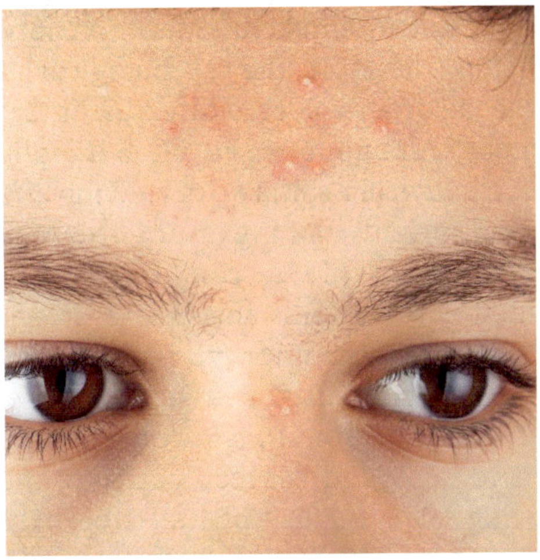

Figure 10.2. Acne vulgaris.

Source: https://ysm-res.cloudinary.com/image/upload/ar_1:1,c_fill,dpr_3.0,f_auto,g_faces:auto,q_auto:eco,w_500/v1/yms/prod/dfb3cf17-c47e-40d9-a330-2dfdcd5de408.

It has been revealed through studies that microbial population imbalance leads to the disruption of the immune response, resulting in chronicity and severity of disease. The intricate interactions between microbiomes and skin and gut health highlight the potential for a holistic approach to treatment modalities. Dietary effects on the gut microbiome are relevant to skin disease, including acne vulgaris, and suggest that dietary control may benefit skin health. Because dermatologists and researchers seek new therapeutic strategies, the microbiome's function offers new avenues to develop preventive and therapeutic remedies that not only address the symptoms but also address the etiology of acne vulgaris (Callewaert et al., 2021) (Figure 10.2).

Definition of Rosacea

Rosacea is an inflammatory, chronic skin disorder characterized by facial erythema, papules, and pustules. It is more common in adults, particularly those with fair skin, and typically presents with flushing on the central face, followed by chronic redness, visible blood vessels, and thickened skin on occasion. Unlike acne vulgaris, which is primarily brought about by clogged pores and overproduction of sebum, the pathophysiology of rosacea is less well understood and is considered to be a resultant effect of genetic propensity, environmental irritation, and immune factors. The diagnostic difficulties in rosacea stem from the overlap of its symptoms with those of other diseases, so physicians must conduct extensive assessments to distinguish it from related skin disorders. Rosacea is typically classified into subtypes, with each subtype possessing its own set of symptoms and clinical manifestations. The four main subtypes are erythematotelangiectatic rosacea, facial flushing and chronic redness; papulopustular rosacea, akin to acne vulgaris with papules and pustules; phymatous rosacea, leading to skin thickening with irregular nodularity of the skin surface; and ocular rosacea, with manifestations affecting the eyes, such as dryness and irritation. It is helpful to be familiar with these subtypes because treatment may be adjusted based on the specific features of the condition. Other than that, lifestyle factors such as emotional stress, climatic factors, and food intolerance may trigger rosacea symptoms, thus the need to implement a holistic approach to managing patients, taking into consideration both the medical and psychosocial aspects of the disease. Pharmacologic and nonpharmacologic therapeutic interventions are largely combined in treating rosacea, depending on patient preference. Topical treatments, such as metronidazole and azelaic acid, address inflammation and bacterial factors, whereas systemic treatments, such as oral antibiotics, are used in more severe cases. Non-pharmacologic therapy, such as mild skin care products and lifestyle changes, also plays a crucial role in reducing flare-ups. In some cases, therapy such as laser treatment can help ease vascular lesions of rosacea. Given the multifactorial etiology of rosacea, there is a need for ongoing research into its mechanisms and treatment, with a specific emphasis on the necessity to develop potent, well-balanced treatment regimens to maximize patient outcomes and quality of life for those affected (Figure 10.3).

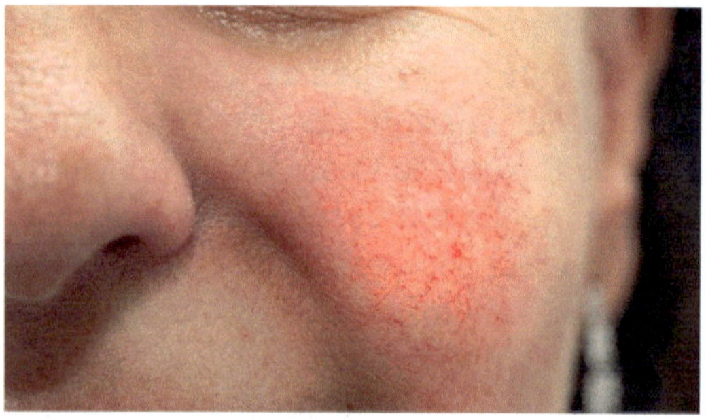

Figure 10.3. Rosacea.

Source: https://images.everydayhealth.com/images/skin-beauty/skin-conditions-you-should-know-about-02-rosacea-1440x810.jpg?w=768.

Importance of Studying These Skin Conditions

Realizing the importance of studying dermatological diseases such as acne vulgaris and rosacea is not only important for individual health but also for larger public health policy. Dermatological diseases have a high global prevalence and affect a large percentage of the population. A study of 27 European countries found that nearly 43.35% of the population had one or more dermatological disorders in the past year, with acne the most common condition, affecting around 5.4% of the population (Richard et al., 2022). Such widespread occurrence of skin disease makes effective dermatological management a priority. Health policies seeking to improve the accessibility of dermatological services must consider these numbers to address the needs of millions of individuals suffering from painful skin infections, thereby raising overall community well-being. Acne vulgaris and rosacea are also known to result in psychosocial effects. These conditions significantly impact a patient's quality of life as they result in embarrassment, anxiety, and depression. Therefore, the psychological burden of these disorders necessitates an integrated system of treatment based on both physical and psychological health. By reviewing effective treatments and management techniques, healthcare providers can then institute combined care systems that not only address symptoms but also improve patients' mental status. Being addressed is a key to addressing the multidimensional aspects of concerns related to acne and rosacea patients, thereby improving their quality of life. Moreover, the exploration of underlying pathophysiological processes generates important knowledge that can have the potential to improve therapeutic strategies for treating acne vulgaris and rosacea. Chronic inflammation is a major driver of the initiation and worsening of such skin disorders, highlighting the need for targeted anti-inflammatory treatments (Rahman et al., 2021). By defining the molecular mechanisms underlying inflammation and its relationship to healthy skin, specialists can formulate new therapeutic interventions that not only suppress symptoms but also address the root causes of these disorders. This awareness provides the potential for new therapies with phenolic acids and other anti-inflammatory agents. For this reason, the pathophysiologic basis of acne and rosacea is essential to understand for the development of effective therapies that translate into better patient outcomes and benefit the dermatologic community at large.

10.1. Causes of Acne Vulgaris

Learning Outcome

1. Illustrate how hormonal changes act as a significant trigger of acne vulgaris
2. Understand the bacterial involvement in acne vulgaris
3. Know the environmental factors of acne vulgaris

The pathogenesis of acne vulgaris is multifactorial, with intrinsic and extrinsic factors both contributing to the clogging and inflammation of the pilosebaceous unit. Among the primary contributors is hypersecretion of sebum, an oily secretion produced by sebaceous glands. Hormonal fluctuations, especially during puberty or menstruation, increase androgen levels, which induce sebum secretion. This excess oil, combined with hyperkeratinization—skin cells that fall away sooner than usual—provides a setting in which plugging of the hair follicles is likely. This plug provides an ideal medium for *Cutibacterium acnes*, a bacterium that typically inhabits the skin, to proliferate and elicit an inflammation response. Understanding these processes underscores the seriousness of acne vulgaris and the necessity of therapies that target both hormonal and microbial processes to curb symptoms and recurrence. The second important area of appreciation of acne vulgaris is the role of the skins microbiota and its interaction with the immune response. The skin's microbiome is not a fixed entity; it is determined by several factors that encompass environmental exposure and diet. Disruption of skin microbial populations, known as dysbiosis, has been implicated in several inflammatory dermatoses, including acne vulgaris. Because the microbiome cooperates with the immune system, alteration leads to a deranged immune response, again contributing to acne. The relationship between gut health and skin disease also highlights the systemic nature of acne vulgaris, in which alterations in the gut microbiome lead to cutaneous pathologies. This realization presents an opportunity for holistic treatment modalities that target microbial health in skin and gut to intercept acne formation and severity (Callewaert et al., 2021). In addition to hormonal and microbiome factors, external host features such as dietary intake, stress, and environmental stimuli also play a significant role in the exacerbation of acne vulgaris.

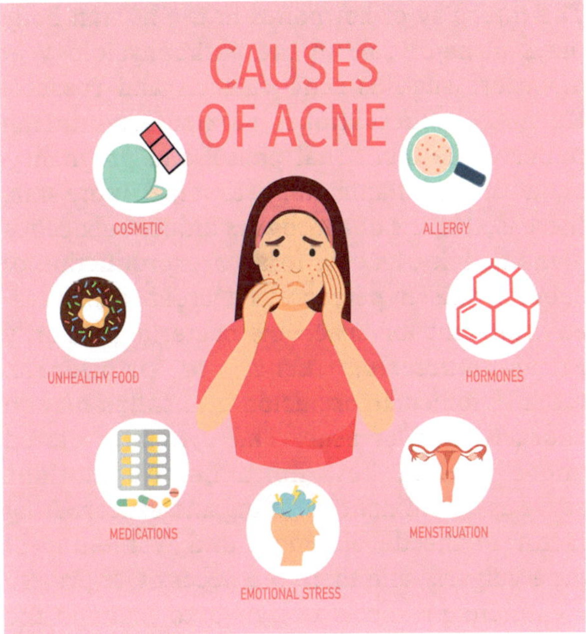

Figure 10.4. Causes of acne.

Source: https://cdn.shopify.com/s/files/1/0591/2988/8965/files/causes-of-acne.jpg?v=1725536129.

Dietary patterns high in refined carbohydrates and dairy products have been associated with an increased prevalence of acne, suggesting that specific food intake may modulate hormonal responses involved in the pathogenesis of acne. Stress has also been identified as a causative factor, as it can activate the hypothalamus-pituitary-adrenal (HPA) axis, which is involved in sebaceous gland function and inflammation (Clark et al., 2020). The effects of these extrinsic influences on individual biological tendencies reflect the multifactorial etiology of acne vulgaris, highlighting the need for an integrated strategy for its management and treatment (Figure 10.4). By taking internal and external factors into consideration, scientists and clinicians are better able to design interventions that address the specific conditions of individuals with this common dermatosis.

10.1.1. Hormonal Changes

The interplay of hormones in the human body plays a major role in the pathophysiology of disorders such as acne vulgaris and rosacea. Hormonal fluctuations, particularly during puberty, the menstrual phase, and pregnancy, enhance the inflammatory response in the skin. Increased levels of androgens induce sebaceous gland activity, leading to an overproduction of sebum. This hypersecretion creates an ideal environment for anaerobic bacteria, primarily *Propionibacterium acnes,* to proliferate, causing follicular occlusion and inflammation characteristic of acne. The dynamics stated above explain how hormonal fluctuations serve as a dominant initiating and exacerbating factor in the development and worsening of acne vulgaris, and therefore necessitate precise treatment protocols designed to manage the underlying hormonal effects on skin well-being. In addition to acne, hormonal effects also appear to have a key role in rosacea pathogenesis, although the mechanisms behind this are not known. Newer evidence has highlighted the inflammatory nature of rosacea, with typical features being erythema and inflammatory lesions. Endocrine changes, particularly in the hypothalamus-pituitary-adrenal (HPA) axis, may exacerbate the manifestations of rosacea, although the precise pathogenesis remains unclear. This interaction is underscored by the skin's ability to respond to stress hormones, which may trigger inflammatory pathways that lead to dilated vessels and erythema that last. Such hormonal interactions illustrate the multifactorial etiology of rosacea, which may require the successful therapy to include an in-depth understanding of both hormonal effects as well as the inflammatory mechanisms that drive the disease (Korting et al., 2009). Also, the skin is an endocrine organ itself, complicating how hormonal changes are connected to conditions like rosacea and acne. The cutaneous HPA-like axis allows localized steroidogenesis in response to systemic stressors as well as environmental stressors and modulates inflammatory skin disease. The pilosebaceous unit is the major site for the synthesis and metabolism of various steroid hormones, including androgens and glucocorticoids, with immediate implications for the pathogenesis of acne and rosacea (Clark et al., 2020). Treatment modalities targeting hormonal pathways, such as hormonal therapy or certain anti-inflammatory agents, may help reduce the severity and frequency of episodes. Recognition of the subtle interrelations between hormones and dermatologic disorders thus provides a vital direction both for clinical research and treatment in dermatology (Figure 10.5).

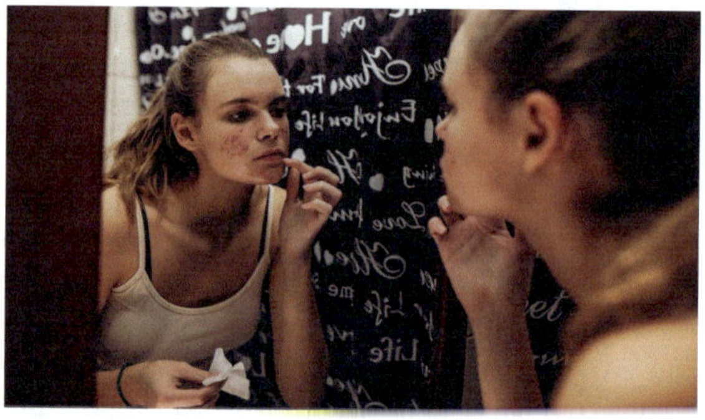

Figure 10.5. Hormone changes in adolescents and young adults.

Source: https://www.grxstatic.com/4f3rgqwzdznj/t5mkStm3KbGEyTkCj2FP1/0ccd86e80117e699748240d66aa1500e/teen_girl_looking_at_acne_in_mirror_1260651280.jpg?format=pjpg&auto=webp&width=704.

10.1.2. Bacterial Involvement

The relationship between bacteria and skin diseases such as acne vulgaris and rosacea is multifaceted and complex. The most direct association is with *Propionibacterium acnes*, a gram-positive anaerobic bacterium. This bacterium flourishes in sebaceous follicles where it triggers a cascade of inflammatory processes. The proliferation of *P. acnes*, along with enhanced production of sebum, results in the blockage of hair follicles and the production of comedones subsequently. As the follicular contents oozes into the immediately adjacent dermis, a non-specific inflammatory reaction ensues, consisting of lymphocytic and neutrophilic infiltrates, which increase inflammation and cause lesions characteristic of acne vulgaris. This bacterial inflammation is not limited to a local phenomenon; it plays a universal role in maintaining skin health and underscores the need for specific antimicrobial therapy in the treatment of acne. In rosacea, too, the bacterial role is similarly important but different from that in acne vulgaris. Although the definitive etiopathogenesis of rosacea remains unclear, recent studies lend support to the belief that inflammation plays a central role in the pathogenesis and worsening of rosacea symptoms. Tetracycline analogs such as doxycycline have been found useful in the management of rosacea and acne, largely because of their anti-inflammatory effects rather than their direct antibacterial action against demodectic mites or other infectious forms. These agents control inflammatory cascades by inhibiting matrix metalloproteinases and suppressing pro-inflammatory cytokines, so facilitating increased skin homeostasis in subjects with rosacea. The complexity of the bacterial role is reflective of the more diffuse inflammatory character of rosacea, warranting deeper exploration of the function of different microbial flora in the development and responsiveness to treatment of the disease (Korting et al., 2009). Even acneiform eruptions can manifest from varied etiologies, including drug-induced causes and secondary infection, well demonstrating the complex interaction of bacterial involvement in cutaneous conditions. Acneiform dermatoses are secondary to an inflammatory response to precipitants like medications, leading to follicular eruptions that can clinically mimic classic acne vulgaris. The eruptions tend to be sudden in onset and are often accompanied by systemic evidence of toxicity, suggesting an underlying substrate of bacterial or viral interaction. Gram-negative folliculitis can complicate acne presentations in some cases, thereby underscoring the usefulness of microbiological testing in the differential diagnosis. The need to distinguish the conditions is paramount in informing appropriate treatment modalities that not only address the symptomatic presentation but also potential bacterial involvement and its contribution to inflammation (Jansen et al., 1998).

10.1.3. Environmental Factors

The relationship between environmental factors and skin well-being is important in the context of rosacea and acne vulgaris. External factors such as pollution, climate, and UV radiation can potentially precipitate the conditions. For instance, exposure to urban air pollutants has been implicated with increased oxidative stress and inflammation, both of which are involved in the exacerbation of symptoms of rosacea and acne. The effects of environmental pollutants extend beyond local skin irritation; sustained exposure can alter the skin's barrier function and microbial flora. Insight into how they are interdependent is hence critical to effective management of patients with these conditions. Discussion of how environmental insults result in skin disease supports the need for holistic measures, not just attention to treatment protocols, but also lifestyle changes to prevent exposure to carcinogenic environmental agents. The reaction of the skin to environmental insult highlights the need for holistic skincare routines tailored to particular conditions like acne vulgaris and rosacea. Other variables such as changes in temperature and humidity can influence sebum secretion, which is a factor in the causation of acne. Conversely, abnormally dry environments can irritate the skin and exacerbate rosacea. All this encourages individuals to cultivate awareness of customized skin care routines, prompting them to adjust their practices according to seasonal variations and local climatic conditions. Improved understanding of such interactions underscores the need for complex treatment regimens, in which environmental adaptations may serve as adjunctive therapies to pharmacological management. The recognition of the role the environment plays in maintaining skin health promotes integrated care, enabling one to actively take measures to manage their conditions successfully. Additionally, the correlation between environmental stressors and the gut-skin axis underscores a dynamic system in which extrinsic stressors may affect intrinsic microbiome health. New research suggests that imbalances in the gut microbiota may play a role in inflammatory dermatological conditions, including acne vulgaris and rosacea. The relationship between the gut, the skin, and the environment is deserving of more in-depth investigation, since altering diets and exposure to toxins have the ability to impact the microbial diversity of the gut. For instance, a diet composed of pre-prepared food can aggravate gut and skin inflammation. Thus, integrative strategies that focus on dietary patterns along with environmental factors could elucidate new avenues for the reconstitution of skin health. Although studies support the intricate interconnectedness among environmental conditions, intestinal microbiome homeostasis, and skin pathology, there is an urgent need to explore integrative therapies that incorporate lifestyle and environmental factors into management to achieve better results (Acharjee et al., 2022; Błaszczyński et al., 2024) (Figure 10.6).

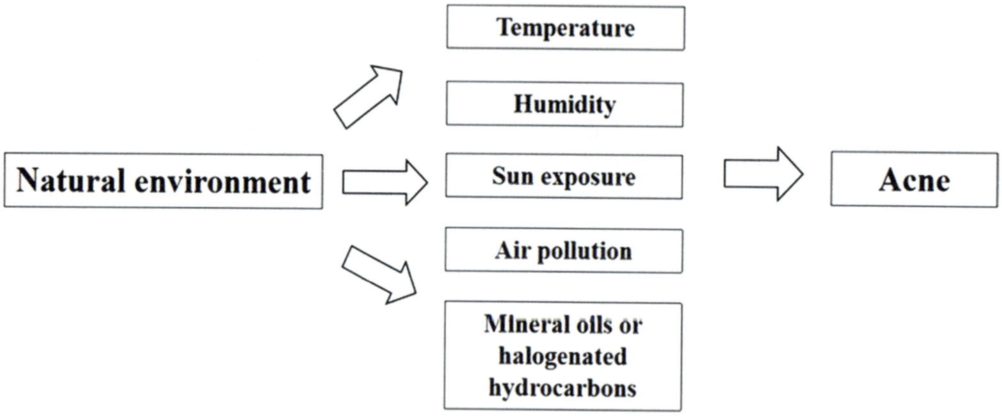

Figure 10.6. Factors of natural environment affecting acne.

Source: https://www.researchgate.net/publication/344375865/figure/fig3/AS:11431281242225212@1715402884131/Factors-of-natural-environment-affecting-acne.tif.

Test Your Knowledge

1. What role do androgens play in the development of acne vulgaris?
2. Which bacterium is predominantly associated with acne vulgaris?

10.2. Causes of Rosacea

Learning Outcome

1. Understand the genetic predisposition in the manifestation of \rosacea
2. Understand the triggers and exacerbating factors associated with rosacea
3. Describe the immune system response of rosacea

The pathogenesis of rosacea is multifactorial and encompasses numerous varied genetic, environmental, and psychosocial variables that together contribute to its etiology. Genetic susceptibility plays a significant role, as the condition has been observed to occur in clusters within families, suggesting an inherited basis. The heritability may be due to a number of polymorphisms that modulate vascular and immune function, thereby causing the characteristic flushing and inflammatory responses of rosacea sufferers. Furthermore, environmental triggers such as ultraviolet light, temperature, and certain dietary elements can precipitate exacerbation of symptoms, illustrating the interplay between intrinsic and extrinsic factors in the etiological explanation of the disorders. Based on understanding these causative factors, treating physicians can respond more effectively with individualized treatment protocols for patients, underscoring the value of extensive evaluation of each patient's trigger profile. Psychological stress becomes a major underlying mechanism in rosacea, adding yet another level of complexity in its etiology. Emotional and psychological stressors can increase cortisol and other stress hormone release, further inducing vascular hyperreactivity in susceptible individuals. The role of the skin as an endocrine organ, functioning in a hypothalamic-pituitary-adrenal (HPA)-like axis, underscores the interconnection between systemic stress responses and cutaneous disease (Clark et al., 2020). Specifically, this axis permits the skin to respond to stress and modulate steroidogenic activity, which can manifest itself as inflammatory dermatoses, for example, rosacea. On this basis, stress management and counseling may therefore be an important element of holistic treatment protocols designed to alleviate symptoms and prevent relapse. Lastly, one cannot ignore the function of microbiomes, with new findings pointing to a potential role of changes in skin microbiota in the etiology of the conditions.

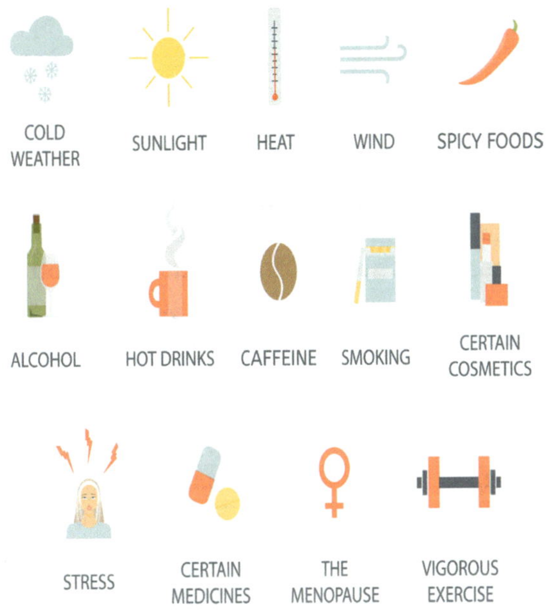

Figure 10.7. Causes of rosacea.

Source: https://www.esteva.com.ua/wp-content/uploads/2021/11/prichiny-rozaczea-angl-1536x864.jpg.

In focus is the potential function of Demodex mites, a cutaneous commensal organism linked to rosacea. High populations of these mites have been identified in patients with the disease, and a potential pathogenic mechanism involving microbial imbalance and dysregulation of the immune system has been proposed. Besides, interaction between the skin's inflammatory reaction and outside microbial threat could be the factor why certain individuals develop rosacea and not others. With growing understanding of the skin's ecological climate, more research into the microbiome's role is crucial to creating bespoke therapies aimed at addressing the causes and manifestations of rosacea (Adaskevich et al., 2006) (Figure 10.7).

10.2.1. Genetic Predisposition

Genetic susceptibility is a key determinant in the onset of skin conditions such as Acne Vulgaris and Rosacea. Experiments have proved that individuals with a family history of such disorders are highly susceptible to developing similar conditions, which points towards a genetic component. A number of genetic contributors have been identified through research that influence the skin's barrier function, immune response, and inflammatory pathways. This genetic influence is best evidenced by changes in sebum constitution and production, both of which are central to the pathogenesis of Acne Vulgaris. Genetic variation can also affect skin pH and microbial colonization, which are central determinants of acne lesion initiation, as seen in the contribution of skin pH to maintaining epidermal barrier integrity and antimicrobial protection (Abeck et al., 2006). In contrast, Rosacea also has its genetic basis. Hereditary tendencies, though not fully understood, suggest that individuals with a history of Rosacea in their family are more likely to have the condition. It is possible that genetic predisposition interacts with environmental stimuli, such as ultraviolet radiation and exposure to heat or cold, to trigger increased inflammatory processes in Rosacea. The condition is characterized by recurrent flushing and facial redness, a symptom of an aberrant immune response caused by hereditary factors (Dogan et al., 2017). Additionally, research has confirmed that vascular reactivity and inflammation gene mutations that control these pathways could be the foundation for the characteristic facial flushing and telangiectasia found in patients with Rosacea, emphasizing the multidetermined nature of the illness. The interplay between hereditary susceptibility and environmental factors is a highly fascinating area to explore further in the management of Acne Vulgaris and Rosacea. Elucidation of the hereditary components may allow more personalized treatment regimens. For instance, understanding that certain patients are genetically susceptible to heightened inflammatory responses or abnormal sebaceous gland function might encourage medical practitioners to adjust their approach accordingly. Along with clinical significance, patient education regarding the hereditary nature of these disorders is also important in facilitating understanding of their disease etiology and course. Additionally, ongoing research into the genetic etiology of Acne Vulgaris and Rosacea will continue to identify new therapeutic targets, ultimately leading to improved patient outcomes for these prevalent skin disorders (Figure 10.8).

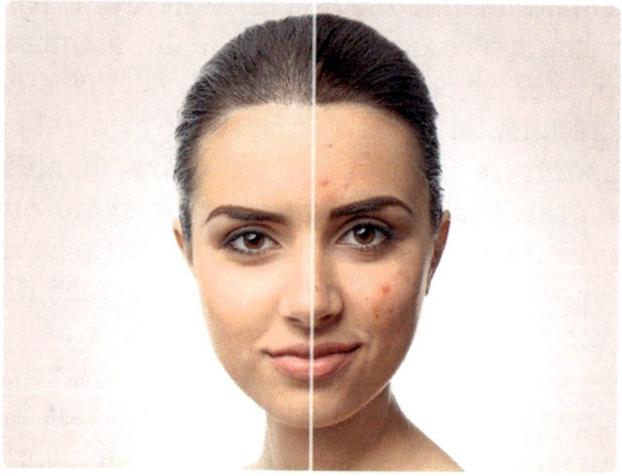

Figure 10.8. Genetics of acne.

Source: https://d2jx2rerrg6sh3.cloudfront.net/image-handler/picture/2018/11/By_Africa_Studio.jpg.

10.2.2. Triggers and Exacerbating Factors

The triggers and exacerbating factors of Rosacea and Acne Vulgaris need to be understood to treat and manage them effectively. It has been identified that emotional stress is a significant factor, and research indicates that stress can lead to the aggravation of acne lesions. The emotional factor can very well influence hormonal changes, which have been known to contribute significantly to acne development. In addition, external conditions such as humidity and temperature can exacerbate the two ailments by inducing excessive sebum production and sweating, thereby providing an environment for bacterial growth. The combination of the stimuli makes it even more difficult to control the two skin diseases, as people have to address both psychological and environmental factors to actually relieve their conditions. Diet also plays a significant role in triggering the eruption of acne vulgaris. There have been reports that some foods, particularly those with high amounts of sugar and unhealthy fats, will cause flare-ups in acne patients. On the other hand, eating diets with a high content of fruits and vegetables is said to have a positive impact on the skin. While the precise mechanisms remain under study, it has been theorized that such dietary consumption influences the gut microbiome and the immune system. A changed gut microbiome can lead to dysbiosis and, hence, exacerbate skin conditions like acne vulgaris and rosacea. The association validates the contribution of dietary elements and encourages a deeper understanding of the impact of nutrition and the microbiota on skin health, suggesting potential therapeutic directions. The presence of specific bacteria in the skin microbiome has also been directly correlated with the severity of acne vulgaris. Research has identified a common occurrence of *Propionibacterium acnes* within lesions, in conjunction with other bacteria such as *Staphylococcus epidermidis* and *Staphylococcus aureus*. Local pressure and hyperhidrosis due to exercise have been reported in research to be causative, demonstrating a synergy between environmental and microbial factors in skin health. The dysbiosis of the skin, as well as possibly the gut microbiomes, not only supports an altered immune response but also suggests interactive pathways that lean toward the development of acne and rosacea. This multifactorial aspect of causative factors and triggers necessitates a holistic treatment strategy that considers the patient's microbiome, lifestyle, and emotional well-being (Abu-Nabaa et al., 2016; Callewaert et al., 2021) (Figure 10.9).

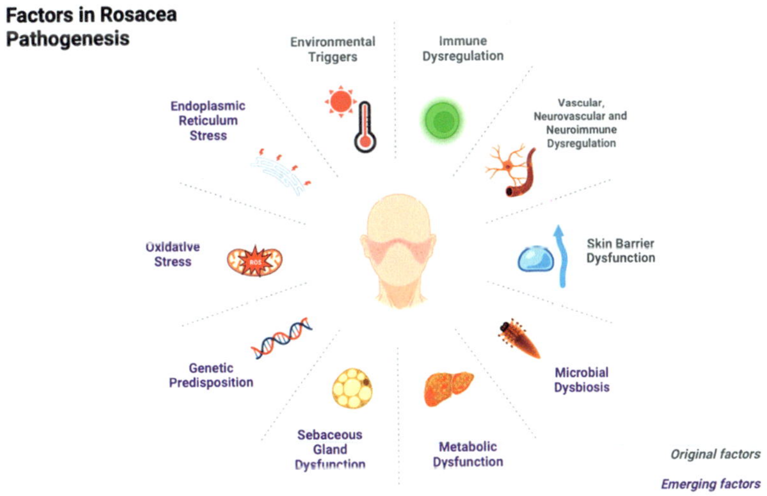

Figure 10.9. Schematic diagram illustrating the original and emerging factors implicated in the pathogenesis of rosacea.

Source: https://www.mdpi.com/biomedicines/biomedicines-11-02153/article_deploy/html/images/biomedicines-11-02153-g001.png.

10.2.3. Immune System Response

The immune response is a key element in the pathogenesis of acne vulgaris and rosacea, two common inflammatory dermatoses. In acne, excess sebum, often due to hormonal imbalances, creates an environment in which *Cutibacterium acnes*, a known pro-inflammatory trigger, can thrive. This triggers activation of components of the innate immune system, which in turn recruits neutrophils and macrophages to the site. This production of pro-inflammatory cytokines worsens the condition and results in the characteristic lesions of acne. Awareness of such an immune response is important for designing targeted therapies to modulate the inflammation and reestablish homeostasis in the skin in patients with acne vulgaris. Similarly, rosacea is not merely characterized by vascular dysregulation but also by an overactive immune system. Studies have demonstrated that rosacea patients are likely to have altered levels of antimicrobial peptides (AMPs), which are critical components of the skin's native defense. Small AMPs, which are typically involved in combating microbial invaders, may become dysregulated and contribute to inflammatory disease associated with rosacea. In addition, studies have revealed to the forefront that AMPs play a crucial role in the therapeutic mechanisms of inflammatory skin diseases, suggesting a possible therapeutic avenue for treating patients with rosacea. The complex interplay between immune responses and skin disease necessitates therapies that re-educate the immune system to combat the etiologic agents of rosacea effectively (Albiol Matanic et al., 2012). The role of the cutaneous hypothalamus-pituitary-adrenal (HPA)-like system also complicates the immune response in conditions such as acne and rosacea. This system enables the skin to respond to stress by secreting hormones that regulate both inflammatory responses and sebum output. Shifts along this dimension can exacerbate inflammatory dermatoses, suggesting that psychological stressors may be increasing the severity of acne and rosacea eruptions. The interplay between hormonal dynamics and inflammation and stress illustrates the symbiotic relationship between the endocrine and immune systems in cutaneous health. As research into the mechanisms of such interactions continues, opportunities to design innovative treatments that target both symptoms and the fundamental hormonal determinants of acne vulgaris and rosacea will become ever more promising (Clark et al., 2020).

Test Your Knowledge

1. Which genetic factor is critical in maintaining the skin's antimicrobial defense?
2. Which climatic conditions are known to worsen acne vulgaris and rosacea symptoms?

10.3. Symptoms of Acne Vulgaris

Learning Outcome

1. Describe the types of lesions
2. Understand the classification of severity in acne vulgaris
3. Know the psychological impact of acne vulgaris

The symptoms of acne vulgaris are very wide-ranging, and they can significantly affect physical appearance and one's well-being. The primary ones are comedones, which are further subdivided into open comedones (blackheads) and closed comedones (whiteheads). Inflammatory lesions, such as papules and pustules, may develop as the condition progresses. These are firm, red bumps filled with pus. The more severe types of the condition can also lead to nodular acne, which manifests as deep, painful acne lesions that cause severe scarring. The severity and occurrence of these symptoms can lead to psychosocial complications of shame and embarrassment, as the public associates clear skin and beauty with social acceptance. There is a requirement to assess the full spectrum of symptoms to provide appropriate management and treatment for the affected. Apart from physical manifestations, the emotional consequences of acne vulgaris are also important and are not usually given attention. Research indicates that patients with this condition usually have increased anxiety levels and rates of depression, mainly due to the observable disfigurement and associated stigma of their skin. The psychological anguish caused by acne can be compounded by unrealistic beauty ideals propagated by media presentation and societal expectations. Clearly, the psychological factors are entrenched as a part of the patient experience of acne vulgaris, further affirming the importance of addressing both dermatology and mental health in the approach to treatment. A recognition of the interface between cutaneous and emotional health highlights the importance of well-designed interventions capable of improving quality of life in the affected. Acne vulgaris affects not only personal experience but also interpersonal relations and social interactions. People may withdraw from social contacts and avoid social interactions due to fear of being judged based on their skin, ultimately causing them to become isolated and further negatively impact their self-esteem. Furthermore, the long-term condition of acne can affect activities of daily living and satisfaction with life. Psychological impacts of the condition are compounded by the risk of side effects from treatments, such as those experienced after the use of isotretinoin, known to have been linked with mood shift. This complex interplay lends credence to using multidisciplinary treatment methods to address not just the physical treatment of the acne vulgaris but also psychological counseling and support. Addressing these symptoms holistically will help minimize both the dermatological and affective impacts of this pervasive disorder, producing a more holistic recovery experience for patients (Dubravka Šimić et al., 2009; Calabrese et al., 2024) (Figure 10.10).

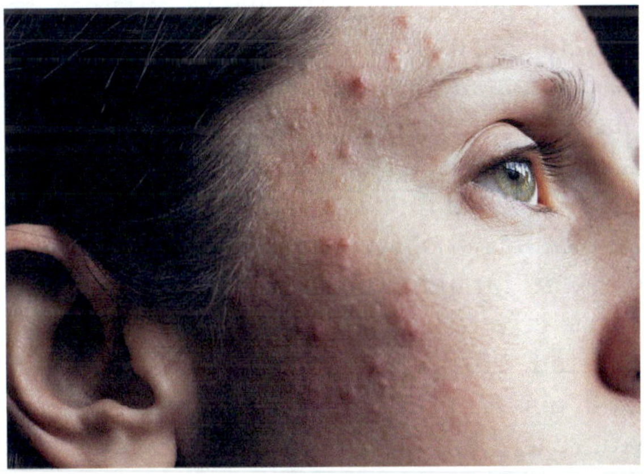

Figure 10.10. Symptoms of acne vulgaris.

Source: https://www.health.com/thmb/M97lm60na0ix41eCtfli4D9NefE=/1500x0/filters:no_upscale():max_bytes(150000):strip_icc()/Health-GettyImages-1390356588-f5c3a87b335a43238d4ef3eff16aa0fe.jpg.

10.3.1. Types of Lesions

The lesion expression is the fulcrum of the diagnosis and understanding of rosacea and acne vulgaris, as they share distinct forms that can significantly affect patient outcomes. For acne vulgaris, the lesions predominantly consist of comedones, papules, pustules, nodules, and cysts. Comedones are open or closed, non-inflammatory lesions and represent the initial phase in the formation of acne. These can eventually become inflammatory lesions in the papular and pustular forms, characterized by swelling and pus, respectively. Nodules and cysts are usually more established forms of acne, and they eventually become scarred, causing the patient ongoing distress. The various types of lesions not only determine treatment regimens but also provide a hint at the severity and longevity of the condition, which is important in clinical practice and warrants accurate evaluation. In contrast, rosacea has a specific set of lesions, such as erythematous papules, pustules, and telangiectasia that affect the mid-face. Chronic flushing and erythema, with the development of these lesions, are other specific features of rosacea. Superficial inflammation may manifest as erythematous papules, while pustules are morphologically similar to acne pustules but are accompanied by unique vascular changes specific to rosacea. Also, telangiectasia or dilated blood vessels can appear, adding to the chronic nature of facial redness. These lesions highlight the complexity of the disease of rosacea, where both the inflammatory and vascular aspects of the condition have to be addressed in a targeted therapeutic approach, leaving no doubt about the distinctions from acne vulgaris with regard to pathophysiology and treatment. The management of acne vulgaris lesions and rosacea can be supported by emerging therapeutic approaches, such as antimicrobial peptides (AMPs) and photodynamic therapy (PDT). AMPs have been gaining attention as potential therapeutic agents for inflammatory dermatoses, including acne vulgaris, due to their resistance-free antimicrobial activity. Besides, PDT has emerged as an appealing therapy not only for acne but also for rosacea, capitalizing on its ability to erase targeted lesions with minimal loss of surrounding tissue. By using a light-activatable photosensitizer, PDT demonstrates efficacy in reducing lesions and rejuvenating the skin, thereby offering the prospect of long-term management of both diseases. These advances highlight the importance of being aware of lesion types in designing effective treatment regimens that account for the unique characteristics of acne vulgaris and rosacea (Figure 10.11).

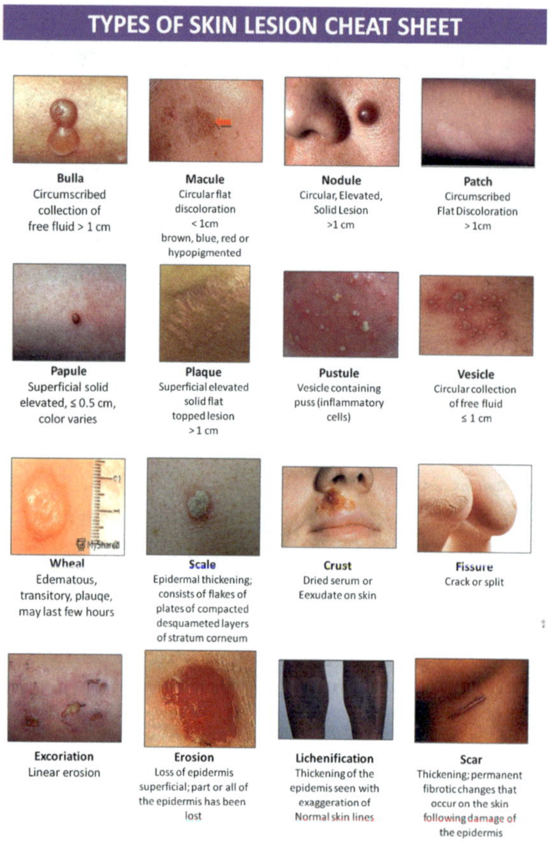

Figure 10.11. Types of skin lesion.

Source: https://cdn.medizzy.com/i4E5NfHcqgL_Ekelr1VUP_CYd70=/800x1149/https%3A%2F%2Fs-media-cache-ak0.pinimg.com%2F736x%2F33%2Fdf%2F2a%2F33df2a01aa165067437e03befb113708--medical-coder-medical-billing.jpg.

10.3.2. Severity Classification

Severity classification of acne vulgaris and rosacea is a critical framework for clinicians to select appropriate treatment modalities and to monitor patient outcomes. Acne vulgaris is typically classified as mild, moderate, or severe based on criteria such as lesion count and type, scarring, and severity of inflammation. Mild acne, for instance, may be found with few comedones and isolated papules, whereas severe forms consist of numerous inflammatory nodules and cysts, causing extensive physical and psychological disability. A nuanced appreciation of these gradations allows dermatologists to aim interventions accordingly, aligning treatment measures with the condition's severity to optimize patients' quality of life and minimize risk of long-term complications. Similarly, severity grading in rosacea is important, as this disabling disorder presents in variable forms, affecting physical appearance, social life, and mental status. Rosacea is most often classified into four subtypes: erythematotelangiectatic, papulopustular, phymatous, and ocular rosacea, each characterized by distinct clinical manifestations that can deteriorate over time. Grading of rosacea severity often incorporates patient questionnaire-based symptoms and objective parameters of facial erythema and lesion types. Characterization of the different subtypes assists in making a more accurate diagnosis, guiding therapeutic interventions, and predicting the course of the disorder. This practice highlights the need for clinicians to observe rosacea's progression in order to prevent exacerbations as well as improve the treatment of affected patients. Incorporating severity classification into practice is not only essential for effective treatment but also underscores the importance of early intervention. Studies have shown that patients with severe rosacea and acne are more likely to harbor psychosocial burdens of anxiety and depression. As such, an established classification of severity enables early referral and counseling that can address the underlying causes. A case in point is a patient with severe inflammatory acne who requires intensive medical intervention and psychological counseling, enabling an integrated approach to care that includes all of these. In addition, continuing education on the classifications and their ensuing clinical implications, as emphasized by Adaskevich et al. (2006), is essential for best practice in dermatology. By integrating severity classification into their diagnostic and treatment frameworks, healthcare providers can significantly enhance the management of acne vulgaris and rosacea, resulting in improved patient health outcomes.

10.3.3. Psychological Impact

The psychological impact of acne vulgaris and rosacea is significant, often extending beyond their physical features. Individuals with acne may experience a range of emotional disturbances, including anxiety, depression, and social withdrawal. As indicated by research, the outward appearance of acne can increase self-awareness of how one looks, leading to body dissatisfaction and low self-esteem. This conflict within oneself can manifest in many ways, ranging from avoiding social events or activities that attract attention to the skin, thus increasing feelings of loneliness. Furthermore, the stress associated with healing a chronic skin disorder has the unintended consequence of intensifying the severity of acne itself, thereby producing a debilitating cycle on psychological and physical health. This subtlety underscores the necessity of holistic care that addresses not only the dermatological concerns but also the psychological dimensions of such disorders. Even in combination with acne vulgaris, rosacea possesses profound psychological dimensions that cannot be ignored. The unpredictable flare-ups and facial redness that characterize rosacea can cause significant emotional distress. Individuals afflicted with it may feel stigmatized and judged by society, further contributing to feelings of shame or embarrassment.

Social stigma is then further reinforced when individuals perceive the condition to be caused by personal hygiene or lifestyle factors, further destroying their self-perception. The chronic nature of rosacea causes many to feel trapped and frustrated by navigating through a condition that is described as being difficult to treat. This makes it all the more important that mental health treatment be a part of the treatment plan for individuals diagnosed with rosacea, as these patients must navigate the whole context of their experience, not the symptoms alone. New therapeutic modalities of treatment for rosacea and acne vulgaris, as the use of botulinum toxin, are indicative of evolving perceptions of these illnesses, including their psychological impact. Favorable results have been demonstrated for the therapeutic efficacy of botulinum toxin in reducing not only the physical manifestations of acne and rosacea but also the psychological morbidity of these patients. As the outward signs of these conditions diminish, individuals experience increased self-esteem and overall quality of life. However, from the literature, further research is still needed to optimally ascertain the long-term effects of such therapy on both the psychological status and skin health. This highlights the need for multidisciplinary therapy that incorporates both dermatological treatment and psychological guidance to treat patients on multiple levels (Clark et al., 2020; Chmiel et al., 2025) (Figure 10.12).

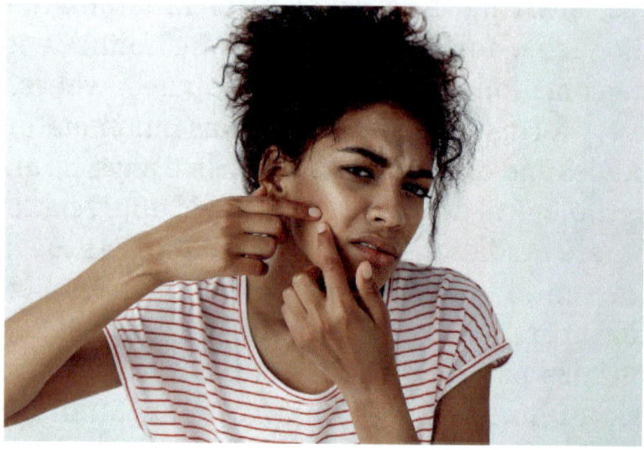

Figure 10.12. The psychological impact of acne on mental health.

Source: https://kulanispa.com/wp-content/uploads/2023/05/The-Psychological-Impact-of-Acne-on-Mental-Edit.jpg.

Test Your Knowledge

1. What are the three types of lesions?
2. What is the classification of acne by severity?

10.4. Symptoms of Rosacea

Learning Outcome

1. Understand the common signs and symptoms of rosacea
2. Know the variability in presentation of rosacea
3. Describe the impact of acne vulgaris and rosacea on quality of life

Rosacea is a long-term inflammatory cutaneous disease characterized by a range of symptoms that can affect a person's quality of life. Most often, patients experience intermittent facial erythema (redness) that may present as flushing or blushing, becoming an ongoing feature over time. To this, telangiectasia, or the prominence of blood vessels, is often seen, contributing to the overall facial redness. In others, papules and pustules may also occur, which are akin to acne vulgaris but with variations in their pathology. Such an inflammatory nature of rosacea, although not fully understood, highlights the complexity of its signs and symptoms and further necessitates a critical examination of its etiology and treatment on account of the predominance of evidence indicating substantial inflammation present in the condition's manifestation (Korting et al., 2009). In addition, ocular symptoms are frequently associated with rosacea, thereby complicating the clinical presentation and affecting patients' general well-being. Dryness, itching, and burning of the eyes, which is termed ocular rosacea, may be experienced by patients. Blepharitis, inflammation of the eyelids, may also affect patients, leading to significant discomfort and complications if left untreated. The association between the skin and ocular symptoms suggests a systemic inflammatory response that transcends the localized cutaneous character, and thus, an in-depth understanding of rosacea is essential for its management and treatment. Finally, the similarity in association between the signs further reinforces the argument for continued research into the pathophysiology of rosacea to formulate targeted treatments that address both the dermatologic and ocular manifestations of the disease (Albiol Matanic et al., 2012). The fluctuating course of rosacea can have extensive psychosocial implications, influencing the patient's mental and emotional well-being. The visible nature of the condition has a tendency to lead to stigma and low self-esteem, hence social avoidance and reduced quality of life. The patient can also become self-conscious about their appearance, particularly when they withdraw from social interactions and, in the long term, become isolated. Also, the variable and constant nature of rosacea symptoms may develop frustration and hopelessness, which contribute to the psychological effect of the disease. Physicians should not only underscore the physical management of rosacea but also detect and address patients' emotional issues. Recognition of this emotional burden is crucial in formulating a comprehensive treatment plan that includes both the physical effects and the psychological health of those suffering from this condition (Korting et al., 2009) (Figure 10.13).

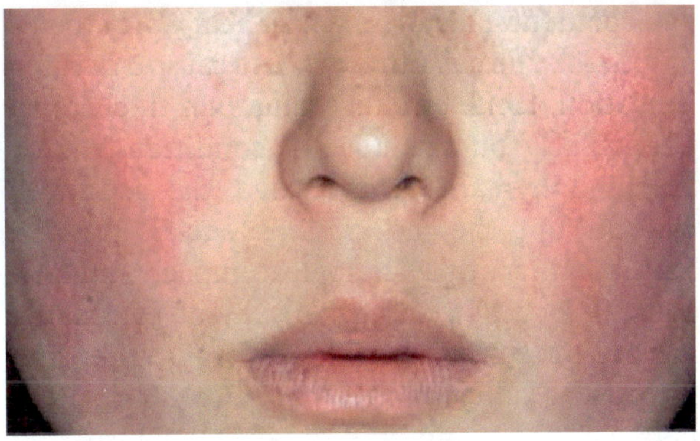

Figure 10.13. Symptoms of rosacea.

Source: https://www.yourgreatskin.com/wp-content/uploads/2023/11/Feature_Rosacea.jpg.

10.4.1. Common Signs and Symptoms

Presentation of Acne Vulgaris is accompanied by a range of typical signs and symptoms that can significantly impact the quality of life for sufferers. Primarily, acne appears as comedones, either closed (whiteheads) or open (blackheads). Inflammatory lesions, such as papules, pustules, and nodules, also exist, which tend to cause distress and risk of scarring if not addressed in a timely manner. These lesions target essentially the sebaceous gland-abundant areas, including the face, back, and shoulders, which tells its own story regarding the relationship between hormonal instability and the severity of acne. Not only is it damaging to one's physical appearance, but it can also be a cause of emotional suffering and anxiety to individuals, particularly young people, and their overall mental health and self-worth, as testified by research works on the psychological impacts of the disease. While Acne Vulgaris has typical signs and symptoms, Rosacea also has typical signs and symptoms, often including facial erythema, visible blood vessels, and acne-like papules and pustules. However, what distinguishes rosacea from other forms of acne is that it is progressive and chronic, with recurrent episodes of flushing or flare-ups triggered by environmental factors such as heat, spicy foods, or alcohol. The condition can also cause a burning sensation, facial swelling, and skin thickening, particularly on the nose, a condition known as rhinophyma. If progressive, the condition can disrupt the individual's social life and have significant psychological impacts, making early recognition and management of rosacea important to prevent symptom progression and improve quality of life. The level of overlap between the symptoms of Acne Vulgaris and Rosacea complicates diagnosis and requires careful evaluation by clinicians. Although the two diseases share some similarities, correct differentiation requires distinguishing them by clinical presentation to use appropriate treatment regimens. Age, lesion pattern, and the presence of other symptoms differentiate the two. Management styles also vary, with Acne Vulgaris often requiring drug therapy, either topical or systemic, while Rosacea may be managed with laser therapy or even some topical preparations aimed at suppressing inflammation and erythema. Addressing the common signs and symptoms, as well as the psycho-emotional effects they have, underscores the necessity of a holistic approach to treatment that considers the physical and emotional well-being of victims of such skin diseases (Kaptanoglu et al., 2017; Błaszczyński et al., 2024).

10.4.2. Variability in Presentation

Presentation variability is a conspicuous feature of both rosacea and acne vulgaris, underscoring their complex nature as skin diseases. Acne vulgaris is typically noted as an array of lesions, including comedones, papules, pustules, and cysts, of varying severity and distribution. Age, endocrine alterations, and hereditary factors are significant determinants of this variation. For instance, while adolescents may have extensive severe inflammatory acne on the face, adults may experience more circumscribed flare-ups or chronic lesions, particularly in the perioral distribution. Its clinical presentation may also change in response to environmental influences or secondary to certain drugs, highlighting the need for diverse treatment approaches that take these polyvariant presentations into account. Similarly, rosacea has a wide range of clinical appearances, which can make diagnosis challenging. Patients can present with chronic facial erythema, flushing, and papules and pustules on the face, but these vary in severity and nature across patients. Some patients have ocular manifestations such as burning or dryness, while others may have phymatous changes, particularly in severe cases. Of note, environmental factors such as temperature fluctuations, food, and emotional stress can trigger rosacea symptoms, leading to variability.

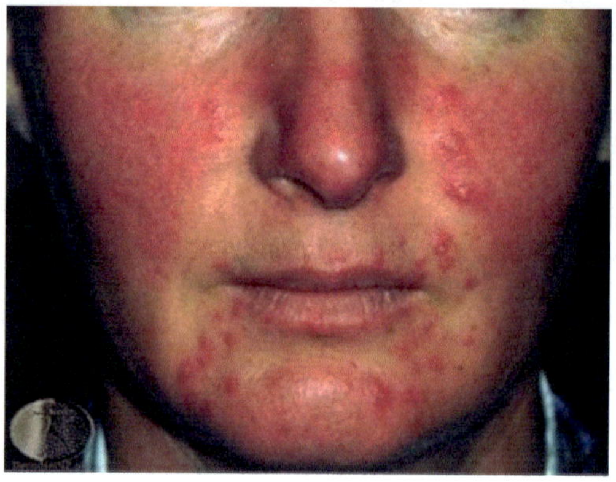

Figure 10.14. Rosacea clinical presentation.

Source: https://img.medscapestatic.com/pi/meds/ckb/86/101186tn.jpg.

Identification of these variations is crucial for clinicians, who need to formulate individualized treatments to address each patient's unique symptomatology and precipitants to optimize management outcomes. The impact of psychological disturbances on the clinical presentation of both rosacea and acne vulgaris complicates their clinical presentations even further. Research has established sadness, anger, and anxiety as significant producers of changes in the severity and duration of skin disease. For example, greater emotional distress may exacerbate inflammatory processes in acne or make rosacea patients develop flushing episodes, creating a cycle of deterioration in skin and emotional well-being. Moreover, the lack of attention to specific emotional states, such as disgust, in recent literature suggests a lack of investigation into the full spectrum of psychosocial factors influencing such conditions (Rizzo et al., 2020). Subsequent studies exploring such correlations can provide insight into enhancing therapy, enabling a more comprehensive understanding and treatment that address both physical manifestations and psychological well-being in patients with acne vulgaris and rosacea (Figure 10.14).

10.4.3. Impact on Quality of Life

Acne vulgaris and rosacea's impact on quality of life is profound, affecting many times beyond mere physical consequences. Such patients usually suffer a lot of psychological morbidity in the form of depression, anxiety, and social withdrawal. Studies show that the visible appearance of skin lesions directly leads to a degraded sense of self-esteem and body image in association with a degraded quality of life. The psychological burden is further added by societal beauty standards, which typically require clean skin, thereby adding to the sense of inadequacy and isolation in victims. For this purpose, the management of the psychological effects of rosacea and acne is the most significant concern, as mental well-being is a very important aspect of general health, and thus multidimensional treatment approaches involving both physical and psychological management become essential. Moreover, chronicity of acne vulgaris and rosacea can significantly compromise everyday functioning as well as interpersonal relations. Most affected individuals report avoiding social interactions, such as gatherings, meetings, and public speaking, out of fear of being judged for their skin condition. This avoidance may create feelings of isolation and worsen underlying mental health. Furthermore, the cost of treatment options, such as topical treatments and dermatological office visits, can be substantial and also contribute to stress and anxiety. Therefore, the effects of such conditions extend well beyond overt cutaneous manifestations, producing a self-reinforcing cycle of social exclusion and emotional distress. Identification and documentation of these integrated effects are vital in the development of successful treatment regimens. Emerging evidence suggests that the endocrine activity of the skin could be a crucial determinant in the pathogenesis of both rosacea and acne, as discussed in the context of the hypothesis of a cutaneous hypothalamus-pituitary-adrenal (HPA)-like axis. This axis emphasizes the skin's sensitivity to stress and its intrinsic ability to regulate steroidogenic activity in the pilosebaceous unit, thereby placing hormonal instability as a causative factor in such diseases (Clark et al., 2020). Moreover, the function of antimicrobial peptides (AMPs) as important components of skin defense mechanisms has been increasingly accepted in recent research, offering potential therapeutic avenues for improving the treatment of acne and rosacea (Albiol Matanic et al., 2012). As researchers continue to untangle such intricately complex biological processes, the potential exists to enhance treatment regimens that not only address the physical symptoms but also minimize the total impact on quality of life in individuals afflicted with these prevalent skin disorders.

Test Your Knowledge

1. What are symptoms of rosacea?
2. How does rosacea affect quality of life?

10.5. Treatment Options for Acne Vulgaris

Learning Outcome

1. Describe the topical treatments in the management of acne vulgaris
2. Learn about oral medications for acne vulgaris
3. Understand the lifestyle modifications of acne vulgaris

Acne vulgaris management encompasses a wide range of options, reflecting the multifaceted nature of this common cutaneous disease. Initial therapy typically consists of topical retinoid, benzoyl peroxide, or salicylic acid preparations. Retinoids, such as tretinoin and adapalene, stimulate cell turnover and suppress pore closure, while benzoyl peroxide possesses antimicrobial properties that reduce *Propionibacterium acnes* proliferation. Salicylic acid, a beta-hydroxy acid, is effective for exfoliation and cleansing of the skin. Most patients also respond to a combination therapy approach, as effectiveness is enhanced and side effects are minimized. It's essential that adolescents and young adults are engaged in learning about these treatments, especially since they are a demographic of interest among patients with acne, as evidenced by studies that highlight the ambiguities of treatment decisions made through collaboration between patients and clinicians (Andrews et al., 2015). Severe or moderate cases require systemic treatment. Oral antibiotics such as doxycycline and minocycline are commonly used to minimize inflammation and bacterial colonization. In spite of this, treatment with such drugs must be closely watched since there is the possibility of side effects as well as the development of antibiotic resistance, and hence personalized treatment programs become a must. Hormonal therapy by means of combined oral contraceptives can be effective as well, particularly in females, by regulating androgenic activity, causing sebum excess. Since research unravels significant discrepancies in information on effective management choices, medical practitioners must embark on thorough conversations with patients on such management choices so that they clearly understand the pros and cons of each (Andrews et al., 2015). In addition to pharmacological management, non-pharmacological interventions also play a crucial role in managing acne vulgaris. These may include modifications in behavior, skin care regimen, and diet to reduce precipitants of inflammation. For instance, the utilization of non-comedogenic products and a gentle cleansing routine prevents triggering of exacerbation. Based on certain observations, high-glycemic-index foods and dairy product consumption in certain individuals may induce acne, and the diet needs to be re-evaluated. Furthermore, education of the chronic status of acne vulgaris and the necessity of ongoing management is crucial, as these elements are pivotal in patient activation in their management plan. Utilizing an interdisciplinary approach to intervention, involving pharmacologic and non-pharmacologic modalities, can lead to improved outcomes in patients with acne vulgaris (Figure 10.15).

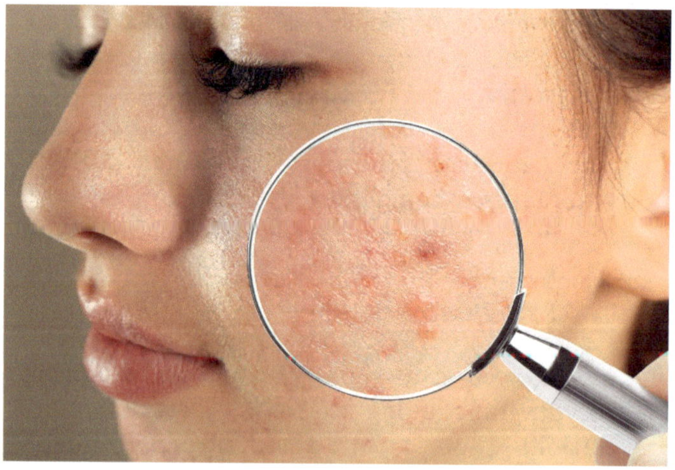

Figure 10.15. Acne vulgaris treatment.

Source: https://drdaesthetics.com/wp-content/uploads/2024/03/0-scaled.jpg.

10.5.1. Topical Treatments

Topical treatments are among the pillars of treatment for acne vulgaris because they directly address both the lesions and the pathophysiology underlying them. The most frequently applied medications are retinoids, benzoyl peroxide, and topical antibiotics, which have all been proven to be effective in reducing inflammation, as well as inhibiting the formation of new acne lesions. Retinoids such as tretinoin cause cellular turnover and therefore inhibit pore plugging, while benzoyl peroxide possesses antibacterial and keratolytic properties. Also, topical antibiotic use, including clindamycin and erythromycin, decreases the number of *Cutibacterium acnes*, the causative bacterium of acne. The synergism that develops from combining drugs tends to yield better outcomes, minimizing side effects and the development of resistance. Overall, the strategic utilization of topical treatment in acne vulgaris has been demonstrated to not only stop the manifestations but also improve the patient's quality of life. While the treatment of acne has often been thought to require a different model, as its inflammatory nature necessitates therapies that act on the inflammation itself rather than merely on bacterial factors, topical medications such as metronidazole and azelaic acid are often recommended for their anti-inflammatory effects. Metronidazole has been found to reduce papules and erythema in rosacea. In addition, azelaic acid has further advantages in diminishing comedonal lesions and hyperpigmentation. Given the increasing incidence of demodicosis, especially in rosacea patients, treatment strategies have lately gained prominence with a focus on antiparasitic actions to treat symptoms. Resolution of etiological factors such as inflammation and bacterial proliferation is important for effectively managing rosacea, as individualized treatment regimens become evident. New modalities, including photodynamic therapy (PDT), are gaining popularity as topical treatments for acne and rosacea, offering options for nonresponsive patients. PDT includes photosensitizers, which, when activated by light, induce cell damage and immunomodulation and therefore target inflammatory lesions effectively. The technique has been shown to be useful in the treatment of inflammatory diseases and is being utilized as an invaluable new tool for dermatology. The flexibility of PDT allows it to be used to move beyond cosmetic procedures, benefiting patients with sun damage and precancerous lesions. Its clinical utility remains to evolve, and additional research is necessary to establish optimal protocols and patient selection criteria with PDT. With continued advancements in topical treatments, the integration of traditional and new treatments will enhance the management of acne vulgaris and rosacea, ultimately improving patient outcomes (Figure 10.16).

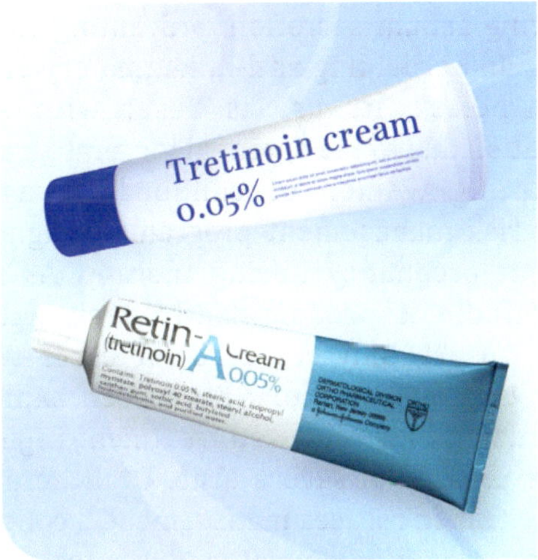

Figure 10.16. Topical treatments for acne vulgaris.

Source: https://miiskin.com/wp-content/uploads/2024/02/prescription-tretinoin-online-540x540.jpg.

10.5.2. Oral Medications

Treatment for Acne Vulgaris is typically in the form of oral medications, especially where topical treatments are inadequate. One of the most common oral therapies is antibiotic treatment, which targets the bacterial component of acne. Tetracyclines such as doxycycline and minocycline have been widely used due to their anti-inflammatory properties and ability to reduce *Cutibacterium acnes*, the etiologic bacteria. Oral contraceptives can also be a significant component in females as they regulate hormonal fluctuations that exacerbate acne. The preferred oral drug should be individualized to the patient, based on the severity of the acne, the patient's history, and potential side effects that may arise from the long-term administration of such drugs, and thus need careful monitoring by medical professionals. In individuals with severe cases of Acne Vulgaris, isotretinoin is a potent oral retinoid drug treatment. This treatment is an excellent choice for nodulocystic or cystic acne that is unresponsive to other forms of treatment. Isotretinoin acts by significantly reducing sebum secretion, preventing clogged pores, and providing anti-inflammatory effects. Nevertheless, its use is beset with strict regulation due to the potential for teratogenicity, prompting women of childbearing age to enter risk management programs designed to prevent pregnancy during therapy. As such, isotretinoin is predominantly dealt with as a last resort, only reserved for cases where other treatment options have been explored, prioritizing individualized treatment regimens in the therapy of severe acne. Oral therapy is also critical in rosacea management, a condition that is a chronic inflammatory dermatosis. While topical medications are usually the first-line treatment of choice, oral antibiotics such as doxycycline and minocycline can be used when patients are resistant to topical therapy. Oral antibiotics provide not only anti-inflammatory benefits but also address any concurrent bacterial factors involved in rosacea flares. Recent studies have also demonstrated the efficacy of alternatives such as oral nicotinamide, which has been shown to improve clinical outcomes in seborrheic dermatitis and may also influence rosacea symptoms (Cantelli et al., 2014). Consequently, a multidisciplinary approach combining both topical and oral medications enables healthcare clinicians to tailor treatment regimens that effectively improve symptoms without compromising safety and efficacy for the patient (Figure 10.17).

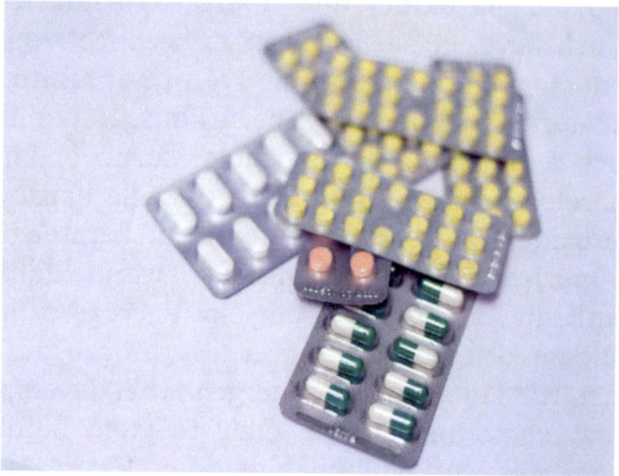

Figure 10.17. Oral medications for treating acne.

Source: https://ensoulclinic.b-cdn.net/wp-content/uploads/2022/10/melany-tuinfosalud-com-QACp304EIR0-unsplash-scaled.jpg.

10.5.3. Lifestyle Modifications

Acne vulgaris and rosacea treatment involves more than standard dermatological care, necessitating recognition of lifestyle modifications that can significantly impact skin health. Dietary choices are particularly significant. Scientific research has indicated that high-glycemic index foods, such as white bread and sweet foods, may aggravate acne by stimulating insulin release, leading to increased sebum secretion and skin cell growth (Sieradocha et al., 2024). Alternatively, eating a balanced diet rich in whole grains, fruit, vegetables, and omega-3 fatty acids may help inhibit inflammatory responses and keep the skin in good condition. In addition, adequate hydration is important; drinking the appropriate amount of water not only maintains skin flexibility but also aids detoxification, reducing the incidence of breakouts. Dietary management is thus a central aspect of lifestyle change for patients with rosacea and acne vulgaris. Apart from dietary changes, psychological well-being is another commonly overlooked element in the context of lifestyle change for patients with rosacea and acne. Psychological distress, such as anxiety and lower self-esteem, can complicate the management of these conditions (Pethani et al., 2025). Mindfulness practices such as meditation and yoga have been documented to alleviate stress and improve resilience. Additionally, maintaining a regular skincare routine in line with one's dermatology guidance not only keeps the skin healthy but also helps bolster feelings of control and normality among individuals with acne or rosacea. For this reason, emotional and psychological care, as well as healthy lifestyle habits, play a pivotal role in the management of the conditions overall. Also, skincare routine and external factors are critical to avoiding the impact of acne vulgaris and rosacea. The day-to-day skincare must be performed with sensitive, non-comedogenic products to avoid irritation and pore clogging. Patients need to be aware of environmental triggers, such as pollution, extreme weather, and allergen exposure, which exacerbate skin manifestations (Sieradocha et al., 2024). Regular cleaning and maintenance of makeup devices and airy clothing help maintain healthy skin. Daily exercise also helps the skin look healthier by improving circulation and evening out hormone levels. All these lifestyle adjustments offer an integrated approach to managing acne vulgaris and rosacea, addressing both their physical appearance and the causative agents responsible for their aggravation.

Test Your Knowledge

1. How do topical antibiotics, such as clindamycin and erythromycin, help in managing acne vulgaris?
2. Which class of antibiotics is most commonly prescribed for moderate to severe acne vulgaris?

10.6. Treatment Options for Rosacea

Learning Outcome

1. Understand the role of topical therapies in the management of rosacea
2. Describe the use of oral antibiotics in treating rosacea
3. Describe the laser and light therapies for rosacea

Management of rosacea requires a good understanding of its chronic nature and treatment modalities in patients. Lifestyle modification is typically the first step, since eliciting and avoiding precipitating factors can go a long way toward reducing flare-ups. Common exacerbating factors include very cold or very warm weather, particular foods, and cosmetics. A daily skincare routine with mild cleansers and moisturizing agents is recommended to maintain the patient's skin integrity. Both lid hygiene and unpreserved artificial tears are also advised, especially in ocular cases, which present in a large percentage of rosacea patients. Thus, instructing patients in these prevention measures not only assists in symptom control but enhances quality of life in general as they manage their condition (Dogan et al., 2017). Where lifestyle modification is not sufficient, local and systemic pharmacologic therapy plays an essential role in the management of rosacea symptoms. Local treatment agents, i.e., metronidazole and azelaic acid, possess anti-inflammatory properties and are commonly used to treat localized symptoms. In more severe lesions, oral antibiotics such as doxycycline are typically given because, in addition to combating inflammation, they target underlying bacterial components in certain patients. These medications can significantly reduce redness and pus formation and lead to prolonged remission. However, patients should be monitored by practitioners for side effects of long-term antibiotic use to maintain a balance between the medication's safety and efficacy in management (Dogan et al., 2017). In more serious cases, particularly those involving widespread ocular manifestations or widespread structural alterations in the skin, more intensive treatment modalities are necessary. Surgical techniques, including lasers and light therapies, are effective in treating vascular lesions and erythema of rosacea. These modalities promote skin renewal and address resistant symptoms to conventional therapy. Further, an interdisciplinary model that includes dermatologists and ophthalmologists is warranted for integrated care, especially when ocular rosacea is present, given the severity of vision problems that may develop in untreated cases. Utilizing a multidimensional treatment model and implementing patient-specific interventions, healthcare workers can maximize therapeutic effects and improve the quality of life for people with rosacea (Dogan et al., 2017) (Figure 10.18).

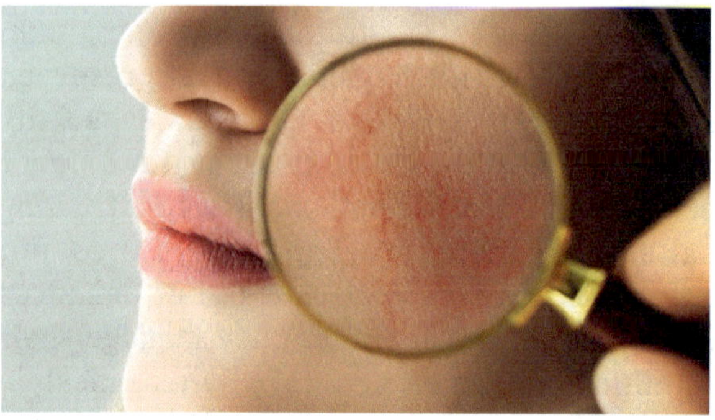

Figure 10.18. Treatment options for rosacea.

Source: https://www.esteva.com.ua/wp-content/uploads/2021/11/03-2-1536x845.jpg.

10.6.1. Topical Therapies

Topical treatments hold core importance in the management of Acne Vulgaris and Rosacea in the management of the multifactorial etiology of the two conditions. In Acne Vulgaris, an estimated 80% of adolescents and young adults are affected, with a variety of skin lesions associated with inflammation of pilosebaceous units. The cornerstone of effective treatment is usually topical agents such as retinoids, which help normalize skin cell shedding and maintain open pores. Antibiotics, when applied topically, can reduce bacterial load on the skin, further reducing inflammation. With the high prevalence of these conditions and their ability to cause psychological distress, early intervention with topical therapies is paramount in the avoidance of such complications as hyperpigmentation and scarring, which have long-term effects on the patients' self-esteem and quality of life (Chmiel et al., 2025). The use of topical therapy is also effective in the management of Rosacea, a chronic inflammatory disorder characterized by erythema, papules, and pustules. While the etiology is not specific, various types of topical agents have been developed to effectively address signs. Agents such as azelaic acid and metronidazole are often employed because they exhibit anti-inflammatory and antimicrobial properties that help reduce the inflammatory process in Rosacea. More recently developed agents, such as brimonidine, have proved promising in quickly reducing redness, one of the hallmark features of the disease. Inclusion of these topical treatments not only addresses physical symptoms but also helps to reduce the mental impact of Rosacea, which otherwise likely to aggravate the condition. Thus, an integrated approach that includes effective topical treatments can greatly enhance management outcomes among affected individuals (Chmiel et al., 2025). New advancements in topical treatments have expanded treatment options for both Acne Vulgaris and Rosacea. Recent studies on the applications of botulinum toxin have shown promise as a potential adjunct therapy, offering new hope for the treatment of acne lesions and inflammation. Studies have shown that botulinum toxin may affect the functioning of sebaceous glands, thus potentially aiding in the control of oiliness and acne eruptions. However, with the advent of new treatment modalities, it is important to conduct comprehensive research to assess their effectiveness and establish appropriate utilization protocols. Progressive developments in topical treatment technologies underscore the importance of individualized treatment protocols, in which medical professionals can tailor techniques to individual patient needs and responses. These developments not only represent progress in dermal procedures but also reflect a greater understanding of the complex nature of conditions like Acne Vulgaris and Rosacea (Bińczyk et al., 2024) (Figure 10.19).

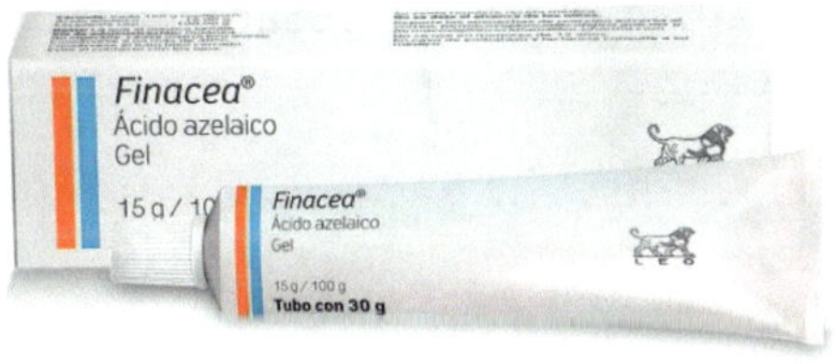

Figure 10.19. Topical treatments of rosacea.

Source: https://resources.claroshop.com/medios-plazavip/s2/62301/4941766/64c15f9b8dba1-a88224fa-ee69-49fd-961e-48c5a8326e25-1600x1600.jpg.

10.6.2. Oral Antibiotics

The use of oral antibiotics in the management of acne vulgaris and rosacea is an old dermatological tradition, primarily due to their anti-inflammatory effect. In moderate to severe acne vulgaris, medications such as doxycycline and minocycline have been used to reduce the number of acne lesions and related inflammation. These tetracycline analogs, however, have already been shown to inhibit a variety of inflammatory processes involved in the pathophysiology of acne. By downregulating cytokines and inhibiting matrix metalloproteinases, these antibiotics resonate so well with the inherent processes that exacerbate acne that they seek not only to heal its presentations but also to attack their inflammatory roots. This multi-dimensional approach supports the therapeutic benefits for patients with acne vulgaris, and oral antibiotics are thus a cornerstone of dermatologic therapy for this condition. In treating rosacea, the inflammatory nature of its course underscores the role of oral antibiotics in management. Evidence indicates that erythema, telangiectasia, and inflammatory lesions in rosacea can be markedly enhanced by antibiotic treatment. Tetracyclines, particularly doxycycline, have been recognized for their unique ability to affect a number of inflammatory mediators that make this skin disease problematic. By inhibiting the migration and proliferation of inflammatory cells, oral antibiotics can reduce the intensity of rosacea attacks, providing patients with significant relief and improved skin texture. However, it is important to note that, although antibiotics are an indispensable part of the therapeutic strategy, they must be supported by other therapeutic approaches for optimal management of rosacea manifestations, as highlighted in the latest dermatological guidelines (Adaskevich et al., 2006). While being effective, prolonged oral use of antibiotics is questionable with regard to side effects and drug resistance. Dermatologists must balance the therapeutic benefits of these medications against the risk of resistance to bacterial strains. Overuse of antibiotics in the treatment of acne and rosacea has led practitioners to a more conservative prescribing approach. Careful monitoring and proper treatment duration are necessary to minimize side effects while best achieving the therapeutic response desired. In addition, alternative therapies, such as topical treatments and lifestyle changes, must be included in multimodal treatment regimens to avoid having patients be solely dependent on oral antibiotics. Such a polypharmacy policy is consistent with the dynamic clinical course of acne vulgaris and rosacea therapy, prioritizing both efficacy and safety in dermatology (Korting et al., 2009) (Figure 10.20).

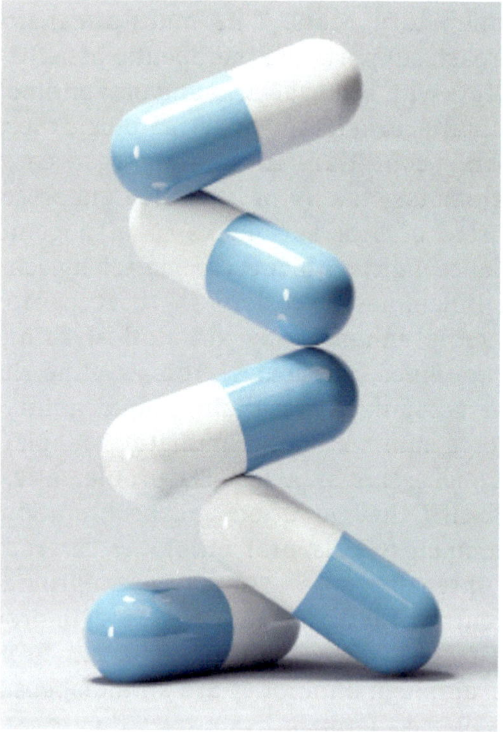

Figure 10.20. Oral antibiotics for rosacea.

Source: https://www.dermatica.co.uk/skinlab/wp-content/uploads/2024/01/Q1-24-Blog-3-Under-the-microscope-Oral-Antibiotics-for-Acne-Rosacea-and-Pigmentation.png.

10.6.3. Laser and Light Therapies

Laser and light therapies are currently prominent adjunct therapies for acne vulgaris and rosacea, addressing issues that conventional treatments cannot fully address. Both modalities use light at various wavelengths to target causative skin diseases, promoting healing and reducing inflammation. For acne vulgaris, for instance, blue light therapy specifically targets *Propionibacterium acnes*, the causative bacteria of acne. This therapy operates by generating reactive oxygen species that effectively kill bacteria on the skin surface, thereby minimizing inflammation and lesion formation. The addition of laser therapy to the treatment of acne can maximize patient outcomes, especially in patients who are resistant to standard pharmacologic approaches, thereby achieving a more holistic management strategy over time, as dictated by newer guidelines (Al-Niaimi et al., 2024).

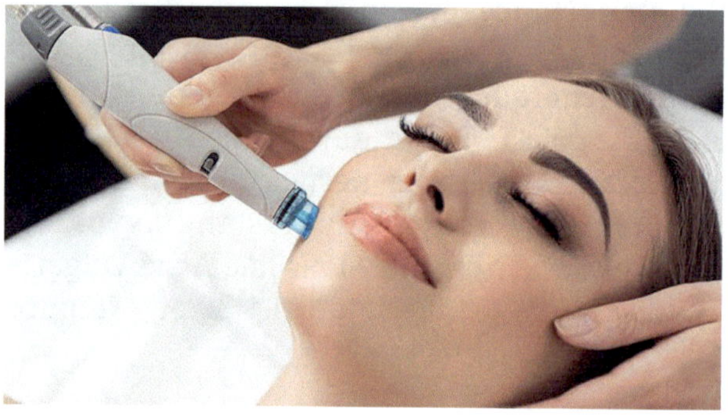

Figure 10.21. Treating rosacea with laser & light therapy.

Source: https://www.westlakedermatology.com/wp-content/uploads/2022/08/rosacea-laser.jpg.

In rosacea, laser and light therapy have complementary but distinct roles. In most individuals with rosacea, there is persistent erythema and visible vessels that can be effectively treated with pulsed dye lasers and intense pulsed light therapy. These treatments are designed to selectively target and coagulate the affected blood vessels while avoiding damage to the surrounding skin tissue, resulting in less redness and an improved skin appearance. Besides this, laser therapy can also aid in reducing the inflammatory components of rosacea, providing symptomatic relief along with cosmetic benefits. As a result of advances in technology, these treatments are constantly evolving and are more convenient and effective for patients with chronic rosacea (Marai et al., 2015). While laser and light therapy for acne and rosacea have been very promising, their administration should be determined after considering individual patient factors. Not all are ideal candidates, and potential contraindications—i.e., skin type, history of photosensitivity, and concurrent medications—must be assessed. Adequate dermatologist pre-treatment counseling and patient education on realistic expectations and possible side effects are crucial. Furthermore, when these treatments are combined with conventional therapies, e.g., topical or systemic medication, better outcomes can be obtained, emphasizing multimodal therapy. As the research continues to clarify the safety and efficacy of laser therapy, concerted efforts in patient management can lead to optimal outcomes in patients with acne vulgaris and rosacea (Marai et al., 2015; Al-Niaimi et al., 2024) (Figure 10.21).

Test Your Knowledge

1. What topical treatment is used for rosacea?
2. What is the best laser treatment for rosacea and acne?

SUMMARY

In bridging the intricate implications of Rosacea and Acne Vulgaris, the significant link between skin disease and hormonal regulation must be appreciated. The skin acts as an active endocrine organ that can perceive physiologic stressors through a cutaneous hypothalamus-pituitary-adrenal (HPA)-like axis. The mechanism not only regulates steroidogenic activity but is also pivotal to the pathogenesis of inflammatory diseases such as rosacea and acne. Identification of these mechanisms provides valuable information for developing individualized treatment modalities to address these diseases appropriately. Novel therapies designed to address hormonal imbalances and systemic stress responses can yield better outcomes for affected patients, a departure from traditional treatment paradigms that often neglect these underlying biological mechanisms (Clark et al., 2020). Furthermore, the advent of treatments such as PDT has altered the treatment of both Rosacea and Acne Vulgaris. PDT employs photosensitizers, which, upon light exposure, initiate selective cell death and immunomodulation. This new form of therapy can be an option for patients with resistant acne and other inflammatory dermatoses. By facilitating focused interventions, PDT not only alleviates apparent symptoms but also ensures a general sense of skin health and patient well-being. The growing body of evidence in support of PDT underscores the importance of integrating new technologies into current practice to achieve optimal treatment efficacy (Lin et al., 2014). In summary, a complete understanding of acne vulgaris and rosacea necessitates an integrated approach that considers both pathophysiologic mechanisms and the constantly evolving therapeutic options available. These cutaneous conditions are not just dermatological illnesses but also interfaces with larger endocrine and inflammatory processes in the body. Future clinical use and research must concentrate on trying out novel treatments that harness the intricacy of the skin's endocrine pathways without excluding cutting-edge technologies like PDT. Ultimately, a multidimensional treatment model with a focus on hormonal balance, targeted therapy, and patient-oriented care will be crucial in maximizing the quality of life of those afflicted with these widespread skin disorders.

Acne vulgaris and rosacea are the most challenging dermatological complications. Acne vulgaris is a very frequent condition that predominantly affects adolescents and young adults with sebum overproduction, clogged follicles, and inflammation, leading to multiple lesions. Topical therapy with good response has been demonstrated in many studies, and especially with trifarotene 50 µg/g cream, which is designed to treat facial and truncal acne. Trifarotene showed considerable improvement in lesion counts and overall skin appearance during phase III clinical studies, indicating its potential as a therapy for the treatment of acne vulgaris. The clear improvement in treatment indicates an important shift in acne management, where understanding the divergent treatment processes and how they work in clinical practice becomes imperative (Ahmad et al., 2019). In contrast, rosacea has a specific set of issues, including flushing, persistent erythema, and prominent vasculature, which are largely observed on the central face. It can be found in adults, particularly fair-skinned individuals. Rosacea is influenced by genetic predisposition, environmental factors, and microbial etiologies, necessitating a multidirectional treatment strategy. The balance of the skin microbiota is extremely critical for healthy skin; dysbiosis has been linked to many dermatological disorders, including rosacea. Insight into the relationship between the skin microbiome and rosacea can guide appropriate interventions, such as lifestyle changes and dietary modifications, that can potentially alleviate symptoms and improve skin health (Mijakovic et al., 2022). Acne vulgaris and rosacea highlight the complexity of skin health and the changing nature of their treatments. Patients typically must be treated on an individual basis, considering individual symptoms, triggers, and reactions to therapy. Familiarity with the dermatologic complexities of these diseases is useful for creating individualized approaches, ranging from pharmacologic treatments such as retinoids to lifestyle modifications that address microbiota balance. Ongoing research into the pathophysiology of acne and rosacea, the role of the skin microbiome, and treatment innovation is necessary to enable a deeper understanding of these conditions, ultimately leading to improved patient care and outcomes. These comprehensive understandings reflect the rapid pace of dermatology and the worth of an interdisciplinary approach towards skincare (Ahmad et al., 2019; Mijakovic et al., 2022).

KEY TERMS FROM THIS CHAPTER

- Acne vulgaris
- Dermatological science
- Dysbiosis
- Erythematotelangiectatic rosacea
- Ocular rosacea
- Phymatous rosacea
- Rosacea
- Cyclooxygenase
- Dermocosmetics
- Erythema
- Hormonal fluctuations
- Papulopustular rosacea
- Propionibacterium acnes
- Sebaceous gland activity

CRITICAL THINKING QUESTIONS

1. **Which of the following is a primary cause of acne vulgaris?**
   a. Decreased sebum production
   b. Inflammation of the hair follicles and sebaceous glands
   c. Overgrowth of yeast on the skin
   d. Genetic mutations
2. **What is the bacterium most commonly associated with acne vulgaris?**
   a. *Staphylococcus aureus*
   b. *Cutibacterium acnes (Propionibacterium acnes)*
   c. *Streptococcus pyogenes*
   d. *Malassezia furfur*
3. **Which of the following is NOT a common trigger for rosacea?**
   a. Alcohol consumption
   b. Spicy foods
   c. Cold weather
   d. Emotional stress
4. **What type of acne is characterized by large, painful nodules?**
   a. Comedonal acne
   b. Papulopustular acne
   c. Nodulocystic acne
   d. Acne conglobata
5. **Which clinical feature distinguishes rosacea from acne vulgaris?**
   a. Presence of pustules
   b. Flushing and persistent redness on the central face
   c. Comedones (blackheads and whiteheads)
   d. Nodulocystic lesions

Short Answer Questions

1. Define acne vulgaris.
2. What is rosacea?
3. What is the cause of acne vulgaris?
4. What is the main cause of rosacea?
5. What are the symptoms of rosacea?

Answer to Critical Thinking Questions

1. (b); 2. (b) ; 3. (c); 4. (c); 5. (b)

REFERENCES

1. Schmid-Wendtner, M., & Korting, H. (2006). The pH of the skin surface and its impact on the barrier function. *Skin Pharmacology and Physiology, 19*(6), 296–302. https://doi.org/10.1159/000094670Abu-Nabaa, Y., Al-Bishaw, A., Amleh, A., Ardah, R., et al. (2016). Bacteria and risk factors of acne vulgaris in Northern West Bank, Palestine. https://core.ac.uk/download/162594203.pdf (accessed on 21st July 2025).
2. Acharjee, M., Akter, S., Akter, S., Banerjee, S., et al. (2022). Impact of gut microbiome on skin health: Gut-skin axis observed through the lenses of therapeutics and skin diseases. https://core.ac.uk/download/558723039.pdf (accessed on 21st July 2025).
3. Adaskevich, V. P., Katina, M. A., & Valles-Kazlouskaya, V. V. (2006). *Practical Dermatology.* https://core.ac.uk/download/80150438.pdf (accessed on 21st July 2025).
4. Ahmad, F., Alió Saenz, A., Blume-Peytavi, U., Del Rosso, J. Q., et al. (2019). Randomized phase 3 evaluation of trifarotene 50 μg/g cream treatment of moderate facial and truncal acne. https://core.ac.uk/download/213449757.pdf (accessed on 21st July 2025).
5. Albiol Matanic, V. C., Bayerl, C., Berg, M., Blount, B. W., Boguniewicz, M., Bourinbaiar, A. S., Bradshaw, J., et al. (2012). Antimicrobial peptides and skin: A paradigm of translational medicine. https://core.ac.uk/download/16432237.pdf (accessed on 21st July 2025).
6. Al-Niaimi, F., Ali, F. R., Copperwheat, S., Gaillard, E. A., et al. (2024). What's new after NICE acne guidelines. https://core.ac.uk/download/619602331.pdf (accessed on 21st July 2025).
7. Andrews, S., Cowdell, F., Eady, E. A., Fenton, C., et al. (2015). Identifying acne treatment uncertainties via a James Lind Alliance Priority Setting Partnership. https://core.ac.uk/download/30733329.pdf (accessed on 21st July 2025).
8. Bińczyk, W., Dróżdż, O., Lissak, K., Nowińska, A., et al. (2024). Topical treatment and aesthetic procedures in management of acne vulgaris. https://core.ac.uk/download/613694708.pdf (accessed on 21st July 2025).
9. Błaszczyński, G., Nojek, P., Nowotarska, A., Pawlik, M., et al. (2024). Effectiveness of different acne treatment methods: A comparison of pharmacological, procedural and natural therapies. https://core.ac.uk/download/636385987.pdf (accessed on 21st July 2025).
10. Borkowska, A., Ciesielski, R., Izdebska, W., Kaźmierczak, A., et al. (2024). Dermo cosmetics in the management of acne vulgaris. https://core.ac.uk/download/620863349.pdf (accessed on 21st July 2025).
11. Bouillon, R., Marcocci, C., Carmeliet, G., Bikle, D. D., White, J. H., Dawson-Hughes, B., Lips, P., et al. (2018). Skeletal and extra skeletal actions of vitamin D: Current evidence and outstanding questions. *Endocrine Reviews, 40*, 1109–1151. https://doi.org/10.1210/er.2018-00126 (accessed on 21st July 2025).
12. Calabrese, L., Ciaffi, J., Cinotti, E., D'Onghia, M., et al. (2024). Fibromyalgia and skin disorders: A systematic review. https://core.ac.uk/download/618720373.pdf (accessed on 21st July 2025).
13. Callewaert, C., De Pessemier, B., Debaere, M., Grine, L., et al. (2021). Gut-skin axis: Current knowledge of the interrelationship between microbial dysbiosis and skin conditions. https://core.ac.uk/download/395605829.pdf (accessed on 21st July 2025).

14. Cantelli, M., Fabbrocini, G., & Monfrecola, G. (2014). Topical nicotinamide for seborrheic dermatitis: An open randomized study. https://core.ac.uk/download/pdf/55117499.pdf (accessed on 21st July 2025).

15. Chilicka, K., Rogowska, A. M., Szyguła, R., Dzieńdziora-Urbińska, I., & Taradaj, J. (2020). A comparison of the effectiveness of azelaic and pyruvic acid peels in the treatment of female adult acne: A randomized controlled trial. *Scientific Reports, 10*. https://doi.org/10.1038/s41598-020-69530-w (accessed on 21st July 2025).

16. Chmiel, M., Maciaszek, O., Podraza, A., Sacher, A., et al. (2025). Botulinum toxin: An innovative approach to treating acne and acne scars: A systematic review. https://core.ac.uk/download/646080098.pdf (accessed on 21st July 2025).

17. Clark, A. K., Saric-Bosanac, S., Shi, V. Y., Sivamani, R. K., et al. (2020). The role of hypothalamus-pituitary-adrenal (HPA)-like axis in inflammatory pilosebaceous disorders. https://core.ac.uk/download/288432496.pdf (accessed on 21st July 2025).

18. Constantinou, A. (2024). *Bakterielle Dysbiose der Haarfollikel: Ein deutlicher Befund bei Patienten mit entzündlichen Haarerkrankungen*. https://core.ac.uk/download/639037031.pdf (accessed on 21st July 2025).

19. Dogan, A. S. (2017). *Ocular rosacea*. https://core.ac.uk/download/322429040.pdf (accessed on 21st July 2025).

20. Jansen, T., & Plewig, G. (1998). *Acneiform Dermatoses*. https://core.ac.uk/download/16432805.pdf (accessed on 21st July 2025).

21. Kaptanoglu, A. F., & Mullaaziz, D. (2017). Acneiform eruptions and pregnancy. https://core.ac.uk/download/322429544.pdf (accessed on 21st July 2025).

22. Korting, H. C., & Schöllmann, C. (2009). Tetracycline actions relevant to rosacea treatment. https://core.ac.uk/download/16432243.pdf (accessed on 21st July 2025).

23. Kravchenko, A. (2019). Influence of *Demodex* mites on life quality of patients with acne and rosacea. https://core.ac.uk/download/639382337.pdf (accessed on 21st July 2025).

24. Lin, J. Y., & Wan, M. T. (2014). Current evidence and applications of photodynamic therapy in dermatology. https://core.ac.uk/download/28949556.pdf (accessed on 21st July 2025).

25. Marai, M. H. (2015). A clinic-pathological investigation of rosacea with particular regard to systemic diseases. https://core.ac.uk/download/30268245.pdf (accessed on 21st July 2025).

26. Mijakovic, I., Qu, L., Wei, Y., Yang, Y., et al. (2022). Advances in the human skin microbiota and its roles in cutaneous diseases. https://core.ac.uk/download/535015295.pdf (accessed on 21st July 2025).

27. Pethani, N., & Pethani, Y. (2025). Psychological impact of acne on adolescents in Ahmedabad: A cross-sectional study on social interactions, self-perception, and lifestyle changes. https://core.ac.uk/download/640070984.pdf (accessed on 21st July 2025).

28. Rahman, M. M., Rahaman, M. S., Islam, M. R., Rahman, F., Mithi, F. M., Alqahtani, T., Almikhlafi, M. A., et al. (2021). Role of phenolic compounds in human disease: Current knowledge and future prospects. *Molecules, 27*, 233–233. https://doi.org/10.3390/molecules27010233 (accessed on 21st July 2025).

29. Revenko, Z. (2016). The modern approach to the complex therapy of demodicosis. https://core.ac.uk/download/301580732.pdf (accessed on 21st July 2025).

30. Richard, M.-A., Paul, C., Nijsten, T., Gisondi, P., Sălăvăstru, C., Taïeb, C., Trakatelli, M., et al. (2022). Prevalence of most common skin diseases in Europe: A population-based study. *Journal of the European Academy of Dermatology and Venereology, 36*, 1088–1096. https://doi.org/10.1111/jdv.18050 (accessed on 21st July 2025).

31. Rizzo, A., Bruno, A., Mento, C., Muscatello, M. R. A., & Zoccali, R. A. (2020). Negative emotions in skin disorders: A systematic review. https://core.ac.uk/download/572841117.pdf (accessed on 21st July 2025).

32. Sieradocha, K. (2024). The mental health implications of acne vulgaris. https://core.ac.uk/download/636385495.pdf (accessed on 21st July 2025).

33. Šimić, D., Letica, E., Zeljko Penavić, J., Vurnek Živković, M., Šitum, M., & Tomić, T. (2009). Psychological impact of isotretinoin treatment in patients with moderate and severe acne. https://core.ac.uk/download/14422732.pdf (accessed on 21st July 2025).

34. Yang, Y., Qu, L., Mijaković, I., & Wei, Y. (2022). Advances in the human skin microbiota and its roles in cutaneous diseases. *Microbial Cell Factories, 21*. https://doi.org/10.1186/s12934-022-01901-6 (accessed on 21st July 2025).

BACTERIAL SKIN INFECTIONS

11

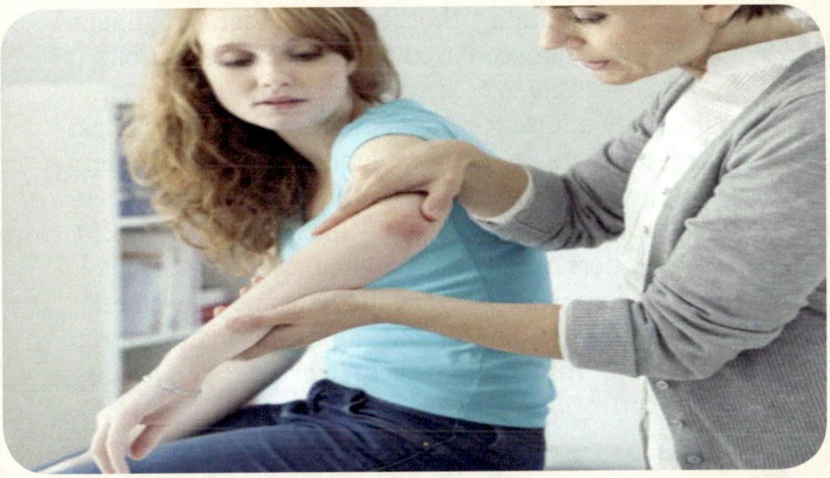

LEARNING OBJECTIVES

After studying this chapter, you will be able to:

1. Describe the types of bacterial skin infections
2. Know the causes and risk factors of bacterial skin infections
3. Describe the symptoms and diagnosis of bacterial skin infections
4. Know the treatment options for bacterial skin infections
5. Understand the complications and consequences of bacterial skin infections
6. Describe the prevention strategies for controlling bacterial skin infections

Introduction

Infection with bacteria on the skin is an issue affecting a number of groups and activities, most notably those in which individuals are repeatedly exposed to particular risk factors. Swimmers are a particularly good example of individuals who are repeatedly exposed to chlorinated water for extended periods, which can soften the skin and lead to dermatoses. They typically result from a multifactorial interaction of causes that involve not only the irritating characteristics of chlorine but also physical stressors such as equipment friction and the humid environment characteristic of aquatic environments. An awareness of these factors is crucial, as they are directly responsible for the incidence and severity of bacterial skin infections among athletes and suggest a need for targeted preventive interventions and effective treatment regimens to mitigate these risks (Patrycja Łazicka et al., 2025). Environmental factors aside, the growing number of resistant bacterial strains also worsens the situation of bacterial skin infections. The case of *Mycobacterium abscessus* illustrates such a conundrum, particularly in relation to cosmetic procedures such as fat grafting. The bacterium has been implicated in post-operative infections, questioning the efficacy of available treatment regimens and the need for ongoing research into its proper treatment. Development of legitimate and standardized animal models for the evaluation of such infections is needed to obtain greater knowledge about bacterial pathogenesis and treatment modalities.

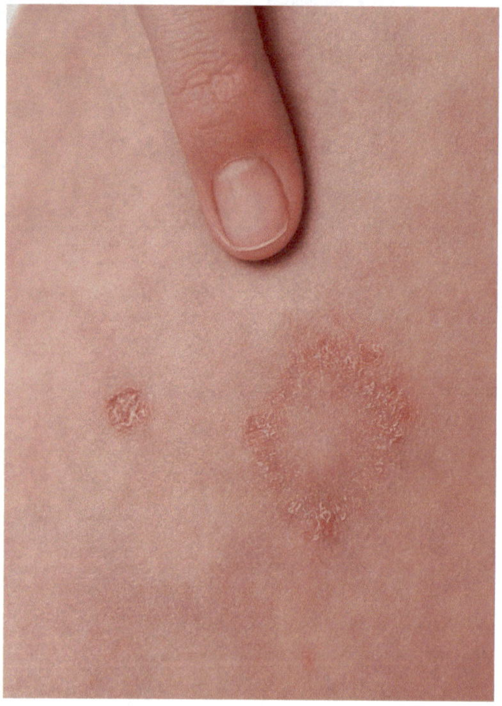

Figure 11.1. Bacterial skin infections.

Source: https://www.thomsonmedical.com/_next/image?url=https%3A%2F%2Fimages.contentstack.io%2Fv3%2Fassets%2Fblt5f400315f9e4f0b3%2Fbltd8403331530f54db%2F66976f6077a78014ee44a4ab%2FBacterial_Skin_Infections_pill_2.png%3Fbranch%3Dprod&w=3840&q=100.

By observing inflammatory responses under controlled conditions, researchers can acquire information vital to developing effective therapeutic strategies and thereby enhancing patient outcomes in both clinical and sporting settings (Diao et al., 2025). Since bacterial dermatoses are complex, an overall approach encompassing prevention, early diagnosis, and therapy is the future. Preventive interventions for high-risk groups, such as athletes, including swimmers, can safely reduce infection rates by applying protective creams, functional athletic wear, and skin care after exposure. Healthcare workers also need to remain vigilant in monitoring new pathogens and resistance patterns that complicate treatment. By combining thorough diagnostic regimens with evidence-based preventive interventions, it is possible to create an enduring system that not only addresses the short-term health problem of bacterial skin infections but also fosters greater awareness of skin health across diverse communities (Patrycja Łazicka et al., 2025). Understanding these dynamics ultimately leads to improved public health outcomes and a better understanding of the importance of bacterial skin infections across various community settings (Figure 11.1).

Definition of Bacterial Skin Infections

Bacterial skin infections are a significant category of infectious diseases in which the development of pathogenic bacteria occurs in the skin or structures related to it. These infections may be caused by numerous bacterial species, usually in the form of localized cutaneous conditions, such as impetigo, cellulitis, or folliculitis. Skin breaches may be the primary site of infection, through which bacteria cross the epidermal barrier. These infections not only inflict extensive morbidity upon the affected individuals but also may potentially elevate to systemic complications unless treated. The clinical presentation can be varied, ranging from trivial irritations to severe skin damage necessitating surgery, and hence the need for early diagnosis and management to prevent adverse outcomes. The impact of bacterial skin infections is further exacerbated by their association with underlying health or environmental conditions, such as immunocompromised states or unsanitary living conditions. Certain segments of the population, such as newborns or people living in poor countries, are extremely prone to dangerous bacterial skin infections that can have serious health consequences, including mortality. For instance, systematic reviews have commented on the heavy burden of infection of pneumonia and sepsis in neonatal groups, hence the need for effective antibiotic therapy to manage these conditions (Bhutta et al., 2011).

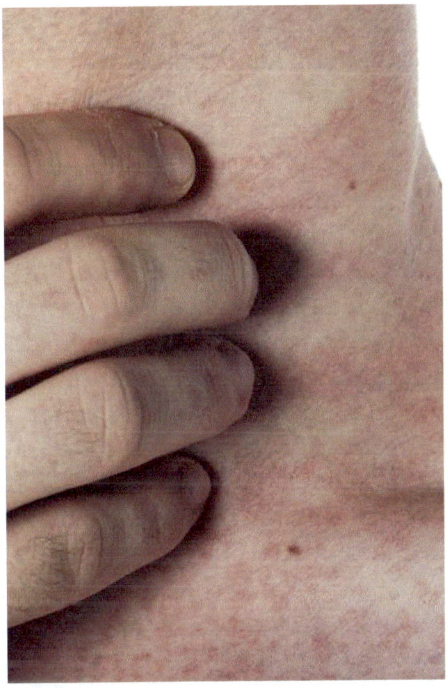

Figure 11.2. Understanding bacterial skin infections.

Source: https://www.novadermnj.com/wp-content/uploads/2019/06/MM6-683x1024.jpg.

It is therefore important to understand the epidemiology, pathophysiology, and risk factors of such infections when developing effective public health interventions and treatment regimens. Treatment of bacterial skin infections usually consists of antimicrobial therapy tailored to the causative bacteria, with alternatives ranging from topical creams to systemic antibiotics. Treatment may also often be confounded by the emergence of antibiotic-resistant organisms and therefore needs cautious microbiological investigation and susceptibility testing. For example, secondary bacterial infections have also been described in Buruli ulcers caused by *Mycobacterium ulcerans*, which are often due to resistant bacteria such as *Staphylococcus aureus* and *Pseudomonas aeruginosa* (Pahlevan et al., 2013). Hence, it is crucial to address the primary bacterial infection and any subsequent complications to prevent long-term morbidity and ensure complete healing. The global control of bacterial skin infections is thus an intricate issue that encompasses an interdisciplinary approach to achieve optimal patient outcomes (Figure 11.2).

Importance of Studying Bacterial Skin Infections

There is a need to study bacterial skin infections to better understand their impact on public health and patient management. As these infections are caused by various pathogens, such as methicillin-resistant *Staphylococcus aureus* (MRSA) and vancomycin-resistant *Enterococcus faecalis* (VREF), determining and comparing their nature and responsiveness to therapy is essential. It helps in imparting proper therapy, reducing complications, and enabling the formulation of preventive strategies. For example, studies have shown that certain natural products, such as honey, have antibacterial properties against pathogens, making them potential alternatives for treating infected wounds and burns (Fidaleo et al., 2015). Therefore, a thorough evaluation of skin bacterial infections not only enhances treatment practices but also facilitates the development of new interventions to address contemporary clinical challenges. In addition to their therapeutic importance, bacterial skin infections also provide a window into the epidemiology and frequency of these diseases, which is valuable for public health monitoring. Skin infection rates can vary substantially by geographic location, climate, and socioeconomic determinants of health, leading to inequities in health outcomes. A proper analysis of such infections allows health workers and planners to identify high-risk groups and implement targeted interventions, such as vaccination interventions or hygiene practice education campaigns. Knowledge of the socio-environmental determinants of these infections can also inform resource planning and health planning. As highlighted in recent studies, organic farming and biological cycles can create conditions conducive to zoonotic diseases; as such, a multidisciplinary approach is necessary for controlling bacterial skin infections (Eijck et al., 2003). Finally, studies on bacterial skin infections are central to advancing our knowledge of antimicrobial resistance (AMR), a global upsurge. Since the bacteria develop resistance to the most commonly used antibiotics and evolve further, it becomes important to study the patterns and mechanisms of such resistance in skin infections. By studying patterns of bacterial resistance and adaptation, researchers can help formulate new antibiotics and treatment strategies that effectively address resistant microbes. Additionally, understanding the relationship between bacterial skin infection and the general immune response can be valuable for optimal prevention and management, particularly in susceptible individuals. Thus, research into these infections is essential not only to improve clinical care but also to resolve broader public health issues concerning AMR.

11.1. Types of Bacterial Skin Infections

Learning Outcome

1. Define the impetigo
2. Understand the bcellulitis
3. Describe the folliculitis

Bacterial skin infections encompass a broad range of diseases, with each condition distinguished by the invading microorganisms responsible. Staphylococcal and streptococcal infections are highly common and may occur in numerous forms, such as cellulitis, impetigo, and folliculitis. *Staphylococcus aureus*, particularly methicillin-resistant (MRSA), is a significant issue in clinical management due to its resistance to several antibiotics, thus making treatment even more complex. Conversely, *Streptococcus pyogenes* is also frequently responsible for skin infections, including erysipelas and impetigo, which are predominantly of childhood. The course of such infection may be remarkably varied, ranging from simple localized erythema and edema to generalized signs of fever and chills, thereby calling for early diagnosis to prevent complications and ensure adequate management of the patient. One of the most relevant bacterial skin infections is caused by Gram-negative bacteria, such as *Pseudomonas aeruginosa*. This pathogen is frequently involved in infections in moist environments, i.e., hospital settings, and can cause diseases such as folliculitis and wound infections, particularly in immunocompromised patients or those with wounds. Pseudomonas infections are quite frequently hard to treat due to their innate resistance to a large number of antibiotics and also due to the fact that they produce biofilms. Clinical management of the infection would typically involve antimicrobial therapy and careful wound care to ensure optimal healing and prevent unnecessary complications. It is essential that clinicians recognize the clinical signs and symptoms of such infections early and initiate appropriate treatment to avert adverse effects. Finally, the characteristic forms of bacterial skin infections, including those associated with cryoglobulinaemia, illustrate the complexity of these disorders. Cryoglobulinaemia can lead to generalized skin manifestations, like rash and lesions, typically secondary to infection, e.g., hepatitis C. In these instances, infection control is paramount not just in the management of the skin manifestations but also in addressing systemic consequences of the offending viral infection. The availability of antiviral therapy offers a potentially causative treatment approach to the cryoglobulinaemic presentation of these cutaneous illnesses, as emphasized in recent therapeutic overviews (Braun et al., 2007). As the medical profession continues to delve deeper into the relationship between bacterial infections and systemic diseases, the success in such complicated cases will depend on the integration of multidisciplinary approaches (Cole et al., 2020) (Figure 11.3).

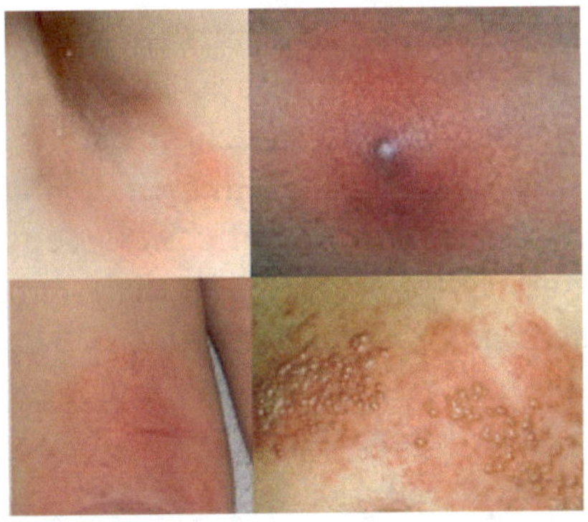

Figure 11.3. Types of bacterial skin infections.

Source: https://drvarsha.com/wp-content/uploads/2021/07/Skin-infections-pic.png.

11.1.1. Impetigo

Impetigo is an extremely contagious bacterial skin infection that primarily affects children but can also occur in adults. This superficial skin infection is most often caused by two bacteria, namely *Streptococcus pyogenes* and *Staphylococcus aureus*. Impetigo is transmitted by direct contact with infected lesions or discharge, and through contact with infested materials such as towels and clothing. Impetigo is clinically characterized by the presence of red lesions that quickly break open, ooze, and form a yellow-brown crust. The contagiousness of impetigo warrants urgent treatment to prevent its spread, especially in group settings such as schools and daycares. Given its pervasiveness, understanding the modes of transmission and early symptoms is crucial for effective prevention and control measures, particularly among children. The management of impetigo focuses on antibiotic treatment and proper hygienic practice. Topical agents such as mupirocin are typically sufficient for localized impetigo, whereas extensive cases may require systemic antibiotics. In addition to pharmacotherapy, educating patients and caregivers on the necessity of keeping clean and not remaining close to infected individuals is a critical aspect.

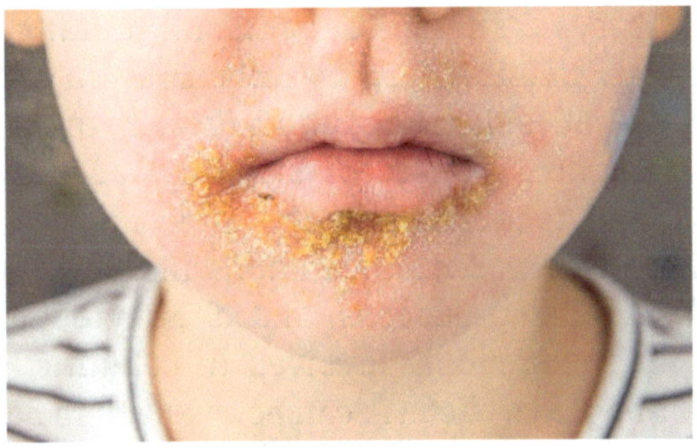

Figure 11.4. Impetigo.

Source: https://images.squarespace-cdn.com/content/v1/61266e982104fd1fe23f9fba/427a43f4-2a1c-4a31-b43a-c31b50085200/Impetigo.jpg.

Proper familiarity with these treatment protocols not only facilitates healing but also prevents secondary bacterial infections in the situation of impetigo. Additionally, schools and community organizations may play an important role in disseminating information regarding impetigo prevention, emphasizing personal hygiene practices and seeking medical attention early when symptoms are present. As public health education has been brought to the forefront by recent research, raising awareness of impetigo in schools is significant. Teachers can use instructional modules to teach students about infectious diseases, such as bacterial skin infections like impetigo. An effective education strategy would entail imparting knowledge on how to prevent and spread impetigo, thereby improving not only students' knowledge but also teachers' competence in teaching health. These initiatives align with the Centers for Disease Control and Prevention guidelines, supporting enhanced knowledge of infectious diseases among young individuals. Through this multifaceted approach, the incidence of bacterial skin infections like impetigo can be reduced, paving the way for a healthier school and community environment (Downie et al., 2006) (Figure 11.4).

11.1.2. Cellulitis

Cellulitis is an acute bacterial cutaneous infection characterized by inflammation of the dermis and subcutaneous tissues. It presents with an acute onset of swelling, erythema, heat, and tenderness in the affected area, as well as systemic manifestations like fever and malaise. Streptococcus and Staphylococcus are most commonly involved in cellulitis, but Gram-negative bacteria can be involved in some cases. The onset is frequently associated with disruption of the skin barrier, which may be due to trauma, incisions during surgery, or dermatologic illnesses such as eczema. Patients with compromised skin integrity are at greater risk of developing cellulitis, and the role of prevention in maintaining skin integrity in high-risk populations cannot be overemphasized. It has been determined through studies that there is a high correlation between existing foot dermatomycosis and the occurrence of cellulitis, particularly acute bacterial leg infection. In a case-control study, mycology-proven foot conditions, tinea pedis and onychomycosis, were found to be major risk factors for acute bacterial cellulitis (odds ratio, OR: 2.4; $p < 0.001$) (Sigurgeirsson et al., 2004). Specifically, interdigital tinea pedis was associated with an even greater risk (OR: 3.2; $p < 0.001$), underscoring the importance of effective treatment of fungal infections as a preventive strategy. Aside from these dermatologic factors, conditions that compromise the cutaneous barrier, such as chronic venous insufficiency and leg edema, also increase the risk of cellulitis. Therefore, treatment of these background diseases can also greatly decrease the risk of infection. Early and adequate treatment of cellulitis is essential to prevent complications, such as abscess formation and spread of infection to deeper tissues. In general, medical practitioners initiate treatment with broad-spectrum antibiotics to cover probable pathogens involved. Even though most uncomplicated cases are appropriately treated in the outpatient clinic, severe or recurrent cellulitis may need hospitalization for intravenous antibiotics and closer monitoring. In addition to antibiotic therapy, management of risk factors—such as treatment of underlying skin disease or good wound care—is vital in reducing recurrence rates. As in literature, management of diseases like tinea pedis and onychomycosis can significantly reduce the risk of acute bacterial cellulitis, and thus multidisciplinary treatment and prevention is vital for optimal patient outcomes (Sigurgeirsson et al., 2004) (Figure 11.5).

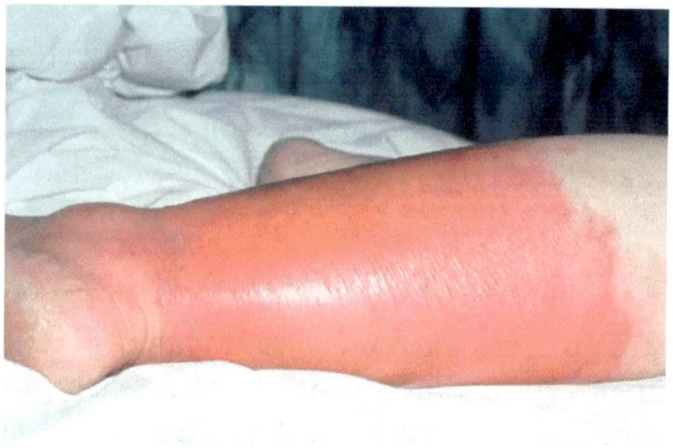

Figure 11.5. Cellulitis.

Source: https://pharmaceutical-journal.com/wp-content/uploads/2023/09/M1300283-Inflammation_due_to_cellulitis_on_the_lower_leg-e1696329391828.jpg.

11.1.3. Folliculitis

Folliculitis is characterized by inflammation of hair follicles, typically caused by bacterial infection, and is a frequent disorder within the broader category of bacterial skin diseases.

The inflammation can appear as small red bumps or pimples around the follicles and is often painful or itchy. The most frequently involved organism is *Staphylococcus aureus*, although other bacteria, such as Pseudomonas aeruginosa, also cause it, particularly in settings like inadequately maintained swimming pools. Aside from its cutaneous manifestations, folliculitis can indicate subclinical conditions such as compromised skin barriers or systemic diseases, showing the link between the outer environment and inner well-being. Detection of folliculitis symptoms is significant, as it can be a sign of more serious infections, particularly in immunocompromised patients, and should be treated promptly. Folliculitis is treated with topical and systemic antibiotics based on the extent of the disease and lesions. In less severe cases, antibacterial soaps or creams may be applied, but in more serious or recurrent cases, oral antibiotics are given in a bid to completely remove the infection. Where the condition is also brought about by shaving or clothing rubbing, changing these activities also helps alleviate and prevent recurrence. Other skin infections may also manifest similarly, as seen in clinical examples, and thus pose a diagnostic challenge. As an example, acneiform eruptions may be mistaken for folliculitis, and it is paramount that clinicians are aware of the distinction to follow appropriate treatment regimens as outlined in accounts of acneiform dermatoses (Jansen et al., 1998). This emphasizes the need for vigilance in clinical presentation of skin infections that require a subtle understanding and individually tailored treatment modalities. While a rather nonspecific issue, folliculitis can also present in association with other dermatologic illnesses, such as eczema. The mention of an itchy, red rash on the face and wrists of a child closely resembling signs of folliculitis is made to highlight the necessity of the correct diagnosis of folliculitis in children. Treatment of both folliculitis and associated conditions, such as atopic eczema, must consider the patient's general health as well as probable external precipitants (Formosa et al., 2007). For instance, when assessing a child's symptoms, healthcare providers must include environmental irritants most likely to induce skin irritation in their assessment, in conjunction with microbial infection issues. Preventive measures like maintenance of skin hygiene and emollient can minimize flare-ups of either the infections or dermatitis. Thus, holistic principles also involve not only the direct treatment of bacterial infections such as folliculitis but also determining the systemic and environmental causes, thereby confirming the relationship between dermatological health and general well-being (Figure 11.6).

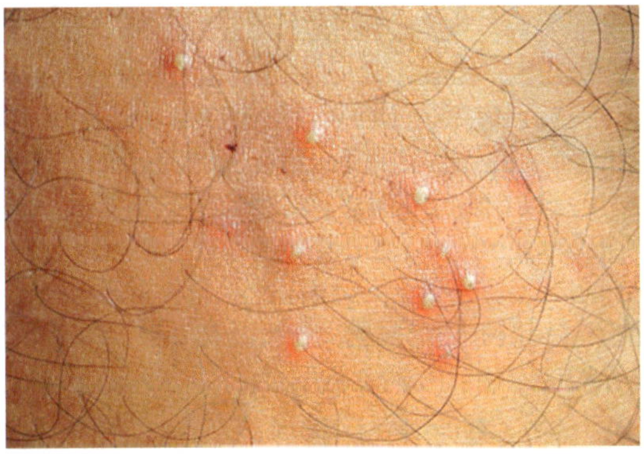

Figure 11.6. Folliculitis.

Source: https://www.arlingtonvaderm.com/wp-content/uploads/2021/02/Arlington-Dermatology-Folliculitis1_1452567668.jpg.

Test Your Knowledge

1. What is cellulitis?
2. What is inflammation of a hair follicle called?

11.2. Causes and Risk Factors

Learning Outcome

1. Describe the bacterial pathogen of the skin
2. Know the pre-existing skin conditions of bacterial skin infections
3. Understand the environmental and lifestyle factors of bacterial skin infections

Bacterial skin infections are caused by a vast array of factors that increase susceptibility. The skin is the largest organ in the body that serves as the first protective mechanism against infection, but can be degraded by several environmental and biological factors. Recurring reasons are due to the presence of gram-positive bacteria, which are most frequently responsible for skin infections since they are capable of penetrating lesions, wounds, or other openings on the skin. Others might have genetic predispositions that make them vulnerable to infections. Diseases like diabetes, obesity, and eczema have been found to further raise the susceptibility to bacterial skin infection, showing how intertwined the interaction between systemic health and local barrier integrity is (AL-hindi et al., 2024). Bacterial skin infections are also strongly influenced by environmental determinants, particularly in developing nations where access to healthcare facilities can be limited. Poor sanitation and unhygienic living conditions can spread pathogens, which tend to lead to outbreaks of infection in clusters of populations. Contamination of water, unhygienic living conditions, and the inability to use clean healthcare facilities can lead to higher skin infection rates. Moreover, the misuse of antibiotics has led to antibiotic resistance, thereby making it harder to offer treatment plans and leading to repeated infections. Awareness of these environmental determinants is necessary to guide public health interventions aimed at diminishing the disease burden of bacterial skin infections in vulnerable populations (AL-hindi et al., 2024). Contact with animals, and particularly through animal-assisted intervention, is another risk factor. While animal-assisted intervention has been found to have a significant emotional and therapeutic value, it also stands to potentially expose individuals to zoonotic pathogens, which can lead to skin infection. Research has indicated that certain pathogens, such as those in the ESKAPE complex, have been present in dogs participating in such therapy sessions and pose a risk of transmission to humans. These zoonotic risks call for proper assessment of hygiene measures while involving animals in healthcare settings. Overall, identification of such varied causes and risk factors is essential for developing an effective prevention against bacterial skin infections to protect vulnerable groups and enhance public health.

11.2.1. Bacterial Pathogens Involved

Bacterial skin infections are most frequently caused by various pathogens, of which *Staphylococcus aureus* is a major contributor. This microorganism is also very famous for producing infections ranging from trivial cutaneous infections such as cellulitis and impetigo to serious conditions in the form of necrotizing fasciitis and abscesses. More precisely, it can produce biofilms, which are very troublesome because they render the organism extremely resistant to antibiotics, making treatment extremely complicated. On top of this, MRSA has also been a public health crisis due to the antibiotic resistance of most drugs used, leading to increased morbidity and medical costs. MRSA's pathogenicity is also enhanced by the ability of the bacteria to evade host immune systems. Interventions against MRSA, such as those containing engineered nanoparticles, have been nicely represented in preclinical reports to have intense antibacterial activity that has the capability to transform the treatment approach for MRSA-induced skin infections (Ye et al., 2024). Other bacterial infections such as *Streptococcus pyogenes* and

Pseudomonas aeruginosa also play an important role in producing skin infections. *Streptococcus pyogenes* also causes erysipelas and impetigo with an acute onset often followed by a tendency towards severe systemic effects. The virulence factors of this bacterium, including toxins and enzymes, enable it to rapidly infect host tissue, causing high morbidity. *Pseudomonas aeruginosa* is largely associated with opportunistic infections of the upper respiratory tract among immunocompromised patients or those with chronic ulcers. Characterized by intrinsic resistance to most antibiotics, Pseudomonas poses a major treatment challenge and underscores the need for novel therapeutic approaches and a more comprehensive understanding of its pathogenicity. Research into newer treatment modalities, such as phototherapy and bioengineering therapy, may be key to preventing infections caused by these pathogens. New evidence implicates other pathogenic agents, such as *Acinetobacter baumannii*, as increasingly significant in bacterial skin infections. Characterized as an opportunistic pathogen, Acinetobacter is best known in the hospital setting, where it can cause complex skin and soft tissue infections. Its capacity to thrive on surfaces and withstand harsh conditions makes infection control even more difficult. Impressive studies have begun to reveal the effects of low-dose UV-A light on bacterial infection, with the potential to inhibit the growth of pathogens like *Acinetobacter baumannii* and *Staphylococcus aureus*. These studies indicate that the therapy with UV-A has the ability to enhance innate immunity through the remodeling of metabolic and regulatory proteins in model organisms like *Caenorhabditis elegans*, revealing promising avenues for upcoming therapeutic treatments against resistant bacterial pathogens (Muthubharathi et al., 2024). This underscores the need for continuous discovery of new therapies to combat the dynamic nature of bacterial skin infections (Figure 11.7).

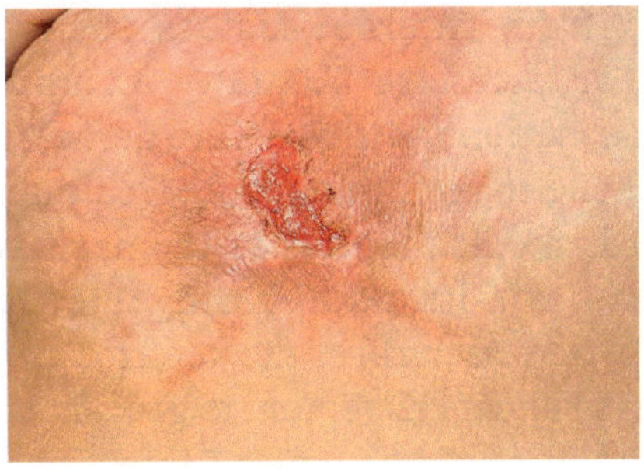

Figure 11.7. Methicillin-resistant *Staphylococcus aureus* (MRSA) skin infections might look like a rash or an area that's red, discolored, painful, swollen, or filled with pus or fluid.

Source: https://my.clevelandclinic.org/-/scassets/Images/org/health/articles/mrsa.

11.2.2. Pre-Existing Skin Conditions

Pre-existing skin conditions play a significant role in individuals' susceptibility to bacterial skin infections. Eczema, psoriasis, and acne cause breakage in the skin barrier, making it easier for pathogenic microorganisms like *Staphylococcus aureus* and *Streptococcus pyogenes* to gain access. Breakdown of the skin's protective system can lead to secondary infection, worsening underlying conditions, and complicating therapy. For example, eczema patients are likely to experience flares after infection, leading to increased itching and inflammation, while patients with psoriasis may observe increased proliferation of psoriatic plaques. Understanding these interactions is relevant to medical practitioners, as they may need to assume a more integrated role in the treatment of both bacterial infection and skin condition. Particularly, immunocompromised subjects, for example, patients undergoing immunosuppressive therapy for conditions like psoriasis, are more likely to be subject to bacterial infections. Such treatment compromises the natural defenses of the skin, which are dependent in large part on the integrity of the immune response. That compromise creates an opportunity for infection, with additional impetus from external factors such as skin trauma or excessive humidity. Compounding this issue, patients with existing dermatological disease tend to require ongoing treatment, such as topical medications that themselves carry the risk of skin irritation during infection. The vicious cycle underscores the need for aggressive monitoring and management to prevent bacterial colonization and subsequent infection in this vulnerable population. Furthermore, new data suggest that systemic disease states comorbid with skin disease tend to affect the severity and frequency of bacterial skin infections.

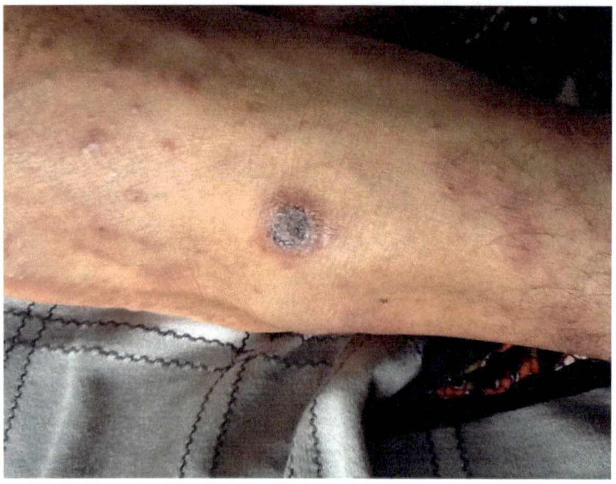

Figure 11.8. Partially healed pre-existing skin lesions.

Source: https://www.researchgate.net/profile/Vadivel-Kumaran-Sivasankaran/publication/263653365/figure/fig4/AS:668508845248518@1536396337609/partially-healed-pre-existing-skin-lesions.jpg.

For instance, conditions such as diabetes or circulatory disease usually have a negative effect on healing and recovery, thus resulting in chronic infection and increased complications. Additionally, individuals who have outbreaks of bacterial infection may actually be worsening their comorbid chronic skin disease by several mechanisms, including stress, hygiene, and side effects of antibiotics. This highlights the multifaceted aspect of the management of bacterial skin infections in existing patients. Hence, a multi-disciplinary treatment involving dermatology, infectious diseases, and patient education is critical to achieving optimal outcomes and overall quality of life in these individuals, particularly in the context of their struggle with skin care amid chronic infection (Figure 11.8).

11.2.3. Environmental and Lifestyle Factors

Lifestyle and environmental determinants are responsible for a significant role in the spread and severity of bacterial skin infections. In urban areas, crowded living conditions are likely to facilitate the rapid transmission of pathogens, thereby increasing the risk of infections such as impetigo and cellulitis. Poor access to sanitation facilities and clean water also tends to exacerbate the problem, particularly among low-income groups. The environmental setting cannot be neglected; the presence of pollutants and allergens also affects the health of the skin, predisposing it to infection. Thus, improving the environmental setting through better urban planning, waste disposal, and public health interventions is vital for reducing bacterial skin infections. Habits of lifestyle also carry a great deal of weight in causing bacterial skin infections. Poor eating habits can compromise the immune system, increasing individuals' vulnerability to infection. Diets with limited consumption of minerals and vitamins, for instance, are bound to hinder the body's defense mechanisms, allowing small cuts or skin irritations to progress to serious bacterial infections. Apart from diet, hygiene practices involving personal cleanliness, such as regular washing of hands and skin care, are crucial in limiting the spread of bacteria. Once individuals adopt active hygiene habits and eat a healthy diet, they significantly reduce the risk of bacterial skin infections, reflecting the contribution of lifestyle to overall skin health. The dynamics of human-animal interactions also contribute to determining the biodiversity of skin microbiomes, which in turn determine the risk of infection. Captured animals, such as domestic pets, have oral and skin microbiomes that differ from those of wild animals. Such variations could reflect the impact of human care on their way of life and health, as demonstrated by studies comparing ancient Egyptian baboons that were kept in captivity and subjected to diet modifications. The impact of alterations in animal microbiomes on the risk of infection could provide insights into prevention strategies for both animals and humans. Thus, the interaction of environmental and lifestyle variables, as illustrated in previous and present environments, plays a vital role in addressing bacterial skin infections fully and enhancing overall health outcomes in diverse populations (Adams et al., 2010; Bramanti et al., 2019).

Test Your Knowledge

1. What is a bacterial pathogen of the skin?
2. What are preexisting skin conditions?

11.3. Symptoms and Diagnosis

Learning Outcome

1. Know the common symptoms of bacterial skin infections
2. Describe the diagnostic methods used by healthcare professionals
3. Differentiate bacterial infections from other skin conditions

The identification of bacterial skin infections relies heavily on identifying the signs of disease typically present. These include erythema, edema, and tenderness at the site of involvement, along with systemic manifestations such as fever and malaise. The nature of the cutaneous lesion can vary widely, from pustules and vesicles to even necrosis, depending on the etiology of the bacteria. Specifically, *Staphylococcus aureus* infection can lead to painful abscesses or boils, while *Streptococcus pyogenes* can yield impetigo or cellulitis, which is covered with a characteristic honey-colored crust. Accurate symptom identification is essential to differentiate bacterial infection from other cutaneous diseases, such as fungal or viral infections, which share a similar clinical presentation, thereby necessitating an ordered diagnostic approach (King et al., 2017). Complete history of the patient and clinical examination are significant factors in diagnosing bacterial skin infections. When evaluating the patient, medical staff usually inquire about recent injuries, e.g., cuts, insect bites, or past dermatoses that may predispose the patient to infection. Laboratory examinations, e.g., wound swabs or skin scrapings cultures, prove useful in identifying the causative microorganism. Also, ancillary tests such as imaging or blood work may be warranted depending on the depth or severity of the infection. In cases of suspected systemic infection, e.g., fever or lymphadenopathy, they may assist in diagnosis and guide appropriate antibiotic therapy. A multicriteria diagnostic approach not only enhances accuracy but also directs the treatment protocol necessary for effective patient management (Al-Wabel et al., 2020). Diagnosis of bacterial skin infection may be challenging in certain situations, though, due to accompanying diseases, and therefore, focus should be on integral clinical assessment. For instance, patients with primary immunocompromised conditions such as diabetes or HIV/AIDS who present with atypical symptoms are often diagnosed inaccurately. In addition, secondary infections due to diseases like scabies can complicate the clinical picture, making diagnosis and treatment even more challenging. The presence of pruritic rashes or burrows associated with scabies, which can occur concurrently with bacterial infections, further emphasizes the need for clinicians to be vigilant in differentiating overlapping symptomatology. Effective management is not just based on awareness of the initial bacterial infection but also on the resolution of basic conditions, which may include infestations or compromised skin integrity. An integrative method that combines symptom awareness and attentive diagnostic procedures is therefore required for optimal treatment outcomes in bacterial skin infections (Al-Wabel et al., 2020) (Figure 11.9).

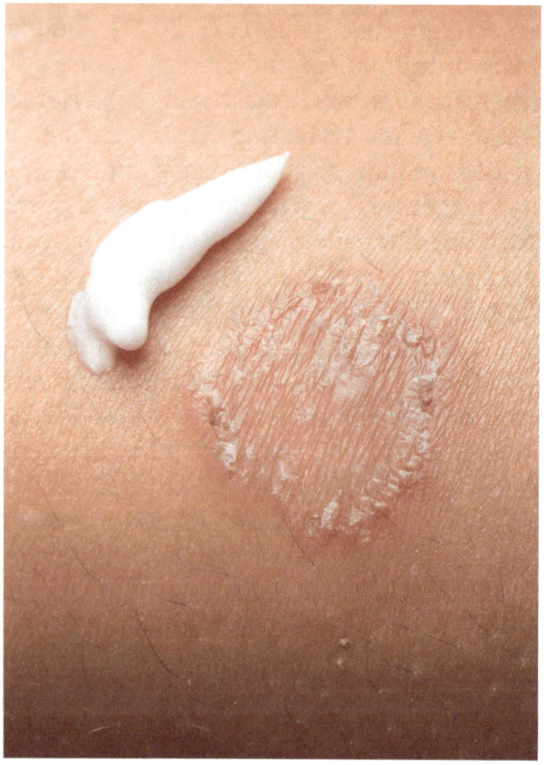

Figure 11.9.

Source: https://www.thomsonmedical.com/_next/image?url=https%3A%2F%2Fimages.contentstack.io%2Fv3%2Fassets%2Fblt5f400315f9e4f0b3%2Fbltce7a12ec30fdd7a3%2F66976f99ec61e9365dbfedca%2FBacterial_Skin_Infections_pill_4.png%3Fbranch%3Dprod&w=3840&q=100.

11.3.1. Common Symptoms of Bacterial Skin Infections

Bacterial cutaneous infections are diverse in their presentation and can manifest with numerous common signs that typically prompt treatment and diagnosis. The most frequent among these signs is local redness and swelling, typically at the site of infection, accompanied by warmth and tenderness. These symptoms exhibit characteristics of inflammation, which are indicators that the body's immune system is attempting to combat the pathogens. Besides these inflammatory signs, one may experience pain or discomfort that might either be mild or severe, depending on the severity of the infection. These initial symptoms play a critical role in guiding healthcare workers to the appropriate course of action, including diagnostic tests and potential treatments. Moreover, pus or discharge typically accompanies bacterial skin infections, and this even signifies the type of infection. This discharge, containing pus, can be yellow, green, or brown in appearance and is typically a mixture of the body's immune cells and bacteria that accumulate at the site of infection. The texture and smell of the discharge can vary, which helps to differentiate between infections. For instance, if there is a foul-smelling discharge, it may indicate anaerobic bacteria, leading to a more complicated clinical presentation. It is important for medical professionals to know how to properly assess and interpret those signs to provide timely interventions that prevent complications and promote healing. Systemic signs may also occur following bacterial cutaneous infections, adding more rationale to urgent treatment. Fever is also a common systemic response, meaning that the body is fighting the infection. Other signs, such as chills, weakness, and malaise, may indicate that the infection is not localized to one area but is affecting the individual's overall health instead.

With certain infections, particularly those with a wide-ranging nature, such as cellulitis, systemic effects can lead to catastrophic outcomes if not managed appropriately. Successful treatments commonly include antipyretics and, if necessary, antibiotics against the resulting bacterial strain. As indicated by current studies, it is relevant to consider the implications of local and systemic symptoms for effective management of bacterial skin infections, providing valuable information for public health programs aimed at controlling their spread (King et al., 2017; Al-Wabel et al., 2020) (Figure 11.10).

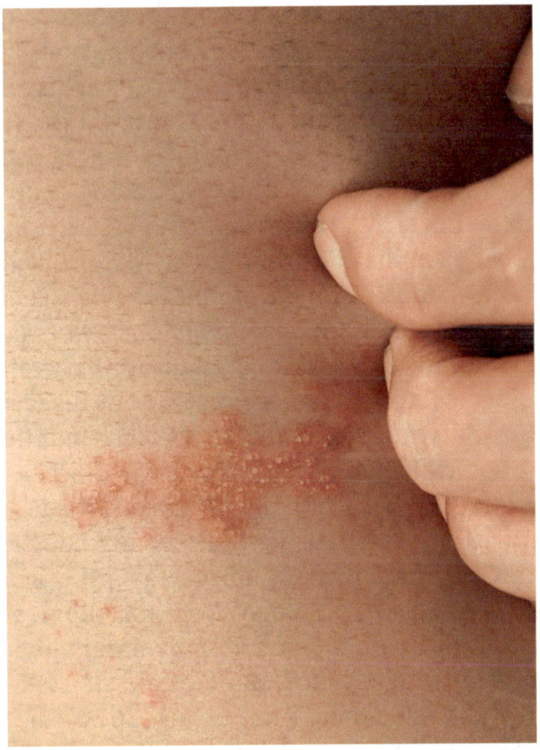

Figure 11.10. Symptoms of bacterial skin infections.

Source: https://www.thomsonmedical.com/_next/image?url=https%3A%2F%2Fimages.contentstack.io%2Fv3%2Fassets%2Fblt5f400315f9e4f0b3%2Fblt32baa5b103b792ea%2F66976f3cd316c77a27b32e43%2FBacterial_Skin_Infections_pill_1.png%3Fbranch%3Dprod&w=3840&q=100.

11.3.2. Diagnostic Methods Used by Healthcare Professionals

The accurate diagnosis of bacterial skin infections is important in establishing effective treatment, largely because of the wide overlap of clinical presentation among various infections. Healthcare professionals use an array of diagnostic methods, including clinical examination, laboratory tests, and imaging studies, to establish a definitive diagnosis. A good clinical examination often precedes additional testing, in which case practitioners assess the usual signs and symptoms, including erythema, swelling, and purulence. However, such clinical signs can be misleading, particularly in polymicrobial infections or in the absence of overt specific symptoms. Hence, laboratory tests such as cultures, polymerase chain reaction (PCR), and serological tests are routinely employed to identify the causative pathogens. This multifaceted strategy enables health clinicians to differentiate between bacterial skin infections and other dermatological presentations in a timely and specific context through focused treatment interventions. Supplementing traditional diagnostic methods, developments in point-of-care testing represent a revolutionary evolution in the diagnosis of bacterial skin infections for healthcare providers. Quick tests can yield results within minutes, enabling earlier intervention and improved patient outcomes. For instance, PCR-based tests can specifically detect bacterial DNA and thus confirm infections caused by notorious pathogens such as *Staphylococcus aureus*. Use of such technology enables more precise detection of resistant bacteria and informs the selection of appropriate antimicrobial therapy. Moreover, rapid tests can prove particularly useful in community clinics where access to advanced laboratory infrastructure may be limited. With these point-of-care diagnostics gaining momentum, they are being utilized by healthcare providers more and more to enhance the accuracy of diagnosis in addition to reducing the time to initiation of treatment, eventually having a significant impact on the right treatment of bacterial skin infections. It is also important that the broader implications of early and precise diagnosis in the public health context be considered. The emergence of multidrug-resistant pathogens highlights the virulence of bacterial skin infection management, which calls for rigorous diagnostic systems. Given the high incidence of such disorders as surgical site infections, the role of diagnostic modalities becomes increasingly significant; Chetter et al. (2015) emphasize the host, environmental, and pathogen factor collaboration in these infections. It is important for medical professionals to rapidly detect causative pathogens so that appropriate treatment and prevention strategies can be implemented. Early detection also helps decrease transmission of skin infections, particularly in shared living environments where conditions are favorable for spreading. The inclusion of high-level diagnostic methods not only improves patient outcomes at the individual level but also supports public health interventions aimed at controlling bacterial skin infections at the community level (Figure 11.11).

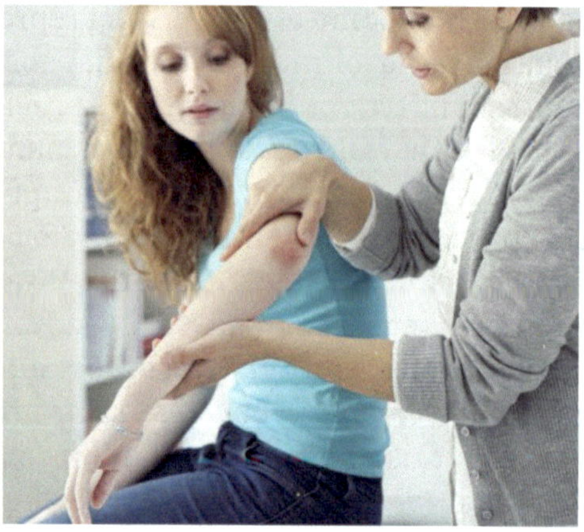

Figure 11.11. Diagnosis of bacterial skin infections.

Source: https://www.skintherapyletter.com/wp-content/uploads/2017/05/8-534x462.jpg.

11.3.3. Differentiating Bacterial Infections from Other Skin Conditions

Differential diagnosis between bacterial infections and other dermatologic disorders is a significant aspect of dermatologic examination, as an incorrect diagnosis can lead to inappropriate treatment and exacerbation of the underlying disease. Bacterial skin infections often present with characteristic signs, such as circumscribed redness, edema, and purulent discharge, which can help differentiate them from noninfectious inflammatory disorders like eczema or psoriasis. Bacterial diseases like impetigo, for instance, are characterized by crusted lesions that are not typically a feature of inflammatory skin disease. By contrast, eczema will be more diffusely distributed and chronic in nature, without acute induration, the sort of thing which one expects with a bacterial infection. Thus, meticulous clinical examination in both the history of the patient and the physical findings is crucial to ensure correct diagnosis so that clinicians recognize the classic findings indicating bacterial etiology compared to other cutaneous diseases. In cases where skin diseases can manifest as bacterial infections, additional diagnostic tests can help clarify the diagnosis. Tests for cultures play a vital role in detecting bacterial pathogens and thereby enabling appropriate intervention strategies. Tests serologically assist in determining underlying immunological conditions that place individuals at risk of recurrent infections. Ailal et al. (2020) direct us to the different implications of congenital errors of immunity (IEI) lying beneath, such as susceptibility to infection, and emphasize the need for careful patient evaluation when bacterial infection returns. Understanding these nuances significantly enhances the clinician's ability to properly differentiate infections from other dermatoses. In addition, when the clinical presentation remains indeterminate, referral to dermatology specialists may be indicated to verify the diagnosis and institute a specific management program. Another important aspect of differentiation is understanding the role of skin microflora and other external factors in skin conditions. Skin harbors a sophisticated microflora that is both protective and pathogenic for the host. Bacterial infection usually follows a broken skin barrier, allowing pathogenic bacteria to flourish. Gall et al. (2025) speak of the action of human skin microflora in special conditions, illustrating how environmental factors, in this instance, occlusion and moisture, may contribute to bacterial growth, mimicking signs of infection. Furthermore, allergens or irritants from outside the body may provoke pre-existing conditions, leading to diagnostic confusion. Hence, recognition of the interaction of skin microflora with the skin barrier and external factors is needed so that bacterial infections can be effectively differentiated from other conditions of the skin, for proper therapeutic measures to be rendered in support of the skin's health.

Test Your Knowledge

1. What are common symptoms of bacterial skin infections?
2. Which diagnostic method is most useful for identifying deep tissue involvement in bacterial skin infections?

11.4. Treatment Options

Learning Outcome

1. Describe the antibiotic therapies in managing bacterial skin infections
2. Understand the role of topical treatments in managing bacterial skin infections
3. Describe the home care and preventive measures in managing bacterial skin infections

The management of bacterial skin infections requires a multi-disciplinary approach that combines pharmacological treatment with other modes of management. Antibacterial therapy is the cornerstone of the management of bacterial skin infections, with antibiotics prescribed based on pathogen sensitivity. The process, however, is hindered by antibiotic resistance. Because bacterial cells are resistant and adaptable, their efficacy can be severely diminished by normal treatments. More specifically, certain pathogens can enter host cells, protecting themselves from antibiotic action and immune detection, which is important in cases of chronic infection. Effective management of such infections, therefore, entails the application not just of existing clinical antimicrobial drugs but also new approaches that enhance drug delivery and efficacy in host tissue to overcome the limitations posed by traditional interventions (Good et al., 2016). In addition to systemic antibiotics, topical interventions also play a significant role in managing localized cutaneous bacterial infections. These preparations can deliver localized therapy, limiting systemic exposure and oral drug-related side effects. They exist as creams, ointments, and solutions and can be supplemented with antibiotics or antiseptics. Evaluation of the specific characteristics of the infection—i.e., severity and presentation—is key in determining the appropriateness of a topically administered treatment. Moreover, studies continue to discover new agents capable of penetrating deeper into skin layers or targeting biofilms produced by bacteria that participate in chronic skin infections. Patient education on the administration of these therapies cannot be overemphasized, as correct use directly affects treatment effectiveness and the prevention of recurrence (Bernthal et al., 2015). Preventive measures also form an essential part of the overall strategy to combat bacterial skin infection. Implementing hygiene measures, particularly in institutions where patients are at risk—hospitals or clinics—will significantly reduce infection incidence. Interventions include promoting hand hygiene among healthcare workers and patients, correcting wound dressings, and educating individuals on the importance of intact and clean skin. Additionally, information regarding risk factors for these infections, such as pre-existing illness or immunocompromised status, allows for the identification of high-risk populations that can be safeguarded by the use of prophylactic therapies. Coordination of treatment regimens not only enhances patient outcomes but also reduces the burden of antibiotic resistance by preserving the effectiveness of currently available drugs. The ongoing risks associated with bacterial infections require dynamic, interactive treatment and prevention strategies, and this calls for consistent research and development in this critical health area (Good et al., 2016) (Figure 11.12).

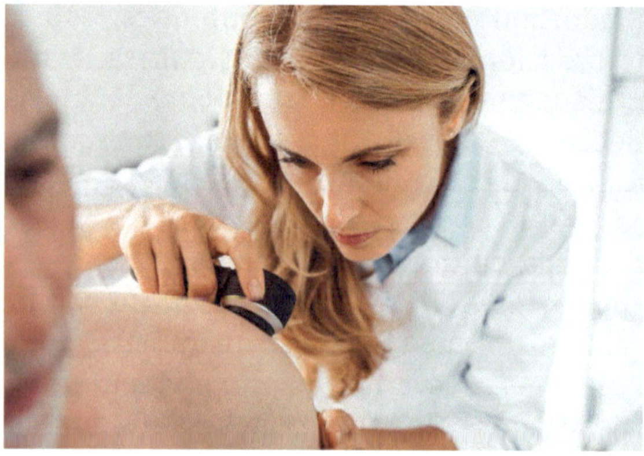

Figure 11.12. Treatment of bacterial skin infections.

Source: https://docsmedicalgroup.com/wp-content/uploads/2024/02/steptodown.com619156-1024x683.jpg.

11.4.1. Antibiotic Therapies

Antibiotic therapy plays an important role in the management of bacterial skin infections, as these infections are often caused by multiple pathogens and thus require specific treatment. The increased emergence of antibiotic-resistant pathogens has made proper selection mandatory to produce desirable patient outcomes. Newer antibiotics introduced in recent years are markedly effective in treating complex skin infections. For instance, dalbavancin, a long-acting lipoglycopeptide antibiotic, is increasingly recognized as a therapeutic option for acute bacterial skin and skin-structure infections (ABSSSI) in pediatric patients. Due to its excellent bactericidal activity against Gram-positive bacteria, including multidrug-resistant strains, dalbavancin is an ideal option for patients who do not respond adequately to standard therapies (Garbo et al., 2024). The therapeutic environment still evolves, with emphasis on the need for ongoing clinical monitoring of these drugs to optimize regimens. As new antibiotic treatments are designed, the need for tailored treatment approaches becomes increasingly clear. Patient-specific characteristics, presumed pathogens, and infection severity must guide antibiotic selection. New developments have ushered in advanced-stage clinical trials a range of contenders, each with new mechanisms of action and antimicrobial activity. These developments signal a shift towards personalizing antibiotic therapy for bacterial skin infections, which is necessary in light of the limitations of existing drugs (Castaldo et al., 2024). Besides, research on the effectiveness of the new drugs in the pursuit of better therapeutic regimens and improved patient outcomes still goes on. This evolution not only improves clinical care but also constitutes a significant response to the growing perils of antibiotic resistance in the treatment of skin infections. The addition of new antibiotic treatments is a revolutionary leap in the therapy of bacterial skin infections. These new agents provide potent alternatives to traditional antibiotics, reducing the potential for resistance and improving patient outcomes. One significant advantage, as illustrated by the dalbavancin case series, is the potential for early discharge from healthcare centers, which has positive implications for patient quality of life and for minimizing healthcare costs (Garbo et al., 2024). However, the introduction of new drugs also calls for greater scrutiny from health workers on the appropriate use of these medications to avoid abuse and the resultant development of drug resistance. The continuous quest for antibiotic therapies, such as those still in trials, will ensure that they address not only the clinical requirements of skin infections but also the broader public health issues with resistance becoming an ever-increasing worldwide phenomenon.

11.4.2. Topical Treatments

Local therapy is a significant treatment for bacterial skin infections, such as superficial bacterial folliculitis, which are frequently caused by Staphylococcus spp. The effectiveness of these treatments is crucial, especially since frequent administration of systemic antibiotics has been a leading driver of antimicrobial resistance. Natural compound discovery, such as propolis, has been studied as a potential natural alternative to conventional antibiotic therapy. Studies indicate that topical gel preparations of propolis extract can deliver active antibacterial components directly to the site of infection, thereby achieving maximum local treatment with minimal systemic side effects. The potential therapeutic application of natural substances such as these addresses urgent clinical needs of patients as well as the larger problem of antibiotic resistance in both human and animal medicine (Dovilė Svetikienė et al., 2025). As the pattern of skin infection changes in dermatology, classical topical antibiotics such as mupirocin become ineffective against emerging strains such as methicillin-resistant *Staphylococcus aureus* (MRSA). The need for novel topical antimicrobial agents is brought to the forefront by the increasing number of treatment failures of employing standard current treatments. Recent research has suggested novel preparations such as arginine undecylenate (GS-1), a product of the combination of L-arginine and undecylenic acid. This drug has exhibited robust antibacterial activity against diverse pathogenic strains, including MSSA and MRSA, without a high likelihood of resistance development under chronic exposure. Such advancements demonstrate the impetus for greater exploration of other topical drugs that can effectively treat bacterial cutaneous infections without sidestepping the challenge of traditional antibiotic resistance (Mayfosh et al., 2025). In addition to efficacy, safety is crucial in the development of topical antibiotics for bacterial skin infections. The compatibility and stability of active medications must be thoroughly tested to preclude patient intolerance and low medication adherence. For instance, drugs like GS-1 have shown satisfactory toxicity profiles in animal models and clinical trials, indicating that such drugs can be safely administered without irritation or sensitization. This is particularly important for treating populations that are more susceptible to skin reactions, such as children and those with existing conditions. Thus, ongoing research into safe and effective topical treatments has the promise to not only enhance patient outcomes but also to be an integral component of a broad strategy to manage bacterial skin infections in an age become increasingly antibiotic-resistant (Dovilė Svetikienė et al., 2025; Mayfosh et al., 2025) (Figure 11.13).

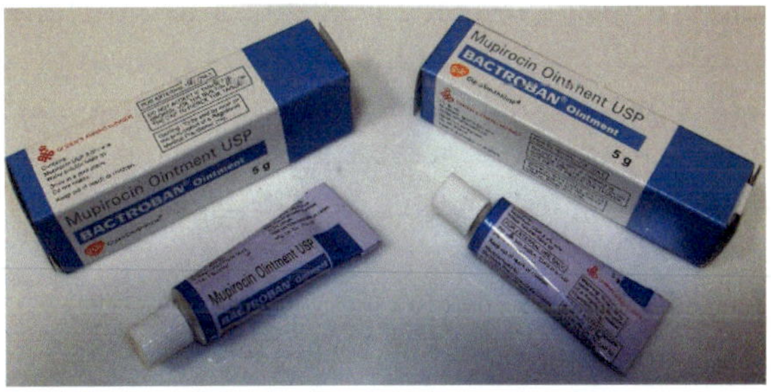

Figure 11.13. Topical treatments.

Source: https://lotusinternational.com/wp-content/uploads/2020/11/BactrobanOintment.jpg.

11.4.3. Home Care and Preventive Measures

Preventive measures and home care are significant in managing bacterial skin infections. A well-designed measure begins with strict observance of hygiene, which is the first line of defense against pathogens. Proper washing of infected areas with antiseptic agents will reduce bacterial burden on the skin. In addition, keeping the skin properly hydrated maintains the skin barrier, lessening the development of cracks that can serve as portals of entry for bacteria. In addition, it is also necessary to inform individuals about the signs and symptoms of bacterial infection, such as redness, swelling, or discharge, so that early diagnosis and treatment can be initiated. By having a positive attitude towards skin health, individuals can also reduce their risk of developing serious complications from bacterial skin infections. In addition to hygiene practices, preventive interventions can include lifestyle changes that promote overall skin health. Proper nutrition plays an important role in maintaining skin integrity, and vitamins A, C, and E directly promote skin healing and immune function. Supplementing a balanced diet with high levels of antioxidants can enhance the body's own protective systems against infection. Proper fluid balance also ensures overall skin hydration and keeps it soft, thereby strengthening defenses against potential weaknesses. Exercise similarly has a beneficial impact on circulation, delivering much-needed oxygen and nutrients to skin tissues. These lifestyle factors, coupled with certain home-care regimens, form a solid foundation for the prevention of bacterial skin infections while ensuring overall health and skin resilience. Apart from lifestyle and basic hygiene modifications, the use of natural remedies and preventive techniques could be employed to complement home care interventions for bacterial skin infections. Certain herbal extracts and essential oils possess antibacterial activity that can be utilized to combat skin infections. For example, plant-based formulations have historically been used in veterinary medicine to support skin health, as noted in manuals on maintaining healthy animal populations (Asseldonk et al., 2011; Groot et al., 2011). Such traditional remedies can be added to standard treatments and provide an overall strategy for controlling infection. Careful research should be undertaken, and, where practicable, professional medical advice should be sought prior to taking new treatments. Through the incorporation of these general measures, one can construct a more robust defense against bacterial skin infection and an environment conducive to healing and skin wellness (Figure 11.14).

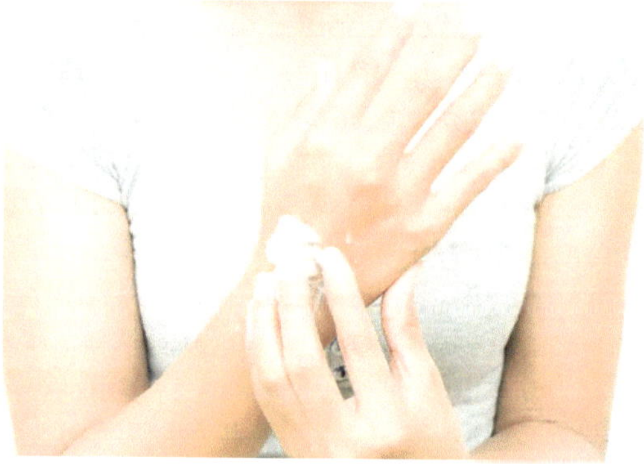

Figure 11.14. Home remedies for skin infection.

Source: https://cdn2.stylecraze.com/wp-content/uploads/2012/08/Home-Remedies-For-Skin-Infection.jpg.webp.

Test Your Knowledge

1. What type of bacteria is dalbavancin most effective against?
2. Which bacteria are commonly associated with superficial bacterial folliculitis?

11.5. Complications and Consequences

Learning Outcome

1. Understand the potential for systemic infection
2. Learn about scarring and skin damage
3. Know the impact of bacterial skin infections on mental health and quality of life

The aftermath of bacterial skin infection extends well beyond outward appearance, leading to a myriad of complications that require urgent medical attention. If left untreated, cellulitis or abscesses can progress to advanced infections with systemic implications. As indicated by research, stress and psychological adjustment disorders have been found to be linked to increased susceptibility to infection, an indication that the existence of co-morbid mental health disorders among patients results in the deterioration of outcomes when there is a bacterial skin infection (Farkas et al., 2020). This interaction requires an integrated treatment approach to address both the physical and psychological needs of patient care. In addition to psychological determinants, the immune system also plays an important role in shaping the courses of bacterial skin infections. Immunocompromised individuals, either due to inherent medical conditions or due to treatments such as immunosuppressive therapy, are particularly susceptible to potentially deadly complications. A report on renal transplant recipients showed a very high incidence of infections caused by reasons like granulocytopenia and hypogammaglobulinemia because of their immunosuppressive treatment (Marchioro et al., 1964). This underscores the importance of close monitoring and infection risk management in immunocompromised populations, as outcomes are lethal when infections go untreated. Thus, serious bacterial skin infection complications underscore the need for effective public health interventions, including prevention and timely treatment. Education and awareness campaigns regarding the hazard posed by bacterial skin infections can be instrumental in altering patient outcomes. Moreover, respect for the complex interplay among psychological, immunological, and environmental variables may lead to more targeted interventions that diminish hazard and enhance patient resilience. Lastly, addressing the intricacies of such infections and their complications is needed to improve overall health outcomes for targeted populations.

11.5.1. Potential for Systemic Infection

Bacterial skin infections such as cellulitis and abscesses can begin as localized infections but can also become systemic. The progression from a cutaneous infection to one that is systemic in nature is a function of numerous factors that encompass the virulence of the etiologic bacteria, the vitality of the host's immune system, and health conditions that predispose to complications. Most significantly, illnesses such as diabetes or obesity have been seen to possess an elevated risk of systemic infection since they impair the body's capacity for defense and pathogen control. The systemic consequences of local bacterial skin infections warrant concern in clinical practice, as early detection and treatment are crucial for preventing progression to more severe states of illness. The modulation of host immunity by the resident microbiota is extensive and intricate, creating an immune barrier against disease-causing microbes. The co-immunity theory indicates that the host immune system, as well as the microbial community, contributes to disease resistance and tolerance. This highlights the potential interaction between local bacterial cutaneous infections and systemic responses. Disruption of this balance, either by antibiotic treatment or by extraneous factors, may lead to a failure of colonization resistance, thereby facilitating the pathogen's entry and spread beyond the primary infection site. Abt et al. (2017) further observe that protective microorganisms not only counteract the effect of pathogens but also engage in restricting them, which is vital in evading the occurrence of systemic infections from a skin breach or a cut. Moreover, understanding the dynamics of treatment for acute bacterial skin and skin structure infections (ABSSSIs) is vital for managing the risk of systemic complications. Retrospective treatment pattern analysis of ABSSSIs revealed that inpatients had more comorbidities and were at higher risk of developing complications (Bookstaver et al., 2018). The correlation between hospitalization and readmission rates reinforces the importance of careful consideration of each patient's factors to determine the optimal treatment plan. Findings highlight that outpatient and inpatient management strategies yield similar outcomes in preventing future emergency visits or readmissions, and that early, appropriate therapeutic management can mitigate the causal harm associated with secondary bacterial skin infections-induced systemic infections.

11.5.2. Scarring and Skin Damage

Bacterial skin infections can lead to severe scarring and skin damage, with far-reaching physical and psychological impacts on the individual. These infections, caused by a variety of bacterial pathogens, commonly lead to inflammation and tissue destruction that can impair the skin's natural healing. As the skin attempts to heal, it may form scar tissue, which is typically more stiff and of a different color from the surrounding skin, resulting in observable blemishes. Infections such as acne vulgaris, which affects a significant proportion of adolescents, can cause permanent scarring due to inflammatory lesions caused by bacterial overgrowth. Scarring not only affects physical appearance but can also lower self-esteem and increase anxiety in participants, further highlighting the importance of treating bacterial infections to prevent such long-term consequences. The role of various treatment modalities in the prevention of the scarring process of bacterial skin infections cannot be overstressed. Routine treatments, such as topical antibiotics and systemic therapy, aim to reduce inflammation and eradicate the etiological bacterial infection, which is crucial for optimal wound healing. Scarring may still occur despite optimal infection control. Other interventions, such as the use of honey on wounds, have been reported to favorably impact healing and scarring. Honey has been shown to possess antimicrobial activity and promote the growth of granulation tissue, thereby enabling a more effective healing environment. Direct evidence reveals honey's potential to decrease the rate of hypertrophic scarring drastically and enhance epithelialization, and, consequently, is a candidate for being part of contemporary wound care management with more traditional modalities (Molan et al., 2006). The psychological impact of scarring from bacterial skin infections further reinforces the need for multiple interventions. Withdrawal from society and negative body image can be triggered by the visibility of scars, particularly in youths with acne and other bacterial skin conditions. While treatments in dermatology may restore the body physically, psychological therapy and support may be essential to address emotional healing from scarring. Additionally, the rising popularity of alternative medicine, including medicinal herbs, reflects a growing search for effective treatments with fewer side effects. In reviewing the clinical evidence regarding these alternatives, their historical use, and established efficacy against a variety of pathogens, as well as the resulting scarring, may provide further avenues for the treatment of bacterial skin infections (Bahmani et al., 2015). An integrated holistic approach that prioritizes both physical and psychological treatment will ultimately improve patient quality of life and outcomes (Figure 11.15).

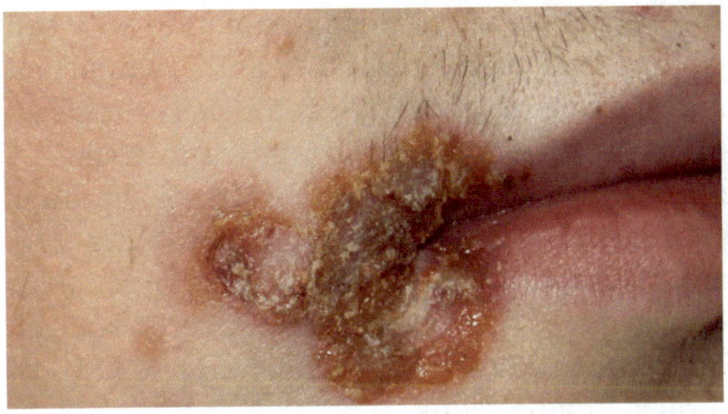

Figure 11.15. Bacterial skin infections lead to significant and skin damage.

Source: https://www.devonshiredermatology.co.uk/wp-content/uploads/2024/09/Screenshot-2024-09-09-at-14.27.17.png.

11.5.3. Impact on Mental Health and Quality of Life

The impact on quality of life and mental health from bacterial skin infection is considerable and widespread. Not only do patients with such infections experience physical distress, but also considerable psychological distress. Pain, itching, and lesions can lead to embarrassment and self-consciousness. Such discomfort may give rise to social withdrawal, decreased participation in daily activities, or social avoidance. Therefore, implications do not stop at basic immediate physical well-being, as mental stress can compound feelings of loneliness and anxiety, leading to a reduced overall quality of life. This interaction highlights the importance of overall treatment tackling both physical symptoms and psychological attention to improve patients' mental health as well as cure the primary infection. Furthermore, social stigmatization of skin-infectious diseases that are visually observable can reinforce mental health problems in the individuals affected. Society creates myths associating skin diseases with unsanitary conditions or infectivity, which supports social exclusion. Such stigmatization not only aggravates loneliness but also causes negative self-concept and low self-esteem. The psychological consequences then manifest in conditions such as depression and anxiety disorders, which further complicate the recovery and healing processes. Integrated care for bacterial skin infections should thus incorporate mental health assessment and interventions to reduce such social problems and build patients' emotional resilience. By acknowledging the intersection between body and mind, physicians can create more effective treatment plans to enhance the well-being of the afflicted. Lastly, research consistently demonstrates that individuals who are chronically ill, including those with repeated bacterial infections of the skin, are more likely to have lower life satisfaction and increased psychological distress. Studies have shown that skin infections left untreated or not treated properly can lead to a cycle of deteriorating mental health because patients find it difficult to deal with persistent symptoms and pain. In addition, the expense of continuous medical treatment can add to stress, affecting an individual's working capacity or ability to build personal relationships. Understanding such dynamics highlights the need for early detection and effective care strategies that address not only the physical state of skin infections but also the psychological impact. Multidisciplinary care models that include dermatological and psychological professionals can be instrumental in facilitating recovery and enhancing the quality of life of patients with bacterial skin infections.

Test Your Knowledge

1. Which health condition is commonly associated with an increased risk of systemic infection from bacterial skin infections?
2. Which bacterial skin condition commonly results in permanent scarring?

11.6. Prevention Strategies

Learning Outcome

1. Understand the hygiene practices in preventing bacterial skin infections
2. Describe the skin care routines in preventing bacterial skin infections
3. Describe the education and awareness campaigns in combating bacterial skin infections

Effective prevention strategies are crucial for controlling bacterial skin infections, particularly in healthcare settings. One of the fundamental strategies includes strict hand hygiene, which has been established to reduce the transmission of pathogens considerably. Evidence indicates that proper hand washing with soap and water or alcohol-based hand rubbing can greatly reduce bacterial carriage on hands and, subsequently, the likelihood of healthcare-associated infections (HAIs) (Delicati et al., 2025). This is a crucial habit in environments with greater contact with infectious agents, as the study reveals that a high percentage of bacteria remain on healthcare-relevant surfaces after incomplete cleaning. Hand hygiene practice, then, must be implemented among caregivers and healthcare providers to ensure a uniform defense against infection transmission. In addition to hand hygiene, environmental sanitation is a basic prevention measure against bacterial skin infections. Proper disinfection of surfaces, particularly those frequently touched or in contact with patients, for example, medical devices and countertops, is essential. The findings of recent research reveal the disparity in bacterial persistence across different surfaces, indicating that Gram-negative infections are more likely to infest laminate surfaces than glass (Delicati et al., 2025). Therefore, procedures must be designed to incorporate frequent cleaning and disinfection to address the material composition of the surfaces. Implementation of these environmental controls not only reduces microbial burden but also eliminates the possibility of cross-contamination between patients and health facilities. Another important intervention of prevention strategies is oriented towards patient education and sensitization, more so in the context of high-risk groups such as individuals with atopic dermatitis, who are at increased risk of secondary infections. Education of the patient in skin care, through daily moisturizing and proper application of topical medications, would ensure adequate maintenance of skin integrity and protection against bacterial invasion. Furthermore, education must touch on early signs of infection and the importance of early use of antibiotics when signs are present. Through practice-integrated education, healthcare providers can facilitate patients to act as partners in their care, thereby reducing the incidence of bacterial skin infections and improving overall skin care management outcomes (Figure 11.16).

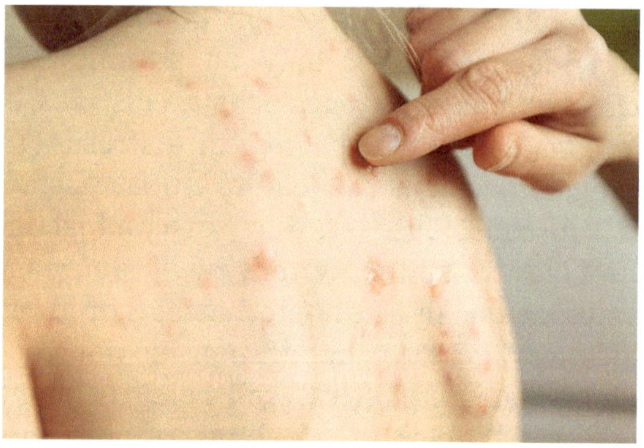

Figure 11.16. Prevent skin infections.

Source: https://www.focusonkidspeds.com/wp-content/uploads/Tips-to-Prevent-Skin-Infections-scaled.jpg.webp.

11.6.1. Hygiene Practices

Good hygiene measures are most important for preventing bacterial skin infections, especially in close-contact settings, such as contact sports. Sportsmen are particularly prone to these infections because the nature of their activities involves direct skin-to-skin contact and the use of shared equipment. Practicing strict hygiene—like frequent handwashing, showering after practice, and using clean towels—fiercely reduces the chances that pathogens like methicillin-resistant Staphylococcus aureus and others will establish themselves. Coaches and players also need to be reminded of the importance of not sharing personal items, such as towels and equipment. Adherence to these hygienic measures not only reduces the incidence but also fosters a health-focused environment, resulting in improved overall athletic performance and participation. Despite advances in medical intervention, bacterial skin infections remain a major public health issue, driven by antibiotic resistance. The widespread use of antibiotics since 1928, when penicillin was discovered, has led to the emergence of antibiotic-resistant bacterial strains, making treatment difficult. In contact sports, poor hygiene is also likely to accelerate this by spreading resistant bacteria among players who may not be well controlled. Good hygiene practice, therefore, is necessary, not only for individual health but also for public health. By establishing a prevention culture through hygiene education and good practices, the transmission of infections and the emergence of resistant bacterial strains can be avoided, thereby safeguarding the health of athletes and the healthcare system. Early detection and prompt action in case of potential skin infections are also key components of a sound hygiene policy. Medical staff and athletic trainers must observe closely for any sign of infection, such as redness, swelling, or pus, in the athletes. Educating athletes to identify these signs can lead to early intervention, greatly reducing the risk of severe infection and transmission. Wound care cannot be overemphasized; it prevents pathogen invasion, making it more significant in sports, where minor injuries such as cuts are frequent. By integrating these habits of hygiene into training schemes and sporting policy, organizations can make possible a proactive culture that not only enhances the safety of competitors but is also a model for wider public health practice and impacts on bacterial skin infection rates directly in the population (Lillestolen et al., 2018; Gaweł-Dąbrowska et al., 2025) (Figure 11.17).

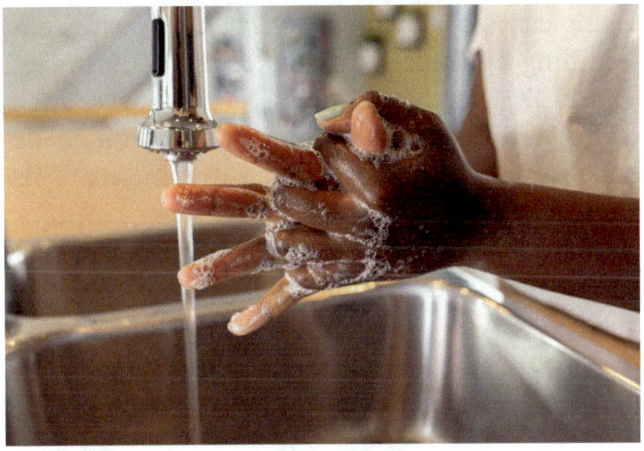

Figure 11.17. Handwashing.

Source: https://domf5oio6qrcr.cloudfront.net/medialibrary/7791/957f06cb-d42f-48fe-b846-13a6749ba516.jpg.

11.6.2. Skin Care Routines

A good skin care routine is essential in preventing bacterial skin infection, which mostly occurs due to the breakdown of the skin barrier. A proper routine entails daily cleansing, moisturizing, and applying products that match one's skin type. Cleansing effectively removes dirt, oil, and bacteria from the skin surface, reducing the risk of infection by pathogens such as *Staphylococcus aureus*. Also, maintaining skin hydration with appropriate moisturizers supports the skin's natural barrier function, which is vital for preventing microbial invasion. Non-compliance with these elementary steps can result in a setting that promotes bacterial proliferation, thus heightened susceptibility to skin infections. Also, inclusion of antiseptic agents in skin care regimens may enhance antimicrobial protection against bacterial infections. Antimicrobial disinfectants and topical products may target pathogenic bacteria without disrupting the skin's normal flora. Information shows that the incorporation of agents such as benzoyl peroxide or salicylic acid can reduce the growth of bacteria that cause acne and inflammation, thus preventing secondary infections. Similarly, in bacterium-infected outbreak scenarios, i.e., rising cases of *Campylobacter jejuni* in chicken-handling settings, as reported by Hansson et al. (2007), heightened hygiene measures, such as repeated use of disinfectants, can also be reflected in personal skin-care regimens. This two-pronged approach not only guarantees personal welfare but also emphasizes the role of environmental hygiene in managing infection risk.

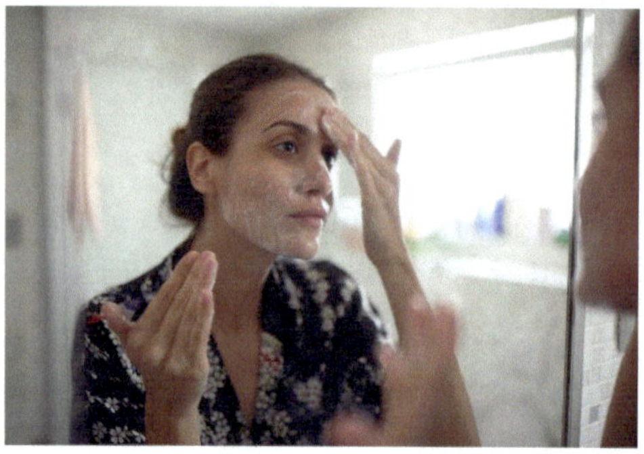

Figure 11.18. Skin care routines.

Source: https://www.health.com/thmb/SdcQB7oWstZFrtyCpl1nUbfBI68=/2119x0/filters:no_upscale():max_bytes(150000):strip_icc()/SkincareRoutine-960b99db9d174754b659f9b546f23502.jpg.

Lastly, awareness of the environment is significant in skin care, particularly in crowded and public places. Washing of hands in a regular basis and being mindful when in contact can significantly reduce the transfer of pathogens that trigger infections. The impact of the COVID-19 pandemic validated the effectiveness of cleanliness procedures, including increased use of personal protective gear and surface disinfection, as seen in Chisari et al. (2020). Performing these skin care routines reinforces the fact that steps to prevent bacterial transmission are necessary. Putting these points into practice enables individuals to more effectively safeguard their skin against bacterial infection, thereby improving overall health (Figure 11.18).

11.6.3. Education and Awareness Campaigns

Educational interventions and sensitization drives are paramount in combating bacterial skin infections, particularly in raising awareness of their causes, prevention, and treatment. Effective drives can de-mystify the character of such infections, which often have their origins in ubiquitous bacteria such as Staphylococcus and Streptococcus. The pathogens have the potential to spread very quickly within communal environments, particularly among the vulnerable populations. By sharing accurate information through various channels, including social media, community workshops, and school-based programs, health authorities can foster preventive behavior. Educational outreach through these activities is essential to instill a culture of hygiene and sensibility, significantly reducing the public health burden and prevalence of bacterial skin infections. The provision of comprehensive awareness campaigns is essential for addressing the factors driving antibiotic resistance in bacterial skin infections. Effective programs not only have to enlighten the public regarding such infections but also emphasize the importance of careful use of antibiotics. Those programs that offer communities education on the potential consequences of indiscriminate or excessive antibiotic use can help prevent drug-resistant strains from developing. As brought to the fore by recent findings, antibiotic resistance results in increased healthcare costs, extended hospital stay, and higher mortality, necessitating a call for action together. Therefore, multidisciplinary education programs, such as the EVADES BUGS framework, have a dual role to play in informing individuals about bacterial infections while simultaneously developing a sense of responsibility for antibiotic stewardship

(Senanayake, 2025). Moreover, education and awareness regarding bacterial skin infections can greatly improve health outcomes and reduce healthcare disparities among populations. By way of illustration, specific population-based campaigns can empower individuals with information focused on their respective risk factors and environmental factors. Interventions targeting rural or underserved populations are likely to have excellent results, such as improved access to adequate medical care and preventive practices. Moreover, these infections are treated at an economic advantage, such as through low-cost interventions that yield long-term returns for populations. Investing in these types of educational programs is not only a public health priority but also a critical part of an effective strategy for preventing both bacterial infections and broader global healthcare challenges (Fenwick et al., 2005).

Test Your Knowledge

1. Which bacterial pathogen is commonly associated with infections in athletic environments?
2. Which bacteria are commonly associated with bacterial skin infections?

SUMMARY

In conclusion, bacterial skin infections are a critical health problem that requires comprehensive understanding and management. The variability in infection types, coupled with their associations with different patient conditions, underscores the importance of patient-specific treatment regimens. For instance, Type 1 diabetic patients have very high risks of varied infections, like cellulitis and osteomyelitis, particularly in the setting of inadequate glycemic control. As explained in recent studies, compliance by patients with insulin therapy is also critical because patients with HbA1c levels over 9% experienced high infection and mortality rates compared to their counterparts with low levels. This emphasizes the importance of self-management in minimizing risks and optimizing patients' outcomes (Salman, 2025). Furthermore, new drugs and antibiotics are required to manage drug-resistant bacteria causing skin infections. Recent evidence on the efficacy of omadacyclines against methicillin-resistant Staphylococcus aureus (MRSA) and other resistant pathogens indicates improved control of acute bacterial skin and skin-structure infections. The results indicate that customized dosing regimens can achieve optimal therapeutic outcomes, characterized by high cumulative fractions of response (CFRs). Such advancements are key to identifying a solution to the acute problem of drug resistance, which complicates infection treatment protocols across various patient populations (Wei et al., 2024). The ultimate outcome is effective management of bacterial skin infections through a multi-faceted approach that includes patient education, adherence to treatment regimens, and ongoing research into therapeutic benefits. The interplay between diabetics' glycemic control and adherence to medications underscores the complexity of infection management. Additionally, new antibiotic medications need to be developed to combat the evolving environment of resistant pathogens. While healthcare faces these challenges, it is imperative that patients and healthcare workers recognize the importance of prophylaxis in preventing and treating bacterial skin infections. Prioritizing measures to prevent such infections, such as ensuring good hygiene and controlling underlying medical conditions, will be key to mitigating their effects across diverse populations (Salman, 2025; Wei et al., 2024).

Bacterial cutaneous infections are of primary interest in dermatological health, owing mainly to their multifactorial etiology and diverse clinical manifestations. *Corynebacterium diphtheriae*, *Staphylococcus aureus*, and *Streptococcus pyogenes* are the primary pathogens in these diseases, and each presents in a unique way clinically. The prevalence of these pathogens is influenced by multiple factors, including microbial load, host immunity, and underlying skin disorders. Interestingly, studies have shown that sexual dimorphism also plays a role in the immune response to such infections, which may contribute to variability in disease severity and outcome between females and males. It is thus necessary to understand such differences when formulating specific therapeutic interventions for the management of bacterial skin infections, as they can maximize treatment regimens and patient outcomes. A very essential part of bacterial skin infections is the dynamic response of the immune system, which varies from individual to individual. Research highlights the significant role of innate immune cells, particularly type 2 innate lymphoid cells (ILC2s), in regulating skin tissue immunity. In females, high numbers of skin-resident T cells, dendritic cells, and ILC2s correlate with heightened immune responses, whereas the androgen-mediated inhibitory influence in males may impair such immune defenses. This sexual dimorphism in the skin's immune environment is important because it influences the body's capacity to respond to bacterial colonization and associated infection. Besides, the relationship between the microbiome and sex hormones further complicates the immune response, underscoring the need for a prudent appreciation of these interactions in determining treatment and prevention measures against bacterial skin infections. Furthermore, the tactics employed by bacteria to evade host immunity must be addressed in the pathogenesis. For instance, *Corynebacterium diphtheriae* produces exotoxins that disrupt host cell signaling and induce inflammation by stimulating the NLRP1 inflammasome, thereby creating a direct link between bacterial virulence factors and immune response activation. The resulting pyroptosis of keratinocytes not only disrupts the skin's barrier function but also locally amplifies tissue inflammation, creating a niche for further bacterial growth. Targeting such interactions, as well as signal transduction pathways associated with the immune response, lies at the core of developing new therapeutic approaches to bacterial skin infections. Through enhanced elucidation of these complex interactions, we are increasingly able to direct future research efforts to mitigate the public health burden posed by such infections.

KEY TERMS FROM THIS CHAPTER

- Antimicrobial resistance
- Cellulitis
- Cryoglobulinaemia
- Fat grafting
- Friction
- Infections
- Pathogenic bacteria
- Bacteria
- Chlorine
- Epidemiology
- Folliculitis
- Impetigo
- Mycobacterium abscessus
- Pseudomonas aeruginosa

CRITICAL THINKING QUESTIONS

1. **Which bacterium is the most common cause of impetigo?**
   a. *Streptococcus pyogenes*
   b. *Staphylococcus aureus*
   c. *Pseudomonas aeruginosa*
   d. *Escherichia coli*
2. **What is the characteristic appearance of lesions in impetigo?**
   a. Vesicles that rupture to form honey-colored crusts
   b. Thickened plaques with silvery scales
   c. Painful pustules with necrotic centers
   d. Red patches with greasy scales
3. **Erysipelas primarily affects which layer of the skin?**
   a. Epidermis
   b. Dermis
   c. Subcutaneous tissue
   d. Stratum corneum
4. **Which bacterial infection involves deep tissues and can rapidly spread, causing necrosis?**
   a. Impetigo
   b. Cellulitis
   c. Necrotizing fasciitis
   d. Folliculitis
5. **Which is a common clinical feature of cellulitis?**
   a. Localized swelling, warmth, redness, and tenderness
   b. Vesicular eruptions with clear fluid
   c. Thickened plaques with fissures
   d. Yellow crusted lesions around the mouth

Short Answer Questions

1. Define the bacterial skin infections.
2. Describe the types of bacterial skin infections.
3. What are the risk factors for bacterial skin infections?
4. What is the best treatment for bacterial skin infection?
5. What is a possible complication of a bacterial infection of the skin?

Answer to Critical Thinking Questions

1. (b); 2. (a) ; 3. (b), 4. (c), 5. (a)

REFERENCES

1. Chiu, L., Bazin, T., Truchetet, M., Schaeverbeke, T., Delhaes, L., & Pradeu, T. (2017). Protective microbiota: From localized to Long-Reaching Co-Immunity. *Frontiers in Immunology, 8,* 1678. https://doi.org/10.3389/fimmu.2017.01678Adams, J., Araujo, M., Araujo, R., Asmah, R. H., Breman, J., Brugman, A., Butler, M., et al. (2010). Allergic disorders in Africa and Africans: Is it primarily a priority? https://core.ac.uk/download/pdf/18410775.pdf (accessed on 21st July 2025).
2. Ailal, F., Al-Herz, W., Bousfiha, A., Casanova, J. L., et al. (2020). Human inborn errors of immunity: 2019 update of the IUIS phenotypical classification. https://core.ac.uk/download/323074666.pdf (accessed on 21st July 2025).
3. Al-Hindi, Z. S., & Al.Dulaimi, T. H. (2024). Review: Microbial skin infections (types, symptoms and methods of diagnosis). https://core.ac.uk/download/599440147.pdf (accessed on 21st July 2025).
4. Al-Wabel, A., Almutairi, B. S., Alsugair, A., Cheng, L., et al. (2020). Scabies: Application of the novel Identify-Isolate-Inform tool for detection and management. https://core.ac.uk/download/287622020.pdf (accessed on 21st July 2025).
5. Asseldonk, T. van, Groot, M., & Puls-van der Kamp, I. (2011). *Natural Poultry Health.* https://core.ac.uk/download/10932085.pdf (accessed on 21st July 2025).
6. Bahmani, M., Moradi Nafchi, A., Nasri, H., Rafieian-Kopaei, M., et al. (2015). Medicinal plants for the treatment of acne vulgaris: A review of recent evidences. https://core.ac.uk/download/143840955.pdf (accessed on 21st July 2025).
7. Bernthal, N. M., Dworsky, E. M., Hu, Y., Loftin, B., et al. (2015). Current animal models of postoperative spine infection and potential future advances. https://core.ac.uk/download/323066862.pdf (accessed on 21st July 2025).
8. Bharatha, A., Kandamaran, L., & Krishnamurthy, K. (2021). Commentary: "Fungal infections of oral cavity: Diagnosis, management, and association with COVID 19". *SN Comprehensive Clinical Medicine, 3,* 2002–2003. https://www.semanticscholar.org/paper/bdf4eb5a0c387e9a515d95953e78fa3f69f5851e (accessed on 21st July 2025).
9. Bhutta, Z. A., Black, R., Cousens, S., Ganatra, H., et al. (2011). Effect of case management on neonatal mortality due to sepsis and pneumonia. https://core.ac.uk/download/13093714.pdf (accessed on 21st July 2025).
10. Bookstaver, P. B., Brown, J., Doron, S., Gllard, G., et al. (2018). Impact of outpatient vs inpatient ABSSSI treatment on outcomes: A retrospective observational analysis of medical charts across US emergency departments. https://core.ac.uk/download/213033349.pdf (accessed on 21st July 2025).
11. Bramanti, B., Guellil, M., Kersten, O., Ottoni, C., et al. (2019). Metagenomic analysis of dental calculus in ancient Egyptian baboons. https://core.ac.uk/download/286075786.pdf (accessed on 21st July 2025).
12. Braun, G. S., Horster, S., Ihrler, S., Schmid, M., et al. (2007). Cryoglobulinemic vasculitis: Classification and clinical and therapeutic aspects. https://core.ac.uk/download/12175185.pdf (accessed on 21st July 2025).

13. Castaldo, N., Vena, A., Limongelli, A., Giacobbe, D., & Bassetti, M. (2024). Emerging treatment options for skin and soft tissue infections tailoring drug selection to individual patients. *Current Opinion in Infectious Diseases, 37*, 80–86. https://www.semanticscholar.org/paper/52899a1221c8f6025687a78c8250ddebdc2a2909 (accessed on 21st July 2025).

14. Chetter, I., & Smith, G. (2015). Infection in prosthetic material. https://core.ac.uk/download/151157240.pdf (accessed on 21st July 2025).

15. Chi, L., Liu, C., Gribonika, I., Gschwend, J., Corral, D., Han, S. J., Lim, A. I., et al. (2024). Sexual dimorphism in skin immunity is mediated by an androgen-ILC2-dendritic cell axis. *Science, 384*. https://www.semanticscholar.org/paper/6ff7d4cc44b6a582fec11598cc814f2f421f14dd (accessed on 21st July 2025).

16. Chisari, E., Krueger, C. A., Barnes, C. L., Parvizi, J., et al. (2020). Prevention of infection and disruption of the pathogen transfer chain in elective surgery. https://core.ac.uk/download/322827646.pdf (accessed on 21st July 2025).

17. Cole, S. A. (2020). Individual and collective identification in contemporary forensics. https://core.ac.uk/download/323082704.pdf (accessed on 21st July 2025).

18. Delicati, A., Marcante, B., Catelan, D., Biggeri, A., Caenazzo, L., & Tozzo, P. (2025). Hand-to-surface bacterial transfer and healthcare-associated infections prevention: A pilot study on skin microbiome in a molecular biology laboratory. *Frontiers in Medicine, 12*. https://www.semanticscholar.org/paper/c3a7a6c229e956ce194016a639d94417cc60e5af (accessed on 21st July 2025).

19. Diao, W., Hu, Y., Chen, X., Li, W., Kpegah, J. K. S. K., Chen, X., Wang, M., et al. (2025). Construction of a subcutaneous fat transplantation model infected with *Mycobacterium*. *Current Medicinal Chemistry*. https://www.semanticscholar.org/paper/e2cdcc0739b15f98f634903b0fd773fec829379b (accessed on 21st July 2025).

20. Downie, D. L. (2006). A model infectious disease curriculum for fourth grade students: Integrating prevention and education concepts in the classroom. https://core.ac.uk/download/12206775.pdf (accessed on 21st July 2025).

21. Edwards, G., Freeman, K., Harward, G., Llewelyn, M., et al. (2020). What diagnostic strategies can help differentiate cellulitis from other causes of red legs in primary care. https://core.ac.uk/download/237942601.pdf (accessed on 21st July 2025).

22. Eijck, I., Groot, M., Kasteel, D., Kijlstra, A., et al. (2003). Analysis of black holes in our knowledge concerning animal health in the organic food production chain. https://core.ac.uk/download/10919416.pdf (accessed on 21st July 2025).

23. Faccin, M., Wiener, D., Rech, R., Santoro, D., & Rodrigues Hoffmann, A. (2023). Common superficial and deep cutaneous bacterial infections in domestic animals: A review. *Veterinary Pathology, 60*, 796–811. https://www.semanticscholar.org/paper/89fd81e7551c58a33ed16bea022faef412580067 (accessed on 21st July 2025).

24. Farkas, D. K., Galea, S., Gradus, J. L., Jiang, T., et al. (2020). Associations between adjustment disorder and hospital-based infections in the Danish population. https://core.ac.uk/download/288432803.pdf (accessed on 21st July 2025).

25. Fenwick, A., Commission for Africa, Molyneux, D. H., Hotez, P. J., *The Lancet*, UNAIDS, et al. (2005). "Rapid-impact interventions": How a policy of integrated control for Africa's neglected

tropical diseases could benefit the poor. https://core.ac.uk/download/pdf/3775709.pdf (accessed on 21st July 2025).

26. Fidaleo, M., Lavecchia, R., & Zuorro, A. (2015). Antibacterial and anti-quorum sensing activities of selected Italian honeys against antibiotic-resistant pathogens. https://core.ac.uk/download/54526147.pdf (accessed on 21st July 2025).

27. Fioretti, A., Menna, L. F., Sansone, M., Santaniello, A., et al. (2020). Systematic review and meta-analysis of the occurrence of ESKAPE bacteria group in dogs, and the related zoonotic risk in animal-assisted therapy, and in animal-assisted activity in the health context. https://core.ac.uk/download/pdf/323188215.pdf (accessed on 21st July 2025).

28. Formosa, M. C. (2007). Atopic eczema. https://core.ac.uk/download/46602108.pdf (accessed on 21st July 2025).

29. Gall, L. S., & Riely, P. E. (2025). Effect of diet and atmosphere on intestinal and skin flora. *Volume II–Literature Survey*. https://core.ac.uk/download/pdf/85249155.pdf (accessed on 21st July 2025).

30. Garbo, V., Condemi, A., Albano, C., Frasca Polara, V., Parrino, R., Macaluso, A., Venuti, L., et al. (2024). Dalbavancin for the treatment of acute bacterial skin and skin structure infections (ABSSSI) in pediatric patients: A case series. *Le Infezioni in Medicina, 32*(2), 231–240. https://www.semanticscholar.org/paper/f2ba5309c593d82e394d7ed43565ce2cf63a1dae (accessed on 21st July 2025).

31. Gaweł-Dąbrowska, D., Jakoniuk, M., Kler, K., Kucharczyk, D., et al. (2025). Infectious skin diseases in contact sports - A literature review. https://core.ac.uk/download/656518080.pdf (accessed on 21st July 2025).

32. Good, L., Kamaruzzaman, N. F., & Kendall, S. L. (2016). Targeting the hard to reach: Challenges and novel strategies in the treatment of intracellular bacterial infections: Targeting intracellular bacteria. https://core.ac.uk/download/76980954.pdf (accessed on 21st July 2025).

33. Groot, M., Kleijer-Ligtenberg, G., & Van Asseldonk, T. (2011). *Natural Swine Health*. https://core.ac.uk/download/10932084.pdf (accessed on 21st July 2025).

34. Hansson, I. (2007). Bacteriological and epidemiological studies of *Campylobacter spp.* in Swedish broilers. https://core.ac.uk/download/11695169.pdf (accessed on 21st July 2025).

35. Jacobs, J. M., & Ottinger, C. A. (2006). USGS/NOAA Workshop on Mycobacteria in Striped Bass, May 7–10, 2006, Annapolis, Maryland. https://core.ac.uk/download/11017969.pdf (accessed on 21st July 2025).

36. Jansen, T., & Plewig, G. (1998). Acneiform dermatoses. https://core.ac.uk/download/16432805.pdf (accessed on 21st July 2025).

37. King, J., Lehrnbecher, T., Pana, Z. D., Steinbach, W. J., et al. (2017). Recognition and clinical presentation of invasive fungal disease in neonates and children. https://core.ac.uk/download/131024549.pdf (accessed on 21st July 2025).

38. Łazicka, P., Jakubowska, E., & Tarnowska, J. (2025). Approaches to the diagnosis of cutaneous diseases among swimmers: Causes, symptoms, prevention, treatment. *Quality in Sport*. https://www.semanticscholar.org/paper/d40bda76f055c87cbba8637171f7c210d571ad77 (accessed on 21st July 2025).

39. Lillestolen, D. (2018). Infections not fought: Antibiotic resistance in underserved communities. https://core.ac.uk/download/158970352.pdf (accessed on 21st July 2025).

40. Lomelí-Valdez, R., Orozco-Covarrubias, L., & Sáez-de-Ocariz, M. (2025). Skin and systemic infections in children with atopic dermatitis: Review of the current evidence. *Frontiers in Pediatrics, 13*. https://www.semanticscholar.org/paper/84163f0d7ec7a2d967f1ddc2cf4e8ac3c68c3854 (accessed on 21st July 2025).

41. Marchioro, T. L., Rifkind, D., Starzl, T. E., Waddell, W. R., et al. (1964). Infectious diseases associated with renal homotransplantation: I. Incidence, types, and predisposing factors. https://core.ac.uk/download/12203488.pdf (accessed on 21st July 2025).

42. Mayfosh, A. J., & Rau, T. (2025). A novel ammonium carboxylate salt of undecylenic acid for the topical treatment of Gram-positive and antibiotic-resistant skin infections. *Experimental Dermatology, 34*. https://www.semanticscholar.org/paper/d42ebec7a5222abdd77073ccd30e1230bd53960f (accessed on 21st July 2025).

43. Molan, P. C. (2006). The evidence supporting the use of honey as a wound dressing. https://core.ac.uk/download/29194784.pdf (accessed on 21st July 2025).

44. Muthubharathi, B. C., Subalakshmi, P. K., Mounish, B. S. C., Rao, T. S., & Balamurugan, K. (2024). Impact of low-dose UV-A in *Caenorhabditis elegans* during candidate bacterial infections. *Photochemistry and Photobiology, 101*, 404–422. https://www.semanticscholar.org/paper/e1300d0307730645f80607618d8516f107c9d687 (accessed on 21st July 2025).

45. Oliveira, A., Resende, F., Santos-Sousa, H., de Sousa, J. P. V., Caires, F., Gonçalves, F., Pinho, A., et al. (2025). IBC Oxford University Poster Abstract 26–Silent threat: unmasking streptococcal toxic shock syndrome post-surgery. *British Journal of Surgery*. https://www.semanticscholar.org/paper/96c9c70ee0602fb7713da37023b12740d9960e0c (accessed on 21st July 2025).

46. Pahlevan, A. A., Wysocki, A. B., Paintsil, A., Shittu, A. O., Shittu, A. O., Bauer, A. W., Anku, B., et al. (2013). Secondary bacterial infections of buruli ulcer lesions before and after chemotherapy with streptomycin and rifampicin. https://core.ac.uk/download/18261879.pdf (accessed on 21st July 2025).

47. Pelton, T. (2009). *Bad Water 2009: The Impact on Human Health in the Chesapeake Bay Region*. https://core.ac.uk/download/80510793.pdf (accessed on 21st July 2025).

48. Robinson, K., Toh, G., Firdaus, M. J., Tham, K., Rozario, P., Lim, C. K., Toh, Y., et al. (2023). *Corynebacterium diphtheriae* causes keratinocyte-intrinsic ribotoxic stress and NLRP1 inflammasome activation in a model of cutaneous diphtheria. *bioRxiv*. https://www.semanticscholar.org/paper/0fa48bb42082c9f92cad48b036b7e504bfe060d7 (accessed on 21st July 2025).

49. Salman, A. S. (2025). Mastering glycemic control in Type 1 diabetes: Revealing bacterial threats and immune defense innovations. *International Journal of Science and Research Archive*. https://www.semanticscholar.org/paper/d7de4abac3071e6e96b3b82966472c5be8c9a387 (accessed on 21st July 2025).

50. Senanayake, S. (2025). Antibiotic resistance: How did we get here and what can we do? https://core.ac.uk/download/pdf/30672479.pdf (accessed on 21st July 2025).

51. Sigurgeirsson, B., Paul, C., Dupuy, A., Guberman, D., Korting, H. C., Kerl, H., Hull, P. R., et al. (2004). Chronic dermatomycoses of the foot as risk factors for acute bacterial cellulitis of

the leg: A case-control study. https://core.ac.uk/download/16432790.pdf (accessed on 21st July 2025).

52. Svetikienė, D., Jokubaite, M., Zamokas, G., Babickaitė, L., Šiugždiniene, R., & Ramanauskienė, K. (2025). Efficacy study of propolis eutectic extract in gel formulations for the treatment of bacterial skin diseases in dogs. *Animals: An Open Access Journal from MDPI, 15*. https://www.semanticscholar.org/paper/aafe726a46b1c779fd565c435e551e1da1d7792e (accessed on 21st July 2025).

53. Wei, X. C., Zhao, M. F., & Xiao, X. (2024). Evaluating omadacycline dosing regimens against drug-resistant pathogens including *Staphylococcus aureus, Streptococcus pneumoniae,* and *Haemophilus influenzae* in adults: A pharmacokinetic/pharmacodynamic analysis using Monte Carlo simulation. *Journal of Chemotherapy, 36*, 532–539. https://www.semanticscholar.org/paper/afd97d9846e534f2259216cb630da5266adb2696 (accessed on 21st July 2025).

54. Ye, Y., Zheng, Q., Wang, Z., Wang, S., Lu, Z., Chu, Q., Liu, Y., et al. (2024). Metal-phenolic nanoparticles enhance low temperature photothermal therapy for bacterial biofilm in superficial infections. *Journal of Nanobiotechnology, 22*. https://www.semanticscholar.org/paper/651fdf62c7dd087e994f278390e7160bc276cf46 (accessed on 21st July 2025).

55. Zegadło, K., Gieroń, M., Żarnowiec, P., Durlik-Popińska, K., Kręcisz, B., Kaca, W., & Czerwonka, G. (2023). Bacterial motility and its role in skin and wound infections. *International Journal of Molecular Sciences, 24*. https://www.semanticscholar.org/paper/12537699d01ca6b0646785eb3831413d006980e5 (accessed on 21st July 2025).

VIRAL INFECTIONS OF THE SKIN

12

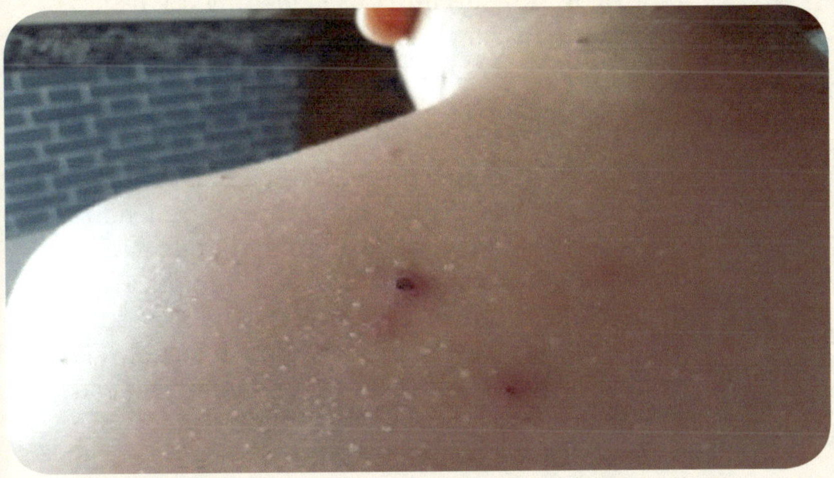

Introduction

Viral dermatoses are addressed in this overview, including herpes simplex virus (HSV), human papillomavirus (HPV), and molluscum contagiosum. Not only do the infections cause physical skin lesions, but they also pose significant psychosocial difficulties for those who have them. Frequent painful outbreaks of herpes, warts, and potential oncogenic complications are caused by HPV. The general implications of these infections warrant in-depth understanding of their transmission patterns, pathology, and potential therapeutic strategies, making them subjects of high research value in dermatology and infectious disease research. The most crucial aspect of combating such viral infections is the research into novel treatment modalities, notably the use of natural bioactive compounds. Research indicates that the compounds possess tremendous potential as antivirals, thereby providing a substitute or complementary approach to conventional therapeutic techniques. Various bioactive compounds, for instance, have been found to inhibit viral replication and mitigate the effects of stressors, such

LEARNING OBJECTIVES

After studying this chapter, you will be able to:

1. Describe the herpes simplex virus (HSV)
2. Understand the human papillomavirus (HPV)
3. Understand the molluscum contagiosum
4. Know the other notable viral skin infections
5. Describe the diagnosis of viral skin infections
6. Understand the impact of viral skin infections on Quality of Life

as inflammation, on the skin. The necessity of effective treatment interventions is underscored by the serious impacts these infections can have on overall health, ranging from mild skin irritation at the local level to severe conditions such as cancer and systemic spread (Sharifi-Rad et al., 2021). In addition, the determination of the immune response to such viral pathogens is significant in finding effective clinical interventions. Type I interferons (IFNs) play a critical role in modulating host defense against viral infection, affecting not only local immune responses but also the organism's systemic capacities. Abnormalities in the interferon signaling pathways have important repercussions that may contribute to the organism's increased vulnerability to infection, such as HSV and HPV, thus highlighting the motivation for exploring further the immunity mechanisms (Meyts et al., 2021). The viral pathogen-host defense interaction highlights the viral nature of viral skin infections and provides a platform for a more nuanced understanding of patient care and therapeutic advancement in this disease group (Figure 12.1).

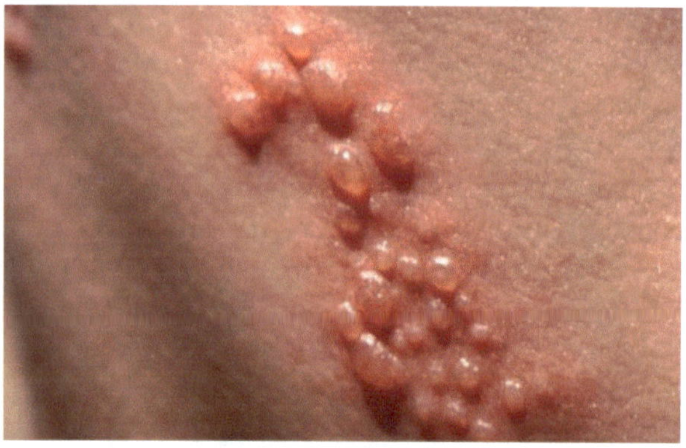

Figure 12.1. Viral infections.

Source: https://static.wixstatic.com/media/2c70ec_1681d32dc62c4219a8b92154ec65ea60.png/v1/fill/w_536,h_286,al_c,lg_1,q_85,enc_avif,quality_auto/2c70ec_1681d32dc62c4219a8b92154ec65ea60.png.

Definition of Viral Infections of the Skin

Viral skin infections are a diverse group of disorders caused by a range of viruses that selectively infect epithelial tissue. These infections take a wide range of forms, ranging from benign lesions to more advanced systemic effects depending on the virus. Common viral infections include HSV, HPV, and molluscum contagiosum. These viruses usually disrupt normal skin architecture, leading to lesion formation such as vesicles, warts, or pustules. Pathogenesis refers to the mechanism by which the virus infects the keratinocytes, leading to local inflammation and cell changes. For instance, HSV often presents as painful vesicular lesions in the genital or oral area, reflecting the virus's tendency to become latent within sensory neurons and thereby complicating the clinical course of infection (Dhume et al., 2023). The impact of viral skin infections is most pronounced in immunocompromised individuals, where the infections are responsible for more serious diseases and greater morbidity. For example, HIV patients are at risk of developing chronic dermatologic presentations of viral infections, including HSV and HPV. The interaction between these sexually transmitted infections and immunosuppression is a concerning epidemiological situation, where viral infections complicate the course of HIV by increasing risk for transmission and treatment (Moorthy et al., 2006). In addition, the frequency of mixed infections further complicates the clinical presentation. HIV-positive patients have atypical presentations of viral infections, which can complicate diagnosis and lead to delayed effective therapy. To investigate viral skin infections, not only is a good knowledge of the viral pathogens themselves required, but also a good knowledge of the host factors underlying the disease process. Viruses such as HSV, HPV, and molluscum contagiosum employ an arsenal of mechanisms to escape the immune system, including manipulation of cellular signaling and regulation of apoptosis in infected keratinocytes.

Moreover, the clinician often needs to treat these infections repeatedly with a multi-disciplinary approach, balancing antiviral therapies against resistance and the risk of recurrence. As studies continue, particularly with respect to the relationship between viral skin infections and illnesses like HIV, more is realized that the treatment of these illnesses will require both a clinical and public health effort in regards to reducing their prevalence and their impact on the suffering populace (Moorthy et al., 2006) (Figure 12.2).

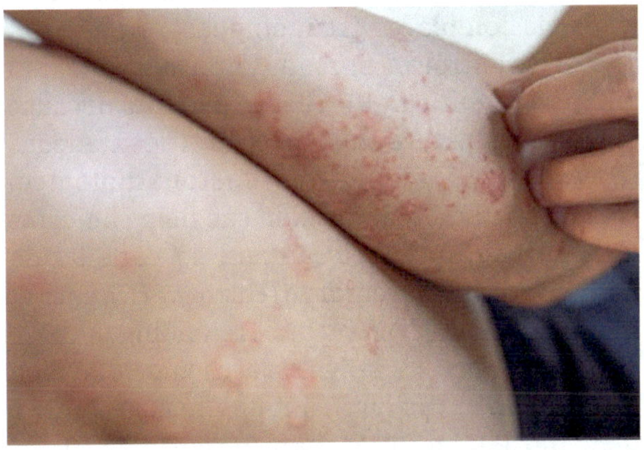

Figure 12.2. Viral skin infections.

Source: https://im.idiva.com/content/2022/Dec/Patient-with-arms-and-legs-covered-in-a-red-rash_639acad352639.jpg?w=938&h=625&cc=1.

Importance of Understanding Skin Viral Infections

The significance of viral skin infections cannot be overemphasized, since they often appear as presenting signs of the underlying illness and immune status. Herpes simplex virus, HPV, and molluscum contagiosum infection frequently manifest as clinically evident rashes on the skin, thereby presenting a unique opportunity for early diagnosis and treatment. Health care providers, particularly dermatologists, must be knowledgeable about these presentations so that they can quickly diagnose associated systemic diseases, e.g., HIV, whose broad spectrum of mucocutaneous manifestations has become a hallmark of the infection. In most cases, the initial presentation of such cutaneous conditions is crucial because it may prompt screening for immunocompromising infections and lead to interventions that significantly reduce morbidity from these conditions (Rajagopalan et al., 2017). Besides, understanding the pathophysiology and routes of transmission of viral infections of the skin is valuable in preventive medicine and public health. Understanding how these viruses are transmitted informs practical ways of reducing transmission rates, in particular for sexually transmitted diseases such as HPV, implicated in cervical neoplasia and other malignancies. By disclosing the risks of such infections, health education interventions can empower people to adopt safer practices, thereby reducing disease prevalence at the population level. Further, identification of the link between viral infection and its cutaneous manifestations can allow detection of outbreaks and inform population-level public health measures. Such an integrated perspective underscores the need for healthcare providers to stay abreast of viral dermatological developments within ongoing medical education (Jakubowska et al., 2024). In addition, the psychosocial impact of skin viral infection also requires a broader understanding on the part of healthcare providers. The observable nature of such infection carries with it the potential to cause immense emotional suffering, social ostracism, and compromised quality of life among infected persons. Thus, the management of the psychological well-being of patients with skin viral infections is equally significant as the management of their physical health. Through the encouragement of a multi-disciplinary framework that considers the psychological in conjunction with medical therapy, clinicians can advance patient outcomes and increase adherence to treatment. Mental health therapy, education on the causative nature of the infections, and the removal of myths about their transmission can effectively eliminate the stigma associated with these diseases. This composite knowledge emphasizes the necessity of understanding skin viral infections not only in the clinical sector but also in maintaining patients' overall health (Jakubowska et al., 2024).

Overview of Common Viral Infections: Herpes, Human Papillomavirus (HPV), Molluscum

Skin viral infections are a significant public health concern, characterized by a range of frequent pathogens infecting millions worldwide. Of these, HSV is the most predominant offender leading to a variety of diseases. These include oral and genital herpes. These diseases typically manifest as painful blisters or ulcers and, in their chronic nature, can lead to recurrent episodes. These are transmitted through direct contact with the site; hence, awareness and precautions are essential. The multifaceted pathogenesis of HSV could involve latency in the neural ganglia, making eradication difficult and causing issues with models of treatment like antiviral medications. Ultimately, understanding the mechanisms and impact of HSV is essential for effective management, as it also helps reduce transmission rates in at-risk populations and overall outcomes. HPV is another viral infection of the skin, but it is known to have an impact on the skin, particularly through its role in anogenital warts and cutaneous lesions. HPV is a diverse group of over 100 related viruses, with some linked to more serious illnesses like cervical carcinoma. HPV dermatoses are most commonly seen as rough-surfaced, raised warts that present in areas of friction. The importance of dermatological examination in differentiating benign from possibly malignant lesions cannot be overemphasized, as early treatment yields positive results. The psychosocial aspect of HPV is also important, with patients anxious or stigmatized about their condition. Accordingly, adequate patient education and open communication can provide the patient with the confidence required to access early intervention and make informed choices to treat their condition (Cannav\uf2 et al., 2020). Molluscum contagiosum, another significant viral dermatosis, warrants mention for its distinctive clinical features and mode of transmission. This poxvirus infection forms small, elevated, dome-shaped papules, termed pearl-like papules. Though benign in most cases, molluscum can pose cosmetic problems, especially in children and sexually active young people, thereby indicating a need for therapeutic intervention in certain instances. Its skin-to-skin mode of transmission places great emphasis on hygiene and self-control of spread. Clinicians can find molluscum difficult to treat in patients because of its benign nature and high rate of spontaneous resolution. Knowing the histopathological characteristics of molluscum can help clinicians identify appropriate treatment so patients do not undergo unnecessary treatment (Dhume et al., 2023). With growing understanding of these viral infections, ongoing research and education will remain at the forefront of efforts to reduce their burden and prevalence (Figure 12.3).

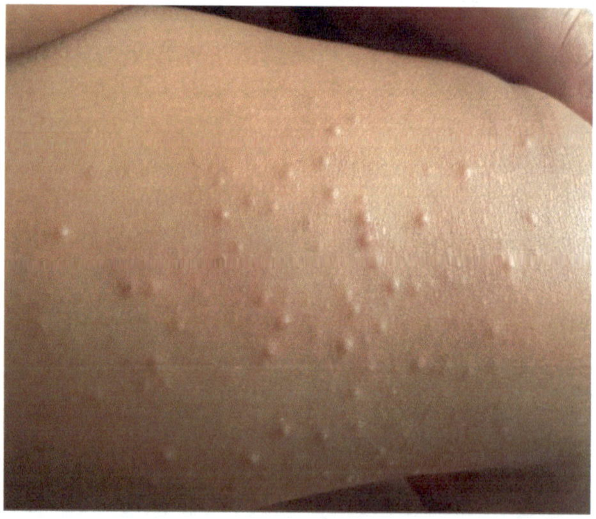

Figure 12.3. Common viral infections.

Source: https://childrenadultskin.com.sg/wp-content/uploads/2018/09/molluscum-contagiosum.jpg.

12.1. Herpes Simplex Virus (HSV)

Learning Outcome

1. Describe the types of herpes simplex virus
2. Understand the symptoms and transmission methods of the herpes simplex virus
3. Know the treatment options and management strategies for herpes simplex virus

HSV, a member of the Herpesviridae family, exists in two broader categories: HSV-1 and HSV-2. While HSV-1 traditionally results in oral herpes, which manifests in the appearance of cold sores or fever blisters on or around the mouth, HSV-2 is primarily associated with genital herpes. Such differences have receded in recent years as both types of HSV can infect oral and genital areas through direct contact. Spread of HSV is mostly through skin-to-skin contact, with an understanding that it is important to understand its mode of transmission in sexually active individuals. From estimates of global prevalence, where there is a very high rate of infection within the population, the burden of HSV on public health is gigantic, and therefore developing education and awareness to decrease its transmission and its associated complications, including psychological distress and social stigma. HSV infection ranges from mild to severe, with the majority of individuals being asymptomatic, spreading the virus to others unaware. Primary infections are typically followed by symptomatic sores, fever, and lymphadenopathy, which are disabling. After the virus has had its initial attack, however, it becomes latent in the nervous system and can be reactivated, leading to recurrent attacks that are themselves frequently less severe. These recurrences are provoked by a myriad of causes, including stress, illness, and immunosuppression. Attainment of knowledge regarding the cyclical nature of HSV is vital to affected persons, as successive recurrences will lead to chronic distress and anxiety about transmission to partners and ramifications on the overall health of the infected person. Knowledge of the nature of HSV and the available management options, including antiviral therapy, is central to promoting quality of life among infected patients. Public health implications of HSV extend into the broader sexually transmitted infections (STIs) domain. The majority of STIs, including HSV, are asymptomatic, with resulting undiagnosed infections that enable ongoing transmission within sexual networks. Preventive intervention utilization, such as regular condom use, STI testing, and vaccination against avoidable viral infections (e.g., HPV), can reduce the incidence of such diseases significantly. In addition, increased awareness of HSV can help to stimulate more informed popular discussion on sexual health and safer sex. Safe-sex education promotion is vital not only for new-infection prevention but also for reducing STI stigma and, in the end, for improved health status for individuals and communities with HSV and other similar infections, hence validating their place in public health policy as part of integrated sexual health education and preventive interventions (Ikokwu et al., 2023; İrem Durusu et al., 2023) (Figure 12.4).

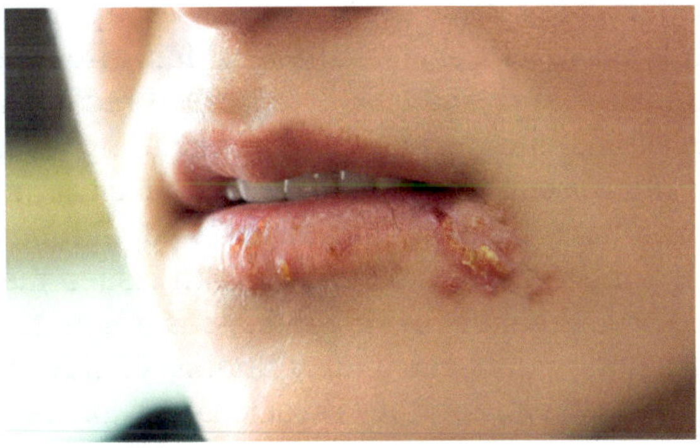

Figure 12.4. Herpes simplex virus (HSV).

Source: https://www.medicalindependent.ie/wp-content/uploads/2022/12/8-12-22-herpes-simplex.jpg.

12.1.1. Types of Herpes Simplex Virus (HSV): HSV-1 and HSV-2

Two types of HSV exist: HSV-1 and HSV-2, and each has distinct features, modes of transmission, and clinical manifestations. HSV-1 is primarily associated with herpetic infection of the oral cavity, causing cold sores or fever blisters on or around the mouth. HSV is commonly spread by oral contact, particularly in childhood, and is common among the global population. Conversely, HSV-2 is nearly completely linked to genital herpes, a sexually transmitted infection that could have a tremendous amount of morbidity in the affected individuals. The effects of these two viruses extend beyond mere skin lesions, and they have grave implications, such as neonatal herpes, which is a public health threat due to its potential for life-threatening infection in newborns. Understanding these forms is critical to the development of targeted prevention and treatment of the diseases caused by HSV. Both HSV-1 and HSV-2 pathogenesis is controlled by complex interactions with the host immune system. Both viruses establish permanent latency in sensory neurons to evade immune surveillance and reactivate in response to numerous stimuli, such as immunosuppression or stress. Their ability to remain latent underscores their evolutionary adaptation and poses extreme challenges for infection control. HSV-1 and HSV-2 can cause recurrent eruptions and periods of viral shedding, even in the absence of disease, thereby facilitating continuous transmission through populations. For this, treating the public health issues that are brought about by HSV infections is a matter of having sufficient understanding of how to transmit them, how they become latent, and how to discuss prevention strategies among sensitive populations. Current research shows that natural products hold great promise for preventing HSV infections, and these findings carry significant implications for treatment. For instance, research has shown that extracts of Vitis vinifera (grape leaf) possess antiviral activity against HSV-1 at very low concentrations, thereby hindering the virus's ability to replicate during the initial stage of infection. The discovery provides a useful avenue for the search for novel antiviral medicines, especially given the increasing resistance to conventional treatments. The plant antiviral research is complemented by recent research to decipher the molecular processes through which HSVs are capable of evading host antiviral immune responses. Emphasized in the literature, such an enhancement of our understanding of HSV-1 and HSV-2 pathogenesis and development of new therapeutic options is crucial to reducing the public health burden of these infections (Tognarelli et al., 2019; Zannella et al., 2021) (Figure 12.5).

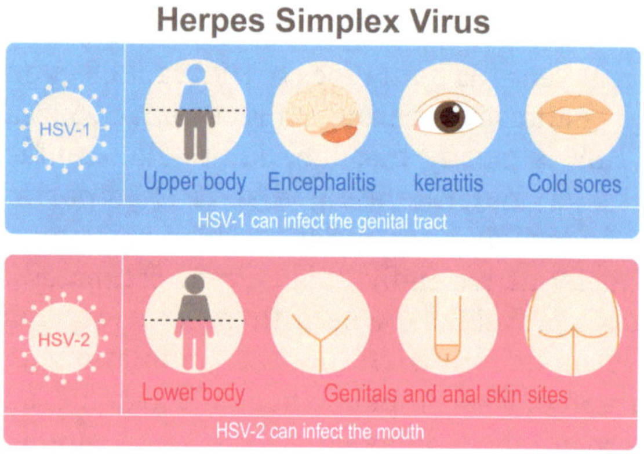

Figure 12.5. Types of herpes simplex virus (HSV).

Source: https://katudermatology.com/wp-content/uploads/2022/06/shutterstock_1342642319-1024x692.jpg.

12.1.2. Symptoms and Transmission Methods

The signs and modes of transmission of viral skin infections such as herpes, Human papillomavirus (HPV), and molluscum contagiosum can vary widely depending on the specific virus. HSV, for instance, is characterized by painful blisters and sores, mainly in and around the oral or genital area. These lesions are likely to recur intermittently, triggered by stimuli like stress, illness, or immunosuppression. HPV infections, however, have the propensity to lead to the development of warts on other parts of the body, including the genital and hands; certain strains also lead to a predisposition to skin cancer. Molluscum contagiosum characteristically has small, shiny lesions with a depressed center, typically located on the trunk and the limbs, especially in children. Identification of such symptoms is vital for early detection and effective treatment of viral skin infections. Modes of transmission of these viral infections are mainly through direct skin contact, and thus identifying these routes is essential for prevention. In herpes, the virus is transmitted during episodes through sexual contact or even when in one's asymptomatic phase. HPV also shares the same mode of transmission, predominantly sexual contact, thus the rationale for preventive measures such as vaccines for high-risk types that lead to cancer. Molluscum contagiosum, while typically acquired by direct contact, is transmissible through fomites or object transfer, such as towels and attire. Current studies have indicated that understanding these transmission dynamics is crucial for managing the spread of these infections, particularly among high-risk groups where immunosuppression may complicate matters. Such a collapse might provide public health with the rationale to disseminate information and education about these viral infections. Alongside the physical manifestations and modes of transmission of these viral infections, there are broader implications for potential socio-economic consequences. The symptomatic presentation differences between each virus can cause significant psychological distress, stigma, and compromised quality of life for infected individuals, particularly for herpes and HPV, where there is a significant social implication to contracting the disease. The economic burden also includes not only healthcare expenses for treatment but also indirect costs related to lost productivity and mental health care. As chronicled, the ongoing replication and resistance trends of such viruses underscore the urgent need to advance antiviral therapy, including potential applications of nanotechnology in drug delivery and therapeutic action (Cojocaru et al., 2020; Rosa et al., 2021). Lastly, finding a solution to the interconnectedness among symptoms, transmission modes, and socio-economic factors is essential for developing holistic management approaches for cutaneous viral diseases (Figure 12.6).

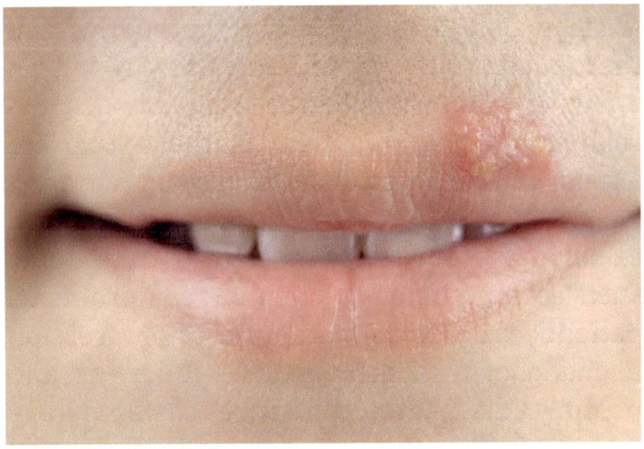

Figure 12.6. Symptoms of herpes simplex virus (HSV).

Source: https://katudermatology.com/wp-content/uploads/2022/06/shutterstock_53580727-2048x1360.jpg.

12.1.3. Treatment Options and Management Strategies

An effective management strategy for skin viral infections, most notably HSV, is based primarily on antiviral medications. The pillars of therapeutics are acyclovir, valacyclovir, and famciclovir, which have the primary consequence of dramatically reducing the duration of illness as well as recurrence frequency. These medications work by interfering with viral replication, thereby allowing the immune system to reassert control over latent infection. In the case of severe or recurrent HSV infection, intravenous acyclovir must be considered. Supportive care is also crucial, as it includes pain management and hydration to minimize discomfort. Education on transmission and trigger points also encourages patients to actively manage their own health, thereby reducing the risk of transmission to others. Strict adherence to regimen therapy not only lessens the symptoms but also plays a crucial role in public health prevention. Human papillomavirus (HPV) is a challenge for treatment due to its varied presentation, ranging from benign warts to the high-risk forms of cervical and other malignancies. Management is currently both preventive and therapeutic. HPV vaccination has proved an effective way to reduce the incidence of HPV-related disease. Treatment of those who are already infected has mostly focused on removing lesions by physical means, such as cryotherapy, excisional procedures, or topical treatments such as imiquimod. In immunocompromised patients, there is a greater risk of progression to malignancy, and thus closer follow-up and possibly adjuvant therapy such as chemotherapy or radiotherapy might be needed (Hewavisenti et al., 2023). New therapies, such as RNA-based therapies, have the potential to target HPV genome sequences specifically, thus increasing the possibilities of eliminating the virus from infected tissue. In general, an approach based on multiple facets is essential for optimal control of conditions associated with HPV. Management of molluscum contagiosum relies predominantly on clinical observation and different intervention methods. Although the infection is generally self-limiting, particularly in healthy patients, treatments are often sought to eliminate lesions more quickly, especially for cosmetic concerns or in immunocompromised hosts. The modalities most commonly used are cryotherapy, curettage, and the application of topical agents such as cantharidin. Immunocompromised patients, in particular, can develop chronic infections that require more aggressive management (Soriano et al., 2018). Public education on modes of transmission, particularly in communal settings such as swimming pools, is also important for preventing outbreaks. Establishing next-generation treatment modalities, including precision therapies that regulate immune responses, is needed to develop improved management strategies. As our understanding of viral persistence and immune escape improves, so too must our treatment and management strategies for molluscum contagiosum and other viral skin diseases (Figure 12.7).

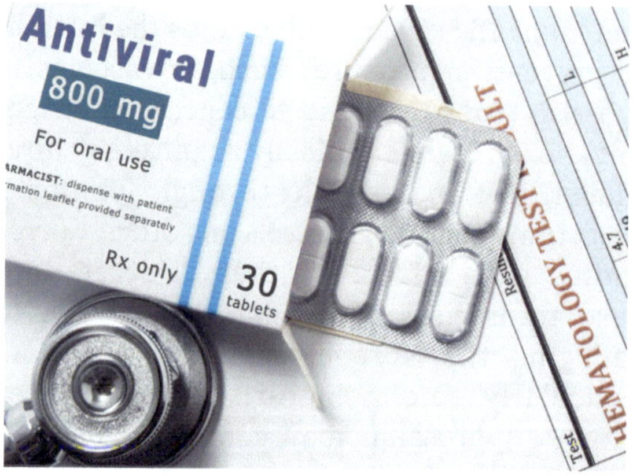

Figure 12.7. Treatment of herpes simplex virus (HSV).

Source: https://katudermatology.com/wp-content/uploads/2022/06/shutterstock_504340591-1536x1021.jpg.

Test Your Knowledge

1. How many types of herpes simplex are there?
2. What is the transmission method for the Herpes simplex virus?

12.2. Human Papillomavirus (HPV)

Learning Outcome

1. Describe the types of HPV and their associated risks
2. Know the symptoms and potential complications of human papillomavirus
3. Describe the vaccination and prevention measures of human papillomavirus

HPV is one of the key viral pathogens, especially because it is linked to several malignancies, of which cervical cancer is of specific note. There are more than 170 types of HPV identified, and they are divided into high-risk and low-risk types, with the latter being involved in cancer formation. High-risk HPV types have been implicated in interfering with normal cellular functions, such as uncontrolled cell growth and subsequent tumorigenesis. This dysregulation is caused by the virus's ability to integrate into the host genome, often disrupting critical regulatory genes. Understanding mechanisms whereby HPV leads to carcinogenesis is crucial in formulating targeted prevention and treatment strategies, especially in high-risk populations for cervical and other cancers caused by HPV. Enhanced awareness and screening can lead to improved early detection and intervention, which are crucial in reducing the burden of HPV-related diseases. Epidemiologically, HPV is an infectious condition that affects both men and women, but it differently affects women's health. Cervical cancer remains a leading cause of cancer deaths in women globally, highlighting the importance of the HPV vaccine and screening interventions in a regular manner. The recent advancement in immunization, particularly the availability of quadrivalent and nonavalent vaccines, has been promising, offering effective protection against the most prevalent high-risk HPV types. These vaccines are especially beneficial if given prior to sexual initiation, and hence, educational activities need to be targeted to young adolescents. Furthermore, the growing incidence of head and neck cancers linked to HPV in men is a novel epidemiological challenge. An understanding of HPV's impact on various populations is essential to develop effective public health policy and intervention strategies that address the specific needs of various populations. The cosmopolitan lifestyle of HPV extends beyond oncology in that the virus also affects dermatologic health as benign warts or condylomata acuminata. These dermatologic manifestations are most commonly observed in sexually active younger individuals and are associated with their own psychological and social morbidity. Importantly, while transient and asymptomatic infections are ubiquitous with most HPV infections, others will experience persistent infections that can lead to further complications if not treated properly. While treatments available range from topical to surgical, their treatment of HPVs with skin disease typically includes multimodal therapy addressing patient education as well as psychosocial support. As HPV remains a clinical problem and a research agenda, its broad implications for health emphasize the need for ongoing studies aimed at elucidating the virus's complex effect on human health, such as its link with chronic inflammation and non-oncogenic disease processes (Sabatini et al., 2019; Zhao et al., 2021) (Figure 12.8).

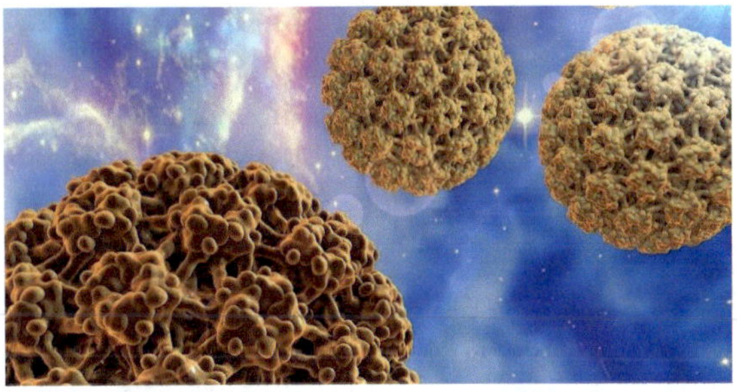

Figure 12.8. HPV (Human papillomavirus).

Source: https://www.nfid.org/wp-content/uploads/bb-plugin/cache/HPV-v1-panorama-7126853789679c126106ce34d14785a8-ifmulep01ros.jpeg.

12.2.1. Types of Human Papillomavirus (HPV) and Their Associated Risks

HPV is a heterogeneous group of viruses, with more than 200 types known to exist to date. Of these, around 40 have been known to infect the genital region, accounting for a substantial portion of sexually transmitted diseases. HPVs of high risk, especially HPV-16 and HPV-18, are well known for their capability to cause malignancies, most importantly cervical cancer. Furthermore, the so-called high-risk types of HPV have also been implicated in other anogenital tract cancers, such as anal and vulvar cancer, which again underscores early detection and vigilance about the vaccine. Low-risk types, HPV-6 and HPV-11, on the other hand, are responsible primarily for benign lesions such as genital warts; yet, in immunocompromised hosts, they can also produce complications, thus equally underscoring the need for close follow-up in all groups. The oncogenic potential of HPV cannot be overstated since it has a very significant role in the pathogenesis of most skin cancers, particularly in recipients of solid organ transplants (OTRs). Studies showed that a significant proportion of OTRs possessed high-risk HPV types with apprising correlations with squamous cell carcinoma (SCC) of the genitalia. Interestingly, of lesions biopsied, a high percentage were positive for high-risk HPV types, particularly in nonwhite OTRs, who were determined to have higher rates of such cancers. Such findings reemphasize the pressing need for heightened awareness and genital lesion screening of this high-risk population, as many patients will remain unaware of risk due to HPV infection and of risk of causative skin cancers (Nadhan et al., 2018). The role of beta-papillomaviruses (βHPVs) in skin cancer is also better understood, notably in the context of actinic keratoses and squamous cell carcinoma. These viruses have been speculated to be involved in carcinogenesis by affecting the skin's cellular architecture and immune system. Evidence shows that βHPV infections, which are stimulated by environmental factors such as ultraviolet radiation, may cause precursors for skin cancer. Both interactions confirm the requirement for integrated prevention strategies involving prevention of HPV and management of environmental risk factors to limit the occurrence of HPV-related skin cancers. By including immunizations and public health interventions aimed at eradicating high-risk HPV types, as well as education on skin protection, healthcare systems are better positioned to address the potential impacts of βHPV on skin carcinogenesis (Hufbauer et al., 2017) (Figure 12.9).

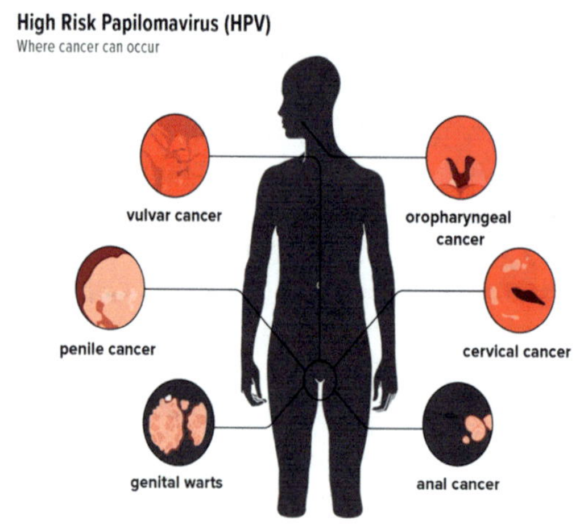

Figure 12.9. Types of high-risk papillomavirus (HPV).

Source: https://i0.wp.com/post.medicalnewstoday.com/wp-content/uploads/sites/3/2022/02/hpv-symptoms-1296x1000-body-1024x793.png?w=1155&h=2137.

12.2.2. Symptoms and Potential Complications

Skin viral infections such as HSV, HPV, and molluscum contagiosum can present with numerous symptoms that significantly impact a person's quality of life. Herpes infections typically manifest as painful blisters or ulcers at the site of infection, typically on the mouth or genitalia. Patients can also experience systemic symptoms, such as fever and lymphadenopathy, during the initial infection. HPV, however, is famous for warts, which can occur anywhere on the body and may be itchy or uncomfortable. Molluscum contagiosum results in small, raised, pearly lesions that can become inflamed or itchy, especially in congenital infections or among immunocompromised patients. Prompt recognition of these signs is vital in order to prevent further skin damage and complications (Gaweł-Dąbrowska et al., 2025; Górska et al., 2024). If left untreated, these viral infections may lead to several complications as they progress. Multiple HSV attacks, for instance, can evolve into more extensive infections that extend beyond the skin to involve mucosal surfaces and eventually lead to secondary bacterial infections. Besides, HPV-positive individuals can develop cancers of the skin, such as squamous cell carcinoma, particularly in the case of high-risk strains of the virus. Molluscum contagiosum also becomes a concern in immunocompromised individuals with widespread lesions, causing significant distress and discomfort. Psychosocial effects of these conditions cannot be ignored because they can result in anxiety, embarrassment, and loss of self-esteem in affected individuals. Early treatment is the most effective preventive measure against these complications, underscoring the importance of access to and knowledge of healthcare (Górska et al., 2024; Gaweł-Dąbrowska et al., 2025). Preventing complications from viral skin infections depends on hygiene and prompt medical care. Good skin care practices, such as avoiding contact with the skin during an outbreak and avoiding sharing personal belongings, can significantly reduce transmission rates. Regular dermatological consultations are required for early detection and management of such infections, particularly among athletes or those who engage in close-contact sports where infection risks are high. Moreover, patient education regarding their condition, the risk of getting its complications, and the appropriate antiviral management will help the patient control their symptoms beforehand. By adopting preventive measures and managing an environment that supports people with viral diseases, the care burden of these diseases can be reduced, leading to improved health and quality of life (Górska et al., 2024; Gaweł-Dąbrowska et al., 2025) (Figure 12.10).

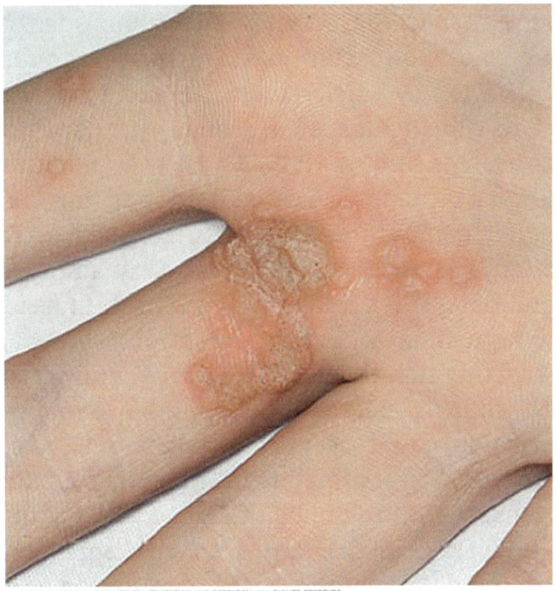

Figure 12.10. Symptoms of human papillomavirus (HPV).

Source: https://www.mayoclinic.org/content/dam/media/global/images/2023/02/10/plantar-warts.jpg.

12.2.3. Vaccination and Prevention Measures

Preventive measures and vaccination are crucial to the battle against viral skin diseases, particularly those caused by molluscum contagiosum, HPV, and HSV. Specific vaccines against HPV have been developed since HPV has a variety of cancers, including cervical and oropharyngeal cancers, associated with it. Widespread HPV vaccination among adolescents can substantially reduce the incidence of these related cancers. Lastly, educational campaigns play a key role in raising awareness regarding the importance of vaccination and informing individuals about the nature of HP transmission and long-term effects. Through a prevention culture, particularly among the young, public health authorities can minimize the threats posed by these viral infections and maximize health benefits globally. Preventive measures beyond immunization must be used to limit the transmission of viral infections such as HSV and molluscum contagiosum. Frequent application of barrier tools, i.e., condoms, can lower the incidence of sexually transmitted diseases, including HSV and HPV, highlighting the significance of safe sex. Testing for HPV regularly, most importantly in sexually active patients, is necessary to detect early and treat potential precancerous lesions. In molluscum contagiosum, a highly infectious disease, restricting skin contact with infected individuals and sharing personal belongings less than advisable could be protective actions. Their incorporation into public health action creates a general culture of health and sensitivity that is important in the control of viral infections and their mitigation in the population. The global outbreak of sexually transmitted diseases, particularly among the youth, calls for combined efforts at vaccination and preventive education when dealing with viral infections in their management. As revealed in studies, the majority of the infections occur asymptotically, resulting in late detection and unchecked spread, particularly among adolescents aged 15-24 years (Wihlfahrt et al., 2023). Thus, it becomes crucial that health care providers also take the initiative to explain the importance of HPV vaccination and regular screening for such conditions. Furthermore, HPVC complications are more likely to develop in immunocompromised patients, underscoring the need for targeted vaccination and personalized preventive interventions among such patients (Hewavisenti et al., 2023). By emphasizing the benefits of preventive care and vaccination, medical practitioners can enable patients to take charge of their own health, thereby reducing morbidity from viral skin infections (Figure 12.11).

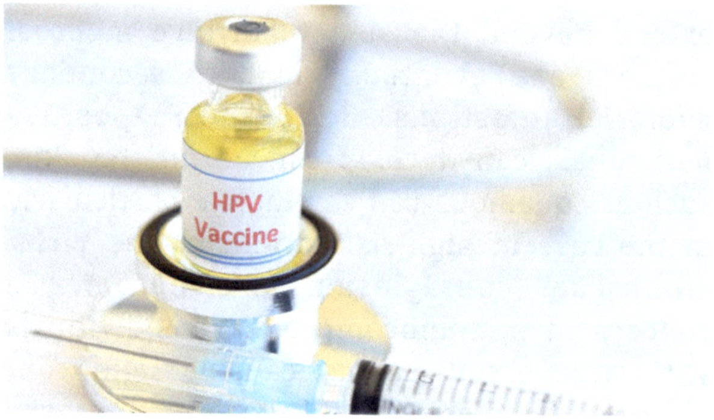

Figure 12.11. Cervical cancer vaccine.

Source: https://d35oenyzp35321.cloudfront.net/Cervical_Cancer_Vaccine_HPV_74e5b9a926.jpg.

Test Your Knowledge

1. What are the three types of HPV?
2. Which preventative measure is most effective in reducing the transmission of sexually transmitted viral infections like HSV and HPV?

12.3. Molluscum Contagiosum

Learning Outcome

1. Describe the characteristics of the molluscum virus
2. Understand the transmission pathways of molluscum virus
3. Know the treatment options and self-care strategies for molluscum virus

Molluscum Contagiosum is a viral skin infection caused by the molluscum contagiosum virus (MCV) that predominantly affects the epidermis, resulting in typical lesions ranging from a few to hundreds. Dome-shaped, umbilicated papules are the hallmark of this infection, which thrives in wet environments and is therefore especially prevalent in children, teenagers, and immunocompromised patients. Molluscum contagiosum is typically a viral infection without systemic symptoms. It rather manifests locally, causing lesions that can itch or become inflamed, with secondary bacterial infection commonly the outcome. Knowledge of the infection's epidemiology is crucial, as it reveals its transmission patterns, which are usually by direct skin-to-skin contact or fomites, making it a very frequent problem in common places such as swimming pools or childcare settings. Treatment of molluscum contagiosum often focuses on conservative measures given its self-limiting nature. In most cases, the lesions resolve spontaneously after a course of 6–12 months, without the need for aggressive therapy. For individuals who wish for a more prompt resolution or are bothered by pain or cosmetic concerns, however, multiple therapeutic options exist. Therapies range from topical therapy, including the use of potassium hydroxide or cantharidin, to procedural therapy the way as cryotherapy or curettage. While these treatments can effectively remove lesions, they may also be painful or result in post-inflammatory hyperpigmentation, particularly in dark skin. Consequently, clinicians often individualize treatments based on the patient's unique needs, and informed consent and realistic expectations become paramount. Recent studies have indicated an association between molluscum contagiosum and infections related to tattoos, highlighting the increasing trend in body art-related skin lesions. Tattooing has become more popular, and the possibility of viral infections in newly tattooed skin is a clinical concern. Descriptions indicate that most tattoo-related infections, though predominantly bacterial, can also include molluscum contagiosum skin lesions, with outbreaks typically localized to the tattoo area. This is coupled with stress on the need for proper aftercare and hygiene during tattooing to minimize infection risk. Along with this, the pathophysiology of such infections should be understood, as immune responses may differ in damaged or inflamed skin. The intersection of skin infection and cosmetic treatment thus necessitates ongoing research to keep public health policy current with developments in body art and skin health (Tampa et al., 2022; Ali et al., 2024) (Figure 12.12).

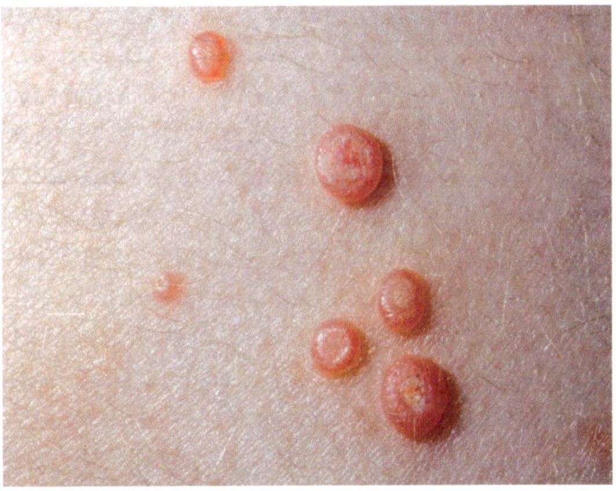

Figure 12.12. Molluscum contagiosum is characterized by small raised lesions often with a central dimple.

Source: https://upload.medbullets.com/topic/120053/images/molluscum.jpg.

12.3.1. Characteristics of the Molluscum Virus

The molluscum contagiosum virus (MCV) is a poxvirus and a significant causative agent of cutaneous viral infections. It consists of small, enveloped, double-stranded DNA, which is crucial for its virulence and reproduction. MCV primarily infects the skin, causing benign epithelial tumors known as molluscum contagiosum lesions. These high, pearl-shaped nodules are typically not painful and can occur in clusters, hence characteristic in appearance. Transmission is via direct skin-to-skin contact, and it is quite prevalent among children, sexually active adolescents, and immunocompromised individuals. The adaptive mechanisms employed by MCV for survival and replication within host cells are a testament to its evolutionary success and explain the challenges involved in developing effective antiviral therapies against it. Immunostimulation triggered by the molluscum contagiosum virus is crucial in unraveling its pathogenicity. MCV is distinct from most other viral infections in that it frequently evades the host's adaptive immune system, leading to persistent infections. Evasion is underpinned by several mechanisms, including inhibition of apoptosis and suppression of pro-inflammatory cytokine production. Interestingly, the presence of molluscum lesions often indicates an underlying immunologic predisposition, particularly in immunocompromised individuals, where lesions are diffuse and multifocal. Furthermore, more recent research has identified that the virus can induce host cell oxidative stress, which plays a multi-functional role in viral replication and disease pathogenesis. In particular, viral infection-induced formation of reactive oxygen species (ROS) has been suggested to trigger pro-inflammatory pathways that are harmful to the host while simultaneously inducing viral replication, establishing a double-edged interaction between the virus and host immune system (Guillin et al., 2019). Molluscum contagiosum lesions have been reported as an opportunistic infection, particularly in immunodeficiency cases. This raises the question of the virus's role in exacerbating other infections and complications among vulnerable populations. Studies have also identified specific molecular markers within the virus linked to pathogenicity, which broadens our knowledge of its infection cycle. Notably, emerging evidence has outlined the role of certain micronutrients, particularly selenium, in modulating viral replication and host immune response. The addition of selenium to the necessary selenoproteins is imperative to provide redox homeostasis, thereby influencing the host's ability to counteract the oxidative stress resulting from viral infections such as MCV. These findings show the intricate relationship between the characteristics of the molluscum contagiosum virus and the nutritional and immunological status of the hosts, necessitating a multidimensional strategy for infection control (Tangye et al., 2022).

12.3.2. Transmission and at-Risk Populations

Knowledge of the routes of transmission of herpes, HPV, and molluscum contagiosum is significant, particularly for groups at greatest risk of developing these diseases. The most common mode of transmission for HSV is direct skin-to-skin contact, i.e., sexual activity, which identifies sexually active young adults and adolescents as being at greatest risk. Furthermore, HPV is primarily transmitted through intimate skin-to-skin contact, and certain forms of it are linked with the causation of cervical and other genital cancers. This is concerning to those who have more than one sexual partner or who participate in sex without a condom, highlighting a crucial need for prevention and education aimed at these populations to limit exposure and improve outcomes. Population-at-risk extends beyond sexually active populations; patients with weakened immune statuses are also at risk for viral infection. Among such populations are

HIV-infected patients, because oral lesions may develop in early stages of disease and serve as key indicators of the process towards acquired immunodeficiency syndrome (AIDS) (Carvalho et al., 2009).

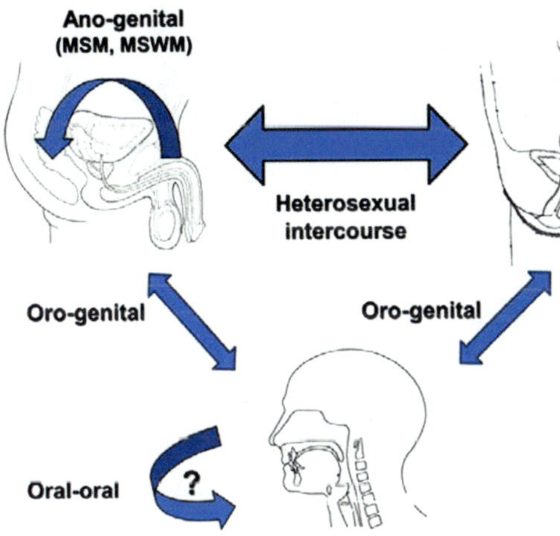

Figure 12.13. Routes and sites of HPV transmission.

Source: https://www.researchgate.net/profile/Singh-23/publication/325554306/figure/fig4/AS:805127820681218@1568968839552/Routes-and-sites-of-HPV-transmission-HPV-being-a-sexually-transmitted-infection.jpg.

To such individuals, the development of viral infections would further exacerbate existing health conditions, exposing them to complications that render morbidity and mortality rates more critical. Such interactions between immunosuppression and viral susceptibility necessitate a multidisciplinary management in healthcare, emphasizing the necessity for regular screenings, preventive measures, and efficacious treatment regimens specifically for such high-risk individuals. Interestingly, the social determinants of age and socioeconomic status are also implicated in the spread of these viral conditions. The young adults, particularly adolescents and young adults, have higher rates of incidence by virtue of factors such as impulsivity and lack of access to healthcare and education regarding safe practices. Disparities in health are even more pronounced among low-income populations where access to care is suboptimal, and education about viral infections is lacking. Public health interventions aimed at educating at-risk groups can enhance awareness, facilitate behavior change, and, eventually, reduce transmission rates and overall public health status. These interventions are crucial in controlling the spread of such infections as herpes and HPV and also in uplifting marginalized groups (Naidoo, 2012) (Figure 12.13).

12.3.3. Treatment Options and Self-Care Strategies

For treatment options for viral skin infections, such as herpes, HPV, and molluscum contagiosum, it is noteworthy to recognize the variety of interventions available. Antiviral therapy, particularly in herpes simplex virus (HSV), has been successful in controlling symptoms and reducing the severity of the attacks. Acyclovir and oral forms thereof are most commonly prescribed, producing healing faster and easing symptoms at flare-ups. In HPV, which has a tendency to appear as warts, treatments include topical agents like imiquimod and podophyllin, and cryotherapy. Treatment focuses on wart destruction, with the viral infection typically located beneath and requiring ongoing care. This therapeutic setting illustrates not only the urgency of individualized pharmacologic intervention but also the need for individual patient evaluations to customize treatments based on unique viral infections and their presentations. In addition to pharmacologic treatment, self-care activities are integral components in managing viral skin infections. Patients are instructed to maintain good hygiene, such as frequent handwashing, especially after handling infected lesions. This can minimize the likelihood of transmitting infections to other areas of the body or to others. Daily washing and drying of the involved area can also help prevent secondary bacterial infection, a common complication of skin lesions. Moreover, instigation of lifestyle modifications, such as stress management and a proper diet, may enhance overall immunity, which is essential against viruses. Self-treatment also includes avoiding exposure to known precipitants of recurrences, particularly in the case of herpes, since food, stress, or hormonal changes can induce recurrences, thus the importance of an aggressive patient-based regimen of skin well-being. Patient education is also responsible for driving treatment for viral cutaneous infections. Understanding the nature of their condition allows patients to respond more favorably to treatment and adhere to self-care practices. For instance, HPV patients can be taught to inform them of the chance that the warts may spontaneously resolve and to ensure regular follow-up to monitor any complications. In herpes, teaching about asymptomatic shedding empowers the patients to prevent transmission risk to sexual partners. Medical practitioners are essential in providing information, as they must adapt to the dynamics of each situation to be successful. A quality management plan that integrates treatment solutions with robust self-care measures is critical for achieving the best health outcomes in patients with skin viral infections, enabling them to maintain a high quality of life regardless of their condition (Figure 12.14).

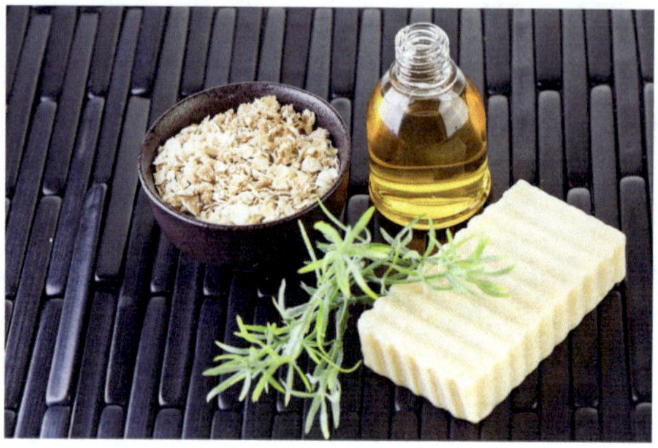

Figure 12.14. Molluscum contagiosum home remedies.

Source: https://cdn-prod.medicalnewstoday.com/content/images/articles/323/323005/molluscum-contagiosum-home-remedy-oatmeal-bath.jpg.

Test Your Knowledge

1. What are the characteristics of molluscum?
2. What is the primary mode of transmission for the herpes simplex virus?

12.4. Other Notable Viral Skin Infections

Learning Outcome

1. Understand the varicella-zoster virus
2. Learn about coxsackievirus
3. Describe the cytomegalovirus (CMV) and its skin manifestations

Among the myriad viral skin infections, molluscum contagiosum (MC) stands out for its unique presentation and mode of transmission. Caused by the molluscum contagiosum virus (MCV), it presents as small, painless, dome-shaped papules on the skin, which are easily confused with other dermatoses. Transmission is most often through direct skin-to-skin contact, hence being prevalent in children and sexually active individuals. Even though MC is typically self-limiting, it can persist for several months and cause cosmetic complications along with secondary infection. Emphasizing the treatments, modalities such as cryotherapy, laser therapy, and topical therapy have been proven effective. Besides, application of cantharidin, a naturally occurring toxin, is now trendy; its therapeutic efficacy in molluscum therapy is particularly enhanced by inducing epidermal acantholysis and enabling lesion clearance, as documented in various clinical reviews of its use in dermatology (Rani et al., 2025). Another such viral infection is the HPV, which spans a wide range of strains—some benign warts and some causing malignancies such as cervical cancer. It is transmitted by direct contact between skin and skin, primarily during sexual activity; however, sexual contact is not required for transmission in settings such as swimming pools.

The warts caused by HPV are painless or may be painful, depending on their size and location. Vaccination is the most effective prevention of the most hazardous HPV types; Gardasil vaccine, which covers a number of HPV types, has been successful in preventing cervical and other anogenital cancers. Public health campaigns persist in advocating vaccination and screening because most infections tend to clear spontaneously, making diagnosis and treatment difficult (Rani et al., 2025). Lastly, HSV is also a prominent viral skin infection worth mentioning.

HSV has two types: HSV-1, most commonly associated with oral ulcers, and HSV-2, which affects predominantly the genital areas. The infections are marked by recrudescence because the virus gets latent in neural ganglia. Stigma and recurrent disease can have negative implications on the mental health of individuals. Antiviral medications, such as acyclovir, have been vital in controlling symptoms and reducing the risk of transmission. But public health interventions, including education regarding the nature of HSV, routes of transmission, and disclosure, have come into prominence in controlling its spread. The dynamics of herpes infections underscore the need for ongoing research into new treatment and prevention methods (Ghali et al., 2025).

12.4.1. Varicella-Zoster Virus (VZV) (Chickenpox and Shingles)

The VZV, a herpesvirus, produces two important clinical syndromes: chickenpox and shingles. Chickenpox, which occurs most frequently in children, consists of an itchy vesicular rash, fever, and malaise. Following primary infection, VZV establishes latency in the sensory ganglia, where it can remain dormant for years. There is a latent period for this; as immunity declines with age or under stress, the virus can reactivate and produce shingles. Reactivation leads to a painful rash limited to single dermatomes, with occasional neurological manifestations, including paresthesia. The duality of VZV's behavior reflects its sophistication and represents the importance of understanding its lifecycle in pediatric and adult groups in describing skin viral infections. Considering the pathophysiology of VZV reveals that the virus exhibits features that influence the immune response. After initial infection, VZV exploits the host's immune processes to evade clearance, preferring to leave a diminished immune response upon latency. This immune escape makes individuals, particularly those with compromised immunity, susceptible to reactivation. In patients with diseases such as Common Variable Immunodeficiency (CVID), for example, there is a strong likelihood of recurrent viral infections, such as those due to VZV, due to impaired humoral immunity. Hence, understanding the immunological processes underlying VZV's behavior is essential in developing effective prophylactic measures, particularly vaccination initiatives that can diminish the chance of both chickenpox and shingles in vulnerable subjects, as reflected in current literature (Al-Hakim et al., 2024). Additionally, the social effects of VZV infections extend beyond the subject patient, highlighting the need for population-level public health interventions. The introduction of the varicella vaccine has substantially reduced chickenpox incidence; however, because fewer people are infected with chickenpox, herd immunity has diminished. Despite vaccination, shingles remains a significant health concern, especially among elderly and immunocompromised individuals. Shingles-related complications such as postherpetic neuralgia have a considerable effect on quality of life, even after vaccination. Furthermore, the association of the cutaneous manifestation and systemic health in certain patient groups, particularly those that are HIV-positive, may indicate the necessity of strict monitoring for viral illness and its cutaneous expression (Du et al., 2024). Hence, ongoing education and public policy interventions focused on vaccination and vigilance are crucial for containing the impact of VZV (Figure 12.15).

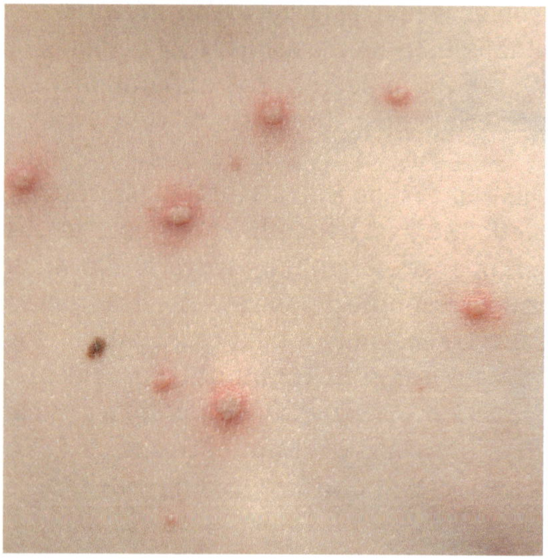

Figure 12.15. Chickenpox is characterized by itchy red spots that turn into fluid-filled blisters.

Source: https://wchh.onlinelibrary.wiley.com/cms/asset/44ce0739-4dff-4dfc-8778-505a2d90ef68/psb1907-fig-0001-m.jpg.

12.4.2. Coxsackievirus (Hand, Foot, and Mouth Disease (HFMD))

HFMD, most commonly caused by Coxsackievirus, is a viral infection that occurs most often in children under 5 years of age. HFMD spreads easily by person-to-person, respiratory droplet, and fomites, and is presented by mouth vesicles or ulcers and rash on the hands and feet. A member of the enterovirus group, Coxsackievirus can cause outbreaks, usually in childcare settings. Understanding the modalities of transmission is crucial in disease prevention, especially since it has a propensity to develop more serious complications if it occurs in immunocompromised hosts or adults. Health education campaigns on hygiene measures such as routine handwashing can also significantly reduce cases and suppress outbreaks in community settings. The clinical picture of HFMD results from the complex interaction between the host immune response and Coxsackievirus. Following infection, the virus invades epithelial cells, inducing cytopathic effects that lead to vesicular lesions. These are typically found on the palms of the hands, soles of the feet, and mucosa of the mouth, and the resulting lesions cause pain and discomfort that may hinder one's routine activities, such as drinking and eating. While HFMD is generally a self-limiting disease, its complications can include viral meningitis or encephalitis, particularly in unusual presentations. The relatively benign character of the disease masks the need for caution on the part of medical professionals; immediate treatment and diagnosis are required to keep symptoms to a minimum and to monitor for potential complications. It highlights the need to rule out HFMD from other dermatological diseases to ensure appropriate and timely treatment. Studies examine various alternatives in the management and control of HFMD, with emphasis on prevention because there is no effective antiviral therapy. Supportive care remains the cornerstone of treatment, managing symptoms to enable increased comfort throughout the illness. Prevention measures against Coxsackievirus are in the early stages of development but offer a potential approach for future prevention. As observed in sexually transmitted disease patterns reported in public health research, such as high rates of unprotected sex leading to heightened transmission (Martínez et al., 2021), viral infection education like HFMD comes into the limelight. Public health programs ensuring infection avoidance are addressed comprehensively and can go a long way in mitigating the burden of HFMD, building healthier communities, and safeguarding vulnerable populations (Barnard et al., 2024) (Figure 12.16).

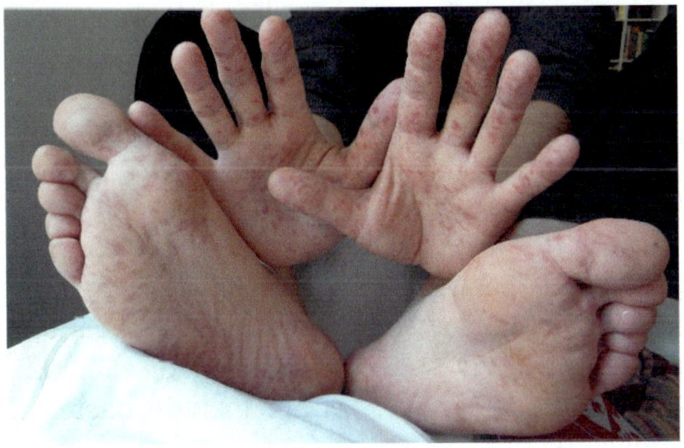

Figure 12.16. Coxsackievirus.

Source: https://upload.medbullets.com/topic/121537/images/handfootmouth.jpg.

12.4.3. Cytomegalovirus (CMV) and Its Skin Manifestations

CMV, a herpesvirus, is known for a wide range of clinical manifestations, with skin manifestations being the most notable. Although often asymptomatic in immunocompetent persons, CMV can cause fatal complications in immunocompromised hosts, particularly solid organ transplant recipients or HIV/AIDS patients. Skin manifestations that appear in association with CMV are usually secondary to systemic infection and can include maculopapular rashes, ulcers, or, in the most severe cases, necrotizing lesions. Due to its opportunistic nature, the formation of skin lesions is most frequently a sign of a general dysregulation of immune system function, and one that underlines the usefulness of CMV as aetiologic for cutaneous expression in host groups prone to such effects. The modulation of CMV infection with autoimmune diseases further complicates the skin lesions in patients. For instance, viral infections such as CMV play a role in triggering autoimmune responses that exacerbate clinical disorders like Primary Sjögren's syndrome (pSS), leading to skin involvement. In pSS, mechanisms such as molecular mimicry or bystander activation may induce autoimmune events that are regulated by infections such as CMV. CMV can provoke the immune system to develop autoantibodies and activate B cells, thereby leading to skin alterations, as is prevalent in individuals with autoimmune diseases.

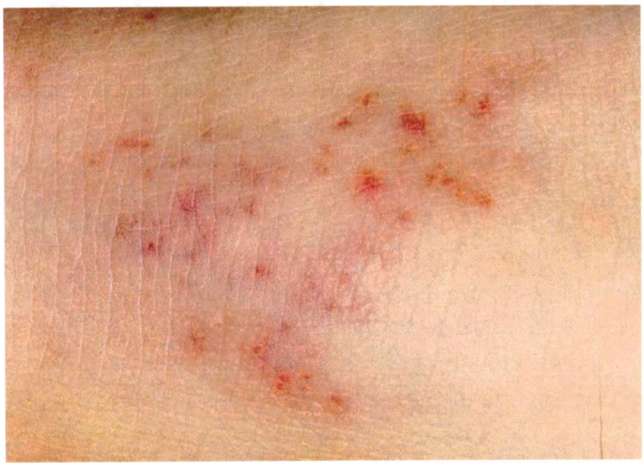

Figure 12.17. Cytomegalovirus (CMV).

Source: https://cdn.open-pr.com/S/b/Sb05870579_g.jpg.

This association underscores the importance of understanding CMV's dual role—as both a direct infectious cause and an inducer of autoimmune skin responses. Moreover, CMV infection implications extend far beyond mere dermatological conditions, frequently correlating with more severe systemic clinical outcomes. In patients with heightened susceptibility, i.e., WHIM syndrome patients, CMV can further compromise the immune function and lead to severe, recurring dermal infections. The challenges of managing these complications are further compounded by graft rejection and immunodeficiency. In hematopoietic stem cell transplantation, immune system recovery is not only crucial but also essential for curing associated skin lesions. Following transplantation, patients exhibit varied immune restoration and resolution of pre-existing infection symptoms, indicating that management of CMV and its cutaneous implications is a multifaceted component of their overall management plan, once again illustrating the convergence of viral infections, immunology, and dermatology in clinical practice (Figure 12.17).

Test Your Knowledge

1. What is the varicella-zoster virus?
2. What is the coxsackievirus?

12.5. Diagnosis of Viral Skin Infections

Learning Outcome

1. Know the clinical evaluation and patient history of viral infections of the skin
2. Describe the laboratory tests and imaging techniques in the diagnosis and management of viral infections of the skin
3. Understand the process of differential diagnosis in viral infections of the skin

Diagnosis of viral skin infections is a crucial aspect of dermatology, particularly for widespread diseases such as herpes simplex virus (HSV), human papillomavirus (HPV), and molluscum contagiosum. Accurate diagnosis generally begins with a thorough medical history combined with a comprehensive physical examination. Clinicians generally assess the distribution, morphology, and evolution of the skin lesions, which can provide significant information about the viral etiology. For instance, the presence of grouped vesicles on an erythematous background is classically observed in herpes simplex infections, whereas HPV is observed as warts with a typical keratotic profile. Here, it is interesting to note that the diagnostic procedure may vary with clinical suspicion; visual inspection may be sufficient for typical presentations, whereas atypical or complex cases may require additional laboratory examinations, including PCR assays or viral cultures for a definitive diagnosis (Beeson et al., 2020). Laboratory diagnosis is especially important in the event of potential complications arising from viral skin infections. For example, differential diagnoses would include bacterial superinfections, eczema herpeticum, or other viral entities that may require alternate treatment modalities. Therefore, in addition to clinical examination, serological tests can be used to detect specific antibodies to HSV or HPV. Ancillary tests are significant in the detection of chronic carrier states or the assessment of vaccination response. Clinical presentation is generally sufficient to diagnose suspected cases of molluscum contagiosum; however, incisional biopsy may be necessary to exclude other viral or neoplastic processes when lesions are atypical. Emphasizing the importance of establishing an accurate diagnosis offers a route to targeted therapeutic interventions that can adequately manage symptoms and prevent transmission (Holmstrup et al., 2018). In addition, the role of consensus documents and clinical guidelines cannot be overstated in diagnosing viral skin infections. In-depth frameworks present clinicians with evidence-based recommendations to guide diagnostic and treatment choices appropriately. Such publications are likely to be syntheses of expert opinion based on a systematic practice overview and are frequently revised to accommodate emerging evidence within the field. Previous classifications of viral infections inform practitioners on the expected progression of each condition and help develop more differentiated care plans. The convergence of the guidelines not only helps strengthen diagnostic accuracy but also warrants treatment interventions that are homogeneous across different healthcare facilities, thus enhancing patient outcomes in the management of viral skin infections (Beeson et al., 2020) (Figure 12.18).

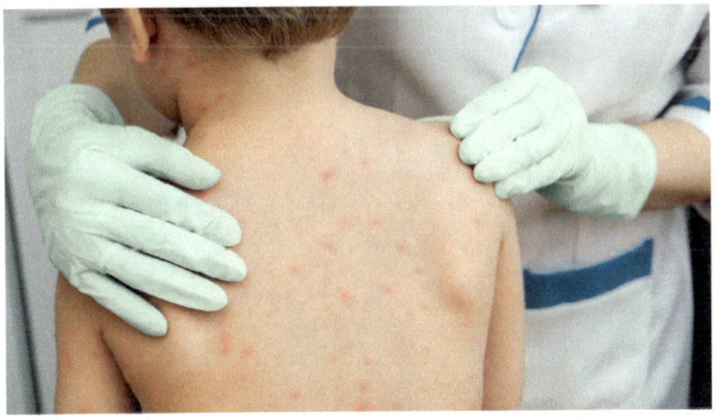

Figure 12.18. Diagnosis of viral skin infections.

Source: https://images.everydayhealth.com/images/2025/what-is-a-viral-skin-rash-00-1440x810.jpg?sfvrsn=bff32fca_3.

12.5.1. Clinical Evaluation and Patient History

Detailed patient history forms a crucial component of the clinical evaluation of viral cutaneous infections such as herpes, HPV, and molluscum contagiosum. The clinicians are required to inquire about the onset, duration, and characteristics of the skin lesions, their location and appearance, and any associated symptoms, such as pain or pruritus. Additionally, a patient's history of medicine—more precisely, any history of immune compromise, current illness, or past viral infections—can help to clarify the possible causes of their present condition. This type of inquiry not only aids in identifying the causative agent but also considers differential diagnoses that may appear similar on the skin, thus facilitating proper treatment without delay and addressing the patient's immediate problems to optimal effect. The clinical value of a complete patient history extends beyond the presenting symptoms themselves; it also encompasses significant lifestyle and behavioral factors. For example, sexual history is relevant in the assessment of HPV-associated lesions since this virus is commonly transmitted through sex, with the most significant being the genital tract. Patients must also be asked about their vaccine status and preventive care. This combined approach is helpful in understanding the mechanisms by which lifestyle choices could influence the outbreak of viral infections, and thereby inform treatment options and public health strategies to reduce transmission levels. An interdisciplinary approach may also be helpful here, with dermatologists and other experts, e.g., infectious disease experts, collaborating. Besides, current research indicates that the clinical examination of cutaneous viral infections should include observation of patients' general health and nutrition. A holistic approach acknowledges that behaviors of life, including diet and skincare habits, influence the integrity and the responsiveness of the skin to treatment. Studies have demonstrated that vitamin and mineral deficiencies can hinder the healing of skin lesions and increase their recurrence (Michalak et al., 2021). Based on this, practitioners can recommend dietary modification or supplements as one component of a comprehensive care plan. This treatment is in line with the aim of promoting long-term health and reducing the risk of skin viral infection, thereby enhancing the patient's quality of life and treatment.

12.5.2. Laboratory Tests and Imaging Techniques

Laboratory tests and imaging techniques play a crucial role in diagnosing and treating viral skin infections such as HSV, HPV, and molluscum contagiosum. Laboratory examination is needed in the diagnosis of viral pathogens as well as differentiating from other cutaneous diseases. As an example, polymerase chain reaction (PCR) is highly effective in detecting HSV from cutaneous lesions with increased sensitivity over traditional culture methods. HPV, however, may be diagnosed by dermal biopsy with subsequent histopathological examination to evaluate for wart morphology and the presence of abnormal keratinocytes. These testing technologies not only enable accurate diagnosis but also guide appropriate clinical intervention, illustrating the integration of laboratory science and clinical dermatology in managing viral skin infections. Advances in imaging technologies have also enhanced the understanding of infectious skin disease. For example, high-frequency ultrasonography is employed to visualize skin lesions and assess their depth, texture, and vascularity, which are critical factors in assessing the severity of viral infection. New imaging modalities, such as dermoscopy, provide specific information on the architecture of warts in viral infections, particularly for differentiating warts due to HPV from other benign/malignant lesions. These imaging modalities support the diagnostic competency of dermatologists with early accurate treatment steps that have a significant impact on patient outcomes. Thus, the integration of imaging with laboratory investigations is a revolutionary idea in modern dermatological practice, as it aims to improve patient care for viral skin infections. Also, the awareness of viral infections with tattooing has suggested laboratory and imaging tests in this field as well. The increased popularity of tattoos as body modification is bringing some particular health problems, such as potential viral infections like HPV and molluscum contagiosum, which can manifest on tattooed skin. Viral conditions have been reported in cases where pigmented tattoos have been applied (Beatrice Bălăceanu-Gurău et al., 2024). The association of tattoo ink detection with an increased risk of viral lesions raises questions about serological evaluation of viral pathogens and follow-up imaging techniques for analysis of lesion development. By identifying and regulating these viral infections associated with tattoos, clinicians can advise patients of potential risks and adopt preventive measures, thereby emphasizing the importance of intensive assessment protocols for addressing dermatological side effects of body art (Cohen, 2021) (Figure 12.19).

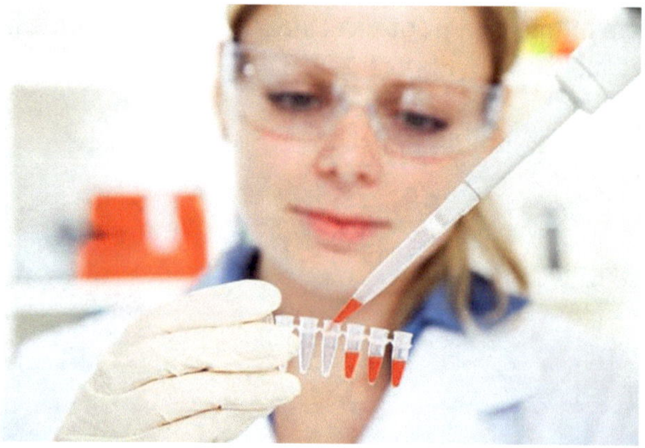

Figure 12.19. Polymerase chain reaction (PCR) testing.

Source: https://genes.co.il/wp-content/uploads/2022/09/PCR-test-Polymerase-Chain-Reaction-.jpeg.

12.5.3. Differential Diagnosis Considerations

The process of differential diagnosis is critical for distinguishing viral skin infections, such as those caused by HSV, HPV, and molluscum contagiosum. Each of these infections can present with overlapping symptoms, posing challenges for clinicians. For instance, both HPV and HSV may have vesicular lesions, but HSV will typically be ulcerating, grouped vesicles with pain, while HPV lesions are painless and manifest as warty growths. Thus, a correct clinical history coupled with an appropriate physical examination is essential for differentiation. Symptomology, including itching, pain, and lesion distribution, assists clinicians in developing a differential diagnosis and determining further testing or therapeutic interventions (Beeson et al., 2023). Familiarity with the epidemiological factors responsible for each viral infection is also important during the differential diagnosis. For example, HSV is most commonly transmitted by direct skin-to-skin contact, whereas HPV is primarily sexually transmitted and associated with certain risk factors such as immunocompromised states. Patient history of recent sexually transmitted disease exposure and history of vaccination may also inform the clinician's assessment. In the case of HPV, there are several risk-related strains; notable among these are certain types of which are referred to as high-risk due to their oncogenic potential, demonstrating the importance of exact diagnosis. Further, the ability to recognize immunocompromised patients who may present in atypical fashion is essential for accurate diagnosis and management of skin lesions (Magalhães et al., 2020). Finally, laboratory tests supplement the clinical examination in further refining the differential diagnosis. PCR, for example, can confirm HSV by directly detecting viral DNA in lesions, while serologic tests can be helpful for assessing the presence of certain HPV types. Clinical diagnosis is often sufficient for molluscum contagiosum, but histologic testing might be required to exclude other viral infections or skin lesions. These methods serve to document the value of being methodical in the identification of superficial viral skin infections. Effective management is based on recognizing these differences, as improper management, particularly in immunocompromised individuals, may lead to increased complications or mismanagement of primary diseases (Magalhães et al., 2020).

Test Your Knowledge

1. What is a key aspect of clinical evaluation for viral skin infections like herpes, HPV, and molluscum contagiosum?
2. Which imaging modality is most useful for distinguishing HPV-related warts from other benign or malignant lesions?

12.6. Impact on Quality of Life

Learning Outcome

1. nderstand the physical symptoms and discomfort in viral infections of the skin
2. Know the psychological effects and social stigma arising from viral infections of the skin
3. Describe the economic burden and healthcare costs linked to viral infections

UViral skin infections such as herpes, HPV, and molluscum contagiosum have manifestations beyond the physical and significantly affect patients' quality of life. Psychological distress is also a significant part of the broader life experience of those who co-exist with such infections. The patients feel embarrassed, anxious, and isolated, particularly regarding the stigmatized dimension of sexually transmitted diseases. Psychological distress might interfere with their social activities and lower their self-esteem, with individuals fearing to be criticized or rejected by friends and even prospective partners. The need for effective management and support systems is evident; these emotional issues must be addressed to improve individuals' quality of life. Beyond psychological effects, viral cutaneous infections can impose physical restrictions that affect daily functioning. For instance, herpes simplex virus recurrence can cause a great deal of distress and pain, compromising an individual's ability to engage in daily activities, such as work or social activities. HPV may result in genital warts and, in certain cases, serious health conditions like cervical cancer, contributing to an individual's health situation. The physical manifestations of such infections could also result in seeking medical assistance, which is time- and cost-intensive, ultimately decreasing patients' welfare. The infectious and chronic characteristics of such diseases can foster feelings of helplessness, and hence, comprehensive healthcare interventions should be ensured.

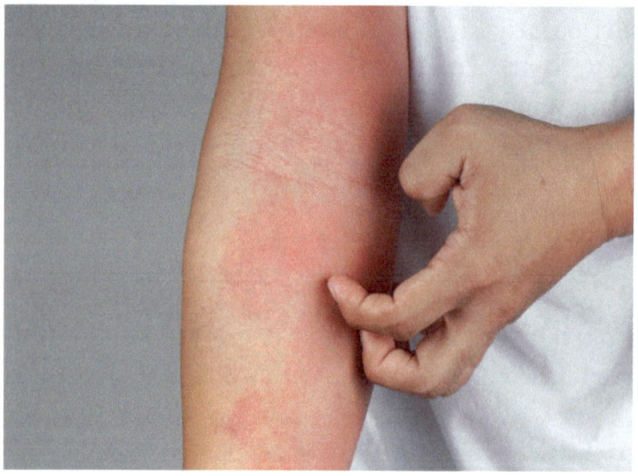

Figure 12.20.

Source: https://ai-care.id/photos/Healthpedia%20Kulit/6256bbbe3bd24.png.

The effect of such viral infections is worse in risk populations, where social, economic, and health factors exacerbate their quality-of-life concerns. Groups with limited access to healthcare resources might have additional barriers to managing these infections effectively. For example, patients will avoid medical treatment out of fear of stigma, as has been noted from resistance to reporting penile diseases among men based on embarrassment and fear (Cannav\\\\uf2 et al., 2020). Further, the fact that such infections are associated with severe diseases—such as in the case of HIV-positive patients, where ocular complications are many more times more common—is an added complication to deal with (Wani et al., 2016). Collectively, these features illustrate the necessity for interventions specifically tailored to meet both the physical and psychological care requirements of individuals with viral skin infections, as fulfilling these elements is imperative to enhancing their quality of life (Figure 12.20).

12.6.1. Physical Symptoms and Discomfort

Physical discomfort and skin symptoms in viral infections, such as herpes, HPV, and molluscum contagiosum, are critical considerations in the impact of these infections on patients. For instance, HSV frequently results in outbursts of painful blisters, itchiness, and inflammation. These lesions can have a serious effect on the quality of life as they not only create physical discomfort but also bring about emotional distress due to their visibility and attendant stigma. In addition, the persistence of the outbreaks means the emotional burden is even greater, putting individuals in a cycle of fear about future recurrences. The acute phase of such infections underscores the need for sensitivity and management techniques to alleviate both physical and mental symptoms associated with these viral skin infections. In the instance of HPV, although many are asymptomatic, the development of genital warts or, in the worst instances, lesions that can put the patient at risk for malignancy introduces a twofold level of unease. Their visible appearance causes significant bodily discomfort in the shape of itchiness and irritation, while their psychological effect will be that of embarrassment and fear regarding sexual health. On top of that, the latent nature of HPV makes individuals worry more as they are unsure about passing it to their partners or possibly getting diseases later on. Awareness of the frequency of the physical manifestations of HPV emphasizes the importance of early diagnosis and education as a part of coping with discomfort and preventing further complications. Molluscum contagiosum, yet another viral dermatosis, again points to the struggle with physical manifestations and discomfort. It is characterized by firm, nontender papules on the skin and can lead to secondary infection due to scratching and pruritus. Although molluscum itself is typically self-resolving, concerns about its infectivity and visibility can have a tremendous impact on one's self-esteem and interpersonal relationships. This is particularly true in children and adolescents, who may be bullied or excluded due to the observable lesions. Thus, effective treatment modalities, in addition to targeting the elimination of lesions, also consider psychotherapy to mitigate social stigma and anxiety due to infection. Lastly, recognition and response to the multidimensional nature of symptoms and pain in viral skin infection are critical for holistic patient care (Figure 12.21).

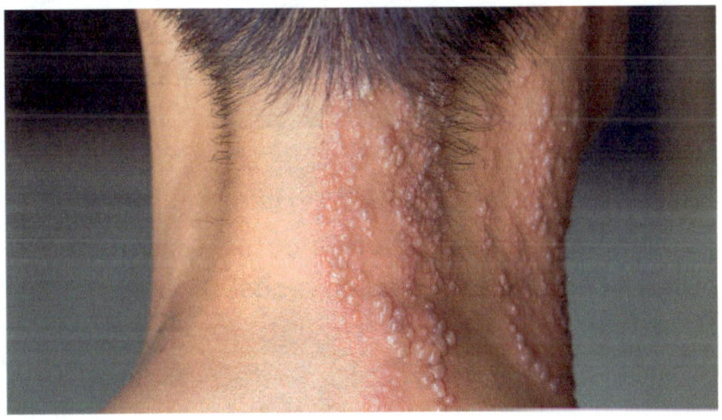

Figure 12.21. Physical symptoms of viral infections of the skin.

Source: https://dermskinhealth.com/wp-content/uploads/2022/05/shingles-herpes-zoster-hero.jpeg.

12.6.2. Psychological Effects and Social Stigma

The psychosocial effects of viral skin infections, particularly herpes, HPV, and molluscum contagiosum, run deep and debilitating. Patients with such infections often have difficulty with depression and anxiety, fueled by transmission fears and concerns regarding their sexual relationships. The intangible quality of most symptoms contributes to vulnerability and, hence, increased psychosocial distress. For instance, the chronic nature of herpes may entail recurrent attacks that disrupt not only the patient's physical wellness but also their mental wellness. The necessity of ongoing medical treatment and psychological strain of having a chronic condition may have an intensified effect on mental health; thus, the importance of addressing integrated medical and psychological care for the afflicted (Ikokwu et al., 2023). The shame related to these viral infections is also a primary causal factor in worsening the psychological effects endured by the afflicted. Tended to be viewed as evidence of promiscuity or irresponsibility, herpes and HPV can provoke societal condemnation that causes individuals to withdraw from society and their peer groups. Such shame might prevent individuals from even seeking the necessary medical care and from openly discussing their condition, generating more embarrassment and shame. The rejection stigma of interpersonal relationships also looms large, as the person can hide their diagnosis from their partners for fear of what they might do. Stigma and mental illness can thus create a vicious cycle, as stigma worsens psychological distress, precipitating more withdrawal and avoidance behavior that diminishes quality of life (Ikokwu et al., 2023). Identification and treatment of the social stigma and psychological effects of viral skin infection are important in maintaining health and well-being. Health education to destigmatize the infection would help individuals cope with such conditions. Sexually transmitted illnesses, such as those caused by viral skin lesions, must be underlined as something natural and never a flaw in a person or their value by public health. Increased awareness of the epidemiology of such infections and their prevalence has the potential to alter attitudes at the public level, encouraging more individuals to seek treatment without fear of stigmatization. In parallel, healthcare professionals must be equipped with skills to deliver compassionate care that addresses the physical and emotional aspects of such infections, thereby facilitating a holistic approach to patient well-being and minimizing the stigma that pervades so many.

12.6.3. Economic Burden and Healthcare Costs

The economic cost of viral skin infections, such as herpes, HPV, and molluscum contagiosum, is a significant concern for health care systems worldwide. These infections impose a significant cost not only to patients but also to preventive and treatment initiatives by the public health. The direct costs include doctor visits, laboratory tests, and, in most cases, prolonged treatments that add to the cost burden. There is also an indirect cost in the form of lost productivity due to workdays lost, further exacerbating the economic burden on patients and the healthcare system. While healthcare expenses continue to rise, the economic impacts of these viral infections necessitate sustainable investment in research and preventive interventions to mitigate their economic effects on society (Scasso et al., 2018). One of the most characteristic aspects of such healthcare expenses relating to such viral infections is the long-term care, as well as the comorbidities caused. For instance, HPV patients have a greater risk of developing certain cancers, and this produces significant healthcare expenses to manage and treat. Herpes simplex virus also produces reactivations that require continuous doctor visits and antiviral treatments. There is evidence that proper control of these infections can reduce total healthcare costs by preventing complications, treatments, and hospitalizations. There has also been reported interaction between chronic conditions and immune response, indicating that viral infections, if left untreated or poorly treated, could result in increased health risks and, consequently, greater healthcare spending (Vega-Ram Hírez et al., 2015). Prevention, exemplified by the HPV vaccines, has potential to mitigate future costs. Immunization not only decreases the frequency of infection but also turns off related expenses, including the treatment of advanced disease stages like cancer operations. By investing in robust public health promotion initiatives aimed at enhancing vaccination rates, communities are capable of incurring fewer healthcare fees in the long run. Thus, linking public health goals with economic needs is required for creating sustainable healthcare models that can respond effectively to the cost of viral skin infections. Addressing such subtleties could lead to more policymaking and research focused on achieving improved health outcomes with lower spending (Scasso et al., 2018).

Test Your Knowledge

1. What physical symptoms are commonly associated with herpes simplex virus (HSV)?
2. What psychological conditions are frequently associated with viral skin infections such as herpes and HPV?

SUMMARY

In general, viral skin diseases, such as herpes, HPV, and molluscum contagiosum, represent major public health issues since they are frequent and potentially capable of producing chronic sequelae. An understanding of pathogenesis and immune response to these infections is valuable in the treatment of both acute presentations and potential sequelae. Viral persistence and the immune system interact most characteristically in immunocompromised patients, who are at heightened risk of severe manifestations and malignancies caused by these viruses. As reflected in growing HPV-related cancers and herpes infection complications, prevention, cure, and awareness efforts are urgently needed to lower the burdens imposed by these infections on healthcare systems and on persons. Moreover, new therapeutic advances suggest promise for future treatments that can battle such infections. For instance, advances in RNA therapies, such as targeting the HPV genome, and novel approaches, such as CRISPR technology, have the potential to revolutionize patient management plans, particularly for immunocompromised individuals. The promise of therapeutic vaccine effectiveness, however, under investigation, carries hope for renewed optimism regarding the HPV disease burden. This underscores the need for ongoing research and clinical trials to optimize treatment regimens and improve quality of life for infected populations, while delineating the public health implications of these viral diseases. In addition, the COVID-19 pandemic has provided additional impetus for thinking about viral skin infections, with the description of SARS-CoV-2 infection-associated oral ulcers emphasizing the need for extensive investigation in patients diagnosed with the virus. Such fresh thinking is in tune with the understanding that viral infections present in complex forms and can affect one another in immunocompromised persons. These findings call for an interdisciplinary approach, such as dermatological assessment in the management of systemic infections, thereby enabling overall patient care. As a result of the shifting epidemiology of viral diseases, ongoing education of healthcare professionals and the general population remains vital to ensuring an informed response to viral skin infections and to minimizing their contribution to global health outcomes (Hewavisenti et al., 2023; Rosa et al., 2021).

The prevalence of viral cutaneous infections, such as HSV, HPV, and molluscum contagiosum, reflects the severity of the public health issue they represent. They occur with a variety of symptoms, producing inflammation and potential morbidity. For instance, herpes simplex virus has produced painful lesions and is noted for recurrences, and HPV produces warts and is of significance in the causation of skin cancers. Molluscum contagiosum most frequently affects children, presenting as pearly, raised lesions. Awareness of such diseases contributes to accurate diagnosis and treatment, further illustrating the importance of constant research and education in dermatovirology. The interplay between viral infection and the immune system is evidence of the complexity of disease management. Some viruses, such as skin infection viruses, may provoke autoimmune reactions that stimulate mechanisms that weaken overall health. For instance, it has been proven that viruses are potential triggers for autoimmune diseases, influencing B-cell hyperactivation and causing primary Sjögren's syndrome and other illnesses. The influence is not localized to the skin, as these infections may reflect systemic immunological events. This dialogue between the skin and the immune system points to the necessity of treating the disease overall, with not just the visible manifestations, but also addressing underlying immune responses that may be implicated. New treatment modalities are being researched for the management of virally-induced skin diseases, including nanotechnology and antiviral studies. Recent studies focus on nano-based drug delivery systems, enhancing the therapeutic effectiveness of antiviral medicines by improving their bioavailability and specificity of delivery. The problem is particularly important today with drug resistance in viral infections. Nanomaterials, such as nanoparticles and liposomes, may improve therapeutic regimens for viral skin infections. The power of nanotherapeutics, as reported in the current literature, will likely transform clinical practice, providing new avenues for the management of long-standing dermatological viral issues (Cojocaru et al., 2020). Furthermore, knowledge of the relationship between treatment protocols and viral pathophysiology remains vital to informing extensive management regimens in infected individuals.

KEY TERMS FROM THIS CHAPTER

- Antiviral therapy
- Fever
- Herpesviridae
- Inflammation
- Molluscum contagiosum
- Neural ganglia
- Public health
- Cancer
- Herpes simplex virus
- Human papillomavirus
- Lymphadenopathy
- Nervous system
- Psychological distress
- Sexually transmitted infections

CRITICAL THINKING QUESTIONS

1. **Which virus is responsible for causing herpes simplex infections?**
   a. Varicella-zoster virus
   b. Human papillomavirus (HPV)
   c. Herpes simplex virus (HSV)
   d. Epstein-Barr virus
2. **What is the hallmark clinical feature of herpes zoster (shingles)?**
   a. Symmetric red, scaly plaques
   b. Unilateral vesicular rash in a dermatomal distribution
   c. Widespread pustules with necrotic centers
   d. Persistent nodules with purulent discharge
3. **Which of the following is a common characteristic of warts caused by HPV?**
   a. Painful ulceration
   b. Hyperkeratotic growths with a rough surface
   c. Vesicular lesions that rupture and crust
   d. Fluid-filled blisters
4. **Molluscum contagiosum is caused by:**
   a. Herpes simplex virus
   b. Poxvirus
   c. Varicella-zoster virus
   d. Human papillomavirus
5. **Which viral infection of the skin is commonly associated with a "slapped cheek" appearance in children?**
   a. Herpes zoster
   b. Fifth disease (Erythema infectiosum) caused by parvovirus B19
   c. Hand, foot, and mouth disease
   d. Measles

Short Answer Questions

1. Define the viral infections of the skin.
2. What is the most common viral infection?
3. What is the herpes simplex virus?
4. What is human papillomavirus (HPV)?
5. What is molluscum contagiosum?

Answer to Critical Thinking Questions

1. (c); 2. (b) ; 3. (b); 4. (b); 5. (b)

REFERENCES

1. Agoues Martínez, J., Atela Azpuru, J. I., & Carbajo Laorden, K. (2021). Sexually transmitted diseases (STDs). https://doi.org/10.2307/j.ctv2pfq2s5.17 (accessed on 21st July 2025).
2. Al-Hakim, A., Kacar, M., & Savic, S. (2024). The scope and impact of viral infections in common variable immunodeficiency (CVID) and CVID-like disorders: a literature review. *Journal of Clinical Medicine, 13*(6), 1717. https://doi.org/10.3390/jcm13061717Ali, A. S., Madani, F. H., Baqasi, A. M., Alshammari, S. M., Aldogil, S. O., & Alaeq, R. A. (2024). A review on viral skin infections in children: Types, clinical picture and outcomes. *Journal of Healthcare Sciences.* https://www.semanticscholar.org/paper/66eb1f3ac8a2b343aa6d98c3170fe6e2f83c5428 (accessed on 21st July 2025).
3. Anitha Rani, A., Ruhani, R., Rangarh, S., & Kumar, A. (2025). Hepatoprotective effect of the *Santalum album Linn.* seeds against high fat diet induced non-alcoholic fatty liver disease in Wistar rats. *IJSAT, 16*. https://doi.org/10.71097/ijsat.v16.i1.1415 (accessed on 21st July 2025).
4. Bălăceanu-Gurău, B., Apostol, E., Caraivan, M., Ion, A., Tătar, R., Mihai, M. M., Popa, L. G., et al. (2024). Cutaneous adverse reactions associated with tattoos and permanent makeup pigments. *Journal of Clinical Medicine, 13*, 503–503. https://doi.org/10.3390/jcm13020503 (accessed on 21st July 2025).
5. Barnard, C. C., & Carpenter, E. (2024). A classification for medical and veterinary libraries. https://doi.org/10.56920/lshtmp-1 (accessed on 21st July 2025).
6. Beeson, M. S., Ankel, F., Bhat, R., Broder, J., Paradise, S., Gorgas, D. L., Spencer Jones, J., et al. (2020). The 2019 model of the clinical practice of emergency medicine. *Journal of Emergency Medicine, 59*, 96–120. https://doi.org/10.1016/j.jemermed.2020.03.018 (accessed on 21st July 2025).
7. Beeson, M. S., Bhat, R., Broder, J., Gaeta, T. J., Janssen, A., Karl, E. R., Lo, B., et al. (2023). The 2022 model of the clinical practice of emergency medicine. *Journal of Emergency Medicine, 64*, 659–695. https://doi.org/10.1016/j.jemermed.2023.02.016 (accessed on 21st July 2025).
8. Cannavò, S. P., Colli, C., Conforti, C., Deinlein, A., et al. (2020). Benign dermatoses of the male genital areas: A review of the literature. https://core.ac.uk/download/343623547.pdf (accessed on 21st July 2025).
9. Carvalho, A. A. T., Frezzini, C., Leao, J. C., Porter, S., et al. (2009). Oral complications of HIV disease. https://core.ac.uk/download/pdf/8295373.pdf (accessed on 21st July 2025).
10. Cohen, P. R. (2021). Tattoo-associated viral infections: A review. *Clinical Cosmetic and Investigational Dermatology, 14*, 1529–1540. https://doi.org/10.2147/ccid.s284796 (accessed on 21st July 2025).
11. Cojocaru, F. D., Botezat, D., Gardikiotis, I., Urîtu, C. M., Dodi, G., Trandafir, L. M., Rezuș, C., et al. (2020). Nanomaterials designed for antiviral drug delivery transport across biological barriers. *Pharmaceutics, 12*, 171–171. https://doi.org/10.3390/pharmaceutics12020171 (accessed on 21st July 2025).
12. Dhume, M. S. M., & Dias, C. P. (2023). Named cells and inclusion bodies in bacterial and viral infections associated with oral cavity. https://core.ac.uk/download/596246883.pdf (accessed on 21st July 2025).

13. Du, T. D., Diep, Y. N., Bùi, T. H. H., Diep, Y. L., Phan, N. P. T., Tran, T. M. L., & Dang, T. N. (2024). Dermatologic manifestations in HIV: Unveiling opportunistic infection. *Tạp chí Truyền nhiễm Việt Nam, 4*, 102–112. https://doi.org/10.59873/vjid.v4i44.338 (accessed on 21st July 2025).

14. Durusu, İ. N., Şen, E. T., Soylu, S., Bozkurt, F., Eren, B., Keleş, İ., Karalar, M., et al. (2023). Cinsel yolla bulaşan hastalıklara multidisipliner yaklaşım. https://doi.org/10.37609/akya.2637 (accessed on 21st July 2025).

15. Gaweł-Dąbrowska, D., Jakoniuk, M., Kler, K., Kucharczyk, D., et al. (2025). Infectious skin diseases in contact sports–A literature review. https://core.ac.uk/download/656518080.pdf (accessed on 21st July 2025).

16. Ghali, H., Smith, L. R., Krenitsky, A., Joseph, A., Aung-Din, D., Hennessy, K., Moore, S., et al. (2025). Topical cantharidin use in dermatology: An updated review. *Dermatology Online Journal, 30*. https://doi.org/10.5070/d330664680 (accessed on 21st July 2025).

17. Górska, M., Kmak, B., & Szot, A. (2024). The most common dermatoses of athletes. https://core.ac.uk/download/620863890.pdf (accessed on 21st July 2025).

18. Guillin, O., Vindry, C., Ohlmann, T., & Chavatte, L. (2019). Selenium, selenoproteins and viral infection. *Nutrients, 11*, 2101–2101. https://doi.org/10.3390/nu11092101 (accessed on 21st July 2025).

19. Hewavisenti, R., Arena, J., Ahlenstiel, C., & Sasson, S. C. (2023). Human papillomavirus in the setting of immunodeficiency: Pathogenesis and the emergence of next-generation therapies to reduce the high associated cancer risk. *Frontiers in Immunology, 14*. https://doi.org/10.3389/fimmu.2023.1112513 (accessed on 21st July 2025).

20. Holmstrup, P., Plemons, J., & Meyle, J. (2018). Non–plaque-induced gingival diseases. *Journal of Periodontology, 89*. https://doi.org/10.1002/jper.17-0163 (accessed on 21st July 2025).

21. Hufbauer, M., & Akgül, B. (2017). Molecular mechanisms of human papillomavirus induced skin carcinogenesis. *Viruses, 9*, 187–187. https://doi.org/10.3390/v9070187 (accessed on 21st July 2025).

22. Ikokwu, G. M. M., Osegbale, I. D., Ralph-Okhiria, O. H., & Ighile, E. F. (2023). Protecting your health: A comprehensive review of sexually transmitted illnesses. *International STD Research & Reviews*. https://doi.org/10.9734/isrr/2023/v12i1154 (accessed on 21st July 2025).

23. Jakubowska, W., Kiełkowicz, A., Pactwa, F., Pisera, D., et al. (2024). Skin and mucosal lesions in the course of HIV infection. https://core.ac.uk/download/597985244.pdf (accessed on 21st July 2025).

24. La Rosa, G. R. M., Libra, M., De Pasquale, R., Ferlito, S., & Pedullà, E. (2021). Association of viral infections with oral cavity lesions: Role of SARS-CoV-2 infection. *Frontiers in Medicine, 7*. https://doi.org/10.3389/fmed.2020.571214 (accessed on 21st July 2025).

25. Laberko, A., Деордиева, E. A., Kriván, G., Goda, V., Bhar, S., Kawahara, Y., Rao, K., et al. (2021). Multicenter experience of hematopoietic stem cell transplantation in WHIM syndrome. *Journal of Clinical Immunology, 42*, 171–182. https://doi.org/10.1007/s10875-021-01155-8 (accessed on 21st July 2025).

26. Magalhães, G. M., Vieira, É. C., Garcia, L. C., Carvalho-Leite, M. L. R., Guedes, A. C. M., & Araújo, M. G. (2020). Update on human papilloma virus–Part I: Epidemiology, pathogenesis, and clinical spectrum. *Anais Brasileiros de Dermatologic, 96*, 1–16. https://doi.org/10.1016/j.abd.2020.11.003 (accessed on 21st July 2025).

27. Maślińska, M., & Kostyra-Grabczak, K. (2022). The role of virus infections in Sjögren's syndrome. *Frontiers in Immunology, 13*. https://doi.org/10.3389/fimmu.2022.823659 (accessed on 21st July 2025).

28. Meyts, I., & Casanova, J. L. (2021). Viral infections in humans and mice with genetic deficiencies of the type I IFN response pathway. *European Journal of Immunology, 51*, 1039–1061. https://doi.org/10.1002/eji.202048793 (accessed on 21st July 2025).

29. Michalak, M., Pierzak, M., Kręcisz, B., & Suliga, E. (2021). Bioactive compounds for skin health: A review. *Nutrients, 13*, 203–203. https://doi.org/10.3390/nu13010203 (accessed on 21st July 2025).

30. Minooee, A., Wang, J., & Gupta, G. (2015). Sports: The infectious hazards. *Microbiology Spectrum, 3*. https://doi.org/10.1128/microbiolspec.iol5-0014-2015 (accessed on 21st July 2025).

31. Moorthy, R. V. (2006). Prevalence of STD in HIV positive patients. https://core.ac.uk/download/235653786.pdf (accessed on 21st July 2025).

32. Nadhan, K. S., Larijani, M., Abbott, J., Doyle, A., Linfante, A., & Chung, C. L. (2018). Prevalence and types of genital lesions in organ transplant recipients. *JAMA Dermatology, 154*, 323–323. https://doi.org/10.1001/jamadermatol.2017.5801 (accessed on 21st July 2025).

33. Naidoo, S. (2012). Oral health & HIV. https://core.ac.uk/download/322407918.pdf (accessed on 21st July 2025).

34. Rajagopalan, R., & Vedhanayagam, M. (2017). Prevalence of mucocutaneous manifestations in human immunodeficiency infection–Learning from a rural centre in Tamilnadu, India. https://core.ac.uk/download/543136416.pdf (accessed on 21st July 2025).

35. Ruffner, M. A., Sullivan, K. E., & Henrickson, S. E. (2017). Recurrent and sustained viral infections in primary immunodeficiencies. *Frontiers in Immunology, 8*. https://doi.org/10.3389/fimmu.2017.00665 (accessed on 21st July 2025).

36. Sabatini, M. E., & Chiocca, S. (2019). Human papillomavirus as a driver of head and neck cancers. *British Journal of Cancer, 122*, 306–314. https://doi.org/10.1038/s41416-019-0602-7 (accessed on 21st July 2025).

37. Scasso, F., Ferrari, G., De Vincentiis, G. C., Arosio, A. D., Bottero, S., Carretti, M., Ciardo, A., et al. (2018). Emerging and re-emerging infectious disease in otorhinolaryngology. *Acta Otorhinolaryngologica Italica, 38*(Suppl. 1), S1–S106. https://doi.org/10.14639/0392-100x-suppl.1-38-2018 (accessed on 21st July 2025).

38. Sharifi-Rad, J., Quispe, C., Rahavian, A., Carneiro, J. N. P., Rocha, J. E., Leal, A. L. A. B., Morais-Braga, M. F. B., et al. (2021). Bioactive compounds as potential agents for sexually transmitted diseases management: A review to explore molecular mechanisms of action. *Frontiers in Pharmacology, 12*. https://doi.org/10.3389/fphar.2021.674682 (accessed on 21st July 2025).

39. Soriano, V., & del Romero, J. (2018). Rebound in sexually transmitted infections following the success of antiretrovirals for HIV/AIDS. *AIDS Reviews, 20*. https://doi.org/10.24875/aidsrev.18000034 (accessed on 21st July 2025).

40. Tampa, M., Mitran, M., Mitran, C., Matei, C., Amuzescu, A., Buzatu, A., & Georgescu, S. (2022). Viral infections confined to tattoos—A narrative review. *Medicina, 58*. https://www.semanticscholar.org/paper/df38387f14f8df652ed6443efc2669a6f1349198 (accessed on 21st July 2025).

41. Tangye, S. G., Al–Herz, W., Bousfiha, A., Cunningham-Rundles, C., Franco, J. L., Holland, S. M., Klein, C., et al. (2022). Human inborn errors of immunity: 2022 update on the classification from the International Union of Immunological Societies Expert Committee. *Journal of Clinical Immunology, 42*, 1473–1507. https://doi.org/10.1007/s10875-022-01289-3 (accessed on 21st July 2025).

42. Tognarelli, E. I., Palomino, T. F., Corrales, N., Bueno, S. M., Kalergis, A. M., & González, P. A. (2019). Herpes simplex virus evasion of early host antiviral responses. *Frontiers in Cellular and Infection Microbiology, 9*. https://doi.org/10.3389/fcimb.2019.00127 (accessed on 21st July 2025).

43. Vega-Ramírez, H., Velasco Rodríguez, V. M., Cruz, J., Hirata, H., Ferreyra, D., & Rocabert, C. (2015). P021: Impulsivity and depressive symptoms in people with HIV diagnosed with a common mental disorder from an HIV clinic in Mexico City. *Journal of the International AIDS Society, 18*. https://doi.org/10.7448/ias.18.3.20152 (accessed on 21st July 2025).

44. Wani, M. G. (2016). Eye complications of acquired immune deficiency syndrome (AIDS). https://core.ac.uk/download/478462554.pdf (accessed on 21st July 2025).

45. Wihlfahrt, K., Günther, V., Mendling, W., Westermann, A., Willer, D., Gitas, G., Ruchay, Z., et al. (2023). Sexually transmitted diseases—An update and overview of current research. *Diagnostics, 13*, 1656–1656. https://doi.org/10.3390/diagnostics13091656 (accessed on 21st July 2025).

46. Zannella, C., Giugliano, R., Chianese, A., Buonocore, C., Vitale, G. A., Sanna, G., Sarno, F., et al. (2021). Antiviral activity of *Vitis vinifera* leaf extract against SARS-CoV-2 and HSV-1. *Viruses, 13*, 1263–1263. https://doi.org/10.3390/v13071263 (accessed on 21st July 2025).

47. Zhao, H., Wu, L., Yan, G., Chen, Y., Zhou, M., Wu, Y., & Li, Y. (2021). Inflammation and tumor progression: Signaling pathways and targeted intervention. *Signal Transduction and Targeted Therapy, 6*. https://doi.org/10.1038/s41392-021-00658-5 (accessed on 21st July 2025).

INDEX

D

E

F

G

H

I

V

Z